The Wiley-Blackwell Handbook of Psychoneuroimmunology

The Wiley-Blackwell Handbook of Psychoneuroimmunology

Edited by

Alexander W. Kusnecov and Hymie Anisman

WILEY-BLACKWELL

A John Wiley & Sons, Ltd., Publication

This edition first published 2014

Registered Office
John Wiley & Sons Ltd, The Atrium, Southern Gate, Chichester, West Sussex, PO19 8SQ, UK

Editorial Offices
350 Main Street, Malden, MA 02148-5020, USA
9600 Garsington Road, Oxford, OX4 2DQ, UK
The Atrium, Southern Gate, Chichester, West Sussex, PO19 8SQ, UK

For details of our global editorial offices, for customer services, and for information about how to apply for permission to reuse the copyright material in this book please see our website at www.wiley.com/wiley-blackwell.

Library of Congress Cataloging-in-Publication Data

The Wiley-Blackwell handbook of psychoneuroimmunology / edited by Alexander W. Kusnecov And Hymie Anisman.
pages cm
Includes bibliographical references and index.
ISBN 978-1-119-97951-7 (cloth)
1. Psychoneuroimmunology. 2. Nervous system–Diseases–Immunological aspects. I. Kusnecov, Alexander W., editor of compilation. II. Anisman, Hymie., editor of compilation.
QP356.47.W55 2013
612.8′233–dc23

2013021883

A catalogue record for this book is available from the British Library.

Cover image: Blood cells, SEM. © Power and Syred / Science Photo Library
Cover design by Cyan Design

Typeset in 10/12.5pt Galliard by Aptara Inc., New Delhi, India

1 2014

Contents

Preface

Alexander W. Kusnecov[1] and Hymie Anisman[2]

[1]*Department of Psychology, Behavioral Neuroscience Program, Rutgers, The State University of New Jersey, New Brunswick, NJ, USA*

[2]*Department of Neuroscience, Carleton University, Ottawa, Ontario, Canada*

During the past decade the biological and behavioral sciences have become increasingly intertwined, as research continues to reinforce the notion that physical and psychological health are a function of interactive biological systems. Mental ill-health as a reflection of deficits in neural functions is potentially precipitated and/or perpetuated by systemic factors engineered by immunological processes; for these are now understood to be modulators of neural activity, and ultimately the cognitive and emotional life of the organism. Similarly, environmental and physiological events, both prior to and after birth, can impact neurodevelopmental and behavioral processes, as well as endocrine and immunological functions. These circumstances serve as the basis for immunological theories for the formation of autistic spectrum disorders and schizophrenia, as well as potential vulnerabilities that set the stage for how later life events influence physiological and psychological adaptation during adult life and the ageing process. Debilitating neuropathological conditions, such as Alzheimer's like dementia and Parkinsons's disease, in which neurodegeneration progressively destroys the motoric, cognitive and emotional lives of the individual, have resurrected and redefined the meaning of "neuroinflammation." This is a hotly pursued process that involves parenchymal glial cells of the brain, as well as the contributions of systemic inflammatory processes that emanate from the immune system. This area has increased attention on the biological functions of astrocytes and microglial cells, and the recognition that they are as much a part of brain function, as oligdendrocytes, the myelinating cells that expedite communication between neurons. Finally, it has also become clear that nutritional, metabolic and cardiovascular health are intimately linked to inflammatory and/or immunological activities, emphasizing the importance of the immune system as both a contributor and reflection of health status across different provinces of physiological function.

In protecting the organism against infectious disease, the hematopoetic cells that give rise to the heterogeneity of lymphocytes, monocytes and other cellular forms – in short, the immune system – are intimately linked to the activities of the central nervous system. This now is an established fact, as the contents of this handbook make abundantly clear. Furthermore, this relationship has served to emphasize a multifactorial, integrative systems approach to the scientific investigation of disease. Of course, no one involved in this field, and especially the authors assembled for this volume, is surprised by this, since reductionistic approaches that seek unitary explanations for complex phenomena are bound to encounter disappointment. Indeed,

Robert Ader in his 1980 Presidential Address to the American Psychosomatic Society, given on the eve of his seminal publication, *Psychoneuroimmunology* (Ader, 1981), gave eloquent voice to this point:

> Despite the most sophisticated strategies designed to achieve uniformity, variability remains one of the most ubiquitous results of all natural and contrived biological experiments. The biomedical scientist, operating within the conceptual and technical constraints imposed by the disciplinary boundaries of a reductionistic philosophy, attempts to control or minimize (or ignore) variability. For the psychosomaticist, such variability is the starting point of his research; it defines the operation of variables with which to be concerned. (Ader, 1980, p. 307)

The contents of this handbook continue to echo these thoughts, and provide a comprehensive source of information on the history, methodology, and conceptual development of different aspects of research into psychoneuroimmunology. In doing so, a balance between traditional and emerging topics of psychoneuroimmunological research is provided that focuses on the clinical and practical implications of findings from human and animal empirical research. While the specialist reader will appreciate the gains made in psychoneuroimmunology, the newcomer to this field will receive an informed introduction to the field, and some of the prominent approaches that currently are under investigation. Some stratification has been incorporated into the book, with initial chapters providing basic information on the immune system, "hard-wired" innervation of lymphoid organs, and neuroscience approaches to examining effects on immune function. These early conceptual and methodological chapters are followed by material that addresses entry of molecular and cellular elements of the immune system into the brain and spinal cord, and the consequences of this to neural function, nociception, or pain, and feedback regulation of immunological and metabolic processes. Immunomodulation through catecholamine, neuropeptide, and neuroendocrine processes is addressed at a basic level, but then moves on to the effects of stressors on immune function. Many of these and subsequent chapters address methodological issues and potential pitfalls when interpreting the results of human and animal studies.

The second half of the book is focused on material that mixes basic and clinical findings to determine the degree to which neural–immune interactions or disruption of the neural–immune axis contributes to disease. An emerging theme is the operation of neural–immune processes throughout the lifespan.In recognition of this point, chapters are provided on how maternal exposure to immunologic and psychogenic stressors influences neural and cognitive development during the postnatal and early adult years, with special attention given to microglial cells and their emerging role in shaping the development of the central nervous system. This is revisited in a later chapter by a detailed treatment of whether immunologic activity can be considered as a plausible factor in the formation of autism, as well as schizophrenia. Ageing is an ever-present background process that late in life contributes to biological variability, and is given attention in two chapters focused on animal and human studies, respectively. As already mentioned, mental health and behavioral abnormalities are a recurring theme, and this is reemphasized in chapters that cover inflammatory processes in stress, depression, cardiovascular disease, and neurodegenerative diseases, such as Parkinson's and Alzheimer's. Related to this, are cognitive deficits, which have become a dominant theme in psychoneuroimmunological investigations. In the present volume, this literature is discussed with a focus on methodological issues and the interpretation of results from studies involving various immune challenges, as well as those addressing the presence of immune-related transcription factors in the brain. Finally, given the prominence of obesity and eating-related disorders, a chapter is devoted to the role of immunologic processes in regulating food intake, energy regulation and metabolism.

We are indebted to the distinguished group of authors who devoted their time and energy to create this handbook. The excellent level of scholarship displayed in these chapters left very little for us to do, and only left us recognizing how impressive this multidisciplinary endeavor has become over the past three decades. We are, of course, cognizant that the full breadth of psychoneuroimmunology has not been represented in these pages. Important topics such as sleep, cancer and exercise have not been included, and this oversight is something for us to correct in future volumes. However, psychoneuroimmunology has become pleasantly unwieldy. One cannot cram everything into a finite number of pages, and volumes such as this are instruments for inspiration and the generation of ambitious research programs.

In coming to the end of this long process, we sadly acknowledge the loss of some dear friends. Dr Steven Zalcman, a contributor to this volume, unexpectedly passed away. Steve was a close friend and colleague who often shared perceptive thoughts about the field, as well as an encyclopedic knowledge of popular music and stand-up comedy – he was as equally comfortable exhorting about interleukins and the brain, as he was about the merits of the Beatles, Stones, and Monty Python!

Sadly, Dr. Robert Ader, a mentor and constant inspiration to all of us, passed away during the development of this volume, but left the field he helped create, quite fertile and fully alive. We are grateful to his support on this project. One of us (AWK) approached him and picked his brain in the simplest of ways: "Bob, should I do this?" No answer is simple, however, when it comes to Bob Ader, although mercifully, the answer was a resounding yes. This handbook has elements of his suggestions, real and implied. Ultimately, we are grateful that he was able to pen, along with his good friend and long-time colleague, Nicholas (Nick) Cohen, a foreword to the book. To paraphrase something Nick stated in a past correspondence, we note that this foreword not only offers a brief historical overview of the field of psychoneuroimmunology, but also represents the final scientific thoughts of Robert Ader.

The production values of this project owe their special touch to the hard work of the publishers. We are particularly grateful to Andrew Peart, Publisher for psychology books at Wiley-Blackwell, who initially approached us to undertake this project. Andy has been a constant source of encouragement and guidance with our various questions and concerns. We could not ask for a better interpreter of the book publishing process. Additional thanks go to Tori Halliday, Karen Shield, and Mirjana Misina, who queried and guided us – hands stretched across the Atlantic – tolerating the long process of reading and re-reading, copyright-getting and various other important details a forgetful editor rarely remembers to do.

Of course, as editors, we know that the buck stops with us. If there is anything to yell about, we are to blame. But we hope the excitement and proven success of psychoneuroimmunology will drown out the noise. This book may hold some hidden nuggets of thought and fact for the experienced and informed, but we are most hopeful that it may inspire new ambitions and promising careers for students and postdoctoral fellows who have yet to be smitten by the allure of this field. And while this book is dedicated to the memory of Robert Ader, I am sure, he will be the first to agree that this book is for you.

Alexander W. Kusnecov
Hymie Anisman

References

Ader, R. (ed.) (1981). *Psychoneuroimmunology*. New York: Academic Press, 1981.
Ader, R. (1980) Presidential Address. Psychosomatic and Psychoimmunologic Research. *Psychosomatic Medicine*, 42(3), 307–321.

Foreword

Robert Ader[1] and Nicholas Cohen[1,2]

[1]*Department of Psychiatry, University of Rochester Medical Center, Rochester, NY, USA*
[2]*Department of Microbiology and Immunology, University of Rochester Medical Center, Rochester, NY, USA*

Just in case a prospective reader of this book doesn't already know the simple definition of psychoneuroimmunology, it is the study of the interactions among behavior, neural and endocrine function, and immune system processes. The central premise of this interdisciplinary field is that adaptation is the product of a single, integrated network of defenses. Each component of this network evolved to serve specialized functions. These are the parochial interests of the "disciplines" into which we have divided the biological sciences. At the same time, though, each component of this defensive network monitors and responds to information (sometimes presented as shared molecules and/or receptors) derived from the others. Thus, we cannot fully understand immunoregulatory processes without considering the organism and the internal and external milieu in which immune responses take place. Immunoregulatory processes, once considered a self-regulating, autonomous agency of defense, have been revealed by research, most of which has been conducted over the past 35 years, to be, in reality, influenced by the brain; and, conversely, neural and endocrine functions and behavior have been shown to be influenced by the immune system.

Our original study on behaviorally conditioned immunosuppression was published in 1975. We were not aware of it at the time, but Russian scientists had conducted studies on the classical conditioning of immune responses in the 1920s. A conditioned stimulus (e.g., heat, tactile stimulation) was repeatedly paired with injections of foreign proteins. Subsequent exposure to the conditioned stimulus alone was thought to have induced antibody production. These studies attracted little attention outside the Soviet Union. Within the Soviet Union, they provoked heated arguments since some investigators believed (but the scientific community rejected the notion) that an antibody response was the direct result of neural activity (i.e., that the nervous system, by itself, could stimulate antibody production).

Other early indications of CNS influences on immunity came from Andor Szentiványi's studies in the late 1950s showing that hypothalamic lesions could prevent anaphylactic shock in animals. Similar lines of research were initiated sporadically following these findings.

One of the earliest pioneers in the study of behavioral influences on immunity was Fred Rasmussen a virologist intrigued by the possibility that emotional states could influence the course of infectious illness. Rasmussen teamed up with Norman Brill, a psychiatrist and James Marsh, a psychologist – probably the first such collaborative team – to start a program of research on stress and infectious disease. During the 1950s and 1960s, Rasmussen and his colleagues examined the effects of various stressors on mice inoculated with different viruses.[1] Susceptibility to infections was increased or decreased, depending on the nature of the stressor. These studies, with obvious implications for the neuroendocrine modulation of immunity, also failed to attract much attention, although they were forerunners of some of the research on early life experiences and disease susceptibility initiated by Drs George Solomon and Alfred Amkraut and others in the mid 1960s.

George Solomon, a psychiatrist, was one of the real pioneers in the development of psychoneuroimmunology. His initial research examined the life histories and personality characteristics of patients with autoimmune disease. In the best known of their studies, Solomon and Rudolf Moos compared rheumatoid arthritis patients with their "at risk," but healthy, relatives. Their analysis also included the presence or absence of rheumatoid factor, an anti IgG antibody characteristic of rheumatoid arthritis. Compared to the patients, rheumatoid factor positive relatives were psychologically "healthy," lacked anxiety, depression, or alienation and reported good relationships with spouses, relatives and friends. Psychological well-being seemed to have had a salutary effect in the face of a genetic predisposition to autoimmune disease.

Solomon was convinced that experimental research would be more persuasive, so he established a "psychoimmunology" laboratory to study the effects of behavioral, social, and endocrine manipulations in animals on immune function and responses to a bacterial antigen, virus-induced tumors, and adjuvant-induced arthritis. As in other such studies, the results varied depending on the stressor and the outcome measure.

During the 1970s, Hugo Besedovsky, another very prominent figure in the development of psychoneuroimmunology, was beginning to construct a neuroendocrine–immune system network with his studies of the effects of immune responses on neural and endocrine function. If, as he and his colleagues (the most "important" one being his wife Adriana del Rey) believed, immune function was integrated with other physiological processes, exposure to an antigen should evoke changes in neuroendocrine activity that, in turn, should have feedback effects on immunoregulatory processes and host defenses. There followed an innovative program of research that provided dramatic demonstrations that the nervous and endocrine systems could perceive and respond to signals emitted by an activated immune system.

The novel studies of several other figures played critical roles in the growing acceptance of this new discipline. There was the research of Ed Blalock and his colleagues (e.g., Eric Smith) who found lymphocytes could be a source of brain peptides and pituitary hormones. Now, it is accepted that brain peptides and their receptors exist within the immune system and that the products of an activated immune system can function as neurotransmitters. Another critical link was forged by investigators led by David Felten, Susanne Stevens, and Karen Bulloch, who described "hard-wired" connections from the nervous system to the immune system.

At a behavioral level, Roger Bartrop described immunologic changes associated with the bereavement that followed the sudden death of a spouse, and several other laboratories launched studies of the immune changes associated with stressful life experiences and emotional states. Marvin Stein, for example, who had studied the effects of hypothalamic lesions and stimulation on anaphylactic reactions in guinea pigs during the 1960s, returned to psychoneuroimmunology in the 1980s with a program of animal research on the immunologic effects of stressful experiences as well as human studies of the immunologic changes associated with

1 Rasmussen was the chair of the Department of Medical Microbiology and Immunology at UCLA in 1965 when one of us (NC) was there as a postdoctoral fellow in a transplantation immunogenetics lab and was unaware of this line of research.

loss and depression. Another interdisciplinary collaboration between Janice Kiecolt-Glaser, a psychologist and Ronald Glaser, a virologist, developed an extremely productive research program beginning with studies of stress-induced immune function and the reactivation of latent viruses. All the aforementioned research initiated in the 1970s and early 1980s was apparently "the right stuff at the right time!" It is likely that no one research program would have had quite the same impact had it not been for the converging evidence of brain–immune system interactions that was appearing in the literature at the same time. These initial studies legitimized questions that had not been asked before. And if the questions – and, sometimes, the questioners – were disparaged, a common experience, the data were compelling and then, undeniable. Thus, the coalescence of research initiated during the 1970s – and the identity provided by the label, psychoneuroimmunology, a book of the same name, a journal and a society – reactivated latent interests and attracted new investigators from different fields to this hybrid field.

Frequently, we have been asked if we had any idea of what we had "started" with our studies of conditioned alterations in immune function or where our studies would lead. Of course we did know that the concept challenged immunological dogma and could be very important, but we never anticipated how rapidly or how large the field would grow and expand and we continue to be amazed by the number of scientists working in various psychoneuroimmunology laboratories – named as such – all over the world. When the journal *Brain, Behavior, and Immunity* (BBI) was launched in 1987, it was overseen by an Editor-in-Chief (a behavioral scientist) and two Associate Editors (an immunologist and a neural scientist). This was sufficient to handle the topical diversity and number of submitted publications and to assign appropriate reviewers from the 31-member Editorial Board. Twenty-five years later, this high-impact journal is guided by an Editor-in-Chief, six Associate Editors and an Editorial Board of 64 scientists. Eight issues are published each year – twice the number that appeared in 1987. Of course, peer-reviewed publication of new data in psychoneuroimmunology is by no means restricted to BBI; high quality papers appear with regularity in a number of highly ranked journals. [The 20th annual meeting of the PsychoNeuroImmunology Research Society (PNIRS) took place in Stockholm, Sweden,in June 2013.] The book *Psychoneuroimmunology,* first published in 1981, is in its fourth edition. Psychoneuroimmunology is now taught in many colleges and universities in this country and abroad. A few textbooks are now available to guide the novice, although multi-authored collections of chapters still prevail. Our guess is that, now, it is close to impossible for any normal mortal to write a single authored, integrated, and up-to-date inclusive psychoneuroimmunology text book in addition to running a funded productive laboratory.

Some contemporary news releases and numerous websites still refer to psychoneuroimmunology as an emerging field. That descriptor might have been appropriate 25 years ago but today, there can be no doubt that by any set of criteria, psychoneuroimmunology has fully emerged from a veil of skepticism as an exemplar of an integrated field of study. We've been afforded a wonderful and rare opportunity to witness this emergence of a new field of research and to chart, for nearly 40 years, its scientific development and its impact on, and integration into, mainstream scientific and medical thinking.[2] This most recent edited volume, *Handbook of Psychoneuroimmunology,* is an exciting and up-to-date presentation of many of these advances.

2 We have also seen psychoneuroimmunology become an exemplar of mind–body medicine, but have watched, with some dismay, how it is being exploited as a cash cow for some self-styled practitioners of non-scientifically validated approaches to patient care.

List of Contributors

Alfonso Abizaid, Department of Neuroscience, Carleton University, Ottawa, Ontario, Canada

Robert Ader, Department of Psychiatry, University of Rochester Medical Center, Rochester, NY, USA

Hymie Anisman, Departments of Neuroscience and Psychology, Carleton University, Ottawa, Ontario, Canada

Marie-Claude Audet, Department of Neuroscience, Carleton University, Ottawa, Ontario, Canada

William A. Banks, Geriatrics Research Education and Clinical Center, Veterans Affairs, Puget Sound Health Care System and Division of Gerontology and Geriatric Medicine, Department of Internal Medicine, University of Washington School of Medicine, USA

Denise L. Bellinger, Department of Pathology and Human Anatomy, Loma Linda University, School of Medicine, Loma Linda, CA, USA

Hugo O. Besedovsky, Division of Immunophysiology, Institute of Physiology and Pathophysiology, Medical Faculty, Philipps University, Marburg, Germany

Staci D. Bilbo, Department of Psychology and Neuroscience, Duke University, Durham, NC, USA

Robert H. Bonneau, Department of Microbiology and Immunology, The Pennsylvania State University College of Medicine, Milton S. Hershey Medical Center, Hershey, PA, USA

Mary T. Caserta, Department of Psychiatry, University of Rochester Medical Center, Rochester, NY, USA

Sarah M. Clark, Laboratory of Behavioral Neuroimmunology, Department of Psychiatry, University of Maryland School of Medicine, Baltimore, MD, USA

Nicholas Cohen, Department of Psychiatry, University of Rochester Medical Center, Rochester, NY, USA

Angela W. Corona, Department of Neurosciences, Case Western Reserve University, Cleveland, OH, USA

Colm Cunningham, Trinity College Institute of Neuroscience and School of Biochemistry and Immunology, Trinity College Dublin, Dublin, Ireland

Adriana del Rey, Division of Immunophysiology, Institute of Physiology and Pathophysiology, Medical Faculty, Philipps University, Marburg, Germany

Robert Dantzer, MD Anderson Cancer Center, Division of Internal Medicine, Department of Symptom Research, Houston, TX, USA

Noël C. Derecki, Center for Brain Immunology and Glia (BIG), Department of Neuroscience, University of Virginia, Charlottesville, VA, USA

Ashley M. Fenn, Department of Neuroscience, Ohio State University, Columbus, OH, USA

Doina Ganea, Temple University School of Medicine, Philadelphia, PA, USA

Jonathan P. Godbout, Department of Neuroscience, Ohio State University, Columbus, OH, USA

Peter M. Grace, Discipline of Pharmacology, School of Medical Sciences, University of Adelaide, Adelaide, South Australia. Department of Psychology and the Center for Neuroscience, University of Colorado at Boulder, Boulder, CO, USA

Shawn Hayley, Department of Neuroscience, Carleton University, Ottawa, Ontario, Canada

Kathi L. Heffner, Department of Psychiatry, University of Rochester Medical Center, Rochester, NY, USA

Cobi J. Heijnen, Laboratory of Neuroimmunology and Developmental Origins of Disease, University Medical Center Utrecht, Utrecht, Netherlands; MD Anderson Cancer Center, Division of Internal Medicine, Department of Symptom Research, Houston, TX, USA

Deborah M. Hodgson, Laboratory of Neuroimmunology, School of Psychology, Faculty of Science and IT, The University of Newcastle, New South Wales, Australia

Mark R. Hutchinson, Discipline of Physiology, School of Medical Sciences, University of Adelaide, Adelaide, South Australia

Shlomit Jacobson-Pick, Department of Neuroscience, Carleton University, Ottawa, Ontario, Canada

Annemieke Kavelaars, MD Anderson Cancer Center, Division of Internal Medicine, Department of Symptom Research, Houston, TX, USA

Achsah D. Keegan, Department of Microbiology and Immunology, Center for Vascular and Inflammatory Diseases and Program in Oncology, Marlene and Stewart Greenebaum Cancer Center, University of Maryland School of Medicine, Baltimore, MD, USA

Keith W. Kelley, University of Illinois at Urbana-Champaign, Urbana, IL, USA

Jonathan Kipnis, Center for Brain Immunology and Glia (BIG), Department of Neuroscience, University of Virginia, Charlottesville, VA, USA

Willem J. Kop, Department of Medical Psychology and Neuropsychology, Center of Research on Psychology in Somatic diseases (CoRPS), Tilburg University, the Netherlands

Alexander W. Kusnecov, Department of Psychology, Behavioral Neuroscience Program, Rutgers, The State University of New Jersey, New Brunswick, NJ, USA

Alvin Lim, Department of Psychology, University of Pittsburgh, Pittsburgh, PA, USA

Darcy Litteljohn, Department of Neuroscience, Carleton University, Ottawa, Ontario, Canada

Dianne Lorton, Department of Psychology, Kent State University, OH, USA

Giamal Luheshi, Douglas Hospital Research Centre, Department of Psychiatry, McGill University, Montreal, Quebec, Canada

Elyse M. Mallimo, Department of Psychology, Behavioral Neuroscience Program, Rutgers, The State University of New Jersey, New Brunswick, NJ, USA

Anna Marsland, Department of Psychology, University of Pittsburgh, Pittsburgh, PA, USA

Kim Matheson, Departments of Neuroscience and Psychology, Carleton University, Ottawa. Ontario, Canada

Jaclyn W. McAlees, Department of Molecular Virology, Immunology, and Medical Genetics, Ohio State University, Columbus, OH, USA

Robert H. M^c^Cusker, University of Illinois at Urbana-Champaign, Urbana, Illinois, USA

Robyn J. Mcquaid, Department of Neuroscience, Carleton University, Ottawa, Ontario, Canada

Zul Merali, Department of Psychiatry, Royal Ottawa Hospital, University of Ottawa, Ottawa, Ontario, Canada

Urs Meyer, Physiology and Behaviour Laboratory, Swiss Federal Institute of Technology (ETH), Zurich, Swittzerland

Kerry C. Michael, Laboratory of Behavioral Neuroimmunology, Department of Psychiatry, University of Maryland School of Medicine, Baltimore, MD, USA

Veronica M. Miller, Wadsworth Center, New York State Department of Health, Empire State Plaza, Albany, NY, USA. School of Public Health, University at Albany, State University of New York, Albany, NY, USA

Paula M.C. Mommersteeg, Department of Medical Psychology and Neuropsychology, Center of Research on Psychology in Somatic diseases (CoRPS), Tilburg University, the Netherlands

Jan A. Moynihan, Department of Psychiatry, University of Rochester Medical Center, Rochester, NY, USA

Dwight M. Nance, Department of Pediatrics, University of California, Irvine, CA, USA

Thomas G. O'Connor, Department of Psychiatry, University of Rochester, Medical Center, Rochester, NY, USA

Caroline J. Padro, Department of Molecular Virology, Immunology, and Medical Genetics, Ohio State University, Columbus, OH, USA

Michael O. Poulter, Robarts Research Institute, University of Western Ontario, Ontario, Canada

Rachael Racine, Department of Immunobiology, Yale University of Medicine, The Anlyan Center for Medical Research & Education, New Haven, CT, USA

Virginia M. Sanders, Department of Molecular Virology, Immunology, and Medical Genetics, Ohio State University, Columbus, OH, USA

Dipak K. Sarkar, Endocrinology Program and Department of Animal Sciences, Rutgers, The State University of New Jersey, New Brunswick, NJ, USA

Jaclyn M. Schwarz, Department of Psychology, University of Delaware, Newark, DE, USA

Mario Skarica, Temple University School of Medicine, Philadelphia, PA, USA

Luba Sominsky, Laboratory of Neuroimmunology, School of Psychology, Faculty of Science and IT, The University of Newcastle, New South Wales, Australia

Leonardo H. Tonelli, Laboratory of Behavioral Neuroimmunology, Department of Psychiatry, University of Maryland School of Medicine, Baltimore, MD, USA. Veterans Affairs Maryland Healthcare System, Baltimore, MD, USA

Adam K. Walker, Integrative Immunology and Behavior Program, Department of Animal Sciences and Department of Medical Pathology, University of Illinois at Urbana–Champaign, Urbana, IL, USA

Linda R. Watkins, Department of Psychology and the Center for Neuroscience, University of Colorado at Boulder, Boulder, CO, USA

Barbara C. Woodside, Centre for Studies in Behavioral Neurobiology, Concordia University, Montreal, Quebec, Canada

Olivia Wynne, Endocrinology Program and Department of Animal Sciences, Rutgers, The State University of New Jersey, New Brunswick, NJ, USA

Jodi L. Yorty, Department of Biology, Elizabethtown College, Elizabethtown, PA, USA

Steven S. Zalcman, Department of Psychiatry, The University of Medicine and Dentistry of New Jersey, New Jersey Medical School, Newark, NJ, USA

1

Basic Principles in Immunology

Relevance for Studies in Psychoneuroimmunology

Sarah M. Clark,[1] Kerry C. Michael,[1] Achsah D. Keegan,[2] and Leonardo H. Tonelli[1,3]

[1] *Laboratory of Behavioral Neuroimmunology, Department of Psychiatry, University of Maryland School of Medicine, Baltimore, MD, USA*
[2] *Department of Microbiology and Immunology, Center for Vascular and Inflammatory Diseases and Program in Oncology, Marlene and Stewart Greenebaum Cancer Center, University of Maryland School of Medicine, Baltimore, MD, USA*
[3] *Veterans Affairs Maryland Healthcare System, Baltimore, MD, USA*

Introduction

Over the past century our knowledge of the immune system and how it functions has grown exponentially. This is especially true in regard to how it relates to and interacts with various physiological systems, including the central nervous system. An important focus of the field of neuroimmunology is to elucidate the ways that the immune system influences neuronal function and subsequently, behavior and cognition through the modulation of cytokines and hormones, especially stress hormones such as corticosteroids. Since the intimate relationship between the immune system and brain function has come to light, research in this field has broadened into psychoneuroimmunology, which specifically addresses the role of the immune system in the development of psychiatric disorders, including depression and anxiety. The purpose of this section is to provide a general overview of basic immune function, describing both the components of the immune system and the various modes of immunity employed in an immune response. Additionally, we will explore the validity of some of the most widely used methods and models for psychoneuroimmunology applied to the study of interactions between immunological processes and behavior and cognition as they relate to mental disorders in humans.

The Components of the Immune System

To understand how the immune system influences the brain, and subsequently, behavior and cognition, it is vital to understand how the immune system functions. The immune system

The Wiley-Blackwell Handbook of Psychoneuroimmunology, First Edition. Edited by Alexander W. Kusnecov and Hymie Anisman.

comprises two major components: specialized cells that carry out the various functions of the immune process, and the chemical messengers that allow these cells to communicate, not only with each other, but with other cells and tissues within the body. These partners in immune function must perform a precise and complex dance in order to maintain homeostasis and, when necessary, to mediate an inflammatory response. In general, as part of the inflammatory response damaged or infected cells secrete chemical messengers called chemokines that serve to attract specific immune cells, which in turn release various cytokines that influence the types of cells and modes of immunity that will be employed to eliminate any potential pathogens. Once these threats have been neutralized the process continues, as immune cells and their chemical messengers also function to mediate tissue repair and regeneration. A lack of coordination from either partner can result in deleterious consequences, including the development of allergies, as well as autoimmune and immune-deficiency disorders.

Cytokines and chemokines – the immune system's messengers

Cytokines and chemokines are protein and glycoprotein molecules synthesized and secreted by cells as part of the immune response. Chemokines are a specialized class of cytokines that derive their name from their role in chemotaxis; a majority of these soluble factors are chemoattractants that serve to guide immune cells to the site of infection. They are characterized by their small size and the presence of four cysteine residues (named C) which contribute to their tertiary structure. They are divided into four families (C, CC, CXC and CX3C) based upon the location of the first two C residues. Chemokines in the C group differ from the other chemokine families in that they contain only two cysteines; secretion of these chemokines attracts T-cell progenitors to the thymus. The CC chemokines have two adjacent cysteines near the amino terminus, while the relevant cysteines in the CXC chemokines can be found at the N-terminus separated by a single amino acid (X). Similarly, the CX3C chemokines have three intervening amino acids; thus far, fractalkine is the only chemokine with this structure that has been identified. In addition to their role in immune function, chemokines contribute to a variety of biological functions, especially in the brain, as will be discussed later.

The major cytokines consist of interleukins (IL), interferons (IFN) and colony-stimulating factors, as well as various growth factors and eicosanoids, including prostaglandins. Cytokines are mainly produced by immune cells and also by a variety of other cell types including brain cells. The specificity of the elicited immune response is dictated by the expression of cytokine receptors that are widely expressed in tissues and organs. Additionally, some cytokine receptors exist in a soluble form and can act as inhibitors of cytokine activity through competitive binding of their ligands. To differentiate between cytokines' biological activity they are often described as either pro-inflammatory or anti-inflammatory; upon damage to or infection of cells and tissues, pro inflammatory cytokines are produced and secreted to stimulate immune system activation. The induction of cytokine expression tends to occur in a step-wise manner, with the expression of certain cytokines dependent upon the prior expression of others; for example, IL-1 is necessary to induce the production of IL-2, IL-6 and tumor necrosis factor (TNF). Anti-inflammatory cytokines, such as IL-10, are also released during inflammation in order to dampen and eventually terminate pro-inflammatory cytokine activity. In many instances, the cytokines IL-4 and IL-13 are referred as anti-inflammatory because they oppose the effects of inflammatory cytokines IL-2 and IFN-γ. However, many inflammatory processes such as allergic inflammation are mediated by the actions of IL-4 and IL-13. Thus, describing cytokines purely by their pro- or anti-inflammatory properties can be misleading since they are pleiotropic in nature and are involved in many biological processes. Maintaining a balance in cytokine and chemokine signaling is vital for sustaining immune homeostasis and stimulating the appropriate immune cells as part of the immune response.

The cells of the immune system

The circulatory system serves as the main highway for the cells of the immune system, so it is not surprising that immune cells are derived from the same source as the other major components of blood. During prenatal development the spleen and liver are responsible for producing both red blood cells and white blood cells; however, once the skeleton begins to develop and the bone marrow becomes established, this responsibility shifts to hematopoietic stem cells (HSCs) within the bone marrow. HSCs give rise to the three cell lineages of the blood and immune system: the erythroid lineage, the myeloid lineage, and the lymphoid lineage (see Figure 1.1). Currently, the general consensus for how these lineages arise is that the initial progeny of HSCs are multipotent progenitor cells (MPPs) which in turn give rise to common myeloid progenitor cells (CMPs). Progeny of these CMPs maintain expression of myeloid specific genes, but can undergo further restriction into either erythroid or lymphoid progenitors. Thus, the myeloid lineage may be considered the default fate for CMPs unless directed towards either erythroid or lymphoid lineages through changes within the milieu of the stem cell niche, including alterations in cytokine expression. Ultimately, the erythroid lineage will develop into red blood cells and platelets while the myeloid and lymphoid lineages will give rise to the cells of the immune system.

The myeloid lineage Members of the myeloid lineage include monocytes, granulocytes and mast cells. The primary function of monocytes is to migrate out of the vasculature and into tissues where they mature into macrophages that will monitor the body and destroy potential pathogens through phagocytosis. Macrophages can be further classified into mobile or fixed macrophages. The alveolar macrophages of the lungs and the dendritic cells of the epidermis are examples of mobile macrophages that can freely travel within the interstitial space, whereas the Kupffer cells of the liver remain fixed in place.

The granulocytes, named for the multiple granules found within their cells, comprise three types of cells: neutrophils, eosinophils, and basophils. These polymorphonuclear cells (PMNs) are confined primarily to the blood stream until activation by cytokines and chemokines released by damaged cells and tissues. These messengers prompt the PMNs to migrate into the interstitial space where they will hunt down and destroy invading pathogens. Neutrophils, which make up the greatest proportion of PMNs, are phagocytic cells that are among the first cells recruited to eliminate invading pathogens. In addition to destroying foreign cells by phagocytosis, neutrophils can also degranulate and release anti-microbial chemicals such as gelatinase and cathepsin. Interestingly, neutrophils have also been observed extruding filaments of DNA and associated proteins that can act as nets to entrap microbes; these extracellular structures provide an alternate method of destroying pathogens and may prevent their spread into the surrounding tissue. Lastly, neutrophils also release cytokines and thus can enhance the inflammatory response by recruiting more immune cells to the site of infection. The other two types of granulocytes, the eosinophils and basophils, make up a relatively small proportion of the total leukocyte population, but are vital in mitigating the effects of pathogens, especially

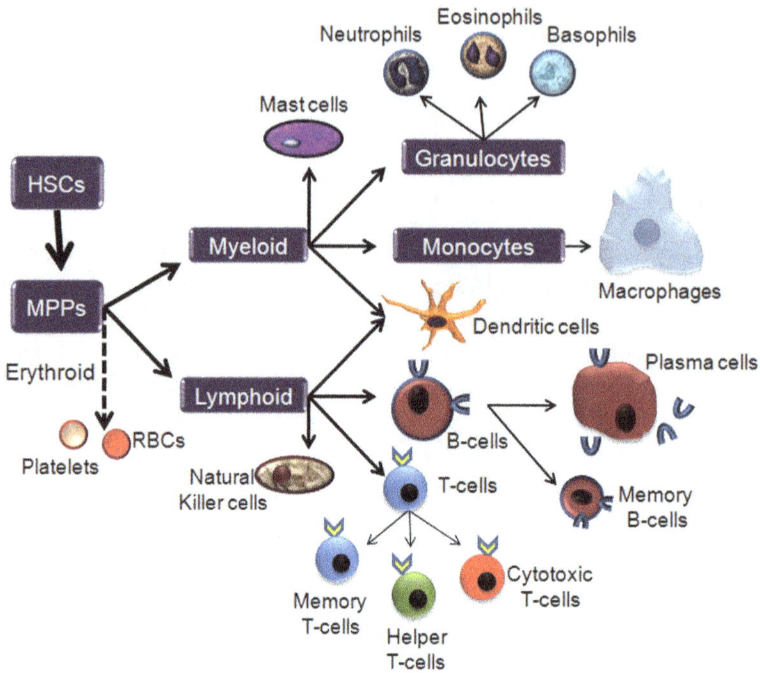

Figure 1.1 Cells of the immune system. Hematopoietic stem cells (HSCs) within the bone marrow are relatively quiescent stem cells whose progeny, multipotent progenitor cells (MPPs), can differentiate into both erythrocytes and leukocytes. There are three potential lineage fates: the erythroid lineage, which gives rise to both red blood cells (RBCs) and platelets, and the myeloid and the lymphoid lineages, which produce the cells of the immune system. Myeloid progenitor cells differentiate within the bone marrow to produce monocytes, granulocytes and mast cells, which then migrate to their target environments within the blood and tissue. Lymphoid progenitors can also be found within the bone marrow, however these cells will differentiate into precursor B-cells that will then migrate into the lymphatic tissues and organs. In contrast, T-cell progenitors leave the bone marrow and migrate directly to the thymus where they will undergo further proliferation and selection for immunocompetency.

for their role in mediating the innate and adaptive immune responses. Although eosinophils and basophils are perhaps best characterized for their anti-parasitical activities, in recent years their role in tissue and immune homeostasis has been further clarified. As part of the adaptive immune response, eosinophils are rapidly recruited to the site of infection by T-helper 2 (T_H2) cells, where they release cytokines and lipid mediators, such as prostaglandin 2, as well as cytotoxic chemicals that can destroy invading pathogens. Additionally, they have the capability of acting as antigen-presenting cells to activate both naïve and memory T-cells. Finally, both eosinophils and basophils have also been implicated in the development of hypersensitivity and allergies, perhaps due to their relationship with T_H2 cells and mast cells.

Mast cells are functionally and morphologically similar to eosinophils and basophils; they play a vital role in the immunity against parasites, and facilitate tissue repair by stimulating angiogenesis, the growth of new blood vessels. However, these myeloid cells are found mainly within tissues adjacent to the external environment, especially within the mucosae of the respiratory and gastrointestinal tracts, and are perhaps best-known for their role in allergic responses. Mast cells are also found in the brain, particularly in some nuclei of the thalamus.

The granules within mast cells store a variety of cytokines and chemokines that facilitate the inflammatory process, as well as histamine which not only dilates blood vessels and is responsible for the pain and itchiness associated with an allergic reaction, but which can also act as a neurotransmitter. Another neurotransmitter, serotonin, has also been found within mast cells, and although the role of these neurotransmitters is not yet clear, they may be involved in cross talk between the immune system and neurons, especially those of the enteric nervous system. Interestingly, in addition to direct damage or the binding of antigens, degranulation of mast cells can also be initiated by various neuropeptides, further supporting the possibility that mast cells represent a link between the immune system and the nervous system.

The lymphoid lineage Lymphocytes derive their name from the fact that they reside primarily within the tissues of the lymphatic system. These tissues include a network of reticular fibers that can be found in virtually every organ of the body; these fibers converge upon the lymph nodes and the two major organs of the lymphatic system: the spleen and the thymus. The main function of the lymph nodes is to filter out and clear lymph as it travels along the lymphatic vessels. Resident macrophages remove and destroy any microbes or cellular debris while lymphocytes monitor the lymphatic stream for the presence of foreign antigens. The lymphocytes include B-lymphocytes, T-lymphocytes and natural killer (NK) cells.

B-cells differentiate within the bone marrow and migrate into the lymph nodes and spleen. Here they will remain in a precursor stage until activated by an antigen, at which time they will undergo rapid proliferation and maturation into antibody-secreting plasma cells. Membrane-bound immunoglobulins (Ig), including IgM and IgD, on the surface of precursor B-cells act as receptors for intact antigens. The binding of the antigen stimulates the production of secretory immunoglobulins, usually referred to as antibodies, including IgM, IgG, IgA and IgE. These antibodies consist of a conserved region and a variable region. It is the conformation of the variable region (the product of the genetic recombination of several genes within the immunoglobulin super-gene family) that makes the antibodies specific for their target antigen. Interestingly, lymphocytes are the only somatic cells that rearrange DNA to produce new protein variants as part of their phenotype.

Once antibodies have been secreted into the extracellular space they can facilitate the removal of pathogens in a variety of ways. By binding to antigens on the surface of pathogens they can make the pathogen more visible to macrophages. That is, the antibody serves as an opsonin (from the latin "to relish"), that marks the pathogen as a target for phagocytosis by macrophages; this will be facilitated by the Fc region of the antibody molecule binding to Fc receptors on the macrophage. Additionally, some immunoglobulins are capable of binding to and activating other effector cells, including granulocytes and mast cells. In the case of IgG, binding to platelets allows for the transfer of immunity across the placenta, which is vital for the development of the fetal immune system. The binding of the Fc region of IgE to the Fc receptor on mast cells results in mast cell degranulation and release of inflammatory mediators such as histamine. The production of IgE antibodies against harmless compounds such as pollen or albumin is responsible for the establishment of allergies.

Although the role of different antibodies in the immune response is quite varied, their primary function is to facilitate the removal of pathogens; however, in order to do so, they must be able to bind to antigens. Individual immunoglobulins are specific for only one or two closely related antigens, though they may be able to bind to other related antigens with lower affinity. However, the immune system cannot sustain an army of B-cells for every possible antigen that the body may encounter. Instead, precursor B-cells expressing a specific antibody monitor the spleen, lymph nodes, and other peripheral lymphatic organs for the antigen that matches its antibody, much like pairing up two pieces of a puzzle. Upon successful binding of the antibody and antigen, the B-cell will undergo a period of rapid proliferation, or clonal expansion, making multiple replicas that will then mature into antibody-secreting plasma cells. Additionally, a subset of B-cells will become memory B-cells, which can rapidly mature into plasma cells should they encounter their specific antigen again.

Unlike the B-cells, T-cells do not differentiate in the bone marrow. Progenitors of T-cells instead migrate to the thymus where they continue to proliferate and undergo thymic selection, a process that ensures that T-cells are immunocompetent. Although initially considered a minor player in the immune response, the importance of T-cells in maintaining immune homeostasis and in modulating the immune response has become abundantly clear. The establishment of their critical role in autoimmune diseases and allergies, as well as immune-deficiency disorders such as HIV/AIDS, has been a major advance in immunology. A naïve T-cell (T_0) has the potential to differentiate into a variety of effector T-cells, which can be distinguished by the expression of recognition proteins known as cluster of differentiation (CD) proteins. Helper T-cells (T_H), also referred to as $CD4^+$ T-cells, modulate both the innate and adaptive immune response; among their many functions, they assist in the maturation of B-cells into plasma cells and memory B-cells, and activate cytotoxic T-cells as well as macrophages. Cytotoxic T-cells (T_c), which are $CD8^+$, attack and destroy virally infected cells as well as tumor cells. The major role of regulatory T-cells ($CD4^+$, $CD25^+$, $FoxP3^+$, T_{reg}), sometimes referred to as suppressor T-cells, is to shut down T-cell mediated immune responses. Finally, memory T-cells are antigen-specific subsets of $CD4^+$ and $CD8^+$ T-cells which have been previously activated and have the capacity to remain viable for long periods of time. Upon re-exposure to the antigen they will rapidly proliferate and activate both T_H and T_C cells so that the immune system can specifically target and destroy the invading pathogen.

The final class of lymphocytes is the natural killer (NK) cells; these cells take part in the innate immune response and act primarily against cells infected by viruses or rogue cells that have become cancerous. Unlike phagocytes, NK cells destroy their targets through the release of perforins, cytolytic enzymes that punch holes in the membrane of the targeted cell. In addition, NK cells discharge a class of proteases called granzymes, which enter the perforated cell and catalyze cell death via apoptosis. Since many of the cells that NK cells target are infected by viruses it is vital that the destruction of the cell is contained; if the cell was merely lysed any viruses that had succeeded in reproducing would be released to infect other cells.

In order to maintain immune and tissue homeostasis myeloid and lymphoid cells work together in a precise and coordinated dance choreographed by cytokines and chemokines. Although each partner is responsible for specific facets of an immune response, they are also dependent upon each other in order to provide the best protection for the host. So as to provide an optimal defense against potential pathogens these components of the immune system employ diverse strategies for identifying and eliminating various microbes.

Modes of Immunity

The immune system must be able to cope with a variety of potential pathogens, as well as tumor cells and other damaged host cells, while mitigating possible damage to healthy cells and tissue. This requires the correct identification of potentially deleterious microbes and cells followed by their targeted elimination. In order to accomplish this the immune system utilizes two distinct, though interdependent, forms of protection which work together in a complex yet highly coordinated assault on pathogens that attempt to invade the body. The innate immune system is a general, non-specific form of defense comprised of anatomical barriers, which serve as a blockade against a majority of microorganisms, and immune cells, including granulocytes, mast cells, macrophages and NK cells, which can recognize and attempt to destroy potential pathogens that breach the barricades of the skin and mucosae. The function of the innate immune system is modulated and enhanced by the adaptive immune system, a specific form of defense which targets and marks pathogens for elimination. However, unlike the innate immune system, a hallmark of the adaptive immune system is that it displays memory, a trait that has been exploited in the development of vaccines. The adaptive immune system evolves in response to the pathogens it encounters over the lifetime of the host, selecting and maintaining a pool of memory B-cells and T-cells specific for antigens the body has been exposed to, so that should the body be invaded by the same pathogen in the future, it can rapidly and specifically target it for destruction.

In order to convey how the immune system contends with the variety of extracellular and intracellular pathogens the host may encounter, the type of defense utilized by immune cells is often described as either cell-mediated immunity or humoral immunity. Cell-mediated immunity is typically modulated by helper T-cell class 1 (T_H1) cells, which orchestrate attacks against intracellular bacteria and viruses, as well as tumor cells. This is often through the release of cytokines, such as interferon, that catalyze the programmed cell-death pathways of infected cells; this process results in the elimination of the pathogen and limits its ability to spread to other cells. In contrast, humoral immunity is targeted against extracellular pathogens, including bacteria, fungi, and helminthes; this form of immunity is mediated by T_H2 and, to a lesser degree, T_H17 cells, which enlist granulocytes and mast cells to facilitate the destruction of these pathogens. Additionally, T_H2 cells can stimulate the release of antibodies from B-cells; these antibodies can then bind to pathogens and mark them for destruction by macrophages.

To function correctly, the immune system must be able to distinguish between healthy host cells and potential pathogens, as well as damaged host cells, including infected or cancerous cells, in order to identify which ones must be destroyed. Members of the innate immune system utilize a set of pattern-recognition receptors (PRRs) that recognize highly conserved motifs that are unique to non-mammalian cells, including components of the bacterial cell wall, such as lipopolysaccharide (LPS) and peptidoglycan, as well as viral nucleic acid structures, such as single-stranded (s.s.) and double-stranded (d.s.) RNA. These molecular structures are referred to as pathogen-associated microbial patterns, or PAMPs; the binding of a PAMP to its receptor triggers signaling pathways that activate transcription factors, such as NF-κB, and induce the expression and secretion of pro-inflammatory cytokines and chemokines. This process initiates an inflammatory response that involves both the innate and adaptive immune systems, with the ultimate goal of eliminating the invading pathogens.

As shown in Figure 1.2, there are four main families of PRRs: Toll-like receptors (TLRs), NOD-like receptors (NLRs), RIG-1-like receptors (RLRs) and C-type lectin receptors (CLRs). Of these, the TLRs are the best characterized; however, ongoing research into the other three classes of PRRs, as well as other lesser-known receptors, indicates that the innate immune system, although non-specific, is efficient at identifying potential pathogens. TLRs are transmembrane proteins with a leucine-rich extracellular domain and a conserved region, the Toll/IL-1 receptor domain, on the cytoplasmic tail. These receptors are expressed in tissues involved in immune function, including the spleen and leukocytes, and on cells within the lungs and gastrointestinal tract, as well as other environments that are exposed to the external environment.

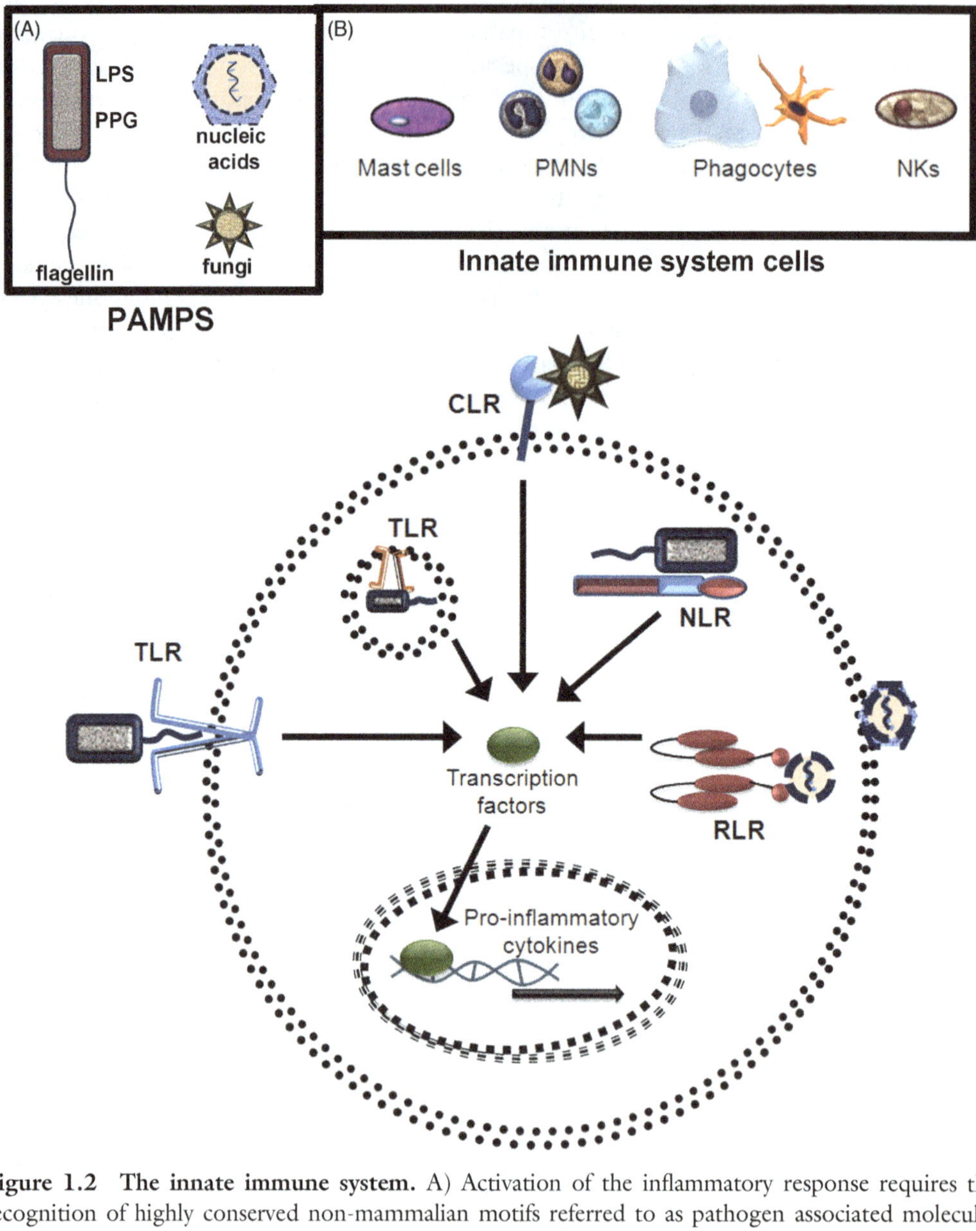

Figure 1.2 The innate immune system. A) Activation of the inflammatory response requires the recognition of highly conserved non-mammalian motifs referred to as pathogen associated molecular proteins (PAMPs). These include bacterial cell wall components such as lipopolysaccharide (LPS) and peptidogylcan (PPG), as well as the protein flagellin, viral nucleic acids (both s.s. and d.s. RNA) and fungal cell-wall components. B) These PAMPs can be identified by a wide assortment of pattern recognition receptors (PRRs) found on a variety of cells, especially those of the innate immune system. The lower panel illustrates how activation of PRRs within the cell by various pathogens initiates signaling pathways that culminate in the production of pro-inflammatory cytokines which will ultimately serve to stimulate the adaptive immune response.

Remarkably, TLRs are also expressed in the brain. Members of the TLR family are found on both the cell surface and within intracellular compartments; this facilitates the detection of pathogens within the extracellular space as well as those that are able to penetrate the cell. The ability of TLRs to recognize a variety of PAMPs is further enhanced by the fact that many exist as heterodimers and/or form associations with various adaptor and accessory molecules that influence their specificity for numerous substrates. TLRs are capable of recognizing all classes of microorganisms, including bacteria, fungi and parasites, as well as viruses. The other three classes of PRRs have a narrower repertoire of PAMPs that they can identify. Recognition of fungal invasion is mediated by CLRs, another transmembrane PRR; interestingly, these receptors bind to carbohydrate structures found in fungi, such as α-glucan and mannan, in a Ca^{2+}-dependent manner. Intracellular PRRs include NLRs and RLRs, which serve to detect pathogens that have penetrated the cell membrane; these PRRs provide a layer of defense in cells that typically do not express TLRs, such as the epithelial cells that line the gastrointestinal tract. NLRs are activated upon infiltration of the cell by bacterial PAMPs, as well as damage-associated molecular patterns (DAMPs) which arise after the integrity of the cell has been compromised. Infection of cells by viruses activate RLRs, which react to the detection of double-stranded RNA; these RNA helicases are vital for anti-viral responses, including the release of IFN-γ, which will not only lead to the destruction of infected cells, but will also serve to activate the T_H1 cells as part of the adaptive immune response.

In contrast to cells that utilize PRRs for the recognition of general motifs expressed by a variety of different pathogens, cells of the adaptive immune system must be able to identify and specifically target pathogens via each pathogen's particular antigens. For example, infection of a cell by influenza will stimulate the innate immune response through the activation of RLRs; however, the optimal immune response would be to destroy the virus before it infected host cells. Here the virus has an advantage because the primary proteins on its surface, hemaglutinin and neuraminidase, are constantly evolving and thus cannot act as PAMPs because different strains express diverse proteins. Nevertheless, they can serve as antigens, unique identifiers of an infection by a specific strain of influenza, and therefore initiate the adaptive immune response.

Nevertheless, any protein or cellular component can potentially act as an antigen, including those on host cells. This requires that lymphocytes be able to distinguish between "self" and "non-self" in order to avoid an autoimmune response. Essentially all cells found within the body express the major histocompatibility complex (MHC) proteins, which act as identifiers of "self"; like fingerprints, MHC molecules are unique to each individual and consequently play a major role in affecting compatibility between donors and recipients of transplanted blood and organs. Additionally, MHC molecules function to alert the immune system of an invasion through the presentation of antigens. Members of the MHC gene family encode two different classes of MHC molecules. Class I MHC proteins are found on virtually all cells and function primarily in "self" recognition, whereas members of Class II MHC proteins are expressed on specialized antigen-presenting cells (APCs); of particular note are the dendritic cells (DCs), which play a vital role in activating T-lymphocytes, and B-lymphocytes, which generate antibodies and target invading cells for destruction.

The stimulation of naïve T-cells by DCs is vital for mounting an offense against invading pathogens (see Figure 1.3). Activation of the T-cell receptor (TCR) requires binding of both an antigen and the MHC, which initiates the maturation of the naïve T-cell; however, polarization (fate specification into T_H1, T_H2, etc.) is dependent upon the milieu of cytokines present in the microenvironment as well as the interaction between the antigen and the T-cell. The first class

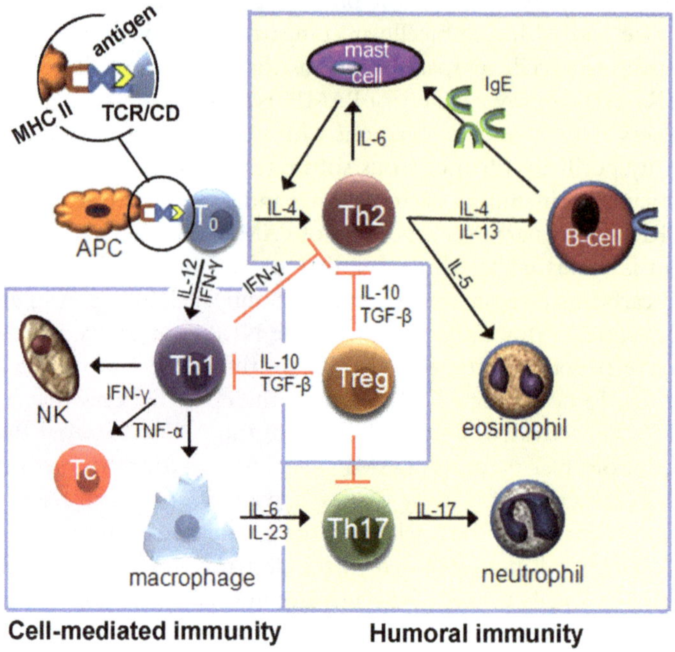

Figure 1.3 The adaptive immune system. In addition to destroying pathogens by phagocytosis, various macrophages and dendritic cells process the pathogen for antigen presentation in order to activate an adaptive immune response. As seen in the upper left corner, the intact antigen is bound to an MHC II molecule on the antigen-presenting cell (APC); this acts as a ligand for the T-cell receptor (TCR) and CD protein on the surface of a naïve T-cell (T_0). Polarization of the T_0 cell depends upon the presence of both the antigen and cytokines. In the presence of IL-12 and IFN-γ cells will assume a T_H1 fate and in turn secrete more IFN-γ as well as TNF-α, which will then modulate both cytotoxic T-cells (T_C) and various cells of the innate immune system. These cells will stimulate the elimination of pathogens through cell-mediated (i.e. intrinsic) processes, such as programmed cell death. On the other hand, if IL-4 is present, T_0 cells will differentiate into T_H2 cells, which modulate the humoral immune response through the activation of assorted innate immune cells. The removal of extracellular pathogens is accomplished by a variety of mechanisms including the degranulation of granulocytes and antibody mediated processes. T_H1 and T_H2 mediated immune responses are downregulated by IL-10 and TGF-β, both of which are secreted by regulatory T-cells (T_{reg}); this action is vital for maintaining immune homeostasis.

of T-cells to be activated is the T_H cells, which will in turn modulate the activity of other T_C cells and B-cells. Various classes of T_H cells specialize in specific forms of pathogens and modes of immunity. Among these classes, the T_H1 and T_H2 cells are the most renowned, however, other T_H cells, including T_H17, follicular T_H (T_{FH}) and inducible regulatory T_H (iT_{reg}) cells, have all recently gained more scrutiny as their roles in the immune response have been further elucidated. The polarization of T_H1 cells occurs in response to IL-12 and IFN-γ, some of which is produced by other mature T_H1 cells. T_H1 cells are characterized by the release of IFN-γ and their role in cell-mediated immunity. Interferons are generally produced in response to viral infections; although an infected cell is not able to protect itself from a virus, it can release interferon which will alert other cells to the presence of the virus and initiate anti-viral measures in those cells, limiting the ability of the infection to spread. Through their release of IFN-γ,

T_H1 cells will also activate T_C and NK cells, thus enhancing an anti-viral immune response. On the other hand, T_H2 and T_H17 cells play vital roles in humoral immunity. T_H2 cells, polarized by the presence of IL-4, specialize in protection against extracellular parasites such as helminths. Similarly to T_H1 cells, T_H17 cells differentiate in response to pro-inflammatory cytokines, including IL-6, IL-21 and IL-23 in combination with transforming growth factor β (TGF-β); these T_H cells aid in the clearance of extracellular bacteria and fungi. The activity of these cells must be tightly regulated, as overstimulation of either T_H1 or T_H17 cells has been shown to elicit autoimmune effects while excessive T_H2 activity has been implicated in the development of allergies and asthma. Subsequently, regulatory, or suppressor, T-cells, as well as iT_{regs} are necessary to dampen and ultimately, terminate the activity of these T_H cells. Finally, T_{FH} cells modulate the maturation of B-lymphocytes into antibody-releasing plasma cells, the second arm of the adaptive immune response.

The Immune System and the Brain

Unlike the peripheral tissues of the body, typical immune cells, such as macrophages, are not commonly found within the brain unless the blood–brain barrier has been compromised. Nevertheless, the brain does have specialized cells with immune-like functions; chief among these are microglia, which are functionally similar to macrophages located in the periphery. Their branching processes make contact with neurons and astrocytes, as well as the endothelial cells of the vasculature. Upon activation, microglia retract their processes and can migrate to sites of injury, where they eliminate apoptotic and necrotic cells through phagocytosis. This function is vital for maintaining homeostasis within the brain. Additionally, both cytokines and chemokines are found throughout the brain, and it has even been suggested that chemokines may act as neurotransmitters or neuromodulators in a variety of brain functions (Rostene *et al.*, 2011; Tonelli, Postolache, and Sternberg, 2005). Chemokines and their receptors are constitutively expressed in regions associated with adult neurogenesis, including the olfactory bulb and hippocampus, where they may modulate cell proliferation and differentiation (Turbic, Leong, and Turnley, 2011). The only member of the CX3C family, fractalkine, is widely expressed in neurons throughout the brain. The role of chemokines in synaptic transmission has gained greater scrutiny as well, as they have been shown to enhance GABAergic function in various brain regions, including the hippocampus (Bhattacharyya *et al.*, 2008) and dorsal raphe nuclei (Heinisch and Kirby, 2009, 2010) and may regulate adenosine receptor activity, subsequently inhibiting glutamatergic neurotransmission (Piccinin *et al.*, 2010). Additionally, astrocytes and microglia secrete both pro- and anti-inflammatory cytokines and, along with neurons, express cytokine receptors, suggesting that even though the brain is sequestered from the peripheral immune system they still communicate with each other.

Over the past few decades it has become abundantly clear that this communication is necessary for the normal functioning of the brain as well as for regulation of the stress response through activation of the hypothalamic–pituitary–adrenal (HPA) axis during times of severe stress and illness (for an exhaustive review please see Yirmiya and Goshen, 2011). The role of T-cells in the modulation of brain function is just beginning to be elucidated; although T-cells are not typically found within the brain parenchyma they do migrate to the meninges and can be found within the blood vessels of highly vasculated regions such as the hippocampus (Brynskikh *et al.*, 2008). Interestingly, although the anti-inflammatory cytokine IL-4 is most often associated with beneficial effects on cognitive function, pro-inflammatory cytokines IL-1, IL-6 and TNF-α have also been linked to maintaining proper brain functioning. These effects are elicited through a variety of mechanisms, not least of which is the secretion of neurotrophic factors such as brain-derived neurotrophic factor (BDNF), nerve growth factor (NGF), insulin-like growth factor-1 (IGF-1), and vascular endothelial growth factor (VEGF) from both brain cells and immune cells. However, excessive release of these cytokines, often as a consequence of severe stress or an inflammatory response, is detrimental and has been linked to impairments in learning and memory, as well as neural plasticity and neurogenesis. Mast cells are also found in the brain and shown to have important modulatory functions including modulating sexual function and emotional states (Nautiyal *et al.*, 2008). These are just a few examples of the importance that immune cells, immune genes, neural-to-immune and immune-to-neural signaling have on brain function and behavior. Due to the relationship between certain inflammatory processes with a variety of cognitive and mental disorders, including depression, schizophrenia and autism, the role of the immune system and immunity on the brain has come under greater scrutiny. Thus, several models have been developed to study the impact of immune system activation on cognition and behavior.

Methods in Immunology with Relevance for Psychoneuroimmunology

The research methodology employed in the study of immune system function is extensive and covers all the aspects of biomedical research, from molecular and cellular to animal models and clinical studies. The present section will focus on some basic and validated methodologies developed in the field of immunology that have relevance for the study of emotional and cognitive effects of immune activation. Most of the experimental models involve the use of whole animals because the study usually demands testing in a behavioral setting aimed at evaluating emotional and cognitive functions. Some of these models have also been employed in human studies, with appropriate modifications for compliance with clinical studies. Furthermore, some *in vitro* cell culture models have also been employed to study specific interactions between immune cells and neurotransmitter systems known to modulate cognition and emotion. Two main methods have been widely used in psychoneuroimmunology to elicit an immune response that may be reflected in changes in behavior and/or mental and cognitive functions. One is using live infectious agents such as viruses, bacteria and parasites that have limited lethality or are capable of establishing permanent infections without resulting in death of the host. Some examples are the use of influenza viruses, neurotropic retroviruses and *Toxoplasma gondii* (*T. gondii*) in schizophrenia research, and the use of attenuated strains of bacteria in depression research. The second method is probably the most often employed: it consists of using molecules that mimic the presence of live infectious agents and therefore elicit an immune response similar to the pathogen. Some examples are the use of polysaccharides such as lipopolysaccharides from Gram-negative bacteria, polyriboinosinic-polyribocytidilic acid (poly I:C) mimicking viral nucleic acid, and proteins with particular antigenic properties such as albumin from chicken egg or myelin basic protein. These models have been complemented by behavioral pharmacological studies using direct administration of cytokines in the brain. The following sections will discuss specific agents commonly used in psychoneuroimmunology, starting with immunostimulatory agents, since they have been the most used in psychoneuroimmunology research.

Lipopolysaccharides

Theoretically, any molecule that is foreign to the organism has the potential to elicit an immune response. Nevertheless, polysaccharides are among the most potent molecules known to be capable of activating a strong immune response that is generally dose-dependent and usually results in death at high concentrations. Unequivocally, the most widely used antigen in psychoneuroimmunology has been lipopolysaccharides (LPS) from Gram-negative bacteria. In particular, a few serotypes obtained from *Escherichia coli* (*E. coli*), serotype O55:B5, serotype O127:B8 and serotype 0111:B4 from Sigma (Sigma-Aldrich, St. Louis, MO), have been employed in a majority of studies. They have been shown to elicit a strong inflammatory response in almost all strains of rats and mice tested so far. An equivalent of LPS from *E coli* obtained from *Salmonella abortus-equi (S. abortus-equi)* has been employed in a landmark clinical study administered intravenously at low concentration in healthy individuals under experimentally controlled conditions (Reichenberg *et al.*, 2001).

Polysaccharides are molecular components of cell walls of bacterial organisms. In particular, *E. coli* is an enterobacteriaceae living in the digestive tract of most mammals. The purified fraction of LPS (the O antigen from the above-mentioned serotypes) from *E. coli* is capable of inducing an immune response when present in systemic compartments of the organism. LPS binds to the soluble lipopolysaccharide-binding protein (LBP) forming the LPS–LBP complex, which in turn binds to CD14 (cluster of differentiation 14) and TLR-4. TLR4 activation leads to a well-described intracellular signaling cascade resulting in activation of the transcription factor NF-κB and production of pro-inflammatory cytokines. As PRRs, the CD14 and TLR4 receptors play critical roles in the innate immune response. Thus, LPS induces a dose-dependent activation of the innate immune response involving macrophages and the production of cytokines such as IL-1β, TNF-α and IL-6 that may ultimately result in death by septic shock if the concentrations are too high. The lethal doses for rats and mice are about 20 to 50 mg/kg depending on the strain and species. Subseptic doses of LPS ranging from 0.1 to 2.5 mg/kg administered peripherally by intraperitoneal (i.p.) injections are capable of inducing the production of cytokines in the brain primarily by microglia and astrocytes, and perhaps even neurons, depending on the dose. Most of the components necessary for the recognition of LPS, including CD14 and TLR4, are expressed in the brain, and mechanisms transducing signals from the periphery to the brain regarding the presence of LPS have been extensively studied. The production of cytokines by brain cells has been associated with the behavioral signs of sickness and other behavioral changes including depressive-like behaviors and cognitive impairments. The mechanisms by which LPS induces neurobehavioral changes are an active area of psychoneuroimmunology research.

The models that have been employed using LPS in the study of behavioral and psychological outcomes relate to the dose and route of administration, number of LPS challenges (single, repeated or chronic) and developmental stage of the challenge. The most common model has been administration of subseptic doses of LPS by i.p. injection. This model of subseptic i.p. LPS intends to mimic an inflammatory process in the periphery involving an increase in circulating cytokines such as IL-1β, TNF-α and IL-6, and it can be interpreted as a model of general systemic inflammation in general. Another model is the direct injection into the brain of low doses of LPS by various methods including a single injection or constant delivery by minpumps. This model has been used to study different mechanisms of interaction between locally produced cytokines and neurons. A less common model employs administration of LPS by intranasal delivery; this model results in an inflammatory process in the respiratory tract that mimics certain types of chronic or seasonal respiratory infections.

Despite the usefulness and validity of these LPS models, certain limitations have been also observed. For example, administration of LPS i.p. and in the brain has been shown to cause tolerance to further LPS challenges, limiting its usefulness as a model of chronic or sustained inflammation. The model has also been questioned due to the lack of evidence that any chronic inflammatory disease or psychological disorder is related to the presence of bacterial LPS. Another problem when using these approaches is the observed variability in the inflammatory response to LPS within individuals of the same species. While the exact reason for this variability has not been fully elucidated, some possibilities have been related to factors such as time of day of the administration, hormonal status, and housing conditions, including hierarchy in the home cage. Despite these limitations it must be recognized that the LPS-challenge model is one of the leading models in psychoneuroimmunology research.

Nucleic acids

Nucleic acids of viral and bacterial origin are also potent activators of the innate immune response. The use of synthetic strands of RNA and DNA to elicit an immune response has proved to be a valid alternative to the use of purified viral and bacterial RNA and DNA. In particular, poly I:C is employed to mimic viral RNA, and phosphorylated and repeated CG sequences oligodeoxynucleotides (CpG ODNs) are used to mimic bacterial DNA in models similar to those described for LPS. Synthetic CpG ODNs activate the immune response by a mechanism engaging Toll-like receptor 9 (TLR9), an intracellular PRR. Thus, the mechanism of immune activation mediated by CpG ODNs is different from that mediated by LPS, yet it also results in activation of the innate immune response and the production of pro-inflammatory cytokines. An important difference is that CpG ODNs are capable of also activating T_H1 responses and the production of interferons in addition to pro-inflammatory cytokines. Briefly, immunostimulatory CpG ODNs initiates a cascade of cellular activation generally starting from B cells and plasmacytoid dendritic cells (pDC) followed by natural killer cells, T-cells and macrophages resulting in the production of pro-inflammatory cytokines and chemokines including IL-1β, IL-6, IL-18, and TNF-α and the T_H1 cytokines IFN-γ and IL-12 (Klinman *et al.*, 2008). They have also been shown to induce cytokine expression in the brain in a manner similar to that of LPS when administered peripherally via i.p. injections. A number of studies have determined the inflammatory and immunostimulatory properties of CpG ODNs in the brain and nervous system, mostly in relation to anti-cancer therapies and infections. However, there has been limited research on the neuropsychological and behavioral effects of CpG challenges. In contrast, poly I:C has been widely employed and is currently one of the leading models for studying immune activation during prenatal and perinatal periods and its effects on the brain and behavior. It also has been employed in models using adult animals that receive repeated administrations in models of chronic fatigue. Poly I:C RNA activates the immune response through a TLR3-dependent-mechanism resulting in the production of pro-inflammatory and T_H1 cytokines. An important role for TLR3 receptors has also been proposed for inducing adaptive immune processes and protective immunity to viruses. Thus, poly I:C challenges are regarded as adequate models of immune activation in response to viruses. Since certain psychiatric diseases, including schizophrenia, are believed to encompass a neurodevelopmental insult possibly involving viruses, poly I:C, rather than LPS, is used in models of maternal immune activation during gestation. In this model pregnant rats or mice are administered i.p. or intravenously with doses around 5 mg/kg over several consecutive days. The offspring is then evaluated on behavior at different developmental stages from early puberty to adulthood. Several neurophysiological and behavioral abnormalities have been documented in these animals that resemble some of the core features of major psychiatric diseases (Meyer and Feldon, 2012). A consideration of this model is that pregnant mothers receiving poly I:C often have reduced litters and/or early mortality depending on the magnitude of the challenge. In addition, the model does not evaluate other important components of a viral infection such as antigen processing of viral proteins and adaptive immune responses. However, the model is extremely useful in showing how activation of the host immune response during critical developmental periods of the CNS results in long-lasting and permanent alterations of brain function and behavior.

Superantigens

Superantigens (SAgs) are a special class of protein toxins that originated from the biological activity of certain viral and bacterial organisms. They are capable of activating T-cells by direct stimulation of the T-cell receptor, leading to a rapid activation and expansion of T-cells. This process increases the production of T-cell cytokines such as IL-2, IL-12 and IFN-γ, and also results in neurobehavioral changes (Urbach-Ross and Kusnecov, 2009). Although SAgs stimulate T-cells to proliferate and produce cytokines, the process does not include the classical mechanisms of antigen processing and presentation of the adaptive immune response. Thus, the name "superantigens" is related to the property of these molecules of "bypassing" this mechanism to directly activate T-cells in a non-specific manner. These molecules bind to or "are recognized" in specific invariable regions of the variable portion of the T-cell receptor (Vβ region). Therefore, they have the ability to stimulate several clones carrying the same invariable gene, resulting in oligoclonal activation and expansion that can constitute up to 10 to 20 % of the T-cell pool of the organism. The most employed SAgs in psychoneuroimmunology research are bacterial enterotoxins secreted from the Gram-positive bacteria *Staphylococcus aureus* (*S. aureus*). They have been characterized by their capacity to activate a number of T-cells in mice, rats, and humans. There are a number of identified superantigenic enterotoxins (SE) from *S. aureus* that have been termed A, B, C, etc., resulting in a serologic classification as SEA, SEB, SEC and so on. In particular, two types, SEA and SEB, have been used in C57Bl/6 and BALB/c mice respectively in psychoneuroimmunology research. SEA and SEB administered by i.p. injections have been shown to result in a complex neurobehavioral mechanism involving activation of specific brain regions and elevations in the cytokines IL-1β, IL-2, IL-6, IL-10, IFN-γ and TNF-α. The behavioral repertoire affected by SEA and SEB has been related to increased anxiety and neophobia (Rossi-George *et al.*, 2005). Remarkably, these effects have been shown to occur without any overt signs of sickness which occur following LPS and poly I:C challenges. Several brain regions have been shown to express the immediate early gene c-fos during SAgs challenge, indicative of neuronal activation. Some of these regions such as the paraventricular hypothalamic (PVH) and arcuate (Arc) nuclei and the central nucleus of the amygdala (CeA) points to neuroendocrine and limbic activation. It also results in elevation of endogenous glucocorticoids and activation of the hypothalamo–pituitary–adrenal (HPA) axis. Another differential feature of this model of T-cell activation with respect to the LPS model is that HPA-axis activation has been shown to be dependent on the cytokine TNF-α alone, as compared to the synergistic actions of IL1-β, IL-6 and TNF-α in the LPS model. The specific activation of T-cells and their cytokines, the absence of malaise, and the engagement of specific brain regions provide an excellent model of T-cell-dependent immune activation that allows for the differentiation of specific mechanisms mediated by T-cells from other non-specific models such as the LPS challenge. This is particularly relevant for human studies because most chronic inflammatory diseases are maintained by the activity of T-cells. Since most chronic inflammatory conditions have been associated with increased incidence of depressive and anxiety disorders, this model is a valid approach in psychoneuroimmunology research.

Proteins

Most protein complexes do not have antigenic properties for their recognition by innate immune cells or PRRs. This implies that a protein complex or a polypeptide that is strange to the organism will require antigen processing and presentation by dendritic cells to lymphocytes, a hallmark mechanism of adaptive or acquired immunity. This process will result in activation of a specific subset of lymphocytes that will initiate an immune process directed at neutralizing and/or clearing the pathogen containing the specific peptide sequence. It usually involves production of antibodies by B-cells and the establishment of immunological memory. The models employing proteins to induce an immune response require a protocol of induction that involves several steps, including a sensitization process by repeated exposure followed by antigen challenge after a period of time. Several proteins have been employed in such models including myelin basic protein (MBP) and albumin from chicken egg or ovalbumin (OVA). MBP is used to model autoimmune multiple sclerosis (MS) in a model initially called experimental allergic encephalomyelitis and later re-named experimental autoimmune encephalomyelitis (EAE), and represents one of the most widely used models to study the initiation and progression of MS. The few studies that have evaluated the emotional, cognitive, and behavioral implications of an active autoimmune and neurodegenerative process in the brain in the EAE model have confirmed that emotional and cognitive disturbances are associated with the inflammatory process of EAE. However, the number of studies addressing emotion and cognition in the EAE model are far less common than those focusing on mechanisms of the disease.

The second most common protein used for inducing and adaptive immune response is OVA, which has been extensively used as a model of protein antigen *in vivo*. The immunization protocol involves sensitization by i.p. injections of OVA solutions coupled to an adjuvant and later exposure to the OVA peptide via respiratory, cutaneous or oral administrations. In general, this model has been employed to induce a T_H2-mediated inflammatory allergic response to OVA that, depending on the route of exposure, may mimic food, respiratory, or skin allergies. Challenge with OVA in sensitized mice and rats results in a complex T_H2-mediated inflammatory reaction that has become one of the standard models of experimentally induced allergies. It includes the clonal expansion of OVA-specific T_H2 lymphocytes and the production of IgE antibodies against OVA by B-cells. This leads to hypersensitivity to OVA that is mostly mediated by mast cell degranulation as the result of binding to and activation of the Fc receptor by the OVA/IgE complex. The inflammatory process triggered by the mediators released by mast cells, such as proteases, leukotrienes, histamine, etc., is amplified by the recruitment of eosinophils and basophils that produce and release more cytokines and inflammatory molecules. A feature of this model is that the magnitude of the inflammatory response depends mostly on the number of challenges rather than the dose of antigen used. Thus, the inflammatory response increases with the number of exposures and not by the single exposure to a higher concentration of the antigen. It has been shown in mice and rats that allergies to OVA are paralleled by increased responses of anxiety in several behavioral tests, and that these responses are related to both early events of the allergic reaction such as IgE-dependent mast cell degranulation and also to later processes such as lymphocyte recruitment. The pattern of cytokine production corresponds to the T_H2 type involving IL-4, IL-5 and IL-13 production mainly by T-cells, eosinophils, and basophils and eventually the release of TNF-α from mast cells. Similarly to the SAgs model, allergies to OVA have been shown to result in c-fos expression in the PVH and CeA, and also in the nucleus of the solitary tract (NTS), suggesting a role for these regions in responding to processes mediated by T-cells (Costa-Pinto *et al.*, 2005). In addition, exposure to OVA in sensitized animals does not result in overt signs of sickness, which is also a feature in the SAgs model. However, no clear evidence of elevations in endogenous glucocorticoids has been reported, pointing to important differences with the previously discussed models (Tonelli *et al.*, 2009). The significance of this model also relies in the opportunity for clinical research since allergies are very common in the population and several human studies have established the link between allergies and anxiety disorders and behavioral responses of anxiety. For instance, state and trait anxiety in allergic individuals have been documented in clinical studies, and increased anxiety and emotional reactivity has been reported after antigen exposure in humans (Buske-Kirschbaum *et al.*, 2008; Rosenkranz *et al.*, 2005). Thus, the OVA model closely represents the emotional alterations associated with allergies – one of the most common chronic inflammatory conditions in the developed world.

Cytokines

The notion that specific cytokines are responsible for eliciting specific neurobehavioral responses through their direct interaction with different neural circuitries has been a major focus of research in psychoneuroimmunology. For instance, cytokines are produced within neural circuitries, and receptors for cytokines are expressed on neurons and other brain parenchymal cells (eg., glia), which can mediate consequent electrophysiological and intracellular responses. Thus, it is easy to understand that a major approach in psychoneuroimmunology has been the direct infusion of cytokines and their antagonists in different brain regions to study behavioral responses to pharmacological doses of cytokines. In addition, peripheral administration of cytokines via intravenous injections has also been extensively employed. These approaches have provided important evidence about the role of several cytokines in mediating behavioral responses associated with immune activation. For example, blocking IL-1β and TNF-α actions in the brain prevents sickness behavior after LPS administration. These studies also showed that elevations of cytokines such as IL-β in the periphery also result in the behavioral changes of sickness, and that blockade of IL-1β in the brain abolished the effect. Thus, these studies provided evidence that immune activation initiated in the periphery that results in the elevation of circulating cytokines is responsible for behavioral changes that are mediated by the actions of cytokines in the brain (Anisman, Gibb, and Hayley, 2008; Dantzer *et al.*, 2008;). An important consideration of studies using direct infusion of cytokines to evaluate behavior is that there are no "true" pharmacological antagonists for cytokines in the classical sense of displacing the ligand from the receptor by competitive binding. Thus, the most employed method for blocking or interfering with cytokine action is by using endogenously produced antagonists such as soluble IL-1 receptor antagonist (IL-1Ra) to prevent the actions of IL-1β. These endogenous cytokine antagonists are often found commercially available from different sources specializing in the production of recombinant proteins. Another method for blocking cytokine action is by using antibodies capable of neutralizing their biological activity, commonly called neutralizing antibodies. Finally, the use of genetically engineered recombinant proteins such as the TNF-α receptor inhibitor Etanercept may become the tool of choice for future pharmacological studies.

Live infectious agents

The live infectious agents, including viruses, bacteria, and parasites, used to study their effects on brain function and behavior can be distinguished by those capable of invading the CNS and establishing permanent infections in the brain and those that proliferate largely in peripheral organs with limited neuroinvasion. Models of chronic CNS invasion mostly involve the use of neurotropic viruses and the parasite *T. gondii*. These models have been employed in studies related to psychiatric diseases such as schizophrenia and autism which have been historically related to viral and parasitic CNS infections. Several studies have provided important insights on the neural and behavioral consequences of permanent or chronic CNS infections. For example, chronic infections in mice and rats with herpes simplex virus (HSV) and Borna disease virus (BDV) have been shown to produce specific alterations in the brain and behavior that relate to higher cognitive function such as learning and memory (Lipkin and Hornig, 2004). The model of chronic infection using *T. gondii* has revealed that the presence of the parasite in brain tissue is capable of influencing specific behaviors of fear and anxiety (Vyas *et al.*, 2007) however the relationship of *T. gondii* infection and schizophrenia remains elusive. These models differ from other models of acute infection using the same and other viruses in the magnitude of the inflammatory response to an acute infection. For example, acute BDV and influenza infections may result in encephalitis with varied damage to the brain. Infections with influenza virus via intranasal instillations in pregnant dams have been employed in models of neurodevelopmental maternal viral insult (Patterson, 2009). The offspring of mice and rats infected with different strains of influenza during pregnancy display deficits in exploratory behavior, social interaction, and recognition of novel objects, and specific deficits in acoustic startle responses, similar to those observed in humans with schizophrenia. In these models the viral infection does not reach the fetus or the developing CNS and thus evaluates the effect of maternal immune activation on the offspring. Experimental infection with the live virus closely represents the course and progression of illness and therefore it may be a better model than poly I:C when studying interactions of maternal immunity and brain development. However, the poly I:C model is more commonly used owing to the more direct set up and implementation of the model. Finally, a model of live bacterial infection has been used by inoculating mice with i.p. injections of an attenuated form of *Mycobacterium bovis*, bacilli Calmette-Guerin (BCG) (O'Connor *et al.*, 2009). Infection of mice with BCG results in a progression of illness characterized by an initial stage during which symptoms of sickness behavior manifest; this is followed by their resolution during the next stage although the mycobacteria are still present in organs such as the lungs, liver and spleen. During this time, cytokine expression and cellular immunity remain activated, offering a window of opportunity to conduct behavioral tests and thus representing a good model of chronic inflammation and/or immune activation.

Immune Processes and their Clinical Consequences on Mental Health

The models presented here have been and continue to be actively employed to evaluate the potential involvement of immunity in initiating, precipitating or perpetuating complex psychiatric diseases of unknown etiology. Although the causes leading to the pathophysiology of mental illness remain unresolved, there is a significant body of evidence implicating the immune system and/or inflammatory processes in some aspects of anxiety and depressive disorders, schizophrenia, and autism as well as in the cognitive and psychological decline of aging. For example, interest in the psychoneuroimmunology of depression was sparked by the observation that cancer patients receiving interferon-alpha (IFN-α) therapy would often develop depressive symptoms. Numerous studies since then have shown that depression in humans is associated with inflammation. Over many studies, researchers have determined a general immunological profile of depression generally characterized by increased acute phase proteins and impaired cellular immunity as well as increased inflammatory cytokines such as IL-1β, IL-6, and TNF-α (Blume, Douglas, and Evans, 2011), and a mild inflammatory response (Kronfol, Singh, and Zhang 1995). Dysregulation of the HPA axis is one of the most consistent physiological findings in major depression; specifically, corticotrophin-releasing hormone (CRH) hypersecretion accompanied by a lowered adrenocorticotropic hormone (ACTH) response to CRH stimulation. Pro-inflammatory cytokines such as IL-1β and IL-6 stimulate the production of CRH and thus may be driving this dysregulation (Maes *et al.*, 1993). Depression in humans encompasses a broad range of symptoms; some of them, including fatigue/hypersomnia, insomnia, weight gain, weight loss, irritability, anhedonia, lack of energy, and decreased libido, are measurable in animals during activation of the innate immune response. The suite of behavioral changes that accompany the LPS model, including social withdrawal, altered sleep patterns, reduced food and water intake, as well as lower activity levels, that collectively are called sickness behavior can be used, with the appropriate considerations, as a proxy for depression. Thus, the behavioral depression induced by the LPS model provides a working model to study mechanisms of neuroimmune interaction leading to the worsening of the motivational state of mammalian organisms (Dantzer *et al.*, 2008).

Another example of the validity of the models discussed previously is the association between T-cell function and anxiety disorders, a large category encompassing a number of distinct disorders, including generalized anxiety, specific phobias, social phobia, post-traumatic stress disorder (PTSD), obsessive–compulsive disorder, and panic disorder. As discussed above, anxiety disorders have been linked to allergic and autoimmune disorders by a significant number of epidemiological and clinical studies. Thus models based on T-cell activation, such as the OVA model, which induce responses of anxiety provide a good working model to study the relationship between allergic inflammation, T-cell function, and anxiety disorders. The SAgs model that involves specific T-cell responses and also affects anxiety provides an additional model to study this relationship. Furthermore, severe anxiety syndromes such as PTSD are accompanied by immunological alterations affecting lymphocyte function. A known long-lasting physiological consequence of psychological trauma is the one observed on T lymphocyte number and function. A number of studies report a higher lymphocyte count in PTSD patients. Findings include increased total lymphocytes (Boscarino and Chang, 1999; Vidovic *et al.*, 2007), higher percentage of cytotoxic $CD8^+$ T-cells (Lemieux, Coe, and Carnes, 2008) and increased overall

$CD8^+$ cytotoxic T-cells (Skarpa *et al.*, 2001). These findings suggest increased production of T-cells with an inflammatory profile (increased cytotoxic and memory-effector T-cells) which last for a considerable time after exposure to psychological trauma and are associated with the permanence of PTSD symptoms (Gill *et al.*, 2009). In addition, natural killer cell activity varies with temporal proximity to trauma, being increased in chronic PTSD and reduced in recent trauma survivors (Vidovic *et al.*, 2007). Circulating inflammatory cytokines, specifically IL-6 and TNF-α, are higher in people suffering from PTSD than in traumatized non-PTSD controls (Maes *et al.*, 1999). Interestingly, this higher circulating IL-6 may be a predisposing factor to the development of PTSD (Sutherland, Alexander, and Hutchison, 2003). In sum, there is a significant parallel between altered lymphocyte function and anxiety disorders that warrants the interest of psychoneuroimmunology.

Further interest in the role of immunity in mental health stems from the evidence of a possible etiology for schizoaffective disorders linked to an infectious agent during development. Studies demonstrated a significant susceptibility in people born in the winter, when rhinoviruses and influenza are most active; population studies have shown that schizophrenia cases also increase after influenza epidemics. Later studies have shown that prenatal exposure to influenza, toxoplasmosis, and herpes viruses like herpes simplex, Epstein-Barr virus, and cytomegalovirus are associated with offspring schizophrenia. These diverse findings indicate that viral infection in general, rather than any one specific pathogen, may be the immune trigger for the long-lasting damage seen in schizophrenia. In this regard, the poly I:C model offers a valuable tool to study specific mechanisms of viral immune activation during pregnancy and their consequences in adulthood on the brain and behavior. It produces schizophrenia-like alterations in the brain, and the associated behavioral symptoms respond to proven anti-psychotic drugs (summarized in Meyer and Feldon, 2012). Additional major psychiatric diseases linked to a developmental immune insult are autism spectrum disorders. A large epidemiological study in Denmark found a significant association between maternal viral infection in the first trimester and autism (Atladóttir *et al.*, 2010). In this case, a role for the production of maternal antibodies against viral or bacterial infections has been proposed. Experiments on antibody transfer provide compelling evidence for this hypothesis. In this type of study, antibodies are collected from mothers who have children with autism, which are then injected into a pregnant animal. In both mice and rhesus monkeys, the resultant offspring have been shown to develop autism-like behaviors, such as hyperactivity, stereotypy, and impaired social interaction (Singer *et al.*, 2009). These fetal-brain-specific IgG antibodies are associated with approximately 15% of human autism cases, and seem specific to the regressive type of autism, in which a child meets developmental milestones until the age of two years, and then begins to miss them.

Concluding Remarks

This chapter presented a brief introduction to some basic aspects of immunity and how it relates to brain function and behavior in the context of mental health research. It also presented some of the models used to study the effects of activation of the immune system on emotional and cognitive function. As these models are dynamic and continue to improve, it is expected that better models of psychoneuroimmune interaction will shed light on complex psychiatric diseases and perhaps provide targets of improved intervention to treat these diseases.

References

Anisman, H., Gibb, J., and Hayley, S. (2008). Influence of continuous infusion of interleukin-1beta on depression-related processes in mice: corticosterone, circulating cytokines, brain monoamines, and cytokine mRNA expression. *Psychopharmacology* (Berlin), 199(2), 231–44.

Atladóttir, H.O., Thorsen, P., Østergaard, L., Schendel, D.E., Lemcke, S., Abdallah, M., and Parner, E.T. (2010). Maternal infection requiring hospitalization during pregnancy and autism spectrum disorders. *Journal of Autism and Developmental Disorders*, 40, 1423–1430.

Baker, D.G., Ekhator, N.N., Kasckow, J.W., Hill, K.K., Zoumakis, E., Dashevsky, B.A., Chrousos, G.P., and Geracioti, T.D. Jr. (2001). Plasma and cerebrospinal fluid interleukin-6 concentrations in posttraumatic stress disorder. *Neuroimmunomodulation*, 9, 209–217.

Bhattacharyya, B. J., Banisadr, G., Jung, H., Ren, D., Cronshaw, D. G., Zou, Y., and Miller, R.J. (2008). The chemokine stromal cell-derived factor-1 regulates GABAergic inputs to neural progenitors in the postnatal dentate gyrus. *Journal of Neuroscience*, 28, 6720–6730.

Blume, J., Douglas, S.D., and Evans, D.L. (2011). Immune suppression and immune activation in depression. *Brain, Behavior, and Immunity*, 25(2), 221–9.

Boscarino, J.A. (2004). Posttraumatic stress disorder and physical illness: results from clinical and epidemiologic studies. *Annals of the New York Academy of Sciences*, 1032, 141–53.

Boscarino, J.A., and Chang, J. (1999). Higher abnormal leukocyte and lymphocyte counts 20 years after exposure to severe stress: research and clinical implications. *Psychosomatic Medicine*, 61(3), 378–86.

Brynskikh, A., Warren, T., Zhu, J., and Kipnis, J. (2008). Adaptive immunity affects learning behavior in mice. *Brain, Behavior, and Immunity*, 22(6), 861–9.

Buske-Kirschbaum, A., Ebrecht, M., Kern, S., Gierens, A., and Hellhammer, D.H. (2008). Personality characteristics in chronic and non-chronic allergic conditions. *Brain, Behavior, and Immunity*, 22(5), 762–8.

Costa-Pinto, F.A., Basso, A.S., Britto, L.R., Malucelli, B.E., and Russo, M. (2005). Avoidance behavior and neural correlates of allergen exposure in a murine model of asthma. *Brain, Behavior, and Immunity*, 19, 52–60.

Dammann, O., and Meyer, U. (2011). Schizophrenia and autism: both shared and disorder specific pathogenesis via perinatal inflammation? *Pediatric Research*, 69, 26R–33R.

Dantzer, R., O'Connor, J.C., Freund, G.G., Johnson, R.W., and Kelley, K.W. (2008). From inflammation to sickness and depression: when the immune system subjugates the brain. *Nature Reviews Neuroscience*, 9(1), 46–56.

Gill, J.M., Saligan, L., Woods, S., and Payge, G. (2009). PTSD is associated with an excess of inflammatory immune activities. *Perspectives in Psychiatric Care*, 45, 262–277.

Heinisch, S. and Kirby, L.G. (2009). Fractalkine/CX3CL1 enhances GABA synaptic activity at serotonin neurons in the rat dorsal raphe nucleus. *Neuroscience*, 164(3), 1210–1223.

Heinisch, S. and Kirby, L.G. (2010). SDF-1alpha/CXCL12 enhances GABA and glutamate synaptic activity at serotonin neurons in the rat dorsal raphe nucleus. *Neuropharmacology* 58(2), 501–514.

Klinman, D., Shirota, H., Tross, D., Sato, T., and Klaschik, S. (2008). Synthetic oligonucleotides as modulators of inflammation. *Journal of Leukocyte Biology*, 84(4), 958–64.

Kronfol, Z., Singh, V.J., and Zhang, Q. (1995). Plasma cytokines, acute phase proteins and cortisol in major depression. *Biological Psychiatry*, 37: 609A.

Lemieux, A., Coe, C.L., and Carnes, M. (2008). Symptom severity predicts degree of T cell activation in adult women following childhood maltreatment. *Brain, Behavior, and Immunity*, 22(6), 994–1003.

Lipkin, W.I., and Hornig, M. (2004). *Psychotropic viruses. Current Opinion in Microbiology*, 7(4), 420–425.

Maes, M., Lin, A.H., Delmeire, L., Van, G.A., Kenis, G., DeJongh, R., and Bosmans, E. (1999). Elevated serum interleukin-6 (IL-6) and IL-6 receptor concentrations in posttraumatic stress disorder following accidental man-made traumatic events. *Biological Psychiatry*, 45, 833–839.

Maes, M., Scharpe, S., Bosmans, E., Vanderwoude, M., Suy, E., Calabrese, J., and Cosyns, P. (1993). Relationship between interleukin-6 activity, acute phase proteins and function of the hypothalamic–pituitary–adrenal axis in severe depression. *Psychiatry Research*, 49, 11–27.

Meyer, U., and Feldon, J. (2012). To poly(I:C) or not to poly(I:C): Advancing preclinical schizophrenia research through the use of prenatal immune activation models. *Neuropharmacology*, 62(3), 1308–1321.

Nautiyal, K.M., Ribeiro, A.C., Pfaff, D.W., and Silver, R. (2008). Brain mast cells link the immune system to anxiety-like behavior. *Proceedings of the National Academy of Sciences of the USA*. 105(46), 18053–18057.

O'Connor, J.C., André, C., Wang, Y., Lawson, M.A., Szegedi, S.S., Lestage, J., Castanon, N., Kelley, K.W., and Dantzer, R. (2009). Interferon-gamma and tumor necrosis factor-alpha mediate the upregulation of indoleamine 2,3-dioxygenase and the induction of depressive-like behavior in mice in response to bacillus Calmette-Guerin. *Journal of Neuroscience*, 29(13), 4200–4209.

Patterson, P.H. (2009). Immune involvement in schizophrenia and autism: etiology, pathology and animal models. *Behavioral and Brain Research*, 204, 313–321.

Piccinin, S., Di Angelantonio, S., Piccioni, A., Volpini, R., Cristalli, G., Fredholm, B.B., Limatola, C., Eusebi, F., and Ragozzino, D. (2010). CX3CL1-induced modulation at CA1 synapses reveals multiple mechanisms of EPSC modulation involving adenosine receptor subtypes. *Journal of Neuroimmunology*, 224(1–2), 85–92.

Reichenberg, A., Yirmiya, R., Schuld, A, Kraus, T., Haack, M., Morag, A., and Pollmächer, T. (2001). Cytokine-associated emotional and cognitive disturbances in humans. *Archives of General Psychiatry*, 58(5), 445–52.

Rosenkranz, M.A., Busse, W.W., Johnstone, T., Swenson, C.A., Crisafi, G.M., Jackson, M.M., Bosch, J.A., Sheridan, J.F., and Davidson, R.J. (2005). Neural circuitry underlying the interaction between emotion and asthma symptom exacerbation. *Proceedings of the National Academy of Sciences of the USA*, 102, 13319–13324.

Rossi-George, A., Urbach, D., Colas, D., Goldfarb, Y., and Kusnecov, A.W. (2005). Neuronal, endocrine, and anorexic responses to the T-cell superantigen staphylococcal enterotoxin A: dependence on tumor necrosis factor-alpha. *Journal of Neuroscience*, 25(22), 5314–5322.

Rostene, W., Dansereau, M.A., Godefroy, D., Van Steenwinckel, J., Reaux-Le Goazigo, A., Melik-Parsadaniantz, S. et al. (2011). Neurochemokines: a *menage a trois* providing new insights on the functions of chemokines in the central nervous system. *Journal of Neurochemistry*, 118(5), 680–694.

Sansone, R.A., and Sansone, L.A. (2011). Allergic rhinitis: relationships with anxiety and mood syndromes. *Innovations in Clinical Neuroscience*, 8, 12–17.

Singer, H.S., Morris, C., Gause, C., Pollard, M., Zimmerman, A.W., and Pletnikov, M. (2009). Prenatal exposure to antibodies from mothers of children with autism produces neurobehavioral alterations: A pregnant dam mouse model. *Journal of Neuroimmunology*, 211, 39–48.

Skarpa, I., Rubesa, G., Moro, L., Manestar, D., Petrovecki, M., and Rukavina, D. (2001). Changes of cytolytic cells and perforin expression in patients with posttraumatic stress disorder. *Croatian Medical Journal*, 42(5), 551–555.

Sutherland, A.G., Alexander, D.A., and Hutchison, J.D. 2003. Disturbance of pro-inflammatory cytokines in post-traumatic psychopathology. *Cytokine*, 24, 219–225.

Tonelli, L. H., Postolache, T.T., and Sternberg, E.M. (2005). Inflammatory genes and neural activity: involvement of immune genes in synaptic function and behavior. *Frontiers in Bioscience*, 10, 675–680.

Tonelli, L.H., Katz, M., Kovacsics, C.E., Joppy, B., Hoshino, A., Hoffman, G., Komarow, H., and Postaloche, T.T. (2009). Allergic rhinitis induces anxiety-like behavior and altered social interaction in rodents. *Brain, Behavior, and Immunity*, 23, 784–793.

Tonelli, L.H., and Postaloche, T.T. (2010). Airborne inflammatory factors: 'from the nose to the brain'. *Frontiers in Bioscience* (Scholar Edition), 2, 135–152.

Turbic, A., Leong, S.Y., and Turnley, A.M. (2011). Chemokines and inflammatory mediators interact to regulate adult murine neural precursor cell proliferation, survival and differentiation. *PLoS One*, 6(9), e25406.

Urbach-Ross, D., and Kusnecov, A.W. (2009). Impact of superantigenic molecules on central nervous system function. *Frontiers in Bioscience*, 14, 4416–4426.

Vidovic, A., Vilibic, M., Sabioncello, A., Gotovac, K., Rabatic, S., Folnegovic-Smalc, V., and Dekeris, D. (2007). Circulating lymphocyte subsets, natural killer cell cytotoxicity, and components of hypothalamic–pituitary–adrenal axis in Croatian war veterans with posttraumatic stress disorder: Cross-sectional study. *Croatian Medical Journal*, 48, 198–206.

Vyas, A., Kim, S.K., Giacomini, N., Boothroyd, J.C., and Sapolsky, R.M. (2007). Behavioral changes induced by *Toxoplasma* infection of rodents are highly specific to aversion of cat odors. *Proceedings of the National Academy of Sciences of the USA*, 104(15), 6442–6447.

Yirmiya, R., and Goshen, I. (2011). Immune modulation of learning, memory, neural plasticity and neurogenesis. *Brain, Behavior, and Immunity*, 25(2), 181–213.

Zuckerman, L., Rehavi, M., Nachman, R., and Weiner, I. (2003). Immune activation during pregnancy in rats leads to a postpubertal emergence of disrupted latent inhibition, dopaminergic hyperfunction, and altered limbic morphology in the offspring: a novel neurodevelopmental model of schizophrenia. *Neuropsychopharmacology*, 28, 1778–1789.

2

Innervation of the Immune System

Denise L. Bellinger,[1] Dwight M. Nance,[2] and Dianne Lorton[3]

[1] *Department of Pathology and Human Anatomy, Loma Linda University, School of Medicine, Loma Linda, CA, USA*
[2] *Department of Pediatrics, University of California, Irvine, CA, USA*
[3] *Department of Psychology, Kent State University, OH, USA*

The brain and the immune system interact by several pathways and mechanisms to affect health and influence disease. The brain regulates immune function via the neuroendocrine system and "hardwiring" of nerves that innervate immune cells in lymphoid organs and tissues. Innervation of immune organs is intimately involved in regulating immune homeostasis, and immune response to challenge. Psychosocial and physical stressors perceived and processed by the brain can affect the immune system through these neural pathways. Neural–immune modulation was first proposed to explain immune effects from behavioral conditioning studies. It is now clear that immune-mediated diseases, including neurodegenerative and cardiovascular disease, cancer, infections, and autoimmunity, can be strikingly influenced by psychosocial factors and behavioral conditions, which can affect morbidity, disease progression, and mortality. Neurally transduced signals to immune cells modulate normal function to maintain immune homeostasis, and regulate host defense to injury or antigen exposure. Peripheral nerves release specific neurotransmitters that bind to selective receptors expressed on immunocytes to affect their function.

The purpose of this chapter is to examine the innervation of lymphoid tissues, and briefly, its regulatory role in immunity. To better understand nerve-to-immune system pathways, we begin with a brief background on the peripheral nervous system as it relates to innervation of the immune system. Next, the innervation of primary and secondary lymphoid organs and mucosal-associated lymphoid tissues is discussed. A brief description of the basic lymphoid organ structure and function precedes each section describing the innervation of each lymphoid tissue in order to provide the basic anatomy needed to understand the nerve distribution, and its importance in immune regulation.

Basic Organization of the Autonomic and Sensory Systems

The nervous system can be subdivided in a very general way into two basic components for study, the central nervous system (CNS) and the peripheral nervous system (PNS) (Figure 2.1).

The Wiley-Blackwell Handbook of Psychoneuroimmunology, First Edition. Edited by Alexander W. Kusnecov and Hymie Anisman.

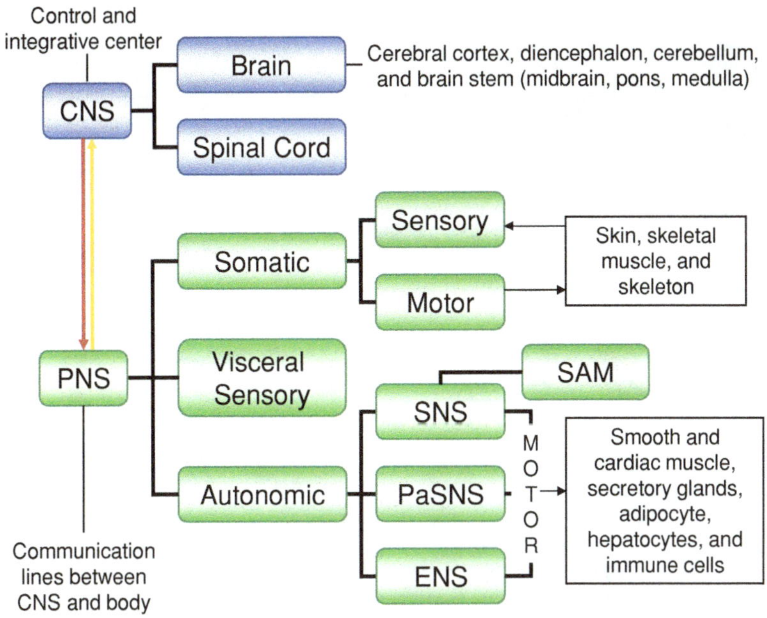

Figure 2.1 The major anatomical and functional divisions of the nervous system. The nervous system is divided into the central nervous system (CNS), consisting of the brain and spinal cord, and the peripheral nervous system (PNS), composed of the spinal and cranial (except I and II) nerves and ganglia (collections of neurons that reside outside the CNS). Sensory information for conscious perception enters the CNS and then ascends (yellow arrow) to the brain for integration. Motor information from the CNS descends to the brain stem and spinal cord, and is conveyed to muscles via the PNS (red arrow). The PNS is anatomically and functionally divided into somatic and autonomic nervous system (ANS) components. The somatic division provides for the sensory and motor functions of the skin, skeletal muscle and skeleton. The ANS regulates the functions of the visceral organs and has two divisions, the parasympathetic and sympathetic nervous systems (PaSNS and SNS, respectively). The sympathoadrenal medullary (SAM) axis is a part of the SNS. The ANS regulates the functions of smooth and cardiac muscle, secretory glands, adipocytes, hepatocytes, and immune cells, and is considered analogous to the motor component for the somatic division, but for involuntary movements. The ANS is an efferent motor system to visceral organs. Visceral sensory afferent nerves provide sensory information from the viscera to the CNS. These neurons are not usually included as a part of the ANS, but form the afferent limb for autonomic reflexes. The enteric nervous system (ENS) is a component of the ANS that resides in the wall of the intestines, and consists of a neuronal network that regulates functions of the gut).

The CNS contains the brain (including the brain stem) and spinal cord, which are protected by the meninges and bones of the skull and vertebrae. The CNS contains anatomically and functionally localized groups of neurons responsible for processing information and providing an appropriate response to different types of environmental and internal stimuli. The PNS is comprised of all the neural elements not in the brain and spinal cord; it is in contact with the external and internal environment. The PNS contains both a somatic and an autonomic component. The somatic component of the PNS consists of sensory receptors, axons, and cell bodies that provide the conduit for sensory input, and the axons of motor neurons and neuromuscular junctions that provide the motor output for controlling the contraction of skeletal muscle. The cell bodies of somatic sensory neurons are housed in dorsal root ganglia

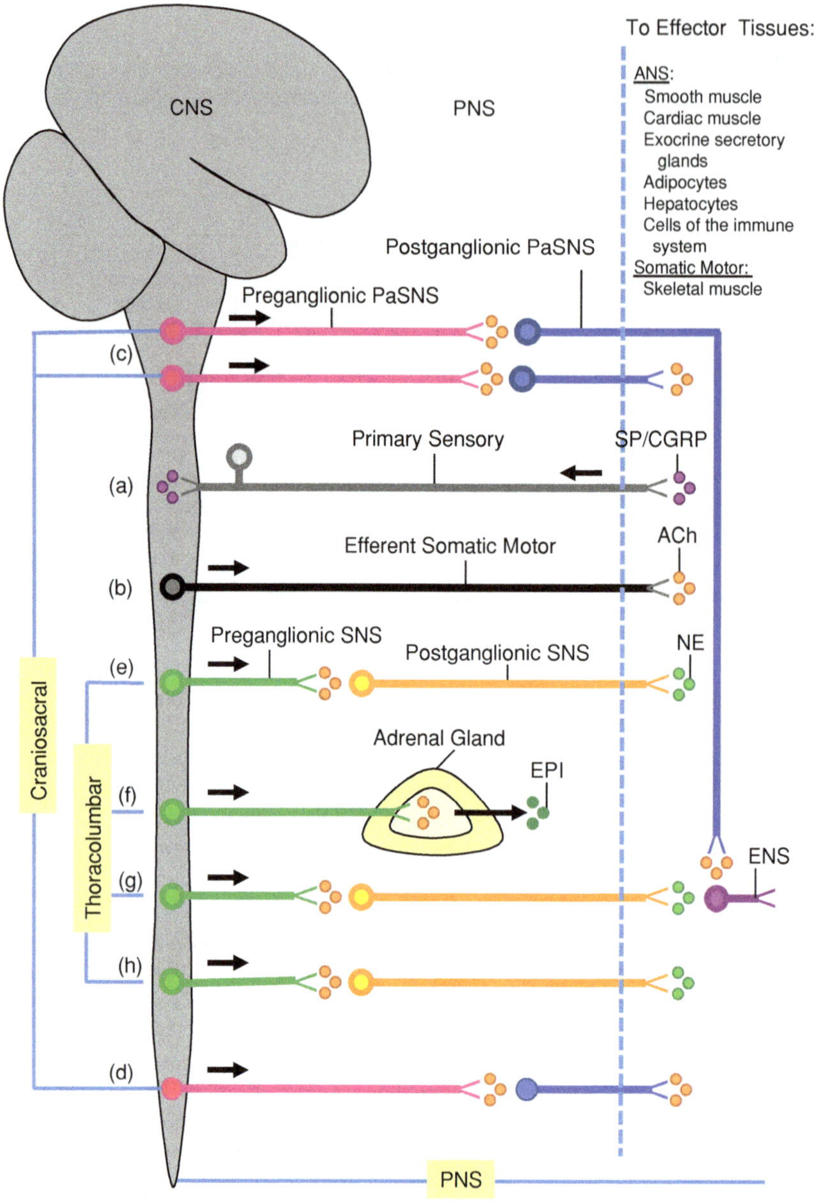

Figure 2.2 Basic features of the autonomic peripheral nervous system (PNS). (a) Afferent nerves from sensory neurons (gray stick neuron) in sensory ganglia convey information sensed from the periphery into the central nervous system (CNS; shown in gray). Primary afferent sensory nerves convey information to the CNS from the body. The viscera afferents or pain fibers shown here have the smallest diameter, are thinly or non-myelinated, and release substance P (SP) and calcitonin gene-related peptide (CGRP) (small purple circles) as their major neurotransmitter both distally and centrally. (b) Efferent nerves of the somatic motor system (black stick neuron) arise from motoneurons in the CNS. Efferent somatic motor nerves signal skeletal muscle via the release of acetylcholine (ACh) that bind to muscarinic receptors. (c–h) The autonomic nervous system (ANS) is composed of the parasympathetic (PaSNS; c–d; pink/blue stick neurons), sympathetic (SNS; e–h; green/yellow stick neurons), and the enteric (ENS; purple stick neurons) nervous systems.

(DRG) or cranial nerve ganglia. Note that the cell bodies of motor neurons are not part of the PNS; they are housed in the spinal cord and brainstem. The autonomic component, referred to as the autonomic nervous system (ANS), controls smooth and cardiac muscle, and exocrine glands, which allows for continuous regulation of basal homeostatic functions, as well as the regulation of stress-related functions of the body. In addition to these classical targets, it is now well established that there are other functional targets of the ANS, including hepatocytes, β-islet cells of the pancreas, fat cells, and cells of the immune system. There are two components of the ANS, the sympathetic (SNS) and parasympathetic (PaSNS) nervous systems. Nerves that supply the immune system derive from two basic divisions of the PNS –sensory and autonomic systems. Sensory nerves or fibers convey information from body regions and organs to the CNS (referred to as afferent fibers), whereas autonomic nerves transmit motor impulses away from the CNS (referred to as efferent fibers).

Overview of the ANS

The ANS is referred to as autonomous because its activities are not consciously controlled. The ANS regulates the functions of visceral organs that are necessary for sustaining life, like the heart and gut, and, relevant to this chapter, immune organs. Anatomically, the ANS is divided into two major components: the sympathetic or thoracolumbar, and the parasympathetic or craniosacral divisions (Figure 2.2). Both divisions originate from neurons in preganglionic nuclei in the brainstem and/or spinal cord. Preganglionic neurons of the SNS are located in the intermediolateral cell (IML) column of the spinal cord from the first thoracic (T1) to the second or third lumbar segment (L2 or L3). Their axons exit the CNS in thoracic and lumbar spinal nerves. The parasympathetic preganglionic neurons are in the intermediate gray matter of the sacral spinal cord (S2–S4) and cranial nerve nuclei in the brainstem (Figure 2.2). Preganglionic parasympathetic nerves leave the CNS in the third, seventh, ninth and tenth cranial nerves, and the second, third and fourth sacral spinal nerves.

Autonomic preganglionic nerves from both subdivisions are thinly myelinated and terminate in autonomic ganglia; however, their anatomical locations differ for the SNS and PaSNS. Generally, sympathetic preganglionic nerves are short and end in autonomic ganglia in the paravertebral chain (on either side of the vertebral column), or in prevertebral ganglia (dorsal

Figure 2.2 (*continued*) The ANS regulates visceral motor functions. The PaSNS and the SNS are two-neuron chain systems. The first-order neurons are central preganglionic neurons (green or pink stick neurons) innervate the second-order postganglionic neurons (blue or yellow stick neurons), whose cell bodies reside in autonomic ganglia and innervate target effector cells. Types of effector cells are listed in the upper right corner. The PaSNS (c–d) arises from the brainstem (c) and sacral spinal cord (d), and therefore is referred to as a craniosacral origin; whereas the SNS (e-h) arises from the thoracic and lumbar spinal cord, and is referred to as a thoracolumbar origin. Postganglionic neurons of the ANS end on effector target cells. All preganglionic and postganglionic parasympathetic nerves signal via ACh (orange circles). Postganglionic sympathetic nerves (yellow stick neurons) use norepinephrine (NE) (light green circles) as its major neurotransmitter. (f) The sympathoadrenal medullary axis is part or the SNS. Preganglionic neurons (green circles) project to the adrenal medulla to regulate the secretion of epinephrine (EPI, dark green circles) and to a lesser extent, NE from adrenal chromaffin cells into the circulation. (g, c) Postganglionic neurons of the PaSNS and the SNS innervate the ENS in the gut.

to the spinal column, usually on the ventral surface of the aorta) (Figures 2.2 and 2.3). The longer, non-myelinated, postganglionic sympathetic nerves exit these ganglia and terminate in their target organs. In contrast, the preganglionic parasympathetic fibers from the craniosacral region are relatively long and end on postganglionic neurons within the walls of, or less commonly adjacent to, their target organs. Short, non-myelinated nerves from postganglionic neurons distribute diffusely, or in networks, to end on effector cells. Therefore, both the SNS and PaSNS exist as a two-motor-neuron chain. Due to the paucity or lack of myelin and their small diameter, pre- and postganglionic axons conduct impulses slowly, and these nerves fire tonically. The distribution of the SNS is widespread, targeting all organs and regions of the body; however, the PaSNS is more limited in its distribution than the SNS, mostly to the head and neck, and the pelvic region (Figure 2.2). Importantly, the terms "sympathetic" and "parasympathetic" are anatomical terms, based on a two-neuron chain, and the locations of first- and second-order neurons in the chain. These terms do not imply any specific type of neurotransmitter release from their terminals, or the type of effect the activation of their nerves will have on organ functions.

In addition to these two divisions, the enteric nervous system (ENS) is considered a third component of the ANS (Figure 2.1). The ENS consists of a large group of highly organized neurons in the walls of the gastrointestinal (GI) system from the esophagus to the distal colon. The ENS has both motor and secretory activities in the gut. Two neuronal networks are included in the ENS, the myenteric plexus (also called Auerbach's plexus) and the submucosal plexus (also called Meissner's plexus). The myenteric plexus is embedded between the outer longitudinal and inner circular muscle layers of the gut, and primarily controls gut motility. In the submucosa, the submucosal plexus controls GI blood flow, regulates epithelial cell function, and serves as a sensor of the lumenal environment. The ENS consists of three types of neurons, sensory, motor, and interneurons. Sensory neurons receive mechanical, thermal, osmotic, and chemical information from sensory receptors in the mucosa and smooth muscle. Motor neurons control GI motility and secretions. Interneurons integrate the sensory information to the motor neurons. While the ENS functions autonomously, normal functioning of the GI system requires bidirectional communication between the ENS, SNS, and PaSNS (via the vagus and sacral nerves). Importantly, the SNS and PaSNS innervate the ENS and the effector cells of the ENS (Figure 2.2). Thus, the ENS functions in a semiautonomous fashion, with modulatory input from the ANS, and has the ability to inform the CNS of its microenvironment by enteric sensory nerves.

The junctions between autonomic nerves and their target cells are called neuroeffector junctions (Figure 2.3). They differ from typical synapses in the CNS, or at the neuromuscular junction, where the nerve ending closely apposes its target and the synapse is enclosed by glial cells to limit neurotransmitter diffusion. Instead, neurotransmitter is released from a chain of varicosities along the postganglionic nerve, which diffuses into a much wider and non-confined cleft between the varicosities and their effector cells (e.g., lymphocytes). Therefore, the released neurotransmitter has a slower onset of the effector cell response and commonly signals many effector cells. Effector cells express receptors to which the neurotransmitters selectively bind, and subsequently affect specific signal transduction pathways to alter cell function.

Traditionally, autonomic nerves have been defined by the primary neurotransmitters they release. Postganglionic parasympathetic, and all preganglionic, neurons release acetylcholine (ACh) as their major neurotransmitter, so they are cholinergic neurons (Figures 2.2 and 2.3). ACh binds to muscarinic and nicotinic receptors in postganglionic neurons. Most postganglionic sympathetic neurons release norepinephrine (NE, also called noradrenaline), so they

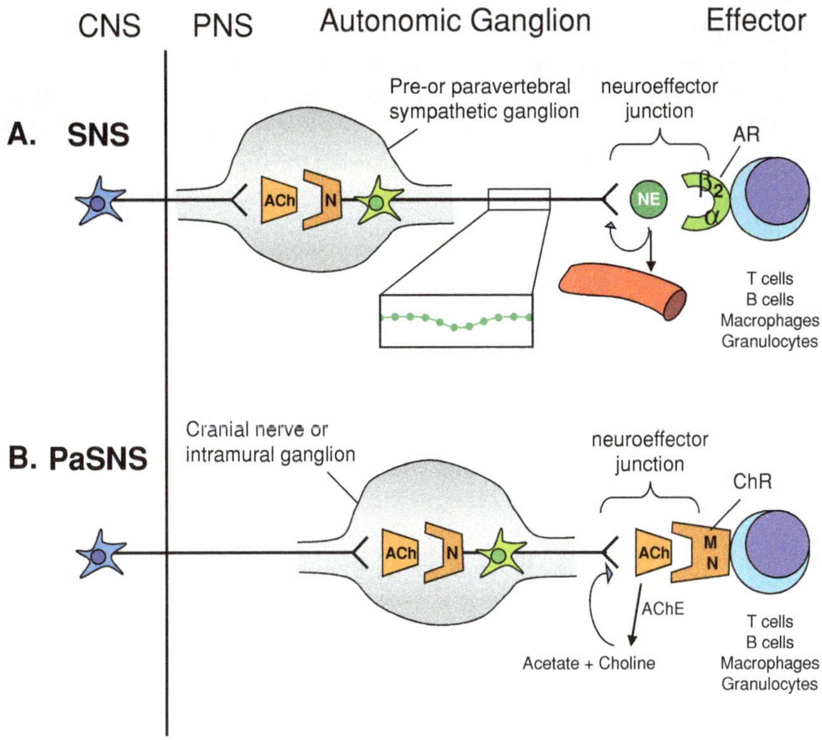

Figure 2.3 Autonomic innervation of target immune effector cells. A. Immune organs are primarily innervated by nerves of the SNS. Preganglionic neurons (blue) innervate postganglionic neurons (green) in pre- or paravertebral sympathetic ganglia. Preganglionic sympathetic neurons release ACh (orange trapezoid) from their nerve terminals that subsequently binds to and activates nicotinic receptors (N) expressed in the cell membrane of postganglionic neurons (green). Postganglionic efferent nerves travel with the blood vessels to reach immune organs. Postganglionic sympathetic neurons form neuroeffector junctions with cells of the immune system. These nerves release NE (green circle) from varicosities present along the length of sympathetic nerves (shown in box). Target immune cells express β- (primarily the β_2-subtype) and α-adrenergic receptors (AR) that bind NE (or EPI from the adrenal medulla) to elicit a functional response. NE is then metabolized, recycled back into sympathetic nerves or enters the circulation. B. Most visceral organs receive a dual innervation from the PaSNS and the SNS; however, strong evidence for PaSNS innervation of lymphoid organs is lacking. However, immune cells express nicotinic (N) and muscarinic (M) acetylcholine (ACh) receptors (ChR). Under certain conditions, immune cells may mobilize to visceral organs innervated by the PaSNS and respond to signals from the PaSNS (e.g., inflammation in the heart). Some visceral organs that house mucosa-associated lymphoid tissue (MALT) are innervated by the PaSNS; however, direct innervation of MALT by the PaSNS needs to be demonstrated. If PaSNS innervation of immune organs does exist, these are the most likely sites. Preganglionic efferent nerves arise from neurons in the brainstem or sacral spinal cord, enter the postganglionic neurons in PaSNS ganglia and release ACh (orange trapezoid) at synapses with postganglionic neurons (green). Postganglionic neurons express nicotinic (N) receptors that bind ACh to elicit an effector response. Postganglionic efferent nerves form neuroeffector junctions with target effector cells. Effector cells express muscarinic (M) cholinergic receptors (ChR) that bind with ACh to elicit an effector cell response. The response is terminated by the degradation of ACh to acetate and choline by acetylcholinesterase (AChE) and these components taken up into the nerve terminal.

are called noradrenergic (NA) or adrenergic neurons. Immune cells express predominantly β_2-adrenergic receptors (ARs), but also α-AR. However, in some target tissues, sympathetic postganglionic neurons are cholinergic (e.g., salivary glands). Additionally, some sympathetic and parasympathetic neurons express neuropeptides or nitric oxide as their major transmitter for signaling effector cells (referred to as non-adrenergic non-cholinergic, or NANC nerves), but so far have not been found in lymphoid organs. Dopamine (DA) is present in all NA sympathetic neurons as a precursor in the synthesis of NE (see Figure 2.6). Some evidence supports DA release by some postganglionic sympathetic nerves, and DA receptors are present in immune cells. In addition to their major neurotransmitter, most autonomic nerves also release several other neurotransmitters (cotransmitters) (see Figure 2.6). Neurotransmitters are synthesized, stored, released, and re-uptaken by autonomic nerves, and each of these processes can be targeted pharmacologically to study the role of the ANS in lymphoid organs.

Overview of the sensory system

The sensory system has visceral and somatic components, but they are not typically subdivided as the motor components historically have been. Some evidence exists for visceral sensory afferent innervation of certain lymphoid organs. However, all body regions that contact the external environment receive a sensory nerve supply, which plays an important role in sensing and responding to foreign substances, microbes, and injury. With one exception, the neuronal cell bodies of all sensory neurons arise from the dorsal root or cranial nerve ganglia, which lie adjacent and lateral to the spinal cord or brainstem, respectively. The sensory axons supplying lymphoid organs have small diameters, and are thinly myelinated or non-myelinated, in contrast to the large-diameter, thickly myelinated somatic axons that end in skin, skeleton and skeletal muscle. Functionally, this means that visceral nerves convey neural impulses more slowly than the large-diameter somatic fibers. Visceral axons in lymphoid organs are linear and punctate, without any apparent specialized sensory receptors. These nerves "sense" and then send information via neurotransmission about their microenvironment to the CNS for conscious perception. Additionally, upon activation they release neurotransmitters from their distal axon that can bind with specific receptors expressed in target cells, such as immune cells. Major neurotransmitters in sensory visceral neurons are substance P (SP) and calcitonin gene-related peptide (CGRP) (Figure 2.2). Nerves immunoreactive for SP and CGRP in some lymphoid organs may be from sensory neurons located in the DRG.

In the CNS, interneurons are interposed between sensory input and motor output (Figure 2.4). Interneurons, which comprise most of the CNS, process and integrate sensory information to affect CNS functioning and motor responses. The most direct and simplest communication between sensory (input) and motor (output) neurons is a *reflex arc* (Figure 2.4). It consists of five components: (1) sensory receptors in or associated with a sensory neuron (detects stimulus); (2) sensory neuron (conducts afferent nerve impulses to the CNS); (3) an integration center (one or more synapses in the CNS); (4) a motor neuron (conducts efferent nerve impulses from integration center to an effector cell; and (5) an effector cell (responds to the efferent impulse, i.e., muscle contraction or glandular secretion). A reflex is a rapid (takes place in milliseconds), involuntary movement or secretion that occurs in response to a sensory stimulus. In a reflex arc, a sensory neuron communicates either directly with a motor neuron (one synapse or monosynaptic as in the knee jerk reflex), or indirectly via polysynaptic connections involving interneurons (as in the withdrawal reflex). Reflexes are not flexible – they

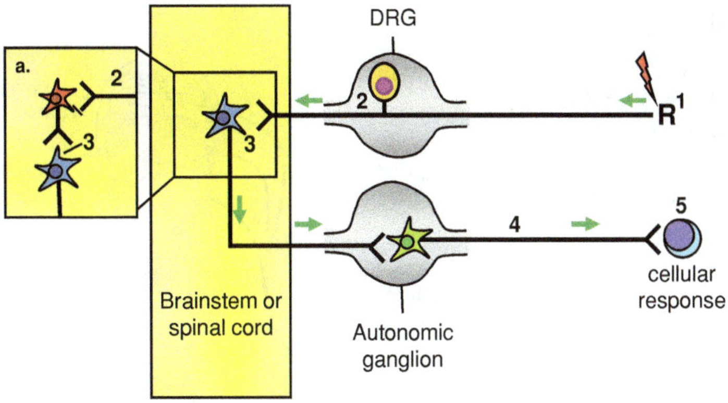

Figure 2.4 An autonomic reflex arc. The basic components of an autonomic reflex arc are (1) a sensory receptor that is associated with (2) the distal terminal of a sensory visceral afferent neuron, (3) one or more synapses in the CNS (multiple synapses shown in (a)) that end on a preganglionic efferent motor neuron whose axon synapses with a postganglionic efferent motor neuron (4) that forms an effector junction with (5) a target effector cell. Activation of this reflex arc (red lightning bolt) sends impulses across this circuit (green arrows) which stimulates a cellular response.

elicit the same behavior every time they are activated. Monosynaptic reflexes do not permit the CNS to "evaluate" or integrate the inciting stimulus with other stimuli. The interposed interneurons between sensory and motor neuron systems allow multiple stimuli perceived by vertebrates to be integrated and processed for a more complex and flexible behavioral response. Somatic and visceral afferents linked via local central connections to autonomic efferent fibers provide the anatomical substrate for reflexes observed in immune regulation. Descending CNS axons impinge on interneurons and/or efferent autonomic motor neurons in the reflex arc to regulate immune function.

Innervation of Lymphoid Organs

Innervation of effector target tissues, like lymphoid organs, implies that the nerves signal target cells via neurotransmission to cause a reproducible response. No single method of study is sufficient to meet all of the criteria for neurotransmission (presence of nerves, release of neurotransmitter(s), interaction of neurotransmitter with specific receptor on target cells, and reproducible functional responses). It is particularly important to understand the limitations of each method and the potential problems in interpreting and evaluating this literature. Here, we report the findings from credible papers investigating sympathetic, sensory, parasympathetic, and peptidergic innervation of lymphoid tissues, where the experimental designs are sound and essential controls were included, and therefore permit reasonable interpretations and conclusions to be drawn from their findings. Figure 2.5 summarizes the sympathetic and parasympathetic innervation of primary and secondary lymphoid organs.

Bone marrow

Structure and function Bone marrow is a primary lymphoid organ that is located in the central cavities of axial and long bones (Figure 2.7), and the major producer of platelets and blood cells

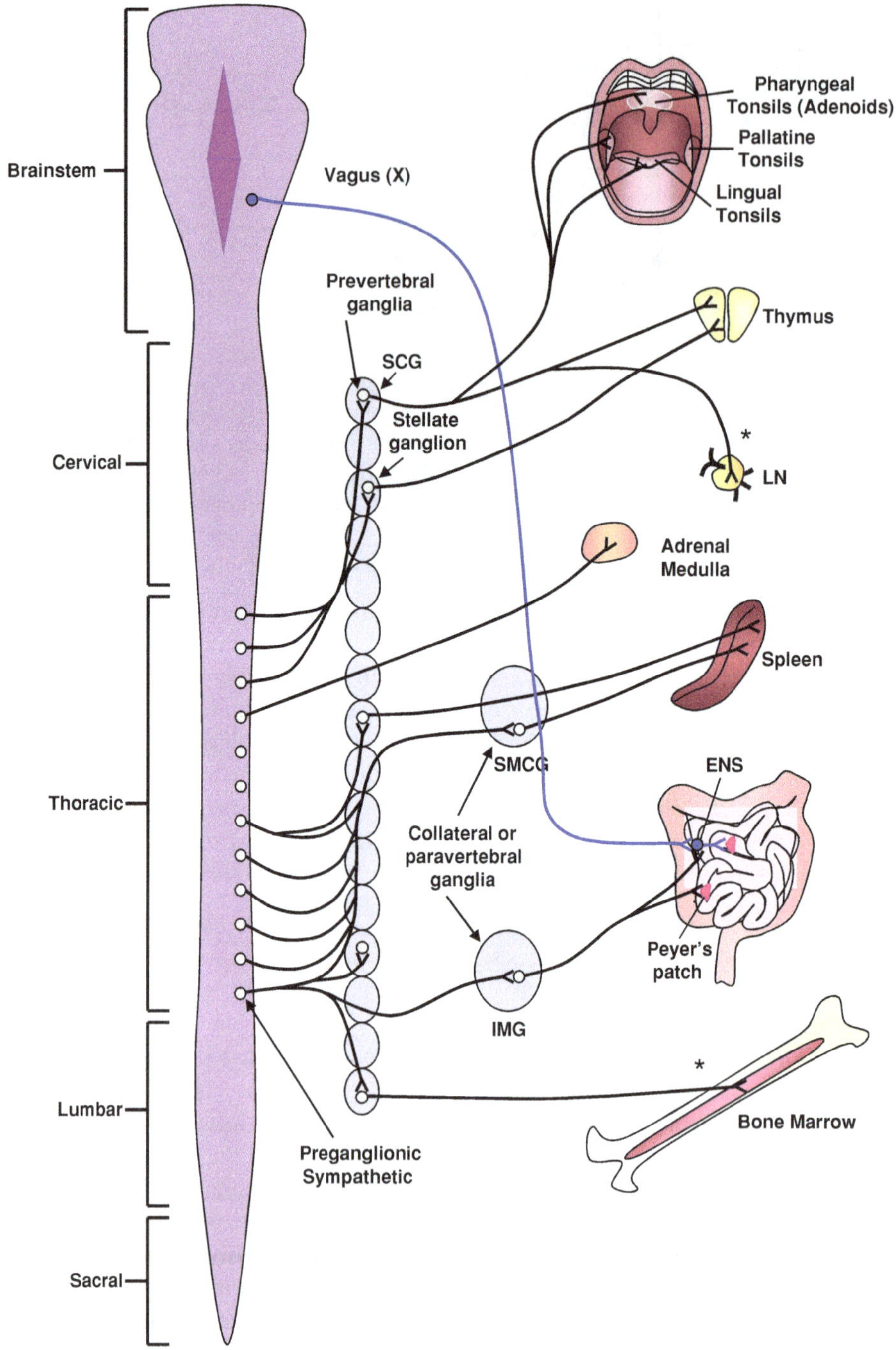

Figure 2.5 Efferent SNS and PaSNS innervation of lymphoid organs and mucosa-associated lymphoid tissue. Black and blue stick neurons illustrates SNS and PaSNS innervation of lymphoid organs, respectively. The source of sympathetic nerves in lymph nodes (LN) and bone marrow is regional. The cervical lymph node and bone marrow in the femur is illustrated (*). ENS – enteric nervous system; SMCG – superior mesenteric–celiac ganglionic plexus; IMG – inferior mesenteric ganglion; SCG – superior cervical ganglion.

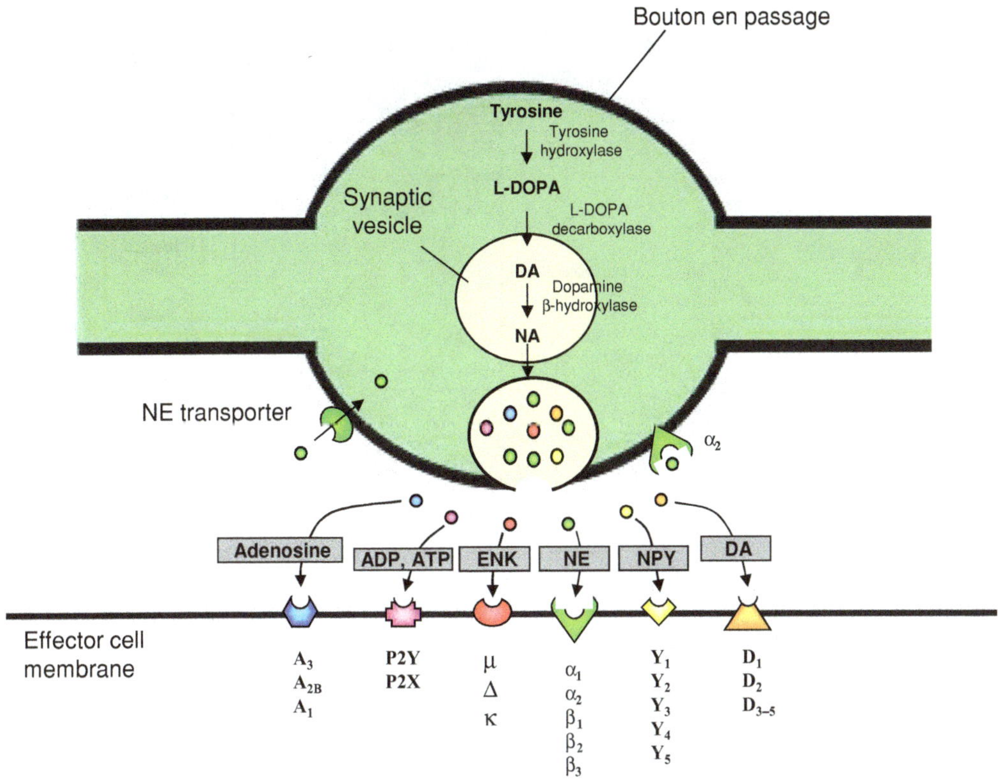

Figure 2.6 Sympathetic bouton en passage and its signaling to an effector target cell. NE is synthesized from the amino acid precursor, tyrosine. Tyrosine is converted to L-3,4-dihydroxyphenylalanine (L-DOPA) by the rate-limiting enzyme, tyrosine hydroxylase, commonly abbreviated TH. L-DOPA is decarboxylated by L-DOPA decarboxylase to form dopamine (DA). DA enters the synaptic vesicle where it is hydroxylated by dopamine β-hydroxylase (DBH) to form NA (=NE). TH, and DBH are used as a marker for NA sympathetic nerves. NE colocalizes with many other neuromediators/neuromodulators, including DA (orange circles), neuropeptide Y (NPY, yellow circles), met- and/or leu-enkephalin (ENK, red circles), ADP and ATP (pink circles), and adenosine (blue circles). At the neuroeffector junction, these mediators, along with NE, are released from the boutons of stimulated NA nerves. They diffuse across the extracellular space and bind with specific receptors (color-coded to match the neurotransmitter) expressed on the cell surface of target cells. Receptor binding affects ion channels and/or activates intracellular signaling cascades to alter cellular functions in target cells. Cellular responses mediated by each neurotransmitter depend on the receptor subclasses expressed in the target cell, the intracellular signaling cascade it is linked to, and the intracellular interactions between the signaling cascades activated by all of the activated receptor classes. NE is inactivated at the neuroeffector junction primarily by reuptake into the nerve terminal, but also by enzyme-mediated degradation and diffusion into the blood circulation. Chronic stimulation down-regulates receptor expression on the cell the surface, which reduces the receptor-mediated signaling by its ligand. Receptors in the post-synaptic membrane of effector cells for NE include β-AR (β_1, β_2 and β_3 subtypes), α-AR (α_1, and α_2 subtypes). α_2-AR expressed on the nerve terminal inhibit NE release (a local negative feedback loop). Post-effector junction receptors for DA ($D_{1\text{-}5}$ subtypes), NPY ($Y_{1\text{-}5}$ subtypes), adenosine (A_1, A_{2B}, and A_3 subtypes), ATP (P2Y, P2X subtypes) and opioids (μ, δ and κ subtypes) are also expressed in the post-synaptic membranes of certain effector cells and can differentially modulate the effects of NE on effector cell function.

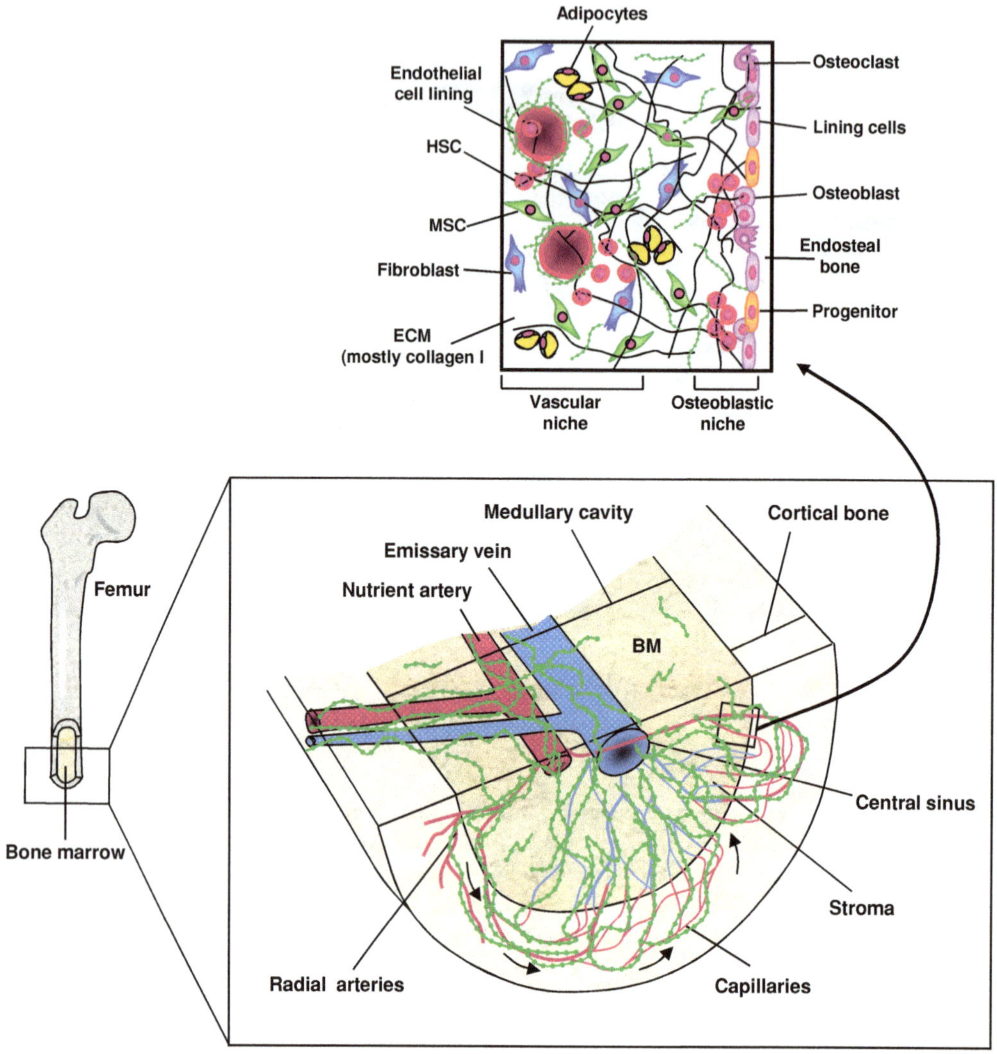

Figure 2.7 Sympathetic innervation of bone marrow. The shaft of the femur has been bisected to reveal the bone marrow in the central cavity (lower left). The region inside the box overlying the shaft of the bone is magnified to reveal the features in the central cavity. NA sympathetic nerves (green varicose linear profiles) travel in neurovascular plexuses with the nutrient artery (shown in red) and one or two nutrient veins (shown in blue). The neurovascular plexus passes through the cortical bone obliquely to enter the bone marrow, and then bifurcates to course parallel to the long axis of the bone shaft centrally in the bone marrow. Sympathetic nerves continue along small arteriole and capillary networks that branch from the nutrient artery and extend outwardly into the cortical bone, and then return to the marrow cavity. Near the bone, the arterioles anastomose with venous sinuses, which are also supplied with NA nerves. Sympathetic nerves innervate the smooth muscle of blood vessels, and also occasionally extend into the parenchyma within both the vascular and osteoblastic hematopoietic stem cell (HSCs) niches (shown upper box), which house a variety of cell types. In the vascular niches, these cells include mesenchymal stem cells (MSCs, green) and HSCs (hot pink), adipocytes (yellow), fibroblasts (blue), macrophages, blood cells and their precursors and adventitial reticular cells of the extracellular matrix (ECM). In the osteoblastic niches they include bone lining cells (osteocytes, oblong lavender), osteoblasts (round lavender), osteoclasts (pink), HSCs, MSCs and blood cells and their precursors.

(lymphocytes, monocytes, granulocytes and erythrocytes). Bone marrow is composed of islands of hematopoietic tissue housed in the hollow interior of axial and long bones, and incompletely separated by trabecular bone. Hematopoietic islands are surrounded by fat cells and vascular sinuses, and contain immature pluripotent cells called stem cells. Stem cells mature into white blood cells (lymphopoiesis and myelopoiesis), red blood cells (RBCs, erythropoiesis), and megakaryocyte-derived platelets. The renewal and differentiation of hematopoietic stem cells (HSCs) into mature blood cells are regulated by the microenvironment, referred to as the HSC niche (reviewed in Ehninger and Trumpp, 2011). HSC niches have varying phenotypes depending on their anatomical location, and dynamically change with blood cell development and immune activation/injury. Components of HSC niches include HSCs, mesenchymal stem cells, reticular cells, endothelial cells, macrophages, osteoblasts (in some types of niches), and sympathetic nerves (Figure 2.7). The microenvironment of the HSC niches is important for regulating HSC retention in the bone marrow, self-renewal of HSCs, and normal development of blood cells. HSCs, mature, and under certain conditions, immature blood cells, and platelets exit the bone marrow into the blood circulation. The bone marrow replenishes the immune system with immunocytes, as well as stem cells for all organ systems, throughout life.

Sympathetic innervation Bone marrow cells are innervated by NA sympathetic nerves (Figure 2.7), forming a brain–immune axis that regulates hematopoiesis and cellular mobilization. Until recently, research investigating the innervation of bone marrow has been limited compared to other primary and secondary lymphoid organs. Both thinly myelinated and non-myelinated nerves are present in the bone marrow (Castañeda-Corral *et al.*, 2011), suggesting autonomic and/or sensory innervation. Neurochemically-specific staining (Tabarowski, Gibson-Berry, and Felten, 1996; Imai *et al.*, 1997; Artico *et al.*, 2002; Imai and Matsusue, 2002) has further demonstrated that NA sympathetic nerves supply the bone marrow (Figure 2.7). In the shaft of long bones, NA nerves travel in neurovascular plexuses with the nutrient artery and one or two nutrient veins. They pass through the cortical bone obliquely to enter the bone marrow. In flat bones, the marrow is innervated by NA nerves that course with several blood vessels of various sizes, entering via large and small nutrient canals or foramina in the bone. After entry, the nerves follow the course of the nutrient artery (Figure 2.7), which bifurcates into branches that course parallel to the long axis of the bone in the central part of the bone marrow. Sympathetic nerves travel along small arterioles and capillary networks that branch from the nutrient artery and extend outwardly toward the cortical bone. The capillary networks extend into Haversian canals, and then return to the marrow cavity. Near the bone, the arterioles anastomose with venous sinuses, which also are supplied with NA nerves. Blood drains from the venous sinuses into collecting venules that lead back to the central longitudinal vein and then into the nutrient veins. Thus, the blood flow pattern is circular. There is no lymphatic drainage in the bone marrow.

NA nerves innervate the smooth muscle of blood vessels, and also occasionally extend into the parenchyma within HSC niches, which house a variety of cell types (Figure 2.7). These cell types include adipocytes, macrophages, adventitial reticular cells, bone lining cells (e.g., osteoblasts), and blood cells and their precursors. Mesenchymal stem cells, HSCs and sympathetic nerves are tightly associated (Ehninger and Trumpp, 2011). NA nerve terminals form neuroeffector junctions with a particular type of stromal cell, the periarterial adventitial cell. These cells are an important source of growth factors, like granulocyte macrophage colony-stimulating factor (GM-CSF), and adhesion molecules. Additionally, sympathetic nerves appose sinus adventitial reticular cells and intersinusoid reticular cells, the latter two cell types communicate via gap junctions. NA nerves in the bone marrow also release neuropeptide Y (NPY). NPY nerves have a similar pattern of distribution in rat bone marrow as those expressing NE; however, NA nerves are more abundant (D. Felten *et al.*, 1985; S. Felten *et al.*, 1988; Bellinger, Lorton, Felten, and Felten, 1992; Bellinger *et al.*, 1992; Tabarowski, Gibson-Berry, and Felten, 1996; Ahmed, Bjurholm, Kreicbergs, and Schultzberg, 1993).

Peptidergic nerves The bone marrow receives a significant innervation by SP and CGRP nerves (Imai and Matsusue, 2002; Kosaras, Jakubowski, Kainz, and Burstein, 2009; Castañeda-Corral *et al.*, 2011; Mach *et al.*, 2002; Jimenez-Andrade *et al.*, 2010). These nerves also express galanin (Gajda *et al.*, 2009). SP and CGRP nerves enter the bone marrow through perivascular plexuses located around nutrient vessels. Most terminate on end plates, but some reach the marrow, where they associate with hematopoietic and stromal cells. SP and CGRP fibers have overlapping distribution in the marrow (Bjurholm, Kreicbergs, Brodin, and Schultzberg, 1998). Vasoactive intestinal polypeptide (VIP) nerves in bone marrow are sparse (Ahmed, Bjurholm, Kreicbergs, and Schultzberg, 1993). The distribution of VIP nerves in the lumbar vertebral bone marrow differs from NA innervation. Nerves containing VIP are not closely associated with the vasculature, and are most abundant in the bone marrow and periosteum.

Origin of innervation Sympathetic nerves in the bone marrow arise from postganglionic sympathetic ganglia (Dénes *et al.*, 2005); their precise location remains to be determined for most of the bone marrow. It is assumed that the nerves derive from the same sympathetic ganglia that supply other structures in that body region (Figure 2.5). The origin of peptidergic nerves other than NPY has not been determined. A sensory origin of SP and CGRP fibers in bone marrow is supported by a loss of normal blood cell production in capsaicin-treated mice, since capsaicin destroys small sensory nerve fibers (Broome and Miyan, 2000; Broome, Whetton, and Miyan, 2000).

Functional significance The intimate NA nerve–HSC–stromal cell relationship provides an anatomical substrate for neural regulation of hematopoiesis that is supported by functional studies (Penn *et al.*, 2010; Elenkov, Wilder, Chrousos, and Vizi, 2000) and the egress of cells from the bone marrow into the blood (Dar *et al.*, 2011; Katayama *et al.*, 2006). The SNS maintains homeostasis of HSC niches, and mobilizes HSCs under stressful conditions. Immunological, physical, and psychological stressors can affect sympathetically-regulated homeostasis of hematopoiesis, and hematopoietic and stem cell release by increasing sympathetic activity in the bone marrow (Tang, Shankar, Gamelli, and Jones, 1999). The SNS's homeostatic role includes maintaining the blood–marrow interface, and controlling peripheral blood cell number by regulating their cell cycle and mobilizing colony-forming cells (Spiegel *et al.*, 2007; Tabarowski, Gibson-Berry, and Felten, 1996; Afan *et al.*, 1997; Dresch, Minc, Poirier, and Bouvet, 1981; Beckman Mirand, and Fisher, 1980; Maestroni and Conti, 1994a, b; Maestroni, Conti, and Pedrinis, 1992; Maestroni *et al.*, 1998; Byron, 1971). The SNS mobilizes HSC in a circadian fashion to regulate circulating HSC numbers (Katayama *et al.*, 2006; Méndez-Ferrer, Lucas, Battista, and Frenette, 2008) by effects on HSC and mesenchymal stem cells (Chow *et al.*, 2011). Granulocyte colony-stimulating factor (G-CSF) is one of the important regulators of HSC efflux from the bone marrow, acting by increasing SNS activity. G-CSF is used clinically to harvest HSCs for bone marrow transplantation (Gertz, 2010). Adrenergic drugs could potentiate the therapeutic effects of G-CSF in mobilizing HSCs for transplantation, and/or attracting stems cells to HSC niches after transplantation. Additionally, adrenergic treatment may be combined with chemotherapies and/or radiotherapies to protect against the myeloablative effects of anticancer treatments (Maestroni, Togni, and Covacci, 1997). Under conditions of sympathetic dysregulation, which commonly occurs in chronic immune-mediated diseases, the regulation of HSC development and egress from the bone marrow may be compromised, as in diabetes (Ferraro *et al.*, 2011).

Thymus

Structure and function The thymus is a primary lymphoid organ, located in the upper portion of the chest cavity, dorsal and superior to the heart and ventral to the sternum (Figure 2.8). In mammals, the thymus consists of two lobes connected by connective tissue called the isthmus. Each lobe is surrounded by a connective tissue capsule from which septae extend into the thymic parenchyma. The septae divide the parenchyma into incomplete, interconnected lobules of variable size. The parenchyma has two anatomically distinct regions, an outer cortex and an inner medulla separated by the corticomedullary zone or junction (CMJ). In the cortex, densely packed immature T-lymphocytes (also called thymocytes) and accessory cells reside in a stroma of reticular epithelial cells (Figure 2.8). Epithelial cells can be divided into distinct populations based on their ultrastructural features, thymic hormone production, staining characteristics, and anatomical location in the thymus. Lymphoblasts proliferate in the cortex next to the capsule; progressively fewer proliferating cells exist towards the CMJ. The CMJ contains immature and mature T-lymphocytes, dendritic cells, perivascular B-lymphocytes and plasma cells. Less cellular than the cortex, the medulla is composed of mature thymocytes, prominent epithelial cells, Hassall's corpuscles (concentrically-arranged epithelial cells), macrophages, dendritic cells, mast cells, eosinophils, B-cells, and infrequently, myoid (muscle-like cells) and neuroendocrine cells.

Another distinct feature of the thymus compared with other lymphoid organs is that the capillary network in the cortex is not fenestrated, forming the blood–thymus barrier (von Gaudecker *et al.*, 1991). This restricts the access of circulating non-self antigens to cortical thymocytes, a functionally critical feature that permits the "education" of thymocyte to discriminate "self" from "non-self". In contrast, capillaries in the thymic medulla are fenestrated and freely permeable to circulating antigens and neural and endocrine regulatory mediators. Blood from the capillary networks drains into the postcapillary venules, and finally returns to the circulation in medullary veins. The thymus has no afferent lymphatic vessels, but does have efferent lymphatic vessels, which drain into an adjacent pair of lymph nodes.

The functional T-cell repertoire forms in the thymus. Briefly, early lymphoid progenitor cells migrate from the bone marrow to the thymus where they differentiate, mature and undergo "T-cell education". These progenitor cells enter the thymic stroma from the circulation through large venules at the CMJ, migrate to the outer cortex (subcapsular zone), and then move toward the medulla as they mature (Figure 2.8). Mature T-cells re-enter the circulation via specialized blood vessels called high endothelial postcapillary venules (HEVs). During intrathymic migration from the outer to inner cortex, they pass through four basic stages of maturation. (1) After entering the thymus, progenitors proliferate, grow in size and begin expressing early differentiation antigens. When they begin their migration from the outer cortex they are triple-negative cells, meaning they do not express CD3 (a marker for the TCR)/CD4/CD8 (Figure 2.8). (2) TCR gene rearrangement occurs next, which is necessary for expression of surface TCRs and T-cell competence, since T-cells recognize foreign antigens

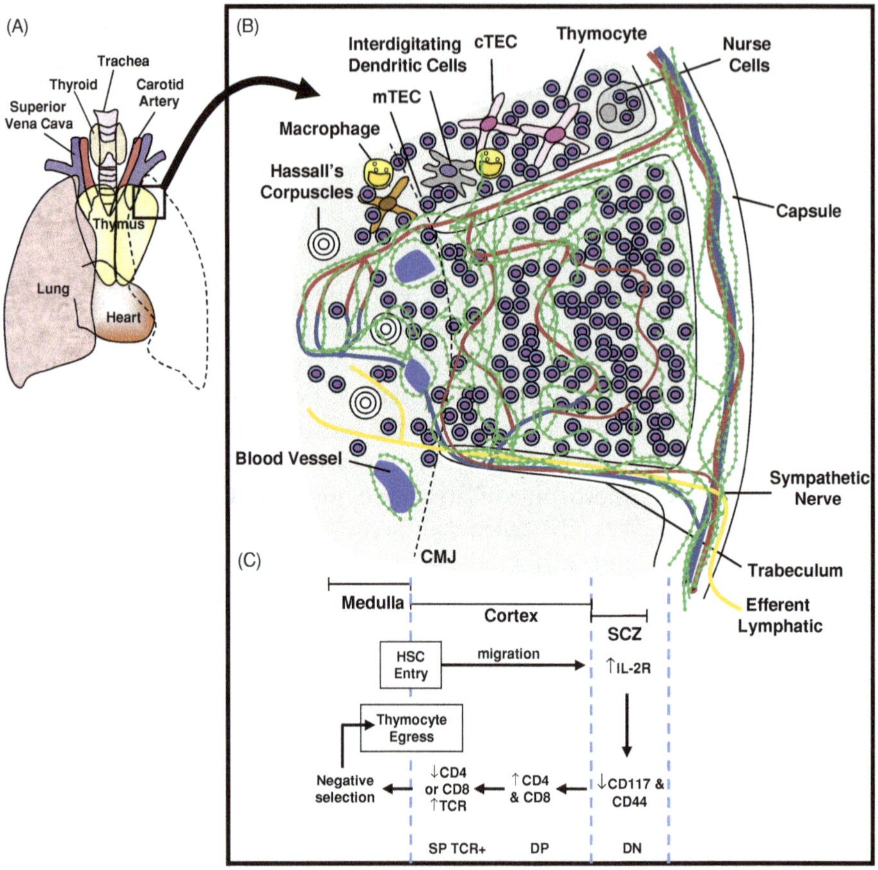

Figure 2.8 Sympathetic innervation of the thymus. The thymus is located in the anterior superior mediastinum, overlying the trachea, anterior to sternum and heart, and posterior to the lungs (A). A portion of the thymic lobe is magnified (on the right side of the figure) to illustrate the anatomy and sympathetic innervation of the thymus (B). After entering into the thymus, NA nerves (green varicose linear profiles) course in association with the blood vessels (red and blue) in the capsule. They continue along the vasculature in intralobular septa, and then radiate from the blood vessels into the parenchyma of the thymic cortex, most prominently at the corticomedullary junction. Sympathetic nerves in subcapsular plexuses associate with blood vessels, but also exit these plexuses and extend into the outer cortical parenchyma among fields of thymocytes. In the medulla, sympathetic nerves are sparse, and primarily associated with the vasculature, particularly the sinuses (blue) near the corticomedullary junction (CMJ). Hassall's corpuscles are found in the medulla in humans, and are formed from concentrically arranged epithelial reticular cells. A role for Hassall's corpuscles in converting naïve thymocytes to a Foxp3 regulatory T-cell lineage has been proposed. Cells located in the vicinity of NA nerves include thymocytes, cortical and medullary thymic epithelial cells (mTEC and cTEC, respectively), nurse cells, dendritic cells, and mast cells in the intralobular septa. NA nerves reside in compartments were thymocytes are "educated" (C). Hematopoietic stem cells (HSCs) enter at the CMJ, and then migrate through the cortex to the subcortical zone (SCZ). Here, they proliferate, upregulate IL-2 receptor (IL-2R) expression, down-regulate HSC surface markers (CD117 and CD44) and lack expression of CD4 or CD8 (double negative, DN). Next, they migrate toward the medulla. During this migration, they first upregulate both CD4 and CD8 (double positive, DP), undergo TCR gene re-arrangement and TCR surface expression for which they are positively selected, and then downregulate either CD4 or CD8 (single-positive, SP). In the medulla, they undergo negative selection (as described in text), and then thymocytes that survive this process migrate from the thymus (at the CMJ) into the blood circulation.

presented on the major histocompatibility complex (MHC) via the TCR (Pearse, 2006). TCR-β rearrangement occurs first. If successful, the cells survive and induce cell surface expression of CD4 and CD8 (double-positive cells). Next, TCR-α rearrangement occurs, with subsequent assembly and surface expression of the TCR (triple-positive cells, $CD4^+CD8^+TCR^+$) (Figure 2.8). Cells that fail to rearrange the TCR-β or -α chain undergo apoptosis. (3) Next, successful engagement of functional TCR with MHC class I or II molecules (MHC I or II) is required for continued maturation of thymocytes. Expression of both CD4 and CD8 is upregulated as coreceptors that bind to MHC II and I, respectively. Cells expressing CD4 and CD8 that bind MHC are positively selected for survival. Failure to bind MHC results in apoptosis. Next, double-positive cells ($CD4^+CD8^+$) make a lineage commitment, by downregulating CD4 and CD8, and then upregulating one of these receptors to become single-positive cells ($CD4^-CD8^+$ or $CD4^+CD8^-$) (Figure 2.8). Single-positive, mature T-cells are located predominantly in the medulla. (4) Negative selection, a process of eliminating autoreactive thymocytes that occurs in the medulla is the next key stage, and it involves the engagement of TCR with MHC II or I and CD4 or CD8, respectively. This leads to the deletion by apoptosis of CD4 or CD8 cells with high affinity for binding "self" peptides. At this stage, some thymocytes are selected to become T-regulatory cells, usually those with intermediate affinity for "self" peptide. Each of these developmental stages occurs in precise compartments in the thymus (Figure 2.8).

The thymus also controls the specificity of T-cells recruited to the circulation by positive and negative selection. Positive selection involves MHC restriction, whereby only T-cells capable of recognizing antigen in the context of host MHC I and II are clonally expanded. The thymic nurse cells, which are cortical epithelial cells that express MHC I and II, internalize immature thymocytes, support their proliferation, and play an important role in positive selection. In negative selection, developing T-cells that express receptors to self antigens undergo apoptosis, and therefore delete potentially harmful autoreactive T-cells.

Sympathetic innervation The SNS innervates the thymus (Figures 2.8 and 2.9) (Williams and Felten, 1981; Williams *et al.*, 1981; Felten *et al.*, 1985; Nance, Hopkins, and Bieger, 1987; Kendall and al-Shawaf, 1991; Weihe *et al.*, 1991; Vizi *et al.*, 1995; Kranz, Kendall, and van Gaudecker, 1997; Cavallotti, Artico, De Santis, and Cavallotti, 1999). NA sympathetic nerves travel in neurovascular plexuses along with the thymic arteries to enter the thymus. The neurovascular plexuses course in the capsule and interlobular septae to enter the thymic parenchyma, largely at the CMJ (Figures 2.8 and 2.9). Therefore, NA nerves are most abundant at the CMJ, surrounding the blood vessels and in the adjacent inner cortical parenchyma. Sympathetic nerves continue along the corticomedullary arterioles, which ramify into capillaries that extend into the cortex. From these neurovascular plexuses, individual nerves extend into the cortical parenchyma, coursing among paracortical thymocytes.

Sympathetic nerves are also abundant in the outer cortex. These nerves form a subcapsular plexus associated with blood vessels, from which they exit and extend into the outer cortical parenchyma among fields of thymocytes (Figures 2.8 and 2.9). In the outer and inner cortex, NA nerves can be distant from blood vessels and smooth muscle cells of the vasculature. In sections of the thymus stained with histofluorescence techniques to visualize catecholamines, sympathetic nerve also form small dense plexuses associated with clusters of yellow autofluorescent cells (Figure 2.9) (Bulloch and Pomerantz, 1984), presumed to be macrophages. NE and NPY colocalize in sympathetic nerves in the thymus, based on their overlapping distribution and selective neurotoxin-induced destruction of sympathetic nerves. NA nerve terminals

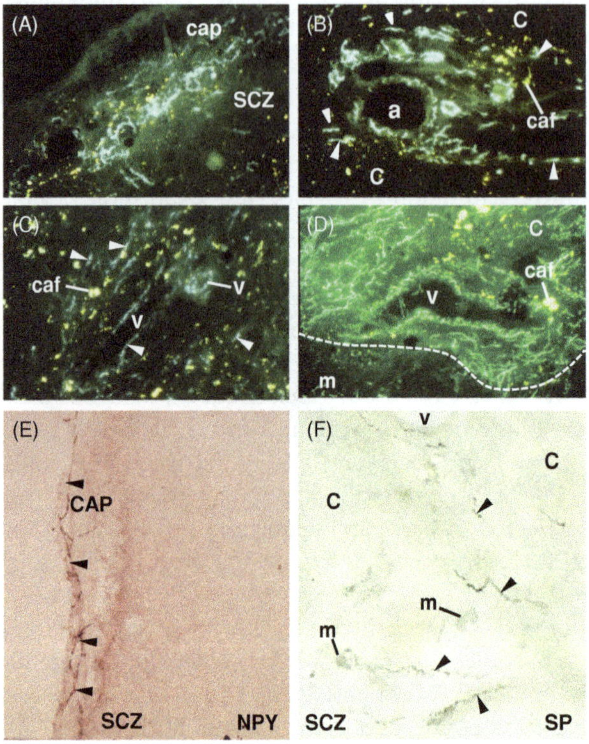

Figure 2.9 Histochemical Staining for Nerves in the Thymus. A. Fluorescently stained sympathetic nerves course in and beneath the capsule in the subcortical zone (SCZ) of the rat thymus. B. A cross sectionally cut vascular plexus in a septum within the thymic cortex (c). Punctate and linear varicose nerve fibers (arrowheads) extend into the surrounding parenchyma where fields of thymocytes, yellow cortical autofluorescent cells (caf), and accessory cells reside. C. Sympathetic nerves surrounding a small cross sectionally-cut blood vessel (v) in cortex of the thymus near the corticomedullary junction. Linear, varicose fluorescent fibers course among thymocytes and yellow cortical autofluorescent cells (caf). D. The density of sympathetic nerves along blood vessels (v) and in the cortical parenchyma of the thymus increase in old rats. m, medulla; c, cortex, caf, yellow cortical autofluorescent cell; corticomedullary junction, dashed line. E. Immunohistochemistry (IHC) reveals neuropeptide Y (NPY)-immunoreactive nerves in the capsule and subcapsular zone in the rat thymus. F. IHC demonstrates substance P (SP)+ nerves (arrowheads) along a blood vessel (v), adjacent to mast cell-like cells (m) usually found in or near the septa, and in the subcortical zone (SCZ) and cortex (c) of the rat thymus.

closely appose thymocytes, mast cells, eosinophils, and other accessory cells, suggesting multiple targets of NA nerves in the thymic cortex. In the medulla, sympathetic nerves are sparse, and primarily associated with the vasculature (Figure 2.9). In mice and rabbits, nerves are not found among medullary epithelial cells; however, NA nerves closely associate with Hassall's corpuscles in the human thymus (de Leeuw *et al.*, 1992).

Thymic NA nerves remodel under physiological conditions and immune stimulation. As the thymus involutes from puberty onward, sympathetic nerve density increases (Figure 2.9D), but not total thymic NE content (Bellinger, Felten, and Felten, 1988). These data suggest that nerves are maintained in the face of diminished thymic mass, which is expected to increase the NE concentration available to interact with target cells under conditions of sympathetic activation. A similar rise in nerve density occurs with antigen stimulation (Novotny and Hsu, 1993) due to a challenge-induced decrease in thymic mass from apoptosis and/or thymocyte egress to secondary immune organs. In contrast, nerve density in the rat thymic cortex declines over the course of pregnancy along with thymic cortical mass. NA nerve density and thymic mass recover to pre-pregnancy conditions at postpartum. Heightened sympathetic activity may be contributory to the nerve loss, since metabolism of NE generates free radicals that can auto-destroy NA nerves.

Peptidergic or cholinergic nerves NPY nerves have an overlapping distribution with NA nerves in the thymus (Figure 2.9E) (Weihe, Müller, Fink, and Zentel, 1989; Kendall and al-Shawaf, 1991; Müller and Weihe, 1991; Weihe *et al.*, 1991; Mitchell *et al.*, 1997; Mignini, Sabbatini, D'Andrea, and Cavallotti, 2011). In contrast with NA nerves, NPY nerve density declines in the aged rat thymus, suggesting reduced NPY concentration in sympathetic nerves. SP and CGRP reside more commonly in the parenchyma than along the vasculature, and in the subcapsular zone and interlobular septa (Figure 2.9F) (Weihe, Müller, Fink, and Zentel, 1989; Bellinger *et al.*, 1990; Müller and Weihe, 1991; Weihe *et al.*, 1991). Septal SP and CGRP nerves enter the cortical parenchyma among immature thymocytes or travel into the medulla (Lorton *et al.*, 1990; Jurjus, More, and Walsh, 1998). SP and CGRP nerves course adjacent to macrophages and mast cells in the capsule, interlobular septum, thymic cortex and at the CMJ (Lorton *et al.*, 1990; Bulloch, Hausman, Radojcic, and Short, 1991; Müller and Weihe, 1991; Jurjus, More and Walsh, 1998). SP fibers represent the bulk of peptidergic nerves in the subcapsular zone (Mignini, Sabbatini, D'Andrea, and Cavallotti, 2011). VIP nerves have a similar distribution as NA and NPY fibers, but are less dense (Bellinger *et al.*, 1997; Mitchell *et al.*, 1997; Mignini, Sabbatini, D'Andrea, and Cavallotti, 2011). They reside within the capsule and interlobular septa. Septal VIP nerves occasionally branch into the thymic cortex. In the deep thymic cortex and medulla, VIP nerves associate with the vasculature or are fine parenchymal fibers. Many of these nerves closely appose VIP-positive lymphoid and accessory cells (al-Shawaf, Kendall, and Cowen, 1991; Müller and Weihe, 1991; Bellinger *et al.*, 1997). In thymoma, peptidergic nerve density declines (NPY, VIP, and SP), suggesting a role in the autoimmune disease, myasthenia gravis (Mignini, Sabbatini, D'Andrea, and Cavallotti, 2011), in which thymoma commonly occurs. Neurotensin nerves widely disperse primarily in the parenchyma rather than the vasculature, and are prominent at the CMJ and medulla. The thymus lacks cholinergic nerves (Nance, Hopkins, and Bieger, 1987; Bellinger *et al.*, 1993).

Sympathetic nerves closely appose smooth muscle and endothelial cells of the blood vessels supplying the thymus. In the capsule and septa, fibroblasts and perivascular mast cells also closely associate with sympathetic nerve terminals. In the thymic cortex, autofluorescent cells, macrophages, eosinophils, thymic epithelial cells, and immature thymocytes commonly reside near NA nerves (D. Felten *et al.*, 1985; Vizi *et al.*, 1995; Kurz *et al.*, 1997). Electron microscopic studies (Novotny, Sommerfeld, and Zirbes, 1990; Vizi *et al.*, 1995) have revealed close proximity of thymocytes, mast cells, fibroblasts, and eosinophils to NA nerves. The close proximity of NA nerves to cell populations that express specific ARs and respond to adrenergic drugs meet most of the criteria for sympathetic neurotransmission. Thymocytes and non-lymphoid cells in the thymus express α_1- and β_2-ARs (Loveland, Jarrott, McKenzie, and Ian, 1981; Marchetti, Morale, Paradis, and Bouvier, 1994; Kavelaars, 2002; Pešić *et al.*, 2009). Additionally non-AR-mediated effects of catecholamines are reported (Bergquist *et al.*, 1997). Intracellular catecholamines transported into the nucleus by specific transporters can interact with steroid receptors and NF-κβ. Through this non-receptor-mediated mechanism, catecholamines can influence transcription processes and modulate apoptosis.

Origin of innervation Sympathetic thymic NA and NPY nerves derive from postganglionic NA neurons in the superior cervical and stellate ganglia in the rat (Figure 2.5) (Nance, Hopkins, and Bieger, 1987; Bellinger *et al.*, 1990; Kendall and al-Shawaf, 1991; Müller and Weihe, 1991; Mitchell *et al.*, 1997). Kendall and al-Shawaf (1991) have found that VIP fibers are not colocalized with NA sympathetic nerves; their origin, and that of SP and CGRP nerves, remains unknown.

Functional significance The thymus is responsible for establishing and maintaining the pool of peripheral T-cells by providing a microenvironment for the proliferation, differentiation and selection of bone-marrow-derived stem cells that seed the thymus. The SNS tightly regulates T-cell development. SNS innervation of blood vessels can affect progenitor cell ingress into and/or T-cell egress from the thymus. These effects may be direct by targeting smooth muscle and/or endothelial cells, or indirect by altering blood flow through the thymus. Altered blood flow can also affect the availability of endocrine mediators for interaction with thymic target cells. The SNS regulates thymopoiesis by altering cell surface antigen expression, like thymus cell antigen-1 (Thy-1) and thymus-leukemia (TL). Thy-1 and TL are important for cell adhesion and signal transduction involved in T-cell differentiation, proliferation and apoptosis. Interactions between SNS and accessory cells influence thymocyte development. AR activation alters thymic epithelial cell function, influencing the thymic microenvironment to affect thymocyte maturation at multiple sites and stages. In this way, the SNS provides an indirect route for "fine tuning" $CD4^+$ and $CD8^+$ T-cell maturation under homeostatic conditions and with immune activation. Sympathetic activation has direct effects in regulating thymocyte proliferation, apoptosis, positive and negative selection, and egress of mature thymocytes from the thymus. Chronic β-AR blockade enhances positive selection, reduces negative selection, facilitates the maturation of selected thymocyte subpopulations, and increases thymocyte production and egress from the thymus (Leposavić *et al.*, 2006; Pešić *et al.*, 2007). In contrast, prolonged α_1-AR inhibition augments thymocyte proliferation and thymocyte yield, and affects lineage commitment (increasing or reducing, respectively, the frequency of $CD4^+CD8^-$ or $CD4^-CD8^+$ expressing TCR-$\alpha\beta^{high}$ (Plećaš-Solarović *et al.*, 2005; Pešić *et al.*, 2009; Leposavić *et al.*, 2010). Collectively, pharmacological studies implicate both AR subtypes in NE-mediated tonic inhibition of thymocyte development, but via different mechanisms (Plećaš-Solarović Bosiljka, Ljubica, and Leposavić, 2004, Plećaš-Solarović *et al.*, 2005; Leposavić *et al.*, 2006; Pešić *et al.*, 2009). Additionally, glucocorticoids can affect sympathetic regulation of T-cell development (reviewed in Leposavić, Pilipović, and Perišić, 2011). Cortical adrenalectomy increases thymic α_1-AR expression; greater α_1-AR activation drives $CD4^-CD8^+$TCR-$\alpha\beta^{high}$ and lowers $CD4^+CD8^-$TCR-$\alpha\beta^{high}$ thymocyte production.

Spleen

Structure and function The spleen is a secondary lymphoid organ that is interposed in the bloodstream and has only efferent lymphatic vessels. The spleen is surrounded by a capsule made up of dense connective tissue and smooth muscle, from which trabeculae incompletely divide the interior (Figure 2.10A and B). It is composed of two basic compartments. The red pulp forms the parenchyma of the spleen and gets its appearance from the blood it filters. The white pulp appears as white dots scattered throughout the red pulp and consists of lymphocytes and accessory cells that form a "cuff" around blood vessels called central arterioles.

The red and white pulps have their own unique functions (Figure 2.10A). The red pulp (1) removes old RBCs and other cellular debris from the blood, (2) recycles iron from the old RBCs, (3) metabolizes hemoglobin (as part of the mononuclear phagocytic system), (4) serves as a reservoir for monocytes and blood, and (5) acts as an immunological filter, capturing foreign materials from the blood that passes through the spleen. The white pulp is involved in developing adaptive immune responses. After injury or antigen exposure, monocytes migrate into the injured tissue to participate in the ensuing immune response. In response to antigen challenge, T- and B-lymphocytes in the white pulp differentiate into effector cells as important components of cellular and humoral immunity. Antigen-presenting cells (APCs) present the antigens to appropriate T- and B-cells in the white pulp. B-cells expand and differentiate into plasma cells in germinal centers of the follicles. The spleen detects blood-borne antigens, and responds to trauma, including heart attacks, gashing wounds, and microbial infections. Splenic monocytes enter the circulation and home to the site of injury or infection.

The red pulp is composed of splenic cords of cells, mostly RBCs and macrophages, bounded by sinuses. The splenic cords filter the blood. The white pulp has three compartments, the periarteriolar lymphatic sheath (PALS), the follicles, and the marginal zone (Figure 2.10B). The PALS is largely composed of T-cells in a loose reticular cell network, which are surrounded by a marginal sinus and zone. The inner PALS is largely composed of $CD4^+$ and $CD8^+$ T-cells, and some dendritic and migrating B-cells. The outer PALS contains T- and B-cells, and macrophages, and is a region important for plasma cell formation. Follicles are continuous with the PALS and are composed primarily of B-lymphocytes but also dendritic cells and $CD4^+$ T-cells. Follicles are transient and depend on immune activation. The follicles may contain germinal centers, sites of clonal B-cell expansion that result from antigenic stimulation.

The marginal zone is situated between the red pulp and the PALS and follicles (Figure 2.10B), and functionally it screens the blood for antigens and pathogens. The marginal zone is separated from the PALS by the marginal sinus, which is lined by a unique subset of metallophilic macrophages. The marginal sinus is a site where lymphocytes and dendritic cells enter the white pulp from the blood. The marginal zone contains reticular fibroblasts, macrophages, dendritic cells, and B-cells. In the marginal zone, dendritic cells and macrophages clear microbes, viruses, and blood-borne antigen, and initiate adaptive immune responses. In response to blood-borne pathogens, marginal zone B-cells differentiate into APCs or rapidly responding plasma blasts (Pillai, Cariappa, and Moran, 2005). Antigen-presenting B-cells mediate both T-independent and -dependent immune responses.

Sympathetic innervation The spleen is abundantly supplied with sympathetic NA nerves (Figures 2.10B and 2.11), comprising ~95–98% of all nerves in the spleen (D. Felten *et al.*, 1985, 1987; Bellinger *et al.*, 2008). These nerves follow the splenic vasculature. NA nerves travel along the branches of the splenic artery that plunges into the spleen at hilar regions (Figure 2.11A). NA nerves then course along capsular and trabecular arteries, which give rise to central arterioles that enter and course in the parenchyma of the spleen. Sympathetic nerves form perivascular plexuses along the central arterioles and extend into the adjacent white pulp. In the PALS, these nerves are closely associated with $CD4^+$ and $CD8^+$ T-cells. NA nerves also enter the marginal and the parafollicular zones adjacent to B-cells and macrophages. Close

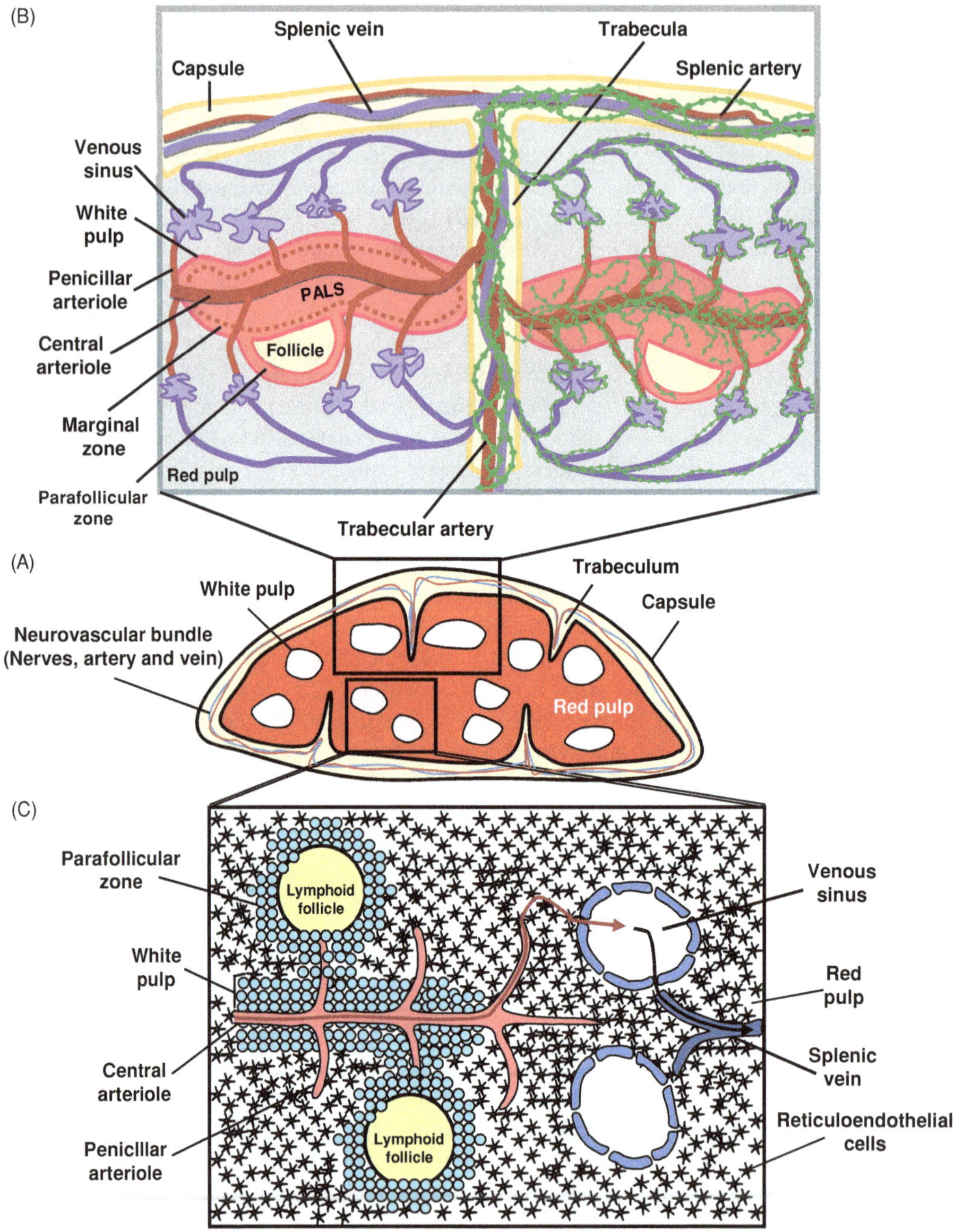

Figure 2.10 Sympathetic Innervation of the Spleen. Illustration of the spleen in cross section showing the organization of the red and white pulp surrounded by an outer connective tissue capsule (A). Trabeculae extend from the capsule into the red pulp (A, B). The left side of figure 10B illustrates the structure of the spleen in the absence of its innervation. Branches of the splenic artery and vein course in the capsule and trabeculae, which are composed of dense fibrous tissue, elastic fibers and smooth muscle. Efferent lymphatic vessels also are found in these compartments. In the red pulp, the central arterioles are surrounded by the white pulp. The white pulp consists of the periarteriolar lymphatic

associations between NA nerves and dendritic cells have not been described but are likely to occur, given the overlapping distribution of these nerves and these cells. Few NA nerves are found in the follicles. At the marginal sinus, central arterioles branch into penicillar arterioles in the marginal zone and red pulp. NA innervation continues along the penicillar arterioles, and subsequent sinusoidal capillaries, venous sinuses, and trabecular, capsular, and splenic veins. These nerves seldom extend from vascular plexuses into the parenchyma of the red pulp. The splenic vein exits the spleen at the hilus, draining into the hepatic portal system. Species/strain differences exist in the extent of parenchymal nerves in the red pulp, and the density of NA nerves in the white pulp can change under certain physiological and pathological conditions. For example, NA nerves in the white pulp are lost in aging (Bellinger, S. Felten, Collier, and D. Felten, 1987), and increased in the red pulp in autoimmune arthritis (Lorton *et al.*, 2005, 2009).

An ultrastructural study has revealed sympathetic nerve terminals in direct contact (~6 nm) with lymphocytes in the PALS and marginal zone (Felten and Olschowska, 1987). No membrane specializations occur at these neuroeffector junctions. Since sympathetic-to-immune cell interaction largely occurs through paracrine release of NE from varicosities of sympathetic nerves, the significance of close nerve–immunocyte contact is not clear. With paracrine release, NE can diffuse large distances from the nerve terminals to interact with target cells that express ARs, so that cells closest to the nerve terminal are exposed to the highest concentrations of NE. Under these conditions, these cells may respond via the lower-affinity α-AR rather than β-AR signaling. The functional significance of NA nerves in the spleen is discussed later, in the section dealing with the lymph nodes.

Peptidergic or cholinergic nerves In rats and guinea-pigs, the distribution of NPY nerves closely mimics that of sympathetic nerves (Figure 2.11E) (Elfvin, Johansson, Höijer, and Aldskogius,

Figure 2.10 (*continued*) sheath (PALS), follicles, and marginal zone. The PALS forms an inner cuff of predominantly T-lymphocytes around the central arteriole. In the outer PALS, interdigitating dendritic cells, migrating B-cells, plasma cells and macrophages are present. The follicle is continuous with the PALS and composed primarily of B-lymphocytes, but also some follicular dendritic cells and $CD4^+$ T-cells. Follicles may contain germinal centers. A band of macrophages and the marginal sinus separate the marginal zone from the PALS and the follicles. The marginal zone contains reticular fibroblasts, macrophages, dendritic cells, and B-cells. The marginal zone blends into the red pulp, and is a site for screening the circulating blood for antigens and pathogens, and antigen processing and presentation. Smaller arterioles branch from the central arterioles, feeding into the capillary beds of the white pulp, some ending in the marginal sinus at the junction between the PALS and the marginal zone. Blood percolates through the marginal zone, and then into the adjacent venous sinus either directly or after passing through the reticular meshwork of the red pulp (B, C). As the white pulp wanes, blood flows through penicillar arteries (surrounded by red pulp) (B, C, red arrow). Blood from the red pulp collects in the venous sinuses which drains into the trabecular veins and converges at the hilus to form the splenic vein (B, C). Blood from the spleen drains into the hepatic portal system. Sympathetic nerves follow the splenic and trabecular arteries into the spleen (right side of panel B), and continue as plexuses associated with central arterioles and their branches. Neurovascular plexuses associated with the central arteriole enter the white pulp to reside among T-lymphocytes and accessory cells in the PALS and marginal zone. NA nerves are rarely observed in the follicles or as free fibers in the red pulp, but are found in association with the venous sinuses and veins that drain blood from the spleen.

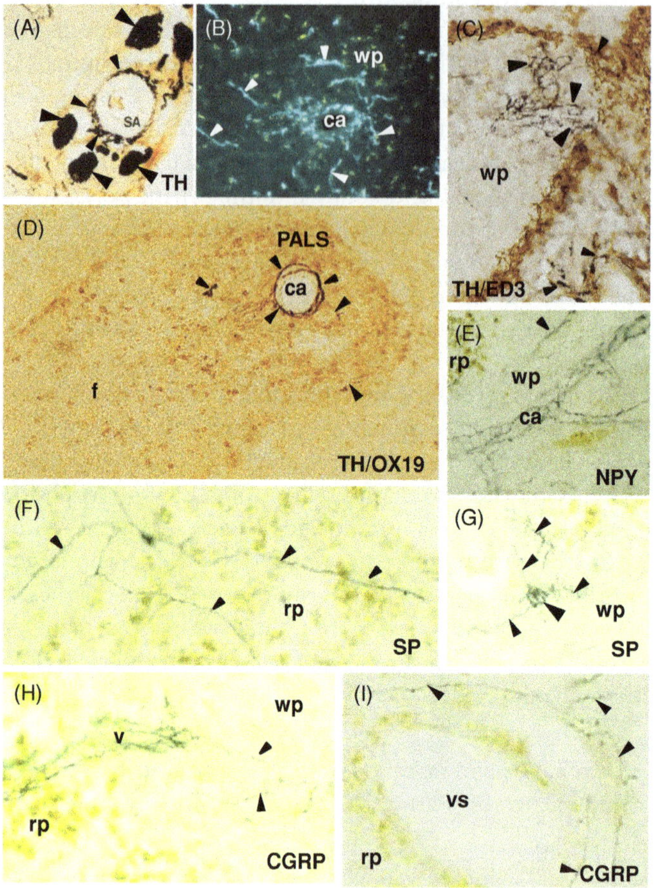

Figure 2.11 Histochemical Staining for Nerves in the Spleen. A. Immunohistochemical (IHC) staining for tyrosine hydroxylase (TH) demonstrates NA nerves (small arrowheads) course along the splenic artery (SA) as well as NA nerve bundles (large arrowheads) robustly stained for TH adjacent to the splenic artery at the hilus of the rat spleen. B. Fluorescence histochemistry for catecholamines reveals a dense plexus of NA nerves along a cross-sectionally cut central arteriole (ca) in the white pulp (wp) of the murine spleen. Fluorescent, punctate and varicose linear nerve profiles (arrowheads) extend from the vascular plexus into the surrounding white pulp. C. In IHC-stained spleen sections, TH+ nerves (black, large arrowheads) are found entering into the marginal zone from an adjacent vascular plexus in the white pulp (wp). In the marginal zone, TH+ nerves (black, small arrowheads) course among the dense inner and diffuse outer band of ED3+ macrophages (brown). D. With dual staining for TH and the T-cell marker, OX19, TH-immunoreactive nerves (black, arrowheads) are visible in close association with the central arteriole and punctate TH+ profiles among OX19+ T-cells in the PALS, but are not seen in the follicle. E. IHC for NPY shows a dense vascular plexus along the length of a central arteriole in the white pulp of the spleen. NPY fibers also are seen in the periphery of the white pulp. F. IHC demonstrates CGRP+ linear, varicose nerves course as individual profiles in the red pulp of the spleen. G. A small vascular-associated nerve plexus positive for SP is present in the white pulp near the red pulp of the spleen. Fine varicose fibers extend radially from the cross-sectionally cut blood vessel. H. CGRP+ nerves travel as a longitudinally-oriented vascular plexus at the junction between the red and white pulp, and extend from this plexus as free fibers into the white pulp. I. CGRP+ fibers (large arrowheads) are present along the venous sinus (vs) in the red pulp (rp) of the spleen.

1994; Jobling, 1994; Weihe *et al.*, 1991), and these nerves are destroyed by treatment with 6-hydroxydopamine (Nagata *et al.*, 1987; Romano, Felten, Felten, and Olschowka, 1991; Stevens-Felten and Bellinger, 1997), indicating that NPY colocalizes with NE in the spleen. Although enkephalin nerves are infrequently observed, their distribution also overlaps with NE and NPY (Fried *et al.*, 1986; Bellinger *et al.*, 1997). VIP nerves also course in the same compartments as NA nerves, but may not be colocalized with NE, NPY, and enkephalin, based on denervation studies using the neurotoxin, 6-hydroxydopamine, to destroy sympathetic nerves (Fried *et al.*, 1986). SP and CGRP nerves are reported in spleens from the rat, cat, guinea pig, cow, and pig (Lundberg, Anggård, Pernow, and Hökfelt, 1985; Fried *et al.*, 1986; Lorton, Bellinger, S. Felten, and D. Felten, 1991; Weihe *et al.*, 1991). These fibers enter the spleen in the splenic nerve, course in the red and, to a lesser extent, the white pulp, along the capsule and trabeculae (Figures 2.11F–I). Somatostatin and cholinergic nerves are not present in the spleen (Nance and Burns, 1989; Chevendra and Weaver, 1992; Bellinger *et al.*, 1993).

Origin of innervation In the rat spleen, the source of sympathetic NA (also NPY and enkephalin) nerves is the superior mesenteric–celiac ganglionic complex, and the thoracic sympathetic trunk (Bellinger, S. Felten, Lorton, and D. Felten, 1989; Nance and Burns, 1989). VIP nerves have been retrogradely traced from the spleen to the superior mesenteric–celiac ganglionic plexus in rats (Chevendra and Weaver, 1992). The origin of SP and CGRP nerves in the spleen remains to be determined.

Lymph nodes

Structure and function Lymph is fluid in the lymphatic vessels that arises from interstitial fluid in the tissue spaces between cells in the body. Approximately 500–600 lymph nodes distribute in clusters throughout the human body, although they reside in seven major regions: the cervical, axillary, inguinal, pelvic, abdominal, thoracic, and supratrochlear regions. Round to bean-shaped in appearance, lymph nodes are interposed between lymphatic vessels (Figure 2.12), and serve two primary functions. First, specialized reticuloendothelial cells and macrophages remove foreign particles, damaged cells, tumor cells, and microbes from the lymph as it slowly percolates through cortical and medullary sinuses of the lymph node. Lymph nodes also provide a microenvironment for antigen presentation to lymphocytes.

The normal structure, function and histology of lymph nodes have been extensively studied and reviewed by Willard-Mack (2006). Reticuloendothelial cells provide the supporting framework for the lymph node. The processes of the reticular cells form channels and interstitial spaces in which antigen-presenting cells (APCs), macrophages and lymphocytes reside. Macrophages cling to the reticular network in the sinuses to capture bacteria and particulates in the lymph, and therefore serve as a filter. The subcapsular sinus lies beneath the capsule except at the hilus, and the trabeculae unevenly divide the lymph node into incomplete lobules (Figure 2.12). The hilus is the site where arteries enter, and veins and the efferent lymphatic vessel exit the lymph node. Several afferent lymphatic vessels, which carry lymph into lymph nodes, enter via the convex surface of the lymph node. Lymph from the afferent vessels drains into the subcapsular sinuses, the trabecular or transverse sinuses, and then into medullary sinuses (Figure 2.12). The medullary sinuses converge at the hilus, where lymph enters the efferent lymphatic vessel to exit the lymph node. After filtering, the lymph leaves via one or two efferent lymphatic vessels.

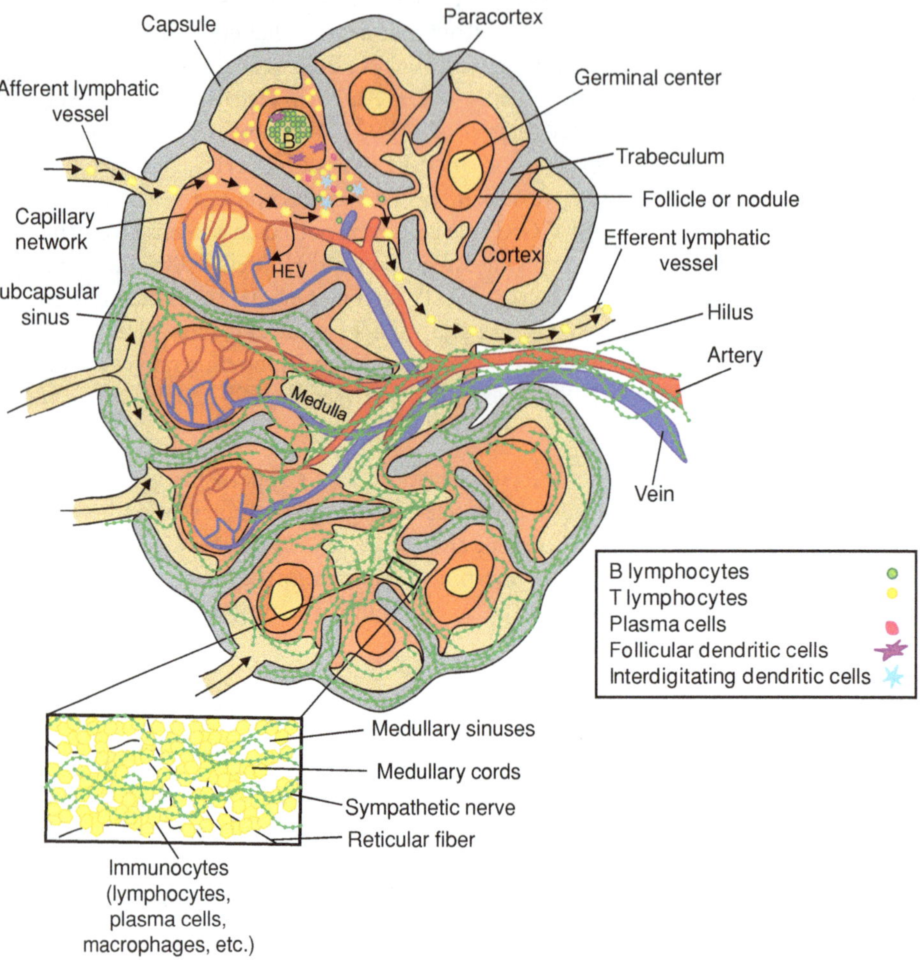

Figure 2.12 Sympathetic Innervation of the Lymph Node. Lymph nodes are surrounded by a fibrous connective tissue capsule, from which trabeculae extend into the parenchyma (gray). Lymph drains from afferent lymphatic vessels into the underlying subcapsular sinus, continues through the cortical and medullary sinuses, and exits the lymph node at the hilus via efferent lymphatic vessels (black arrows). The trabeculae divide the lymph node into incomplete lobules composed of an outer cortex, middle paracortex, and an inner medulla. The cortex contains primarily the follicle, which may contain a germinal center (pale region of activated, proliferating B-cells), surrounded by a mantle zone consisting of naïve B-cells and accessory cells (i.e., macrophages and dendritic cells (purple)). The paracortex contains predominantly T-cells (yellow) and other cells (i.e., interdigitating dendritic cells (blue), plasma cells (pink)). The medulla is comprised of large blood vessels, medullary cords and medullary sinuses. The medullary cords are rich in plasma cells and macrophages. Antibodies produced by plasma cells enter the efferent lymphatic vessel. Sympathetic nerves enter the lymph node in the hilar region in association with the vasculature. NA nerves continue with the blood vessels into the medulla and capsule. From these plexuses, NA nerves enter into the T-dependent regions of the cortex and paracortex. NA fibers extend and branch from the vascular plexuses into the parenchyma among T-lymphocytes and accessory cells that surround the nodules. Sympathetic nerves largely avoid entry into the nodules that are densely populated with B-lymphocytes and supporting cells like follicular dendritic cells. In the medulla, NA nerves course along the medullary cords adjacent to the medullary sinuses (shown in lower left box).

Lymph nodes are composed of many lymphoid lobules encased in a connective tissue capsule, and surrounded by lymph-filled sinuses (Figure 2.12). Trabeculae extend from the capsule to divide the lymph node into lobules. Each lobule is associated with a lymphatic sinus system and a single afferent lymphatic vessel. Lymphoid lobules are the basic anatomical and functional units of the lymph node, and have three basic compartments – an outer cortex, middle paracortex, and an inner medulla. Lobules are arranged side-by-side, with an apex toward the capsule and a base toward the medulla. Superficially, the cortex of each lobule contains spherical follicles surrounded and separated by interfollicular cortex, sometimes called diffuse cortex (Figure 2.12). Each follicle has (1) an outer zone of loosely packed small lymphocytes, macrophages and occasionally plasma cells that extends into the medullary cords, (2) a middle zone of densely packed small lymphocytes (largely B-cells) and macrophages confined to cortex, and (3) an inner zone of large lymphocytes and macrophages, which may include an inner germinal center (secondary follicle). The germinal center contains primarily proliferating B-cells. When a lymphocyte recognizes an antigen, B-cells become activated and migrate to germinal centers where they proliferate (clonal expansion). When antibody-producing plasma cells are formed, they migrate to the medullary cords. The paracortex of each lobule contains a single deep cortical unit or DCU that is divided into a central and peripheral zone (Jia *et al.*, 2012). Adjacent DCUs often converge forming large multiunit complexes. The paracortex lies between the germinal centers and the medulla, and contains predominately T-lymphocytes.

In the lobule, T- and B-cells home to separate areas to interact with APCs, and for clonal expansion. B-cells localize to primary follicles where follicular dendritic cells present antigen. In the follicle, activated B-cells proliferate to form a germinal center (secondary follicles). In contrast, T-cells home to the paracortex and interfollicular cortex to interact with APCs. Activated T-cells proliferate and enlarge the paracortex. Lymphocytes migrate to and from B- and T-cell areas in the peripheral DCU and interfollicular cortex. Precursors of plasma cells migrate to the medullary cords to mature, and subsequently secrete antibodies into the lymph. There are two main compartments in the medulla, the medullary cords and sinuses (Figure 2.12). Lymphoid and myeloid cells form cords of cells in the spaces of the reticuloendothelial network that form the medullary sinuses. Medullary cord cells include mature B-cells, activated T-cells, macrophages and plasma cells. After stimulation, T-lymphocytes migrate first to the medulla, and then re-enter the blood stream through HEVs to home to the appropriate target tissue.

Sympathetic innervation The presence and distribution of sympathetic nerves in lymph nodes had been demonstrated in mice, rats, guinea pigs, cats, and humans (D. Felten *et al.*, 1984, 1985; Fink and Weihe, 1988; Panuncio, De La Peña, Gualco, and Reissenweber, 1999). Sympathetic nerves accompany the vasculature, which enter the lymph node at the hilus (Figures 2.12 and 2.13). NA nerves then course with the straight arterial branches into the medulla, or as subcapsular plexuses in rodents (Felten *et al.*, 1985) (Figures 2.12 and 2.13) but not humans (Panuncio, De La Peña, Gualco, and Reissenweber, 1999). In the medulla, sympathetic nerves reside adjacent to the medullary sinuses (Figure 2.12), lymphocytes, reticuloendothelial cells, macrophages, and plasma cells of the medullary cords (Felten *et al.*, 1984; Fink and Weihe, 1988; Stevens-Felten and Bellinger, 1997). The arteries further divide to form arterioles, and in the cortex, capillary beds (Figure 2.12). Sympathetic nerves remain in close proximity to these vessels. In the cortex, a large number of NA nerves extend from the vasculature into the paracortical and interfollicular zones, but avoid the follicles (Figures 2.12 and 2.13). With histofluorescent staining, these nerves reside among T-lymphocytes and autofluorescent cells,

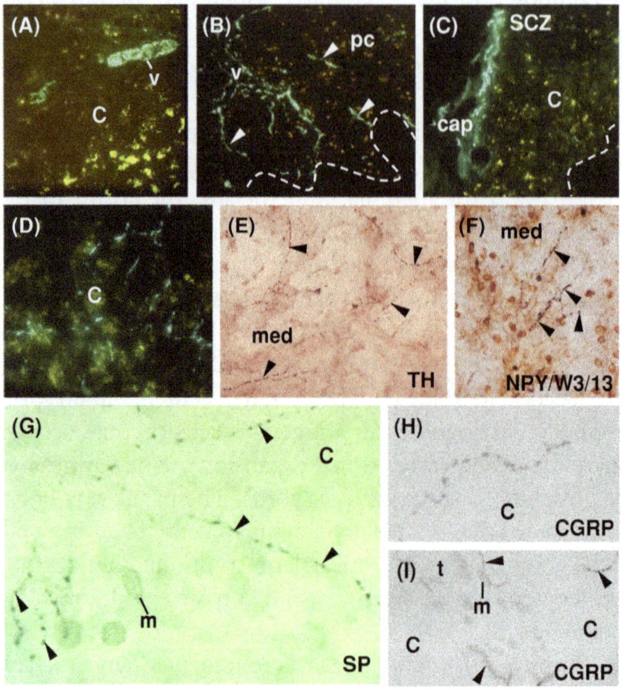

Figure 2.13 Histochemical Staining for Nerves in Lymph Nodes. A. NA nerves travel along a blood vessel (v) in the cortex (c) of a mesenteric lymph node from a mouse. B. In a murine popliteal lymph node, a vascular plexus of NA nerves in the paracortex (pc) near the corticomedullary junction (CMJ; dashed line) extends linear and punctate profiles (arrowheads) into the parenchyma of the paracortex. v, blood vessel. C. NA nerves course in the capsule (cap) of a mesenteric lymph node. D. Fluorescent nerves are present in the cortex (c) of a mesenteric lymph node. E. IHC reveals delicate varicose, tyrosine hydroxylase (TH)+ nerves (arrowheads) coursing in the medulla (med) of a lymph node. F. Double-label IHC shows neuropeptide Y (NPY)-immunoreactive nerves (arrowheads) among T-helper cells (W3/13+) in the medulla (med). G. IHC staining for substance P demonstrates the presence of fine, varicose SP+ nerve profiles (arrowheads) in the cortex (c) among mast cell-like cells (m) in the cortex of a rat mesenteric lymph node. H. Linear varicose nerves positive for calcitonin gene-related protein (CGRP) in a rat mesenteric lymph node. I. CGRP+ fibers (arrowheads) are present in a trabeculum (t), adjacent cortex (c), and in close proximity to mast cell-like cells (m).

assumed to be macrophages (Figure 2.13A–D). Based on electron microscopy, NA nerves in lymph nodes form neuroeffector junctions with vascular smooth muscle, reticular cells, plasma cells, and lymphocytes (Novotny and Kliche, 1986; Novotny, 1988). To a lesser extent, sympathetic nerves supply the postcapillary HEVs in the paracortex, and the veins that exit from the organ at the hilus. Thus, sympathetic nerves innervate T-cell-rich regions (paracortical and cortical zones), with minimal innervation of B-lymphocyte-rich follicles and germinal centers (Felten *et al.*, 1984; Stevens-Felten and Bellinger, 1997). Like the spleen, the density of NA nerves in paracortical and cortical regions is influenced by a number of factors, including the location of the lymph nodes (Li and Novotny, 2001), age (Bellinger, Lorton, S. Felten and D. Felten, 1992; Bellinger *et al.*, 1992), neurotrophic support (Carlson *et al.*, 1995), immune activation (Novotny *et al.*, 1994), and disease processes (Lorton *et al.*, 2005, 2009; del Rey *et al.*, 2006).

Peptidergic nerves Nerves containing dopamine β-hydroxylase (an enzyme marker for DA or NE), NPY, VIP, peptide histidine isoleucine (PHI, a coproduct of the same precursor as VIP), SP, CGRP have been reported in lymph nodes (Fink and Weihe, 1988; Bellinger *et al.*, 1990; Stevens-Felten and Bellinger, 1997). These nerves enter lymph nodes at the hilus with the vasculature. NPY nerves follow the same course and distribution as NA sympathetic nerves (Figure 2.13F) (Fink and Weihe, 1988; Bellinger *et al.*, 1990; Stevens-Felten and Bellinger, 1997), consistent with colocalization with NE in NA nerves. In contrast, SP and CGRP nerves are comparatively sparse and their distribution differs from sympathetic nerves (Fink and Weihe, 1988; Bellinger *et al.*, 1990; Stevens-Felten and Bellinger, 1997). After entry at the hilus, SP and CGRP reside beneath the capsule, as non-vascular fibers in the medulla, CMJ, and between follicles (Figure 2.13G–I). These nerves course among cortical and medullary lymphocytes and accessory cells. VIP nerves are also sparse. They associate with the blood vessels that enter lymph nodes in the rat mesenteric, but not popliteal lymph nodes (Bellinger *et al.*, 1997), suggesting lymph-node-specific differences in VIP nerves based on their body location. In the mesenteric lymph nodes, VIP nerves reside near blood vessels, interfollicular T-cell zones, in the cortex, at the CMJ, and along the medullary cords (Fink and Weihe, 1988; Stevens-Felten and Bellinger, 1997).

Origin of lymph node innervation For most lymph nodes, the ganglia from which their sensory or sympathetic nerves derive has not been determined. Since lymph nodes drain regional structures where they are located in the body, it is assumed that their nerves come from the same ganglion or ganglia as other regional structures (Figure 12.5). Consistent with this assumption, fluorogold injected into the rat submaxillary lymph node retrogradely labeled sympathetic neurons in the caudal portion of the ipsilateral superior cervical ganglion (Romeo *et al.*, 1994). The contralateral superior cervical ganglion has not examined, so it is not known if sympathetic innervation is bilateral. Consistent with these findings, sympathetic nerves in rat cervical lymph nodes disappear after removal of the superior cervical ganglia (Giron, Crutcher, and Davis, 1980). The overlapping distribution of NPY and sympathetic nerves in lymph nodes suggests colocalization, but needs to be demonstrated. Sensory nerves in the tracheobronchial lymph nodes in guinea pigs arise from the cervical DRG (C3-C8) (Kurkowski, Kummer, and Heym, 1990). Further, electron microscopy has revealed fine myelinated nerves in axillary and mesenteric lymph nodes (Li and Novotny, 2001), that are likely sensory nerves, as sympathetic nerves are unmyelinated.

Functional significance of sympathetic innervation in secondary lymphoid organs: lymph nodes and spleen

Lymph from regional body structures drain into their associated lymph nodes. After APCs are activated, they migrate to draining lymph nodes to present antigens to T-lymphocytes. Therefore, lymph nodes are anatomically positioned to direct the immune system to sites of injury and infection. Sympathectomy (sympX) during adjuvant arthritis induction or neonatal sympX reduces the severity of acute disease and flares, and reduces hyperalgesia (Ebbinghaus *et al.*, 2011). SympX lowers interleukin (IL)-2, IL-17 and transforming growth factor-β in supernatants from lymph nodes and/or spleen. These findings are consistent with a role for the SNS in driving T-helper (T_H) 2/ T_H17 responses. T_H cell differentiation in response to an antigen is influenced by local activity in lymph node sympathetic nerves during the early phase of dendritic cell stimulation (Maestroni, 2002). Sympathetic activation in lymph nodes stimulates IL-10 release and inhibits IL-12 by dendritic cells, and reduces their APC capability in a contact hypersensitivity model (Maestroni and Mazzola, 2003; Elenkov, Wilder, Chrousos, and Vizi, 2000). Given that IL-10 promotes differentiation of T_H2 cells and IL-12 promotes differentiation of T_H1 cells, sympathetic nerves in lymph nodes and spleen promote T_H2 cell and inhibit T_H1 cell differentiation, in part, by regulating the production of these two cytokines.

NE released from nerves signal target immune cells via β_2- and α-AR (α_1- and α_2-subtypes) (Sanders, Kasprowicz, Kohm, and Swanson, 2000; Kavelaars, 2002) expressed on their cell surface. T- and B-cells predominantly express β_2-AR, except for T_H2 cells which lack β_2-AR based on findings using murine T_H2 cell clones. B-cells express more β_2-AR than $CD4^+$ T_H1 cells. Pharmacological data suggest that T-cells also express α-AR, but whether B-cells express α-AR is not clear. α_2-AR are also found prejunctionally at the neuroeffector junctions, and function in feedback inhibition of sympathetic nerve firing (Elenkov and Vizi, 1991). Greater nerve activity promotes signaling via α-AR, which have a higher activation threshold than β_2-AR on immune cells. NA sympathetic nerves influence both innate and adaptive immunity, and play an important role in inflammation. They regulate leukocyte proliferation/expansion, leukocyte trafficking, differentiation of lymphocytes, and effector functions, including the production of soluble immune mediators (e.g., chemokines and cytokines) and antigen processing and presentation.

Differentiation and activity of $CD8^+$ and $CD4^+$ T_H1 and T_H2 cells is modulated by the SNS. In general, the SNS reduces cell-mediated immune responses, promotes T_H2 cell-dependent antibody responses, and can promote or suppress T_H1 cell-driven antibody production by affecting the production of interferon-γ by T-cells (Kin and Sanders, 2006). The SNS plays a regulatory role in humoral immunity, differentially affecting antibody production depending on the isotype (e.g., IgG1, IgE, IgA etc.). More recent data support sympathetic regulation of $CD4^+$ T-regulatory and T_H17 cells to affect tolerance and cell-mediated immunity (Bhowmick *et al.*, 2009; Ebbinghaus *et al.*, 2012; Guereschi *et al.*, 2013). Inhibitory SNS actions on cellular immunity occur via the inhibition of cytotoxic T-lymphocyte, natural killer cell, neutrophils, and macrophage activity. In contrast, delayed-type hypersensitivity responses to a contact sensitizing agent (a secondary immune response) are enhanced with SNS activation (Madden, Sanders, and Felten, 1995). The timing of exposure to NE or β-AR agonist relative to the state of $CD8^+$ T-cell differentiation may explain differential functional responses. The SNS generally has a potent anti-inflammatory action by suppressing pro-inflammatory cytokine production (particularly, production of macrophage tumor necrosis factor-α (TNF-α)), an effect mediated largely by β_2-AR stimulation(Elenkov, Wilder, Chrousos, and Vizi, 2000; Bellinger *et al.*, 2008). Although, β_2-AR-mediated anti-inflammatory effects are the most often reported, under certain conditions NE can drive inflammation, promoting TNF-α production by macrophages via an α-AR-mediated mechanism. Thus, the effect of sympathetic activation on inflammation depends on which AR class has the greatest expression in macrophages, and the intensity of SNS activation. In general, effects of the sympathetic to immune cell signaling is reported to be largely inhibitory, however, depending upon the circumstances, can be either inhibitor or excitatory to most immune cell functions. The direction of the response is dependent, at least in part, upon the timing of NE release relative to the activational state of the immune cell, the amount and length of time NE is available for adrenergic receptor interaction, the adrenergic receptor subtypes and the amount of each subtype that the immune cell expresses, and the micro-environment in which different immune challenges and disease states induce (altered cytokine, chemokine, and toll like receptor ligands for example). Finally, rhythmic sympathetic activity can entrain and modulate the molecular circadian clock in natural killer cells and other spleen cells to affect their functional responses across the day (Logan, Arjona, and Sarkar, 2011).

Innervation of Diffuse Lymphatic Tissue or Mucosa-Associated Lymphoid Tissue (MALT)

Structure and function The terminology defining the structure of mucosa-associated lymphoid tissue (MALT) adopted by the Society for Mucosal Immunology Nomenclature Committee in 1997 (Brandtzaeg, Kiyono, Pabst, and Russell, 2008) will be used in this chapter. The structure and function of MALT has been reviewed recently by Cesta (2006). Most of the immune system resides in the mucous membranes (wet epithelia) that line the body surfaces, and that are exposed to the external environment. MALT is subdivided based on its body location. The best described and studied are lymphoid tissues associated with the gut, bronchus, and nasopharynx. The basic cell types in MALT are T- and B-lymphocytes, plasma cells, dendritic cells and macrophages (Figure 2.14). Specialized lymphocytes (predominantly $CD8^+$) called intraepithelial cells or (IELs) reside in the epithelium, but technically are not considered a part of MALT (Brandtzaeg, Kiyono, Pabst, and Russell, 2008). The IELs can expand into memory/effector T-cells in the surface epithelium, and extensive cross-communication occurs between the IEL, epithelium and immune components in the lamina propria. Processes from dendritic cells from the underlying MALT also extend into the wet epithelium. Therefore, MALT is a lymphoepithelial tissue. Underlying the epithelium, the lymphoid tissue that comprises MALT resembles the structure of lymph nodes (Figure 2.14). MALT is composed of B-cell follicles, also called lymph nodules. Lymph nodules are interposed between small, diffuse aggregates of T-cell-dependent zones containing a variety of APCs (e.g., dendritic cells and macrophages) and T-cells (Cesta, 2006). In contrast to lymph nodes, MALT lacks afferent lymphatic vessels. Instead of surveying antigens from lymph, MALT directly samples antigens from the mucosal surface. Regardless of its location in the body, all MALT has this same basic structure and function; however, the lymph nodules are arranged differently depending on the site, species, age, and activational state (e.g., normal vs. chronically inflamed). At some sites the lymphoid nodules may be surrounded by a complete or incomplete connective tissue capsule, such as in the tonsils. The lymphoid nodules usually contain germinal centers at the base of the nodules. MALT is located beneath the epithelial lining in a layer called the lamina propria (Figure 2.14). The lamina propria is composed of immune cells diffusely scattered in connective tissue overlying a smooth muscle layer, but these immune cells are not included as part of MALT (Brandtzaeg, Kiyono, Pabst, and Russell, 2008).

MALT serves as a functional barrier where foreign substances and microbes can selectively pass across the epithelium into the lamina propria for immune surveillance (Brandtzaeg, Kiyono, Pabst, and Russell, 2008). There are two structurally overlapping functional compartments for mucosal immunity, the inductive and effector sites. At inductive sites, antigens are sampled by the mucosal surface, and activation of naïve T- and B-cells is induced. So, lymph nodules, IELs, and lymph nodes that drain the mucosae are sites of B- and T-cells induction. For example, lymphoid follicles in the distal ileum (Peyer's patches) and mesenteric lymph nodes are inductive sites where activated T- and B-cells clonally expand and differentiate into T-effector and IgA-producing plasma cells, respectively. The effector cells preferentially home to effector sites in the gut via site-specific cues. At effector sites, immune cells have ingressed, are retained, and have differentiated into effector cells (e.g., IgA-secreting plasma cells). Effector sites are histologically distinct and include the lamina propria of various mucosae, surface epithelia, and exocrine glands. In the gut, the epithelium that overlies the lymphoid follicles, referred to as follicle-associated epithelium (FAE) contains specialized cells called M cells, named for their microfolded apical cell surface (Figure 2.14). Thin-epithelial M cells transfer soluble and particulate antigens from the gut lumen via distinct mechanisms depending on

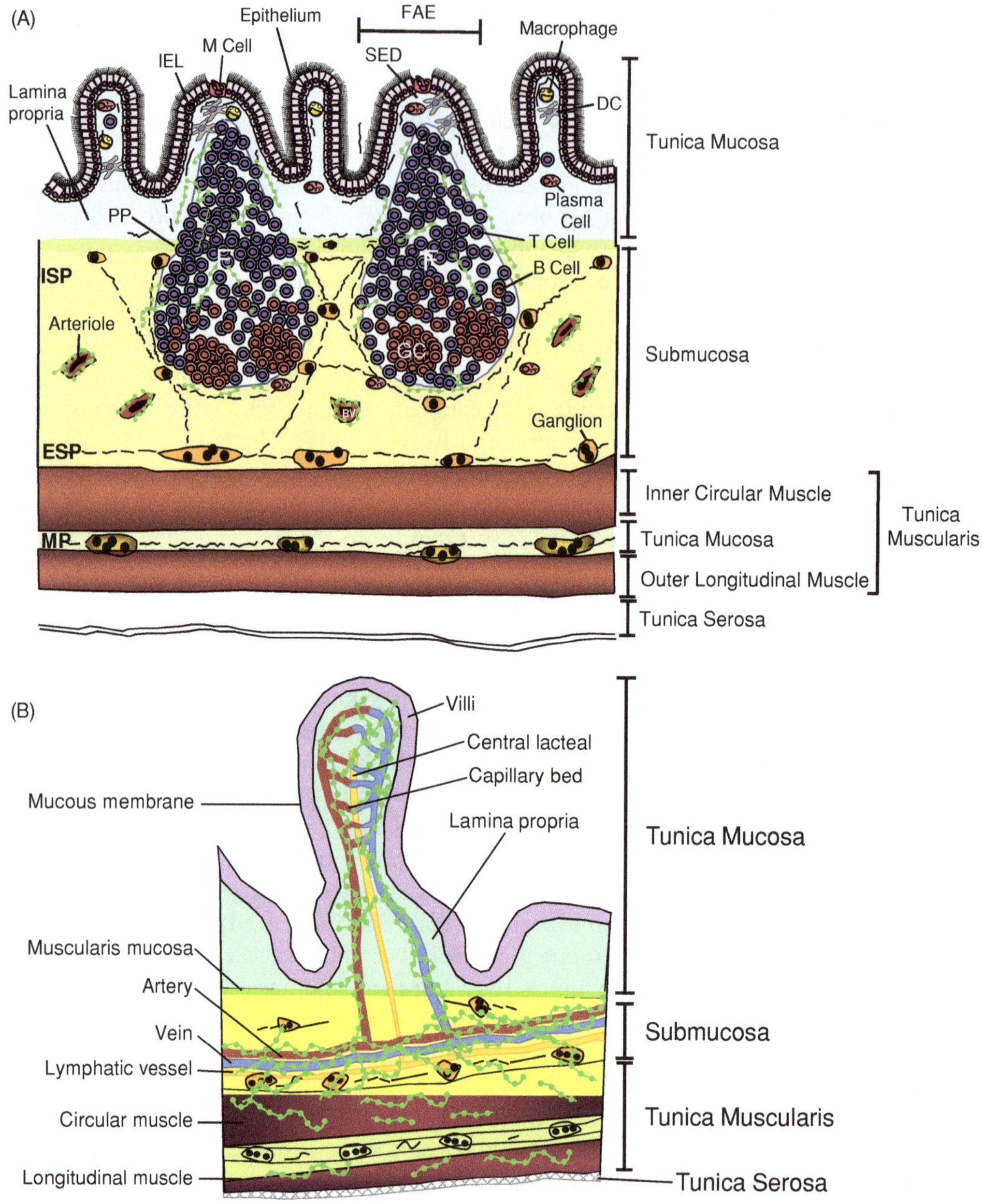

Figure 2.14 Sympathetic innervation of Peyer's patches. A. Peyer's patches (PP) closely associate with a specialized follicle-associated epithelium (FAE), which contains an M cell. The lamina propria (turquoise) beneath the M cell (subepithelial dome (SED)) is rich in antigen-presenting cells (i.e., dendritic cells and macrophages). The lamina propria and epithelium comprise the tunica mucosa. PP are present in the lamina propria and submucosa (yellow), and contain a superficial domal region (rich in T-cells) and basal germinal centers (rich in B-cells). Additionally, the lamina propria contains a large number of plasma cells, T-cells, B-cells, macrophages and dendritic cells, especially in the villi. The types of immune cell types illustrated in the lamina propria and submucosa in Figure 2.14A but are not shown in this Figure 2.14B to better visualize the distribution of nerves. The regions in which they reside are labeled. Intraepithelial lymphocytes (IEL) are often seen in the overlying epithelium. Ganglia (orange and gold) of the enteric nervous system (ENS) include the myenteric plexuses (MP, gold)

their physical properties (e.g., size and lipid solubility). Despite the importance of MALT in host defense, innervation of immune compartments remains understudied compared with other lymphoid organs.

Innervation of gut-associated lymphoid tissue (GALT) The most extensive lymphoid tissue in the body is GALT. GALT is present in the jejunum and ileum as Peyer's patches, the colon as solitary nodules, and the cecum as the appendix (Brandtzaeg, Kiyono, Pabst, and Russell, 2008). In GALT, nerves with specific neurotransmitters have precise distribution patterns; however, information about their relationships with specific types of immune cells is limited. GALT is innervated by sympathetic nerves (Figure 2.14) (Felten, Overhage, S. Felten, and Schmedtje, 1981; Felten *et al.*, 1985; Elenkov, Wilder, Chrousos, and Vizi, 2002; Straub *et al.*, 2006; Bellinger *et al.*, 2008). In the rabbit, sympathetic nerves from collateral mesenteric ganglia travel along blood vessels and penetrate the serosal surface of the large intestine to enter the appendix, and then travel longitudinally in the muscularis interna associated with both the vasculature and enteric smooth muscle (Felten, Overhage, S. Felten, and Schmedtje, 1981; Felten *et al.*, 1985). They course along branching neurovascular plexuses in internodular septae that travel radially towards the lumen, and as they reach the interdomal regions of the lamina propria they enter into the thymus (T-cell)-dependent zones and branch extensively. In T-cell-dependent zones, NA nerves extend beneath the basement membrane of the epithelium and closely apposed to plasma cells and other lymphoid cells in the absence of close contact with blood vessels. NA nerves are also present near presumptive serotonergic enterochromaffin cells. Sympathetic nerves are not found to any appreciable extent in the lymph nodules (Figure 2.14). A similar sympathetic nerve distribution is observed in the Peyer's patches (Figure 2.14) and sacculus rotundus, the distal part of the ileum that transitions into the colon, except that the density of enterochromaffin cells varies depending on the GALT location. Tract-tracing and functional studies clearly demonstrate a sympathetic origin for most NA nerves; however, a small number arise from the ENS (Quinson, Robbins, Clark, and Furness, 2001; Straub *et al.*, 2006)

Ganglionic plexuses of the ENS intimately associate with Peyer's patches. ACh, VIP, SP, somatostatin, galanin, and CGRP nerves from the internal submucous plexus or postganglionic sympathetic neurons surround the domes of the follicles in the T-cell-dependent zones (Kaleczyc *et al.*, 2010). However, very few fibers enter the follicle proper or the germinal

---

Figure 2.14 (*continued*) between the inner and outer circular muscles (red) of the tunica muscularis, and the submucosal ganglionic plexus (orange), which is composed of the internal and external submucosal plexuses (ISP and IEP, respectively). Neurons in the ENS (black circles) contain many different neurotransmitters, as indicated in the text. Nerves from the submucosal plexus (black linear profiles) course around the periphery of the PP and into T-cell-rich zones. Sympathetic nerves (green varicose profiles) course along blood vessels in the submucosa, and in the periphery and dome of the follicle (F), but avoid the germinal centers. B. Sympathetic nerves (green varicose profiles) travel along blood vessels that supply the intestines, penetrating the serosal surface of the intestines to enter the gut (not shown). Then they travel longitudinally in the muscularis interna associated with both the vasculature and enteric smooth muscle. Sympathetic nerves course along branching neurovascular plexuses in internodular septae, coursing radially towards the lumen. As they reach the interdomal regions of the lamina propria they enter into the thymus (T-cell)-dependent zones and branch extensively. Neurons (black dots) of the ENS are shown as black dots within the ganglia of the myenteric plexus (gold; between outer longitudinal and inner circular muscle layers of the gut) and the submucosal plexus (orange; in submucosa). The distribution of nerves arising from these ganglia is illustrated (black lines).

centers (Balemba *et al.*, 1998; Vulchanova *et al.*, 2007). SP and CGRP appear to be colocalized (Vulchanova *et al.*, 2007). SP and CGRP fibers coursed in close proximity to presumptive macrophages (based on their expression of calprotectin). In the subepithelial dome region, peptidergic nerves intermingle with MHC class II-positive cells that resemble dendritic cells. Radial bundles of peptidergic nerves project into a single dome, intersperse around it and between adjacent domes. These nerves are likely to originate from both ENS ganglionic plexuses, providing an anatomical substrate for rapid integration, coordination, and modulation of antigen sampling and processing in different subepithelial domes. Since enteric neurons receive input from both the SNS and PaSNS (via the vagus nerve) systems, autonomic regulation of the gut is both direct and indirect (Figure 2.5).

Functional significance of GALT innervation In addition to their well-defined roles in regulating intestinal motility and active transepithelial ion transport, the ANS and ENS modulate intestinal immune function involved in mucosal protection and defense. GALT maintains tolerance to food antigens and commensal microflora, and initiates innate and acquired immune responses against luminal pathogens. NA and peptidergic (i.e., NPY, VIP, CGRP, and SP) receptors expressed on cells of the immune system, including lymphocytes, macrophages, dendritic cells, granulocytes, and mast cells, regulate their functions. The extent that infection is modulated by the SNS across different regions of the gut in a normal host has not been determined; however current data indicate important SNS–GALT–bacterial interactions that regulate bacterial adherence, uptake into the gut, and bacterial growth (reviewed in Lyte, Vulchanova, and Brown, 2010). *In-vitro* studies support the proposition that the SNS differentially modulates the uptake and adherence of bacteria like *Escherichia coli* (*E. coli*) (enhanced) and *Salmonella* (reduced), in the gut via an α-AR-mediated mechanism (Green, Lyte, Kulkarni-Narla, and Brown, 2003; Schreiber, Price, and Brown, 2007). Whether similar effects of the SNS occur *in vivo* is unknown. Similarly, how the SNS responds to and regulates commensal bacteria and pathogens in the gut is also unclear. Additionally, bacteria detect neurotransmitters like NE via binding to histidine kinases, enhancing their virulence potential at the genomic level, at least for enterohemorrhagic *E. coli*, *Campylobacter jejuni* and *Vibrio parahemolyticus* (Lyte *et al.*, 1997; Cogan *et al.*, 2007; Nakano, Takahashi, Sakai, and Nakaya, 2007; Spencer *et al.*, 2010). Finally, α-AR-mediated bacterial growth has been reported (Lyte *et al.*, 1997; Freestone, Haigh, and Lyte, 2007). Collectively, these studies support SNS–host–microbial interactions in the gut, affecting the growth, virulence, and invasiveness of pathogenic bacteria and host defense.

Current understanding of neurotransmitter effects on immune cells is mainly based on studies *in vitro*, or studies in tissues other than Peyer's patches. However, available data from the gut suggest differential roles for both peptidergic and sympathetic nerves in regulating the barrier function, ingress of antibody-secreting cells (both IgM+ and IgA+), APC functions, lymphocyte and macrophage cytokine production, granulocyte/mast cell degranulation, and effector functions, primary and secondary immune responses, and allergic and inflammatory responses in the intestinal mucosa (Hart *et al.*, 1990; Ohkubo *et al.*, 1994; González-Ariki and Husband, 2000; Sharkey and Mawe, 2002; Straub *et al.*, 2006; Nijhuis, Olivier, and de Jonge, 2010; Keita and Söderholm, 2010; Lyte, Vulchanova, and Brown, 2011). Because immune cell function depends on both the activation status and the specific tissue microenvironment, it will be critical to investigate more thoroughly the functional interactions between immune cells, the ENS, SNS and PaSNS, particularly within immune inductive sites of the gut, like the Peyer's patches.

Rodent models of gut inflammation, like indomethacin-induced gastric ulceration, colitis and inflammatory bowel disease provides support for pro-inflammatory and anti-inflammatory effects of sympathetic nerves in the gut (Straub *et al.*, 2006; Lomax, Sharkey, and Furness, 2010). Pro-inflammatory effects of the SNS are mediated via α_2-AR, whereas anti-inflammatory effects are mediated via β_2- and β_3-ARs (Straub *et al.*, 2006; Vasina *et al.*, 2008). Additionally, through reflex channels, inflammation in one region of the gut alters gut function in other regions. It is clear that the nervous system plays a prominent and complex role in regulating the gut flora, immune surveillance, immune responses to foods and microbes, and gut inflammation via bidirectional cross-talk with cells the immune system that reside in lymphoid compartment.

Innervation of bronchus-associated lymphoid tissue (BALT) Aggregates of lymphoid cells and lymphoid follicles in the mammalian respiratory tract and lungs are referred to as BALT. BALT develops after contact with antigens; it is not preformed like GALT and the tonsils. Single aggregates called bronchus-associated lymphoid follicles randomly distribute along the bronchial tract and at bifurcations beneath the bronchial epithelium. BALT spans across the smooth muscle layer of the mucosa into the submucosa. Primary and secondary follicles associate with adjacent diffuse lymphoid tissue, efferent lymphatic vessels and HEVs (sites for ingress or egress of immune cells). Nerves containing NE, NPY, VIP/PHI, SP, or CGRP are reported predominantly beneath the lymphoid epithelium, associated with smooth muscle, less often in the periphery, and rarely in the center of the follicle (Nohr and Weihe, 1991). SP and CGRP nerves were more abundant in the subepithelium and generally less frequent along blood vessels than NE, NPY, or VIP/PHI nerves. Nerves, regardless of their neurotransmitter phenotype, do not extend into the epithelium. NA and NPY nerves are preferentially perivascular, forming dense plexuses along blood vessels and occasionally extending into the parenchyma near lymphoid cells. VIP-containing fibers display a similar distribution as NA nerves, but occur with lower frequency. Nerves expressing CGRP, SP or met-enkephalin were more abundant in the parenchyma than NPY, TH or VIP/PHI. All nerves containing NE, NPY, VIP, SP, CGRP, or met-enkephalin were found in close proximity to mast cells and ED1+ macrophages, suggesting a role for these neurotransmitters in regulating macrophage and mast cell function. Functional studies support this hypothesis. SP and CGRP nerves are assumed to be sensory; NPY and NA nerves are assumed to be sympathetic. VIP and PHI are often considered transmitters of the PaSNS, but are present in postganglionic sympathetic neurons. Similarly, SP and CGRP are found in non-NA postganglionic sympathetic neurons, and SP in postganglionic parasympathetic neurons. The origin of BALT innervation is not known, although treatment with capsaicin, a selective neurotoxin of small sensory afferents, reduces the number of CGRP nerves in the lung. Innervation of BALT suggests neuroimmune regulation in the respiratory tract.

Innervation of nasopharyngeal-associated lymphoid tissue (NALT) In most species, the nasal passages contain a ring of lymphoid tissue that circle the pharynx and extend to the back of the oral cavity, the oropharyngeal (palatine) and nasopharyngeal (pharyngeal, adenoid) tonsils. Additionally, the tubal tonsils surround the auditory canals, and the lingual tonsils reside in the mucosa of the posterior third of the tongue. Tonsils function in host defense against pathogens that enter the nasal and oral passages and respond to innocuous substances on the mucosal surface. Pathogens and other particulates are actively taken up by M cells in the FAE overlying the lymphoid follicles. Tonsils are composed of the extra-follicular T-cell-region, the outer mantle zones of follicles and the inner germinal centers (called secondary lymphoid follicles).

Very little is known about the types of nerves that supply the tonsils. Innervation of the palatine tonsils is largely provided by sympathetic postganglionic fibers arising from the cranial cervical ganglia and cervicothoracic ganglia. Parasympathetic postganglionic fibers from the pterygopalatine ganglia and afferent fibers from cranial nerves V, IX and X also supply the palatine tonsils, but sympathetic NA nerves are the most abundant. NA nerves associate with blood vessels that encircle the lymphatic nodules (Ueyama *et al.*, 1990; Sirot'áková, Schmidtová, Kocisová, and Kuchta, 2002; Russo *et al.*, 2009). Nerves extend from blood vessels into T-cell zones, avoiding germinal centers. The palatine tonsil is sparsely innervated with peptidergic nerves containing NPY, SP, CGRP, and VIP/PHI (Weihe and Krekel, 1991; Russo *et al.*, 2009). These fibers distribute to the same regions as described for other MALT – in close proximity to blood vessels, beneath the epithelium, and interfollicular T-cell areas, but avoiding the follicle proper and germinal centers. NPY, SP, CGRP, and VIP/PHI nerves end among T-cells and macrophages. SP and CGRP fibers reside near B-cells. Peptidergic nerves represent a small percentage of the total innervation.

No Parasympathetic Innervation of Immune Organs

There is no credible neuroanatomical evidence for parasympathetic (cholinergic) innervation of any organs of the immune system (Nance and Sanders, 2007). This conclusion is further substantiated by the failure to identify definitive markers for cholinergic (parasympathetic) fibers and terminals in any immune organ (Schäfer, Eiden, and Weihe, 1998). The singular source of efferent neural innervation of immune organs is provided by the SNS. So what about the vagus nerve?

The Role of the Vagus Nerve and the Cholinergic Anti-inflammatory Reflex

There is evidence for a functional role of the vagus nerve in immune regulation (Maier *et al.*, 1998; Antonica, Magni, Mearini, and Paolocci, 1991; Rosas-Ballina and Tracey, 2009); however, anatomical data necessitates mediation via indirect pathways. Tracey (2009) uses the term "the cholinergic anti-inflammatory reflex" to refer to the pathway that mediates the functional responses that result primarily from efferent vagal nerve stimulation. However, this term is a misnomer from several standpoints. First, it is unclear whether the pathway mediating this response meets the criteria for a reflex. The specific stimulus initiating the response and the physiological response that results from stimulation have not been defined. Secondly, "cholinergic", in the context of the ANS, implies that the efferent limb of this "reflex" is parasympathetic, which is not supported by the neuroanatomical data.

As emphasized above, the vagus nerve is primarily a sensory nerve with regard to the regulation of the immune system; however, Tracey and colleagues (Borovikova *et al.*, 2000; Saeed *et al.*, 2005) have proposed that the *efferent* vagus nerve plays a powerful role in regulating systemic and localized inflammatory responses, primarily by inhibiting splenic macrophage production of TNF-α (Rosas-Ballina *et al.*, 2008). Electrical stimulation of the cut efferent vagus nerve can inhibit endotoxin-induced sepsis and TNF-α production, as well as localized peripheral inflammatory responses produced in a dermal air pouch. These anti-inflammatory effects of efferent vagal stimulation are all dependent upon cholinergic α7 nicotinic receptors (Wang *et al.*, 2003). However, we have shown that the adrenal medulla and sympathetic nerves inhibit splenic macrophage TNF-α production and systemic inflammation (Meltzer *et al.*, 2004). Likewise, Yoon *et al.* (2006) have shown that inhibition of localized inflammatory responses in the air pouch model is mediated via a sympathoadrenal pathway. Is it possible that both the PaSNS and SNS mediate the same inhibition of splenic TNF-α and inflammation? Tracey (2009) now acknowledges that the efferent vagus nerve does not provide direct efferent cholinergic input to the spleen, and now agrees (see Nance and Sanders, 2007) that, in fact, the sympathetic (NA) splenic nerve is the final and only anti-inflammatory efferent pathway to the spleen. However, to save their vagal-based hypothesis, they now propose that the efferent vagus nerve must connect with prevertebral sympathetic postganglionic neurons that innervate the spleen (Tracey, 2009). Unfortunately, careful neuroanatomical analysis of the innervation of the spleen by retrograde and trans-synaptic tracing studies (Nance and Burns, 1989; Cano *et al.*, 2001) has failed to identify any neuroanatomical vagal–sympathetic–spleen pathway. Recently, the vagal anti-inflammatory neural pathway proposed by Tracey has been examined further electrophysiologically by McAllen and colleagues (Bratton *et al.*, 2012). They have systematically tested for direct synaptic connections between the vagus nerve and the splenic nerve in rats. First, using whole nerve recordings, they show that stimulating the *intact* vagus nerve (sensory fibers present) produces an immediate electrophysiological response in the splenic nerve (inhibition followed by excitation). Most significantly, once the central branch of the vagus nerve is crushed, vagal stimulation produces no responses in the splenic nerve. This shows once more that *the only functional link between the vagus nerve and the splenic nerve is via an afferent reflex through the CNS*, and there is no synaptic efferent vagal pathway to the spleen. Extending their analysis further, they next electrophysiologically identify individual sympathetic postganglionic cell bodies that innervate the spleen, and then try to activate these spleen-specific sympathetic neurons by vagal stimulation. Again, *efferent* vagal stimulation has no effect on the firing rate of identified splenic sympathetic neurons, whereas stimulation of the sympathetic preganglionic splanchnic nerve produces an immediate response in these same identified splenic sympathetic neurons. In a final neuroanatomical experiment, they combine retrograde tract-tracing techniques from the spleen with anterograde tract-tracing from the dorsal motor nucleus of the vagus. They find that the few vagal efferent fibers identified in prevertebral abdominal ganglia are not the ganglia that contained large numbers of cell bodies of sympathetic neurons innervating the spleen. Thus, they find no neuroanatomical contacts between vagal efferent terminals and splenic sympathetic motor neurons, entirely consistent with previous neuroanatomical studies (Nance and Burns, 1989, Cano *et al.*, 2001) and their electrophysiological data. Lastly, a recent analysis of the anti-inflammatory effects of vagal stimulation in α7 nicotinic receptor knockout (KO) mice, (Vida, Peña, Deitch, and Ulloa, 2011) suggests that the requirement for α7 nicotinic receptors is limited, if not peculiar, to "efferent" (cut vagus nerve) vagal stimulation. Although largely ignored and discounted by the authors, they show that stimulation of the intact vagus nerve (afferent vagal stimulation) in α7 KO mice produces a profound suppression in lipopolysaccharide (LPS)-induced TNF-α production, but as shown by others, stimulation of the cut efferent end of the vagus nerve has no effect on TNF-α production in these KO mice. Significantly, they next showed that directly stimulating the splenic sympathetic nerve in the α7 KO mice produced a dramatic suppression in LPS-induced TNF-α comparable to that produced by afferent vagal stimulation. These results illustrate the functional significance of vagal afferents, and not vagal efferents, in the neuroregulation of the immune system. Additional studies by Vida *et al.* (2011) in β_2-AR KO animals further verify that the splenic sympathetic (catecholamine) nerve is the sole efferent anti-inflammatory pathway to the spleen (Nance and Sanders, 2007). Thus, anti-inflammatory effects mediated by the nervous system are mediated entirely by sympathetic β-ARs on immune cells. Thus, the α7 KO story appears to reflect some peculiar or unique aspect of stimulating a cut-vagus nerve, because a primary afferent limb (vagal afferents) and efferent arm (splenic nerve) of the immune regulatory system remain intact in animals that have no α7 nicotinic receptors. Regulatory and immune alterations noted in α7 KO mice are likely due to defects in the SNS already demonstrated for α7 KO animals, as the PaSNS in these animals is normal (Franceschini *et al.*, 2000).

So, given that the anti-inflammatory effects of efferent vagal stimulation requires the spleen, the splenic (sympathetic) nerve, and β_2-ARs (Vida, Peña, Deitch, and Ulloa, 2011; Vida *et al.*, 2011), and the fact that there is no neural connection between the vagus and the splenic sympathetic postganglionic neurons, then the demonstrated effects of efferent vagal stimulation on sympathetic adrenergic-dependent splenic and systemic immune responses must be via an indirect pathway that utilizes a non-neural intermediary. Just as an example, musculocutaneous sensory stimulation produces the release of cholecystokinin (CCK) from the gut via the efferent vagus nerve (Uvnas-Moberg, Lundeberg, and Bruzelius, 1992) and, interestingly, CCK activates the central neuroimmune regulatory system (Verbalis, Stricker, Robinson, and Hoffman, 1991), inhibits inflammatory cytokine production during endotoxic shock (Ling *et al.*, 2001), and TNF-α production in the spleen (Meng *et al.*, 2002). All of these effects are comparable to what is observed with efferent vagal stimulation. In further support of this possibility, the anti-inflammatory effects of a high-fat meal are mediated via fat-induced CCK release that is mediated by the vagus nerve (Luyer *et al.*, 2005). Another possible mechanism is that sustained stimulation of the efferent vagus nerve (guts churning away) would generate sensory signals from the alimentary tract and abdominal viscera which would be detected by vagal sensory fibers if the non-stimulated vagus nerve were left intact, as well as thoracic dorsal root sensory ganglia. This sensory feedback will subsequently activate the sympathetics via established central and peripheral neural pathways. In support of this possibility, sustained sensory stimulation of cutaneous and muscle tissue by a variety of stimuli have the same anti-inflammatory action reported for efferent vagal stimulation. These anti-inflammatory actions include the inhibition of LPS-induced splenic TNF-α production, anti-septic shock, and inhibition of TNF-α in the inflamed air pouch model (Kwon *et al.*, 2003; Aoki *et al.*, 2005; Nance *et al.*, 2005;), all of which are mediated via β-ARs and the SNS – the same as with efferent vagal stimulation. Thus, the mechanism mediating the reported anti-inflammatory effects of vagal stimulation has yet to be identified; however, it can be stated as fact that it is not via a direct neural link with the SNS and the spleen. Lastly, electrical stimulation of the sensory (afferent) vagus nerve produces the same counter-regulatory neuroendocrine and hypothalamic responses that are produced by an inflammatory challenge (Hosoi, Okuma, and Nomura, 2000; see Vida, Peña, Deitch, and Ulloa, 2011). However, stimulation of other nerves or regions of the body have been shown to activate splenic sympathetic nerve activity and inhibit the innate immune system (Sato, 1997). Thus, with regards to the detection and responsiveness to immune-related stimuli, the afferent vagus is not unique and shares this immune-signal-detection function with many afferent nerves distributed throughout the body. Given that activation of β-ARs by the SNS mediates the anti-inflammatory effects of efferent vagal stimulation (Vida *et al.*, 2011), then it is difficult to understand why anyone would choose this indirect and as yet unidentified pathway to activate a sympathetic adrenergic anti-inflammatory pathway (see Nance and Sanders, 2007). There are more efficient means of activating the SNS than cutting the vagus nerve and stimulating the efferent branch. There are adrenergic agonists that suppress inflammation and splenic TNF-α production the same as shown for nicotinic cholinergic agonist and vagal stimulation, which in the end still require the sympathetic catecholamines to do the job. Why use a nicotinic agonist to indirectly stimulate a β-AR-mediated anti-inflammatory response instead of just employing a β-adrenergic agonist? Consistent with this, Vita *et al.* (2011) show that a β-adrenergic agonist could still save animals from septic shock long after vagal stimulation and nicotinic agonists had failed.

Sensory Innervation of Immune Organs

Neuroanatomical studies have shown that the thymus and spleen do not receive any afferent innervation (Nance, Hopkins, and Bieger, 1987; Nance and Burns, 1989; Cano *et al.*, 2001; Trotter *et al.*, 2007). However, there is neuroanatomical evidence that lymph nodes and bone marrow may be innervated by sensory nerves (Kurkowski, Kimmer, and Heym, 1990; Imai *et al.*, 1997). Although the function of sensory nerves in these immune organs has not been established, Lorton *et al.* (2000) has shown that prior treatment of draining lymph nodes with a sensory nerve fiber toxin attenuated the subsequent development of adjuvant-induced arthritis. This limited or complete absence of sensory innervation of organs of the immune system can be contrasted with the afferent innervation of other organs, tissues and body regions. All body surfaces and supporting tissues are innervated by sensory nerves and importantly, these are also primary sites of injury and microbial/antigen exposure. Sensory fibers and terminals that are located at sites of tissue injury, infection, or antigen exposure play a critical role in localized inflammatory responses and the activity of sensory nerves contribute to the development and persistence of inflammatory disease (Neuhuber and Tiegs, 2004).

The Role of Sensory Nerves in Immune Regulation

All regions, organs and tissues of the body receive sympathetic input, and all body surfaces that are potential sites of microbial invasion or antigen challenge (skin, oral and gut mucosa, peritoneum, lungs, etc.) receive an extensive afferent neural innervation whose terminals are often associated with cellular elements of the immune system, such as mast cells. The pro-inflammatory contribution of sensory fibers to the local inflammatory response to microbes and antigens at these body surfaces represents a significant modulator of localized inflammatory (innate) immune responses, and possibly the subsequent adaptive immune response (Shepherd *et al.*, 2005). In addition to sensory nerve terminals modulating the activity and trafficking of immune cells at specific sites of injury, microbial and antigen invasion, these same sensory nerves transmit specific signals to the CNS and a central neuroimmune regulatory network (Nance and MacNeil, 2001) that mediates the coordinated cascade of autonomic, neuroendocrine, and behavioral responses produced by localized and systemic inflammatory challenges. There has been much focus on the sensory component of the vagus nerve in immune regulation since the first report that subdiaphragmatic vagotomy attenuated the central activational effects of intraperitoneal injections of endotoxin (LPS) (Wan *et al.*, 1994). Many studies have shown a fundamental role for the sensory vagus nerve in transmitting neuroimmune afferent information from the abdominal cavity and viscera (Maier *et al.*, 1998). Importantly, this immune-signaling function of vagal afferents is not unique to the vagus nerve, and sensory fibers distributed throughout the body, such as in skin, muscle, mucosal surfaces, can respond to immunological stimuli and transmit this information to the CNS via peripheral and central sensory pathways (see results of Zang *et al.*, 2008).

Summary of Innervation of the Immune System

Sympathetic NA innervation predominates in all immune organs, whereas afferent innervation of the immune system may be limited to lymph nodes, bone marrow, and body regions where the immune system interfaces with the external environment. To date, there is no credible neuroanatomical evidence for efferent vagal or parasympathetic innervation of lymphoid organs; however, lymphoid tissues in the mucosa appear to receive parasympathetic innervation, warranting further investigation. Certain patterns and features of sympathetic innervation are consistently seen across immune organs (Felten *et al.*, 1985, 1987; Elenkov, Wilder, Chrousos, and Vizi, 2000; Bellinger *et al.*, 2008). Sympathetic nerves enter lymphoid tissues in neurovascular bundles in connective tissue, where they course near macrophages and mast cells. Innervation of lymphoid organs is regional and specific. For example, in secondary lymphoid organs, sympathetic NA nerves distribute to T-lymphocyte, macrophage, and plasma cell compartments, and avoid nodular regions where B-lymphocytes develop and mature.

In lymphoid tissue, sympathetic nerves signal to a variety of immune cell types via paracrine, non-synaptic release to regulate vascular functions, leukocyte trafficking, hematopoiesis and lymphocyte maturation, and immune regulation during injury and wound healing, infection, and challenge with foreign substances. Nerves coordinate vascular, stromal and immune cell interactions necessary to maintain homeostasis. Nerves supplying immune organs form neuroeffector junctions with multiple immunocytes and with different phenotypes. Although close contacts (6–20 nm) between nerve terminals and immunocytes occur, junctions of ~200–250 μm prevail. Neuromediators diffuse across the junction to bind with specific receptors on target cells (i.e., paracrine release) that are linked to ion channels and/or second-messenger systems that mediate neurotransmitter effects. Neurotransmission via paracrine release from visceral nerves occurs more slowly than in the somatic sensory system, but is faster than hormonal regulation. Targets of nerves in lymphoid organs are both stationary (i.e., stromal cells) and mobile (i.e., lymphocytes), and NE release from postganglionic sympathetic nerves is regulated at multiple levels of the neuroaxis via short, intermediate and long feedback loops.

The major neurotransmitters of autonomic and sensory nerves colocalize with, and release other neuromediators that modulate the functions of the major neurotransmitters. However, these neuromediators may be present in nerves that lack the classical neurotransmitter in, and whose distribution differs from, autonomic and sensory nerves. Many immunohistochemical markers for cholinergic nerves are not exclusive to these nerves, including ACh and AChE. Sympathetic NA nerves display plasticity – the ability of the brain or nerves to change structurally and/or functionally due to changes in the microenvironment. Both their density and distribution can be affected by many factors, including age, genetic background or mutations, neurotrophic support, drugs, disease processes, health and nutritional status. Altered nerve density and distribution affect their ability to signal to immune cells, and lead to changes in signal transduction mechanisms in target cells that can have significant functional consequences.

References

Afan, A.M., Broome, Caroline, S., Nicholls, Sian, E., Whetton, Anthony, D., and Miyan, Jaleel, A. (1997). Bone marrow innervation regulates cellular retention in murine haemopoietic system. *British Journal of Haematology*, 98, 569–577.

Ahmed, M., Bjurholm, A., Kreicbergs, A., and Schultzberg, M. (1993). Neuropeptide Y, tyrosine hydroxylase and vasoactive intestinal polypeptide-immunoreactive nerve fibers in the vertebral bodies, discs, dura mater, and spinal ligaments of the rat lumbar spine. *Spine (Philadelphia 1976)*, 18, 268–273.

al-Shawaf, Ali, A., Kendall, Marion, D., and Cowen, Timothy (1991). Identification of neural profiles containing vasoactive intestinal polypeptide, acetylcholinesterase and catecholamines in the rat thymus. *Journal of Anatomy*, 174, 131–143.

Antonica, Angela, Magni, Franco, Mearini, Luigi, and Paolocci, Nazareno (1994). Vagal control of lymphocyte release from rat thymus. *Journal of the Autonomic Nervous System*, 48, 187–197.

Aoki, Eri, Kasahara, Takako, Hagiwara, Hisako, Sunaga, Mikako, Hisamitsu, Naoko, and Hisamitsu, Tadashi (2005). Electroacupuncture and moxibustion influence the lipopolysaccharide-induced TNF-alpha production by macrophages. *In Vivo*, 19, 495–500.

Artico, Marco, Bosco, Sandro, Cavallotti, Carlo, Agostinelli, Enzo, Giuliani-Piccari, Gabriella, Sciorio, Salvatore, Cocco, Lucio, and Vitale, Marco (2002). Noradrenergic and cholinergic innervation of the bone marrow. *Internal Journal of Molecular Medicine*, 10, 77–80.

Balemba, O.B., Grøndahl, M.L., Mbassa, G.K., Semuguruka, W.D., Hay-Smith, A., Skadhauge, E., and Dantzer, V. (1998). The organisation of the enteric nervous system in the submucous and mucous layers of the small intestine of the pig studied by VIP and neurofilament protein immunohistochemistry. *Journal of Anatomy*, 192, 257–267.

Beckman, Barbara, Mirand, Edwin, and Fisher, James, W. (1980). Effects of beta adrenergic agents and prostaglandin E1 on erythroid colony (CFU-E) growth and cyclic AMP formation in Friend erythroleukemic cells. *Journal of Cellular Physiology*, 105, 355–361.

Bellinger, Denise, L., Felten, Suzanne, Y., Ackerman, Kurt, D., Lorton, Dianne, Madden, Kelly, S., and Felten, David, L. (1992). Noradrenergic sympathetic innervation of lymphoid organs during development, aging, and in immune disease. In F. Amenta (Ed.) *Aging of the Autonomic Nervous System* (pp. 243–284). Boca Raton, FL: CRC Press.

Bellinger, Denise, L., Lorton, Dianne, Felten, Suzanne, Y., and Felten, David, L. (1992). Innervation of lymphoid organs and implications in development, aging, and autoimmunity. *International Journal of Immunopharmacology* 14, 329–344.

Bellinger, Denise, L., Lorton, Dianne, Romano, Tracy, D., Olschowka, John, A., Felten, Suzanne, Y., and Felten, David, L. (1990). Neuropeptide innervation of lymphoid organs. *Annals of the New York Academy of Sciences*, 594, 17–33.

Bellinger, Denise L, Lorton, Dianne, Hamill, Robert, W., Felten, Suzanne, Y., and Felten, David, L. (1993). Acetylcholinesterase staining and choline acetyltransferase activity in the young adult rat spleen: lack of evidence for cholinergic innervation. *Brain, Behavior, and Immunity*, 7, 191–204.

Bellinger, Denise, L., Felten, Suzanne, Y., Collier, Timothy, J., and Felten, David, L. (1987). Noradrenergic sympathetic innervation of the spleen: IV. Morphometric analysis in adult and aged F344 rats. *Journal of Neuroscience Research*, 18, 55–63. DOI, 10.1002/jnr.490180110.

Bellinger, Denise, L., Felten, Suzanne, Y., Lorton, Dianne, and Felten, David, L. (1989). Origin of noradrenergic innervation of the spleen in rats. *Brain, Behavior, and Immunity*, 3, 291–311.

Bellinger, Denise, L., Lorton, Dianne, Horn, Laura, Brouxhon, Sabine, Felten, Suzanne, Y., and Felten, David, L. (1997). Vasoactive intestinal polypeptide (VIP) innervation of rat spleen, thymus, and lymph nodes. *Peptides*, 18, 1139–1149.

Bellinger, Denise, L., Felten, Suzanne, Y., and Felten, David, L. (1988). Maintenance of noradrenergic sympathetic innervation in the involuted thymus of the aged Fischer 344 rat. *Brain, Behavior, and Immunity* 2, 133–150.

Bellinger, Denise, L., Millar, Brooke, A., Perez, Sam, Carter, Jeff, Wood, Carlo, ThyagaRajan, Srinivasan, Molinaro, Christine, Lubahn, Cheri, and Lorton, Dianne (2008). Sympathetic modulation of immunity: Relevance to disease. *Cellular Immunology*, 252, 27–56.

Bergquist, Jonas, Josefsson, Elisabet, Tarkowski, Andrej, Ekman, Rolf, and Ewing, Andrew (1997). Measurements of catecholamine-mediated apoptosis of immunocompetent cells by capillary electrophoresis. *Electrophoresis*, 18, 1760–1766.

Besedovsky, H.O., del Rey, A., Sorkin, E., Da Prada, M., and Keller, H.H. (1979). Immunoregulation mediated by the sympathetic nervous system. *Cellular Immunology*, 48, 346–355.

Bhowmick, S., Singh, A., Flavell, R.A., Clark, R.B., O'Rourke, J., and Cone, R.E. (2009). The sympathetic nervous system modulates CD4(+)FoxP3(+) regulatory T cells via a TGF-beta-dependent mechanism. *Journal of Leukocyte Biology*, 86, 1275–1283.

Bjurholm, A., Kreicbergs, A., Brodin, E., and Schultzberg, M. (1988). Substance P- and CGRP-immunoreactive nerves in bone. *Peptides*, 9, 165–171.

Borovikova, Lyudmila, V., Ivanova, Svetlana, Zhang, Minghuang, Yang, Huan, Botchkina, Galina, I., Watkins, Linda, R., Wang, Haichao, Abumrad, Naji, Eaton, John, W., and Tracey, K.J., (2000). Vagus nerve stimulation attenuates the systemic inflammatory response to endotoxin. *Nature*, 405, 458–462.

Bratton, B.O., Martelli, D., McKinley, J.J., Travaks, D., Anderson, C.R., and McAllen, R.M. (2012). Neural regulation of inflammation: No neural connection from the vagus to splenic sympathetic neurons. *Experimental Physiology*, 97, 1180–1185.

Brandtzaeg, P., Kiyono, H., Pabst, R., and Russell, M.W. (2008). Terminology: nomenclature of mucosa-associated lymphoid tissue. *Mucosal Immunology*, 1, 31–37.

Broome, Caroline, S., and Miyan, Jaleel, A. (2000). Neuropeptide control of bone marrow neutrophil production. A key axis for neuroimmunomodulation. *Annals of the New York Academy of Sciences*, 917, 424–434.

Broome, Caroline, S., Whetton, Anthony, D., and Miyan, Jaleel, A. (2000). Neuropeptide control of bone marrow neutrophil production is mediated by both direct and indirect effects on CFU-GM. *British Journal of Haematology*, 108, 140–150.

Bulloch, Karen, Hausman, J, Radojcic, T, and Short, S. (1991). Calcitonin gene-related peptide in the developing and aging thymus. An immunocytochemical study. *Annals of the New York Academy of Sciences*, 621, 218–228.

Bulloch, Karen, and Pomerantz, William (1984). Autonomic nervous system innervation of thymic-related lymphoid tissue in wildtype and nude mice. *Journal of Comparative Neurology*, 228, 57–68.

Byron, John, W. (1971). Evidence for a β_2-adrenergic receptor initiating DNA synthesis in haemopoietic stem cells. *Experimental Cell Research*, 71, 228–232.

Cano, Georgina, Sved, Alan, F., Rinaman, Linda, Rabin, Bruce, S., and Card, J. Patrick (2001). Characterization of the central nervous system innervation of the rat spleen using viral transneuronal tracing. *Journal of Comparative Neurology*, 439, 1–18.

Carlson, Sonia, L., Albers, Kathryn, M., Beiting, Daniel, J., Parish, Mark, Conner, James, M., and Davis, Brian, M. (1995). NGF modulates sympathetic innervation of lymphoid tissues. *Journal of Neuroscience*, 15, 5892–5899.

Castañeda-Corral, G., Jimenez-Andrade, J.M., Bloom, A.P., Taylor, R.N., Mantyh, W.G., Kaczmarska, M.J., Ghilardi, J.R., and Mantyh, PW. (2011). The majority of myelinated and unmyelinated sensory nerve fibers that innervate bone express the tropomyosin receptor kinase A. *Neuroscience, 178*, 196–207.

Cavallotti, D., Artico, M., De Santis, S., and Cavallotti, C. (1999). Occurrence of gamma-aminobutyric acid-transaminase activity in nerve fibers of human thymus. *Human Immunology*, 60, 1072–1079.

Cesta, Mark, F. (2006). Normal structure, function, and histology of mucosa-associated lymphoid tissue. *Toxicologic Pathology*, 34, 599–608.

Chevendra, V., and Weaver, L.C. (1992). Distributions of neuropeptide Y, vasoactive intestinal peptide and somatostatin in populations of postganglionic neurons innervating the rat kidney, spleen and intestine. *Neuroscience*, 50, 727–743.

Chow, Andrew, Lucas, Daniel, Hidalgo, Andrés, Méndez-Ferrer, Simón, Hashimoto, Daigo, Scheiermann, Christoph, et al. (2011). Bone marrow CD169+ macrophages promote the retention of hematopoietic stem and progenitor cells in the mesenchymal stem cell niche. *Journal of Experimental Medicine*, 208, 261–271.

Cogan, T.A., Thomas, A.O., Rees, L.E., Taylor, A.H., Jepson, M.A., Williams, P.H., Ketley, J., and Humphrey, T.J. (2007). Norepinephrine increases the pathogenic potential of Campylobacter jejuni. *Gut*, 56,1060–1065.

Dar, A., Schajnovitz, A., Lapid, K., Kalinkovich, A., Itkin, T., Ludin, A. et al. (2011). Rapid mobilization of hematopoietic progenitors by AMD3100 and catecholamines is mediated by CXCR4-dependent SDF-1 release from bone marrow stromal cells. *Leukemia*, 25, 1286–1296.

de Leeuw, F.E., Jansen, G.H., Batanero, E., van Wichen, D.F., Huber, J., and Schuurman, H.J. (1992). The neural and neuro-endocrine component of the human thymus. I. Nerve-like structures. *Brain, Behavior, and Immunity*, 6, 234–248.

delRey, Adriana, Roggero, Eduardo, Kabiersch, Alexa, Schäfer, Martin, and Besedovsky, Hugo, O. (2006). The role of noradrenergic nerves in the development of the lymphoproliferative disease in Fas-deficient, lpr/lpr mice. *Journal of Immunology*, 176,7079–7086.

Dénes, A., Boldogkoi, Z., Uhereczky, G., Hornyák, A., Rusvai, M., Palkovits, M., and Kovács, K.J. (2005). Central autonomic control of the bone marrow: multisynaptic tract tracing by recombinant pseudorabies virus. *Neuroscience*, 134, 947–963.

Dresch, C., Minc, J., Poirier, O., and Bouvet, D. (1981). Effect of beta adrenergic agonists and beta blocking agents on hemopoiesis in human bone marrow. *Biomedicine*, 34, 93–98.

Ebbinghaus, Matthias, Gajda, Mieczyslaw, Boettger, Michael, K., Schaible, Hans-Georg, G., and Bräuer, Rolf. (2011). The anti-inflammatory effects of sympathectomy in murine antigen-induced arthritis are associated with a reduction of Th1 and Th17 responses. *Annals of Rheumatic Disease*, 71(2),253-61.

Ehninger, Armin, and Trumpp, Andreas (2011). The bone marrow stem cell niche grows up: Mesenchymal stem cells and macrophages move in. *Journal of Experimental Medicine*, 208, 421–428.

Elenkov, I.J, and Vizi, E. Sylvester (1991). Presynaptic modulation of release of noradrenaline from the sympathetic nerve terminals in the rat spleen. *Neuropharmacology*, 30, 1319–1324.

Elenkov, Ilia, J., Wilder, Ronald, L., Chrousos, George, P., and Vizi, E. Sylvester (2000). The sympathetic nerve–an integrative interface between two supersystems: the brain and the immune system. *Pharmacological Reviews*, 52, 595–638.

Elfvin, L.G., Johansson, J., Höijer, A.S., and Aldskogius, H. (1994). The innervation of the splenic capsule in the guinea pig: An immunohistochemical and ultrastructural study. *Journal of Anatomy*, 185, 267–278.

Felten, D.L, Overhage, J.M., Felten, S.Y., and Schmedtje, J.F. (1981). Noradrenergic sympathetic innervation of lymphoid tissue in the rabbit appendix: further evidence for a link between the nervous and immune systems. *Brain Research Bulletin*, 7, 595–612.

Felten, D.L., Felten, S.Y., Carlson, S.L., Olschowka, J.A, and Livnat, S. (1985). Noradrenergic and peptidergic innervation of lymphoid tissue. *Journal of Immunology*, 135, 755s–765s.

Felten, D.L., Felten, S.Y., Bellinger, Denise, L., Carlson, Sonia, L., Ackerman, Kurt, D., Madden, Kelley, S. et al. (1987). Noradrenergic sympathetic neural interactions with the immune system: Structure and function. *Immunological Reviews*, 100, 225–260.

Felten, D.L., Livnat, Shmuel, Felten, S.Y., Carlson, Sonia, L., Bellinger, Denise, L., and Yeh, Pamela (1984). Sympathetic innervation of lymph nodes in mice. *Brain Research Bulletin*, 13, 693–699.

Felten, S.Y. and Olschowka, J. (1987). Noradrenergic sympathetic innervation of the spleen: II. Tyrosine hydroxylase (TH)-positive nerve terminals form synaptic-like contacts on lymphocytes in the splenic white pulp. *Journal of Neuroscience Research*, 18, 37–48.

Felten, S.Y., Felten, D.L., Bellinger, Denise, L., Carlson, Sonia, L., Ackerman, Kurt, D., Madden, Kelley, S. et al. (1988). Noradrenergic sympathetic innervation of lymphoid organs. *Progress in Allergy*, 43, 14–36.

Ferraro, Francesca, Lymperi, Stefania, Méndez-Ferrer, Simón, Saez, Borja, Spencer, Joel, A., Yeap, Beow, Y. et al. (2011). Diabetes impairs hematopoietic stem cell mobilization by altering niche function. *Science Translational Medicine*, 3,104ra101.

Freestone, Primrose, P., Haigh, Richard, D., and Lyte, Mark (2007). Blockade of catecholamine-induced growth by adrenergic and dopaminergic receptor antagonists in *Escherichia coli* O157,H7, *Salmonella enterica* and *Yersinia enterocolitica*. *BMC Microbiology*, 7,8.

Fink, T., and Weihe, E. (1988). Multiple neuropeptides in nerves supplying mammalian lymph nodes: Messenger candidates for sensory and autonomic neuroimmunomodulation? *Neuroscience Letters*, 90, 39–44.

Franceschini, Davide, Orr-Urtreger, Avi, Yu, Wei, Mackey, Laura, Y., Bond, Richard, A., Armstrong, Dawna et al. (2000). Altered baroreflex responses in alpha7 deficient mice. *Behavioral Brain Research*, 113, 3–10.

Fried, G., Terenius, L., Brodin, E., Efendic, S., Dockray, G., Fahrenkrug, J., Goldstein, M., and Hökfelt, T. (1986). Neuropeptide Y, enkephalin and noradrenaline coexist in sympathetic neurons innervating the bovine spleen. Biochemical and immunohistochemical evidence. *Cell and Tissue Research*, 243, 495–508.

Gajda, M., Litwin, J.A., Zagólski, O., Lis, G.J., Cichocki, T., Timmermans, J.P., and Adriaensen, D. (2009). Development of galanin-containing nerve fibres in rat tibia. *Anatomia, Histologia, Embryologia*, 38, 112–117.

Genton, Laurence and Kudsk, Kenneth, A. (2003). Interaction between the enteric nervous system and the immune system: Role of neuropeptides and nutrition. *The American Journal of Surgery*, 186, 253–258.

Gertz, M.A. (2010). Current status of stem cell mobilization. *British Journal of Haematology*, 150, 647–662.

Giron, Louis, T., Jr., Crutcher, Keith, A., and Davis, James, N. (1980). Lymph nodes–a possible site for sympathetic neuronal regulation of immune responses. *Annals of Neurology*, 8, 520–525.

González-Ariki, Silva, and Husband, Alan, J. (2000). Ontogeny of IgA(+) cells in lamina propria: Effects of sympathectomy. *Developmental and Comparative Immunology*, 24,61–69.

Green, Benedict, T., Lyte, Mark, Kulkarni-Narla, Anjali, and Brown, David, R. (2003). Neuromodulation of enteropathogen internalization in Peyer's patches from porcine jejunum. *Journal of Neuroimmunology*, 141, 74–82.

Guereschi, M.G., Araujo, L.P., Maricato, J.T., Takenaka, M.C., Nascimento, V.M., Vivanco, B.C., Reis, V.O., Keller, A.C., Brum, P.C., and Basso, A.S. (2013). Beta2-adrenergic receptor signaling in CD4+ Foxp3+ regulatory T cells enhances their suppressive function in a PKA-dependent manner. *European Journal of Immunology*, 43, 1001–1012.

Hart, R., Dancygier, H., Wagner, F., Lersch, C., and Classen, M. (1990). Effect of substance P on immunoglobulin and interferon-gamma secretion by cultured human duodenal mucosa. *Immunology Letters*, 23, 199–204.

Hosoi, Toru, Okuma, Yasunobu, and Nomura, Yasuyuki. (2000). Electrical stimulation of afferent vagus nerve induces IL-1β expression in the brain and activates the HPA axis. *American Journal of Physiology and Regulatory Integrative Comparative Physiology*, 279, R141–R147.

Imai, Shinji, and Matsusue, Yoshitaka (2002). Neuronal regulation of bone metabolism and anabolism: Calcitonin gene-related peptide-, substance P-, and tyrosine hydroxylase-containing nerves and the bone. *Microscopy Research and Technique*, 58, 61–69.

Imai, Shinji, Tokunaga, Yoshimitsu, Maeda, Toshihiro, Kikkawa, Masanori, and Hukuda, Sinsuke. (1997). Calcitonin gene-related peptide, substance P, and tyrosine hydroxylase-immunoreactive innervation of rat bone marrows: An immunohistochemical and ultrastructural investigation on possible efferent and afferent mechanisms. *Journal of Orthopaedic Research*, 15, 133–140.

Jia, L., Xie, Z., Zheng, J., Liu, L., He, Y., Liu, F., and He, Y. (2012). Morphological studies of lymphatic labyrinths in the rat mesenteric lymph node. *Anatomical Records (Hoboken)*, 295, 1291–1301.

Jimenez-Andrade, Juan, M., Mantyh, William, G., Bloom, Aaron, P., Xu, Haili, Ferng, Alice, S., Dussor, Gregory et al. (2010). A phenotypically restricted set of primary afferent nerve fibers innervate the bone versus skin: Therapeutic opportunity for treating skeletal pain. *Bone*, 46, 306–313.

Jobling, P. (1994). Electrophysiological events during neuroeffector transmission in the spleen of guinea-pigs and rats. *Journal of Physiology*, 476, 153–165.

Jurjus, Abdo R, More, Newton, and Walsh, Raymond, J. (1998). Distribution of substance P positive cells and nerve fibers in the rat thymus. *Journal of Neuroimmunology*, 90, 143–148.

Kaleczyc, J., Podlasz, P., Winnicka, A., Wasowicz, W., Sienkiewicz, W., Zmudzki, J., and Lakomy, M. (2010). Characterization of autonomic nerve markers and lymphocyte subsets in the ileal Peyer's patch of pigs infected experimentally with *Brachyspira hyodysenteriae*. *Journal of Comparative Pathology*, 143, 248–257.

Katayama, Yoshio, Battista, Michela, Kao, Wei-Ming, Hidalgo, Andrés, Peired, Anna, J., Thomas, Steven, A., and Frenette, Paul, S. (2006). Signals from the sympathetic nervous system regulate hematopoietic stem cell egress from bone marrow. *Cell*, 124,407–421.

Kavelaars, Annemieke (2002). Regulated expression of alpha-1 adrenergic receptors in the immune system. *Brain, Behavior, and Immunity*, 16, 799–807.

Keita, A.V., and Söderholm, J.D. (2010). The intestinal barrier and its regulation by neuroimmune factors. *Neurogastroenterology and Motility*, 22, 718–733.

Kendall, Marion, D., and al-Shawaf, Ali A. (1991). Innervation of the rat thymus gland. *Brain, Behavior, and Immunity*, 5, 9–28.

Kin, N.W. and Sanders, V.M. (2006). It takes nerve to tell T and B cells what to do. *Journal of Leukocyte Biology*, 79, 1093–1104.

Kosaras, Bela, Jakubowski, Moshe, Kainz, Vanessa, and Burstein, Rami (2009). Sensory innervation of the calvarial bones of the mouse. *Journal of Comparative Neurology*, 515, 331–348.

Kranz, Andrea, Kendall, Marion, D., and von Gaudecker, Brita (1997). Studies on rat and human thymus to demonstrate immunoreactivity of calcitonin gene-related peptide, tyrosine hydroxylase and neuropeptide Y. *Journal of Anatomy*, 191, 441–450.

Kurkowski, Ruth, Kummer, Wolfgang, and Heym, Christine (1990). Substance P-immunoreactive nerve fibers in tracheobronchial lymph nodes of the guinea pig: Origin, ultrastructure and coexistence with other peptides. *Peptides*, 11, 13–20.

Kurz, Bodo, Feindt, Janka, von Gaudecker, Brita, Kranz, Andrea, Loppnow, Harald, and Mentlein, Rolf (1997). Beta-adrenoceptor-mediated effects in rat cultured thymic epithelial cells. *British Journal of Pharmacology*, 120, 1401–1408.

Kwon, Y.B., Kim, H.W., Ham, T.W. Yoon, S.Y., Roh, D.H., Han, H.J. et al. (2003). The anti-inflammatory effect of bee venom stimulation in a mouse air pouch model is mediated by adrenal medullary activity. *Journal of Neuroendocrinology*, 15, 93–96.

Leposavić, G., Arsenović-Ranin, N., Radojević, K., Kosec, D., Pešić, V., Vidić-Danković, B. et al. (2006). Characterization of thymocyte phenotypic alterations induced by long-lasting beta-adrenoceptor blockade in vivo and its effects on thymocyte proliferation and apoptosis. *Molecular and Cellular Biochemistry*, 285, 87–99.

Leposavić, G., Pešić, V., Stojić-Vukanić, Z., Radojević, K., Arsenović-Ranin, N., Kosec, D., Perišić, M., and Pilipović, I. (2010). Age-associated plasticity of α1-adrenoceptor-mediated tuning of T-cell development. *Experimental Gerontology*, 45, 918–935.

Leposavić, G., Pilipović, I., and Perišić, M. (2011). Cellular and nerve fibre catecholaminergic thymic network: Steroid hormone dependent activity. *Physiological Research*, 60 Supplemental 1, S71–82.

Li, Y., and Novotny, G.E. (2001). Regional differences in innervation of lymph nodes in the Wistar rat. *Journal of Anatomy*, 199, 735–739.

Ling, Yi-Ling, Meng, Ai-Hong, Shan, Bao-En, Zhang, Jun-Lan, and Zhang, Xiao-Peng (2001). Effects of cholecystokinin on cytokines during endotoxic shock in rats. *World Journal of Gastroenterology*, 7, 667–671.

Logan, Ryan W, Arjona, Alvaro, and Sarkar, Dipak, K. (2011). Role of sympathetic nervous system in the entrainment of circadian natural-killer cell function. *Brain, Behavior, and Immunity*, 25, 101–109.

Lomax, A.E., Sharkey, K.A., and Furness, J.B. (2010). The participation of the sympathetic innervation of the gastrointestinal tract in disease states. *Neurogastroenterology and Motility*, 22, 7–18.

Lorton, Dianne, Bellinger, Denise, L., Felten, Suzanne, Y., and Felten, David, L. (1990). Substance P innervation of the rat thymus. *Peptides*, 11, 1269–1275.

Lorton, Dianne, Lubahn, Cheri, Engan, Chad, Schaller, Jill, Felten, David, L., and Bellinger, Denise, L. (2000). Local application of capsaicin into the draining lymph nodes attenuates expression of adjuvant-induced arthritis. *Neuroimmunomodulation*, 7, 115–125.

Lorton, Dianne, Lubahn, Cheri, Sweeney, Sarah, Major, Amy, Lindquist, Carl, A., Schaller, Jill et al. (2009). Differences in the injury/sprouting response of splenic noradrenergic nerves in Lewis rats with adjuvant-induced arthritis compared with rats treated with 6-hydroxydopamine. *Brain, Behavior, and Immunity*, 23, 276–285.

Lorton, Dianne, Lubahn, Cheri, Lindquist, Carl, A., Schaller, Jill, Washington, Cathy, and Bellinger, Denise, L. (2005). Changes in the density and distribution of sympathetic nerves in spleens from Lewis rats with adjuvant-induced arthritis suggest that an injury and sprouting response occurs. *Journal of Comparative Neurology*, 489, 260–273.

Lorton, D., Bellinger, D.L., Felten, S.Y., and Felten, D.L. (1991). Substance P innervation of spleen in rats: Nerve fibers associate with lymphocytes and macrophages in specific compartments of the spleen. *Brain, Behavior, and Immunity*, 5, 29–40.

Loveland, Bruce, E., Jarrott, Bevyn, and McKenzie, Ian F.C. (1981). The detection of β-adrenoceptors on murine lymphocytes. *International Journal of Immunopharmacology*, 3, 313–318.

Lundberg, J.M., Anggård, A., Pernow, J., and Hökfelt, T. (1985). Neuropeptide Y-, substance P- and VIP-immunoreactive nerves in cat spleen in relation to autonomic vascular and volume control. *Cell and Tissue Research*, 239, 9–18.

Luyer, Misha, D., Greve, Jan, W.M., Hadfouone, M'hamed, Jacobs, Jan, A., Dejong, Cornelis, H., and Buurman, Wim, A. (2005). Nutritional stimulation of cholecystokinin receptors inhibits inflammation via the vagus nerve *Journal of Experimental Medicine*, 202, 1023–1029.

Lyte, Mark, Vulchanova, Lucy, and Brown, David, R. (2011). Stress at the intestinal surface: catecholamines and mucosa-bacteria interactions. *Cell and Tissue Research*, 343, 23–32.

Lyte, M., Arulanandam, B., Nguyen, K., Frank, C., Erickson, A., and Francis, D. (1997). Norepinephrine induced growth and expression of virulence associated factors in enterotoxigenic and enterohemorrhagic strains of Escherichia coli. *Advances in Experimental Medicine and Biology*, 412, 331–339.

Mach, David, B., Rogers, Scott, D., Sabino, Mary Ann, C., Luger, Nancy M, Schwei, Mathew, J., Pomonis, James, D. et al. (2002). Origins of skeletal pain: Sensory and sympathetic innervation of the mouse femur. *Neuroscience*, 113, 155–166.

Madden, K.S., Sanders, V.M., and Felten, D.L. (1995). Catecholamine influences and sympathetic neural modulation of immune responsiveness. *Annual Review of Pharmacology and Toxicology*, 35, 417–448.

Maestroni, George, J., and Conti, Ario (1994a). Modulation of hematopoiesis via alpha 1-adrenergic receptors on bone marrow cells. *Experimental Hematology*, 22, 313–320.

Maestroni, George, J., and Conti, Ario (1994b). Noradrenergic modulation of lymphohematopoiesis. *International Journal of Immunopharmacology*, 16, 117–122.

Maestroni, George, J., Conti, Ario, and Pedrinis, Ennio (1992). Effect of adrenergic agents on hematopoiesis after syngeneic bone marrow transplantation in mice. *Blood*, 80, 1178–1182.

Maestroni, George, J., Cosentino, M., Marino, F., Togni, M., Conti, Ario, Lecchini, S., and Frigo, G. (1998). Neural and endogenous catecholamines in the bone marrow. Circadian association of norepinephrine with hematopoiesis? *Experimental Hematology*, 26, 1172–1177.

Maestroni, George, J., and Mazzola, Paola (2003). Langerhans cells beta 2-adrenoceptors: Role in migration, cytokine production, Th priming and contact hypersensitivity. *Journal of Neuroimmunology*, 144, 91–99.

Maestroni, George, J. (2002). Short exposure of maturing, bone marrow-derived dendritic cells to norepinephrine: Impact on kinetics of cytokine production and Th development. *Journal of Neuroimmunology*, 129, 106–114.

Maestroni, G.J., Togni, M., and Covacci, V. (1997). Norepinephrine protects mice from acute lethal doses of carboplatin. *Experimental Hematology*, 25,491–494.

Maier, Steven, F., Goehler, Lisa, E., Fleshner, Monika, and Watkins, Linda, R. (1998). The role of the vagus nerve in cytokine-to-brain communication. *Annals of the New York Academy of Sciences*, 840, 289–300.

Marchetti, Bianca, Morale, Maria, C., Paradis, Pierre, and Bouvier, Michel (1994). Characterization, expression, and hormonal control of a thymic beta 2-adrenergic receptor. *American Journal of Physiology*, 267, E718–E731.

Meltzer, Jonathon, C., MacNeil, Brian, J., Sanders, Veronica, Pylypas, Susan, Jansen, Arno, H., Greenberg, Arnold, H., and Nance, Dwight, M. (2004). Stress-induced suppression of in-vivo splenic cytokine production in the rat by neural and hormonal mechanisms. *Brain, Behavior, and Immunity*, 18, 262–273.

Meng, Al-Hong, Ling, Yi-Ling., Zang, Xiao-Peng, Zhao, X.Y., and Zhang, Jun-Lan (2002). CCK8 inhibits expression of TNF-α in the spleen of endotoxic shock rats and signal transduction mechanism of p38 MAPK. *World Journal of Gastroenterology*, 8, 139–143.

Méndez-Ferrer, Simón, Lucas, Daniel, Battista, Michela, and Frenette, Paul, S. (2008). Haematopoietic stem cell release is regulated by circadian oscillations. *Nature*, 452, 442–447.

Mignini, F., Sabbatini, M., D'Andrea, V., and Cavallotti, C. (2011). Neuropeptides of human thymus in normal and pathological conditions. *Peptides*, 32, 920–928.

Mignini, F, Streccioni, V, and Amenta, F. (2003). Autonomic innervation of immune organs and neuroimmune modulation. *Autonomic and Autacoid Pharmacology*, 23, 1–25.

Mitchell, Barry, Kendall, Marion, Adam, Elizabeth, and Schumacher, Udo (1997). Innervation of the thymus in normal and bone marrow reconstituted severe combined immunodeficient (SCID) mice. *Journal of Neuroimmunology*, 75, 19–27.

Müller, S., and Weihe, E. (1991). Interrelation of peptidergic innervation with mast cells and ED1-positive cells in rat thymus. *Brain, Behavior, and Immunity*, 5, 55–72.

Nagata, M., Franco-Cereceda, A., Saria, A., Amann, R., and Lundberg, J.M. (1987). Reserpine-induced depletion of neuropeptide Y in the guinea-pig: Tissue-specific effects and mechanisms of action. *Journal of the Autonomic Nervous System*, 20, 257–263.

Nakano, Masayuki, Takahashi, A., Sakai, Yuko, and Nakaya, Yutaka (2007). Modulation of pathogenicity with norepinephrine related to the type III secretion system of *Vibrio parahaemolyticus*. *Journal of Infectious Diseases*, 195, 1353–1360.

Nance, Dwight, M., and Burns, Joan (1989). Innervation of the spleen in the rat: Evidence for absence of afferent innervation. *Brain, Behavior, and Immunity*, 3, 281–290.

Nance, Dwight, M., and Sanders, Virginia, M. (2007). Autonomic innervation and regulation of the immune system (1987-2007). *Brain, Behavior, and Immunity*, 21, 736–745.

Nance, D.M., Luczy-Bachman, G., Min, P., Lee, Y-B., and Cho, Z-H. (2005). The immunomodulatory effects of counter-irritation are mediated via the sympathetic nervous system. *Brain, Behavior, and Immunity*, 19, 4, S1, e52–e53.

Nance, Dwight, M., Hopkins, David, A., and Bieger, Detlef (1987). Re-investigation of the innervation of the thymus gland in mice and rats. *Brain, Behavior, and Immunity*, 1, 134–147.

Nance, Dwight, M. and MacNeil, Brian, J. (2001). Immunoregulation by the sympathetic nervous system. *Neuroimmune Biology*, 1, 121–139.

Neuhuber, Winfried, L., and Tiegs, Gisa (2004). Innervation of immune cells: Evidence for neuroimmunomodulation in the liver. *The Anatomical Record Part A*, 280A, 884–892.

Nijhuis, Laurens E, Olivier, Brenda J, de Jonge, Wouter, J. (2010). Neurogenic regulation of dendritic cells in the intestine. *Biochemical Pharmacology*, 80, 2002–2008.

Nohr, D. and Weihe, E. (1991). The neuroimmune link in the bronchus-associated lymphoid tissue (BALT) of cat and rat: Peptides and neural markers. *Brain, Behavior, and Immunity*, 5, 84–101.

Novotny, G.E. (1988). Ultrastructural analysis of lymph node innervation in the rat. *Acta Anatomica (Basel)*, 133, 57–61.

Novotny, G.E., Heuer, T., Schöttelndreier, A., and Fleisgarten, C. (1994). Plasticity of innervation of the medulla of axillary lymph nodes in the rat after antigenic stimulation. *The Anatomical Record*, 238, 213–224.

Novotny, G.E., and Kliche, K.O. (1986). Innervation of lymph nodes: A combined silver impregnation and electron-microscopic study. *Acta Anatomica (Basel)*, 127, 243–248.

Novotny, G.E., Sommerfeld, H., and Zirbes, T. (1990). Thymic innervation in the rat: A light and electron microscopical study. *Journal of Comparative Neurology*, 302, 552–561.

Novotny, G.E., and Hsu, Y. (1993). The effect of immunostimulation on thymic innervation in the rat. *Journal für Hirnforschung*, 34, 155–163.

Ohkubo, Nobuyuki, Miura, Soichiro, Serizawa, Hiroshi, Yan, Han, J., Kimura, Hiroyuki, Imaeda, Hiroyuki et al. (1994). In vivo effect of chronic administration of vasoactive intestinal peptide on gut-associated lymphoid tissues in rats. *Regulatory Peptides*, 50, 127–135.

Panuncio, A.L., De La Peña, S., Gualco, G., and Reissenweber, N. (1999). Adrenergic innervation in reactive human lymph nodes. *Journal of Anatomy*, 194, 143–146.

Pearse, Gail (2006). Normal structure, function and histology of the thymus. *Toxicologic Pathology*, 34, 504–514.

Penn, Angela, Mohr, Alicia M, Shah, Salil G, Sifri, Ziad C, Kaiser, Vicki L, Rameshwar, Pranela, and Livingston, David, H. (2010). Dose-response relationship between norepinephrine and erythropoiesis: Evidence for a critical threshold. *Journal of Surgical Research*, 163, e85–e90.

Pešić, V., Kosec, D., Radojević, K., Pilipović, I., Perišić, M., Vidić-Danković, B., and Leposavić, G. (2009). Expression of alpha(1)-adrenoceptors on thymic cells and their role in fine tuning of thymopoiesis. *Journal of Neuroimmunology*, 214, 55–66.

Pešić, V., Plećas-Solarović, B., Radojević, K., Kosec, D., Pilipović, I., Perisić, M., and Leposavić, G. (2007). Long-term beta-adrenergic receptor blockade increases levels of the most mature thymocyte subsets in aged rats. *International Immunopharmacology*, 7, 674–686.

Pillai, Shiv, Cariappa, Annaiah, and Moran, Stewart, T. (2005). Marginal zone B cells. *Annual Review of Immunology*, 23, 161–196.

Plećaš-Solarović, Bosiljka, Lalić, Ljubica, and Leposavić, Gordana (2004). Age-dependent morphometrical changes in the thymus of male propranolol-treated rats. *Annals of Anatomy*, 186, 141–147.

Plećaš-Soloravić, B., Hristić-Živković, I., Radojević, K., Kosec, D., and Leposavić, G. (2005). Chronic alpha(1)-adrenoreceptor blockade produces age-dependent changes in rat thymus structure and thymocyte differentiation. *Histology and Histopathology* 20, 833–841.

Quinson, N., Robbins, H.L., Clark, M.J., and Furness, J.B. (2001). Locations and innervation of cell bodies of sympathetic neurons projecting to the gastrointestinal tract in the rat. *Archives of Histology and Cytology*, 64, 281–294.

Romano, Tracy, A., Felten, Suzanne, Y., Felten, David, L., and Olschowka, John, A. (1991). Neuropeptide-Y innervation of the rat spleen: Another potential immunomodulatory neuropeptide. *Brain, Behavior, and Immunity*, 5, 116–131.

Romeo, Horacio, E., Fink, Thorsten, Yanaihara, Noboru, and Weihe, Eberhard (1994). Distribution and relative proportions of neuropeptide Y- and proenkephalin-containing noradrenergic neurones in rat superior cervical ganglion: Separate projections to submaxillary lymph nodes. *Peptides*, 15, 1479–1487.

Rosas-Ballina, M., and Tracey, K.J. (2009). Cholinergic control of inflammation. *Journal of Internal Medicine*, 265, 663–679.

Rosas-Ballina, Mauricio, Ochani, Mahendar, Parrish, William, R., Ochani, Kanta, Harris, Yael, T., Huston, Jared, M. et al. (2008). Splenic nerve is required for cholinergic antiinflammatory pathway control of TNF in endotoxemia. *Proceedings of the National Academy of Science U.S.A.*, 105, 11008–11013.

Russo, D., Fantaguzzi, C.M., Di Guardo, G., Clavenzani, P., Costerbosa, G.L., Ligios, C., and Chiocchetti, R. (2009). Characterization of sheep (*Ovis aries*) palatine tonsil innervation. *Neuroscience*, 161, 813–826.

Saeed, Rubina, W., Varma, Santosh, Peng-Nemeroff, Tina, Sherry, Barbara, Balakhaneh, David, Huston, Jared, Tracey, Kevin, J. et al. (2005). Cholinergic stimulation blocks endothelial cell activation and leukocyte recruitment during inflammation. *Journal of Experimental Medicine*, 201, 1113–1123.

Sanders, V.M., Kasprowicz, D.J., Kohm, A.P., and Swanson, M.A. (2000). Neurotransmitter receptors on lymphocytes and other lymphoid cells. In R. Ader, D.L. Fenten and N. Cohen (Eds.) *Psychoneuroimmunology, Edition 3* (pp. 161–169). San Diego, CA: Academic Press.

Sato, Akio (1997). Neural mechanisms of autonomic responses elicited by somatic sensory stimulation. *Neuroscience and Behavioral Physiology*, 27, 610–621.

Schäfer, M.K., Eiden, L.E., and Weihe, E. (1998). Cholinergic neurons and terminal fields revealed by immunohistochemistry for the vesicular acetylcholine transporter. II. The peripheral nervous system. *Neuroscience*, 84, 361–376.

Schreiber, Kristin, L., Price, Lisa, D., and Brown, David, R. (2007). Evidence for neuromodulation of enteropathogen invasion in the intestinal mucosa. *Journal of Neuroimmune Pharmacology*, 2, 329–337.

Sharkey, Keith, A., and Mawe, Gary, M. (2002). Neuroimmune and epithelial interactions in intestinal inflammation. *Current Opinion in Pharmacology*, 2, 669–677.

Shepherd, Andrew, J., Downing, James E, Miyan, Jaleel, A. (2005). Without nerves, immunology remains incomplete – in vivo veritas. *Immunology*, 116, 145–163.

Sirot'áková, Maria, Schmidtová, Katarina, Kocisová, Monika, and Kuchta, Milan (2002). Adrenergic and acetylcholinesterase-positive innervation of palatine tonsils in mammals. *Acta Histochemica*, 104, 349–352.

Spencer, H., Karavolos, M.H., Bulmer, D.M., Aldridge, P., Chhabra, S.R., Winzer, K. et al. (2010). Genome-wide transposon mutagenesis identifies a role for host neuroendocrine stress hormones in regulating the expression of virulence genes in Salmonella. *Journal of Bacteriology*, 192, 714–724.

Spiegel, Asaf, Shivtiel, Shivtiel, Kalinkovich, Alexander, Ludin, Aya, Netzer, Neta, Goichberg, Polina et al. (2007). Catecholaminergic neurotransmitters regulate migration and repopulation of immature human CD34+ cells through Wnt signaling. *Nature Immunology*, 8, 1123–1131.

Stevens-Felten, S.Y., and Bellinger, D.L. (1997). Noradrenergic and peptidergic innervation of lymphoid organs. *Chemical Immunology*, 69, 99–131.

Straub, R.H., Grum, F., Strauch, U., Capellino, S., Bataille, F., Bleich, A. et al. (2008). Anti-inflammatory role of sympathetic nerves in chronic intestinal inflammation. *Gut*, 57, 911–921.

Tabarowski, Z., Gibson-Berry, K., and Felten, S.Y. (1996). Noradrenergic and peptidergic innervation of the mouse femur bone marrow. *Acta Histochemistry*, 98, 453–457.

Tang, Y., Shankar, R., Gamelli, R., and Jones, S. (1999). Dynamic norepinephrine alterations in bone marrow: Evidence of functional innervation. *Journal of Neuroimmunology*, 96, 182–189.

Tracey, Kevin, J. (2009). Reflex control of immunity. *Nature Reviews Immunology*, 9, 418–428.

Trotter, R. Nicholas, Stornetta, Ruth, L., Guyenet, Patrice, G., and Roberts, Margo, R. (2007). Transneuronal mapping of the CNS network controlling sympathetic outflow to the rat thymus. *Autonomic Neuroscience*, 131, 9–20.

Ueyama, Teizo, Kozuki, Kageyuki, Houtani, Takeshi, Ikeda, Michiko, Kitajiri, Masanori, Yamashita, Toshio et al. (1990). Immunolocalization of tyrosine hydroxylase and vasoactive intestinal polypeptide in nerve fibers innervating human palatine tonsil and paratonsillar glands. *Neuroscience Letters*, 116, 70–74.

Uvnas-Moberg, K., Lundeberg, T., and Bruzelius, G. (1992). Vagally mediated release of gastrin and cholecystokinin following sensory stimulation. *Acta Physiologica Scandinavica*, 146, 349–356.

Vasina, V., Abu-Gharbieh, E., Barbara, G., de Giorgio, R., Colucci, R., Blandizzi, C. et al. (2008). The beta3-adrenoceptor agonist SR58611A ameliorates experimental colitis in rats. *Neurogastroenterology and Motility*, 20, 1030–1041.

Verbalis, Joseph, G., Stricker, Edward, M., Robinson, Alan, G., and Hoffman, Gloria, E. (1991). Cholecystokinin activates c-fos expression in hypothalamic oxytocin and corticotropin-releasing hormone neurons. *Journal of Neuroendocrinology*, 3, 205–213.

Vida, Gergely, Peña, Geber, Deitch, Edwin, A., and Ulloa, Luis (2011a). α7-Cholinergic receptor mediates vagal induction of splenic norepinephrine. *Journal of Immunology*, 186, 4340–4346.

Vida, Gergely, Peña, Geber, Kanashiro, Alexandre, del Rocio, Maria, Thompson-Bonilla, David, P., Deitch, Edwin, A., and Ulloa, Luis (2011b). β2-Adrenoreceptors of regulatory lymphocytes are essential for vagal neuromodulation of the innate immune system. *The Federation of American Societies for Experimental Biology Journal*, 25, 4476–4485.

Vizi, E. Sylvester, Orso, E., Osipenko, O.N., Hasko, G., and Elenkov, I.J. (1995). Neurochemical, electrophysiological and immunocytochemical evidence for a noradrenergic link between the sympathetic nervous system and thymocytes. *Neuroscience*, 68, 1263–1276.

von Gaudecker, Brita (1991). Functional histology of the human thymus. *Anatomy and Embryology (Berlin)*, 183, 1–15.

Vulchanova, Lucy, Casey, Melissa, A., Crabb, Gwen, W., Kennedy, William, R., and Brown, David, R. (2007). Anatomical evidence for enteric neuroimmune interactions in Peyer's patches. *Journal of Neuroimmunology*, 185, 64–74.

Wan, Weihua, Wetmore, Lisa, Sorensen, Craig, M., Greenberg, Arnold, H., and Nance, Dwight, M. (1994). Neural and biochemical mediators of endotoxin and stress-induced c-fos expression in the rat brain. *Brain Research Bulletin*, 34, 7–14.

Wang, Hong, Yu, Man, Ochani, Mahendar, Amella, Carol, A., Tanovic, Mahira, Susarla, Seenu et al. (2003). Nicotinic acetylcholine receptor α7 subunit is an essential regulator of inflammation. *Nature*, 421, 384–388.

Weihe, E. and Krekel, J. (1991). The neuroimmune connection in human tonsils. *Brain, Behavior, and Immunity*, 5, 41–54.

Weihe, E., Müller, S., Fink, T., and Zentel, H.J. (1989). Tachykinins, calcitonin gene-related peptide and neuropeptide Y in nerves of the mammalian thymus: interactions with mast cells in autonomic and sensory neuroimmunomodulation? *Neuroscience Letters*, 100, 77–82.

Weihe, E., Nohr, D., Michel, S., Muller, S., Zentel, H.J., Fink, T., and Krekel, J. (1991). Molecular anatomy of the neuro-immune connection. *International Journal of Neuroscience*, 59, 1–23.

Willard-Mack, Cynthia, L. (2006). Normal structure, function, and histology of lymph nodes. *Toxicologic Pathology*, 34, 409–424.

Williams, John, M., and Felten, David, L. (1981). Sympathetic innervation of murine thymus and spleen: A comparative histofluorescence study. *The Anatomical Record*, 199, 531–542.

Williams, J.M., Peterson, R.G., Shea, P.A., Schmedtje, J.F., Bauer, D.C., and Felten, D.L. (1981). Sympathetic innervation of murine thymus and spleen: Evidence for a functional link between the nervous and immune systems. *Brain Research Bulletin*, 6, 83–94.

Yoon, Seo-Yeon, Kim, Hyun-Woo., Roh, Dae-Hyun, Kwon, Young-Bae, Han, Ho-Jae, Beitz, Alvin, J., and Lee, Jang-Hern. (2006). Intrathecal clonidine suppresses zymosan-induced peripheral leukocyte migration in a mouse air pouch model via activation of spinal muscarinic type 2 receptors and sympathoadrenal medullary activity. *Neuropharmacology*, 51, 829–837.

Zang, H., Ching, S., Chen, Q., Li, Q., An, Y., and Quan, N. (2008). Localized inflammation in peripheral tissue signals the CAN for sickness response in the absence of interleukin-1 and COX-2 in the blood and brain. *Neuroscience*, 157, 895–907.

3

In Vitro and *In Vivo* Assessment of Immune System Modulation of Brain Function and Neurochemistry

Michael O. Poulter[1] and Zul Merali[2]

[1]*Robarts Research Institute, University of Western Ontario, Ontario, Canada.*
[2]*Department of Psychiatry, Royal Ottawa Hospital, University of Ottawa, Ottawa, Ontario, Canada.*

Overview

It is clear that the immune system is not dissociated from brain function, but rather a dynamic interaction exists between the two, as well as with neuroendocrine systems and autonomic system functioning. As such, there has been considerable attention devoted to brain neurochemical and functional analysis to better understand these interactions. In the following chapter, we will focus on some of the methods currently available to study neural–immune interactions. Specifically, we will consider methods that allow us to assess how an immune challenge may come to influence the neurochemistry of the brain and how nerve cell activity is modified by immune system signaling. This description will, hopefully, serve as an introduction to these techniques as well as indicating new avenues of investigation that arise from them.

Approaches to Assessing Brain Changes Associated with Immune and Cytokine Challenges

There are several neurochemical methods available to measure changes in the activity of specific neuronal systems within the central nervous system, and they fall into two general categories: those that assess static or steady state conditions, and those that assess dynamic changes. Postmortem tissue analysis has been used for several decades to assess endogenous levels of neurotransmitters, metabolites and/or neuropeptides in the steady-state condition, which provide a 'snapshot' in time. For these studies, brain tissue can be harvested via brain dissection to assess relatively large brain regions such as aspects of the cortex, hippocampus, pons, medulla, brain stem, cerebellum, and hypothalamus. For a more localized approach, a micropunch technique can be used. In this method, brain tissue is first sectioned (approx 300–1000 μm) using either a commercial matrix (fresh tissue) or cryostat (frozen tissue) and then discrete regions or individual nuclei are dissected from the sections using micropunch needles. Tissue

The Wiley-Blackwell Handbook of Psychoneuroimmunology, First Edition. Edited by Alexander W. Kusnecov and Hymie Anisman.

is then typically homogenized in acid and samples analyzed for transmitter/peptide content using one of many available methods for quantification. These techniques are still common practice, as it is often easier to assess the impact of drugs, stressors, or immune challenges on tissue levels of neurochemicals using a postmortem micropunch approach. Indeed, there are studies dating back to the 1980s showing activation of brain regions during an immune challenge based on analysis of postmortem tissue (Dunn, 1988).

Postmortem analyses have several drawbacks, especially as the effects of immune challenges on brain neurochemical changes can be expected to vary over time, but postmortem tissue only allows for the analysis of the biochemical levels that had existed at a predetermined moment in time. This problem may be particularly important in the case of immune challenges, as these entail a cascade of variations (witness the time-dependent changes that occur with respect to cytokine changes in response to an inflammatory challenge). Although more complex than postmortem analyses, there are techniques, such as *in vivo* microdialysis, that allow for the determination of chemicals that have been released from neurons, and this can be achieved at intervals of 2–10 minutes, depending on several technical factors, including the amount of the substrate being assessed.

Immune system mediators have also been known for some time to have acute effects on neuronal activity, and receptors for immune system mediators are expressed throughout the brain on nerve and glial cells (Cartier, Hartley, Dubois-Dauphin, and Krause, 2005). The best-characterized are the actions of interleukins on hypothalamic activity that regulate body temperature (Hori *et al.*, 1992). Studies using electrophysiological techniques have revealed numerous responses indicating that neuronal excitability, neurotransmission, and long term plasticity can be influenced by cytokines. The techniques used for these studies include extracellular, intracellular, and patch clamp electrophysiological recordings. In addition, imaging of brain activity has been carried out using dyes that detect calcium ion movement (Pita, Jelaso, and Ide, 1999). Another imaging technique which has been used recently to follow cytokine activity is voltage-sensitive imaging of voltage fluctuations in brain slices (Ikeda, Tsuda, Inoue, and Murase, 2007). The information obtained by these studies varies according to the technique used. *In vitro* electrophysiology (on cultured neurons for example) provides detailed information such as concentration–response relationships. More "intact" preparations like brain slices provide information on how the neurocircuitry may be affected, while *in vivo* recordings may provide insight on how the affected brain function influences whole-body responses. The choice between which of these techniques is used is dependent on the needs of the experimenter. A rule of thumb is that there is a trade-off between getting detailed pharmacological and/or biophysical information about neural function versus gaining insight into how the altered brain function affects the physiological outputs of the neural circuit or whole animal behavior.

Below, we discuss how the neurochemistry of the brain may be altered by immune function, outlining how cytokines may alter neurotransmitter content. We then outline some of the strategies that have used electrophysiological techniques to gain insight into how brain circuits "work" and how the immune system may affect these behaviors.

Analysis of brain neurochemistry

Using several biochemical techniques that gauge the content of various neurotransmitters, it has been shown that cytokines can have profound affects on brain neurochemistry. For example, it was observed that interleukin (IL)-1β administered systemically increased the concentrations of the norepinephrine (NE) metabolite, 3-Methoxy-4-hydroxyphenylglycol (MHPG), which is thought to reflect increased transmitter utilization, in several brain regions, but most prominently within the hypothalamus (Dunn, 1988; Kabiersch, del Rey, Honegger, and Besedovsky, 1988). Likewise, levels of 5-Hydroxyindoleacetic acid (5-HIAA), a major metabolite of serotonin (5-HT), also increased across many regions following IL-1β administration (Dunn, 1992; Zalcman *et al.*, 1994). Using a micropunch technique, it was also shown that IL-1β increased the concentrations of MHPG and the dopamine (DA) metabolite, 3,4-Dihydroxyphenylacetic acid (DOPAC), at specific hypothalamic regions, including the arcuate nucleus plus median eminence and increased MHPG levels at the paraventricular nucleus (PVN) as well as at extrahypothalamic sites, including the locus coeruleus and medial prefrontal cortex (Lacosta, Merali, and Anisman, 1999a). Regional changes in the content of monoamines and/or their metabolites have also been observed following adminstration of other cytokines (IL-2, IL-6, and tumor necrosis factor (TNF)-α) or the bacterial endotoxin, lipopolysaccaride (LPS; Lacosta, Merali, and Anisman, 1999b; Zalcman *et al.*, 1994), suggesting widespread action of immune challenges on CNS functioning.

However, interpretations of such changes in postmortem tissue are not always straightforward, as changes in transmitter/peptide content at a single point in time do not necessarily reflect the dynamics of the system. In the case of amines, some insight can be gained by the concomitant measurement of neurotransmitters and their metabolites, providing an index of utilization. A case in point involves the examples already mentioned in which elevated metabolites were thought to reflect increases in neurotransmitter utlization/release. But, even then, interpretation can be ambiguous, as it is often the case that more than one catabolic pathway exists, and thus changes in metabolites may not always reflect changes in transmitter release. Further, transmitter release and metabolism do not always co-vary, and the uncertain fate of amine metabolites over lengthy periods following cytokine treatment may not permit an accurate assessment of utilization rate. Even more complicated is the interpretation of changes of peptidergic content (e.g., that of corticotropin releasing factor; CRF) derived from postmortem tissue. Elevated tissue levels could reflect increased synthesis, diminished release, diminished degradation or increased release accompanied by an increase in synthesis. Furthermore, lack of change of peptide concentrations does not necessarily mean no effect; if peptide release is enhanced, but is matched by increased rate of synthesis, tissue levels remain constant (in the case of amines one may measure catabolites as an index of utilization, but this cannot be done with respect to peptides). Similarly, in situ hybridization studies can often reflect altered peptidergic activity. However, increased levels of peptide mRNA often occur some time after the event, and might not necessarily translate into increased production and/or release of the peptide. As such, like others, we invested significant effort in establishing techniques that permit the monitoring of dynamic changes in neuropeptide and/or transmitter utilization.

In vivo *neurochemical techniques* Despite their inherent technical difficulties, *in vivo* studies often provide clearer answers about the potential role of various neurotransmitter systems compared to those obtained through other approaches. When one measures the release of transmitters/peptide(s) *in vivo*, it is known with a degree of certainty whether a system is activated or not in terms of interstitial availability of the transmitter/peptide. Yet another distinct advantage of such a sampling technique is that one can concurrently measure neurotransmitter availability with an ongoing behavioral or functional state.

Three main techniques have been developed and refined over the years to measure dynamic changes in extracellular levels of transmitters and/or peptides in intact animals: voltammetry, push–pull perfusion, and microdialysis. Voltammetry, an electrochemical method used for the *in vivo* monitoring of neurotransmitters within extracellular fluid of the brain, has limited use due to low sensitivity of the biosensors and the fact that it can only be used to detect readily oxidizable species (i.e., DA, NE and 5-HT). However, an advantage of this technique is the higher temporal resolution (if assessment of momentary changes is the aim), as measurements of neurochemicals can be carried out at intervals as short as 100 ms (Stevenson and Gratton, 2003).

By a great margin, *in vivo* microdialysis is the most popular technique for the measurement of dynamic transmitter or peptide changes. This method was developed in the 1980s, but has evolved significantly over the past 30 years. Microdialysis, as its name implies, involves the introduction of a small dialysis membrane (typically 1–4 mm in length) to the tip of a probe separating the extracellular fluid from a perfusion medium within the probe. Once the probe is inserted into a site of interest, a perfusion medium is slowly and continuously infused (via an infusion pump; typically at a rate of 0.3 to 3 μl/min) through the dialysis probe and into outflow tubing where it can be collected for analysis. Molecules that are small enough to diffuse through the dialysis membrane will do so readily, passing from the high concentrations of the extracellular space to the low concentration within the membrane's lumen, whereas proteins and larger molecules are excluded. Most of the advantages of microdialysis are directly related to the membrane. Essentially, the membrane acts as a filter that partially purifies samples prior to analysis, and prevents enzyme-catalyzed degradation of the sample. In addition, the membrane minimizes the possibility of tissue damage because there is no net efflux of fluids from the probe into the tissue. Finally, it also offers some technical advantages, as the size of the active membrane can be customized, thus controlling the size of the area to be perfused. However, the probe membrane is also responsible for one of the main caveats/limitations of microdialysis, in that the pore size of the membrane will dictate the extent to which larger molecules will be able to pass through it. Thus, while amino acids and monoamines readily diffuse through the membrane, larger molecules, such as peptides and cytokines, pass through with difficulty, if at all.

Nonetheless, microdialysis is a highly robust technique, and has been employed, albeit sparingly, to shed light on the dynamics of monoamine release following an immune challenge. Indeed, using *in vivo* microdialysis, interpretation of the data from the various postmortem studies of increased levels of monoamine metabolites reflecting increased transmitter utilization/release has been confirmed. For example, peripheral or central administration of IL-1β increased the release of NE at the medial and anterior hypothalamus, PVN, as well as at extrahypothalamic sites, such as the medial prefrontal cortex (Kaur, Cruess, and Potter, 1998; Shintani *et al.*, 1993; Smagin, Swiergiel, and Dunn, 1996). We have also shown increased interstitial levels of 5-HIAA and homovanillic acid (HVA) at the nucleus accumbens, and 5-HIAA at the hippocampus, following peripheral IL-1β administration (Merali, Lacosta, and Anisman, 1997; Song, Merali, and Anisman, 1999). Interestingly, the transmitter release profiles following cytokine administration were distinct from those elicited by a neurogenic stressor (airpuff), suggesting a different mechanism of action. Microdialysis studies have further revealed cytokine-specific transmitter release profiles. Indeed, IL-2 (but not TNF-α) administration increased release of 5-HT and 5-HIAA at the hippocampus (Pauli, Linthorst, and Reul, 1998), and IL- 2 and IL-6 administration (but not IL-1β) reduced DA release at the nucleus accumbens (Anisman, Kokkinidis, and Merali, 1996). Similarly, LPS perfused into the striatum decreased the release of DOPAC, but not HVA at this site (Maurino, Machado, and Santiago, 2010).

Overall, the data derived from studies using microdialysis have made it clear that challenges, including cytokines and stressor events, influence monoamine release, and that these effects occur at multiple brain sites. Moreover, many of these amine variations have been consistent with the view that illnesses such as depression might be related to monoamine variations elicited by inflammatory challenges, although it is equally clear at this point that attributing complex illnesses simply to monoamines is short-sighted (see the extensive literature supporting a role for peptides such as CRF and growth factors like BDNF in depressive illness). Nevertheless, when combined with other approaches to assess the link between immune functioning and psychopathology, microdialysis can be an exceptionally powerful technique.

While considerable knowledge has already been gained through the use of microdialysis, it should be recognized that in recent years several refinements and improvements have been made to the technique, making it an even more powerful tool to monitor release *in vivo* of transmitters and/or peptides in freely behaving animals. One area of significant improvement has been in probe design and availability. Whereas years ago microdialysis probes were custom-made, today they are commercially available, and probes can be selected in different sizes and with different membranes. For example, thinner probes are now available to sample in mice or from small brain regions in rats (i.e., PVN) that were previously limited to push–pull perfusion technique. Moreover, membranes with higher molecular weight cut-offs (MWCO) can be purchased that have much better permeability for transmitters and, in particular, peptides. Even cytokines have been measured in the brain using probes with very high MWCO membranes, however, recovery for these macromolecules is still very low, and the source of cytokine release recovered within the extracellular space remains a source of controversy (Summy-Long, Hu, Long, and Phillips, 2008). Another area of improvement has been in the analytical methods used for detection. While monamine levels in dialysates are typically assessed using high performance liquid chromatography (HPLC), significant improvements have been made to this methodology which has resulted in increased sensitivity through an optimization of detection limits. These improvements primarily include the 'miniaturization' of HPLC component (i.e., cell detectors and columns) and the subsequent reduction in sample volumes required for analysis – down from micro- to nanolitres. The net result of these improvements has been a significant reduction in sampling time, from the traditional 15- to 30-minute intervals, although temporal resolution remains a crucial factor when trying to assess the rapid changes in transmitter/peptide levels which likely underlie physiological and/or behavioral responses associated with stress/immune challenges.

The third approach that can be employed for *in vivo* sampling, which is related to microdialysis, is that of a push–pull perfusion. One of the major differences between this technique and microdialysis is the absence of membrane on the probe. For push–pull, a prototypic probe consists of two concentric cannulae, one with an outer (pull part) and an inner infusion cannula (push part). A perfusion medium is continuosly infused into a target site throught the 'push' cannula and then withdrawn through the 'pull' cannula using two peristaltic pumps. A major advantage of this method is the high recovery of the released transmitter/peptides (greater than 80% recovery rates compared to the less than 20% with microdialysis), which permits detection of neurochemicals that may be present in low concentrations. Another factor that often necessitates the use of this technique (which is a lot more demanding, as the rate of infusion and withdrawal have to be matched perfectly and a slight obstruction of the flow can inflict tissue damage rapidly and irreversibly) is when the target site is anatomically small. The push–pull assembly is highly localized, extending just slightly (approximately 0.3–0.5 mm) into a target site, and therefore more appropriate for small loci such as the median eminence, arcuate nucleus, and PVN.

While advantageous in some regards, in general, the push–pull perfusion technique is not popular owing to the technical challenges associated with it. Nevertheless, there are several published reports based on push–pull perfusion (largely from two groups of researchers) demonstrating the increased release of NE, CRF and arginine vasopressin from hypothalamic sites, including the PVN and median eminence following IL-1β administration (systemic and central) (MohanKumar and MohanKumar, 2005; Watanobe and Takebe, 1993, 1994). Moreover, this technique has enabled measurement of the central release of cytokines, which is typically very difficult, if not impossible, using standard microdialysis procedures. Indeed, Kakizaki, Watanobe, Kohsaka, and Suda (1999) showed the release of IL-6 and TNF-α at the PVN in response to systemic LPS administration.

Recent improvements have been made to the push–pull perfusion technique that have greatly reduced the likelihood of transmitter/peptide deletion and/or tissue damage (both due to very high flow rates which can be up to 20 μl/min) through the 'miniaturization' of the probes and subsequent reductions of flow rates down to nanolitre concentrations (Slaney *et al.*, 2011). This has been further enabled with the advent of more sensitive detection methods (i.e., micro-liquid chromatography coupled with mass-spectrometry).

Analysis of Neuron Function Alterations by Cytokines

As discussed earlier, immune system mediators have profound effects on the neurochemistry of the brain; however, these techniques only infer the functional impact that may occur. In order to evaluate how brain function may be changed it is necessary to employ techniques that assay the ways that both acute stimuli and chronic adaptations alter nerve cell and/or neural circuit behavior. Conventional electrophysiological techniques (extracellular, sharp electrode, and patch electrode) have been employed only relatively recently to investigate this question, and much needs to done in order bring the field up to the level of knowledge that other physiological and pharmacological investigation have achieved. Below, we provide a brief overview of the action of cytokines and provide a description of current knowledge of how brain circuits "work." Finally, we suggest future lines of inquiry that seem necessary to understand fully how immune function alters brain function, in order to understand the relations between cytokine signaling and behavior.

The activity of both pro- and anti-inflammatory cytokines has wide-ranging effects on neuronal activity. For example, IL-1β at femtomolar concentrations has been shown in rat subfornical organ neurons to have profound excitatory effects. In the range of 100–500 fM it transiently activates a non-specific cation channel which greatly increases the frequency of action potential generation. At higher concentrations (1 pM) it causes a more sustained depolarization, while at still higher concentrations (100 pM) it produces a biphasic response. The initial depolarization is followed by a sustained hyperpolarization that reduces excitability (Desson and Ferguson, 2003). Another study, using extracellular recordings, found similar changes in activity in higher (cortical) structures (Lukats, Egyed, Lenard, and Karadi, 2005; Tancredi *et al.*, 2000). Lukats and colleagues found that microiontophoretic application of IL-1β into the orbital frontal cortex of rats increased the firing rate of neurons. In hippocampus, IL-6 and LPS administration have been shown to reduce long-term potentiation (LTP). IL-6 mediated this by inhibition of the mitogen-activated protein kinase (MAP kinase, ERK) (Tancredi *et al.*, 2000) while LPS effects were mediated by activating Caspase 1 (Vereker *et al.*, 2000). Further, IL-8, which is released by glial cells, has been shown to reduce calcium currents in neurons by interacting with G protein coupled chemokine receptors, CXCR 1 and 2 (Puma *et al.*, 2001).

Long-term effects on neuron function may occur as well, as chronic exposure to LPS has been shown to alter the excitability of inhibitory (GABAergic) neurons in culture. This includes lower input resistance; reduced amplitude of GABA mediated synaptic transmission and an elevated threshold for action potential generation. Further, once the cells did fire the action potentials produced were substantially fewer. Co-administration of LPS and the IL-1β antagonist IL-1ra prevented the effects on reduced inhibitory (GABA) transmission, but not the reduction in intrinsic neuronal excitability (Hellstrom, Danik, Luheshi, and Williams 2005). Although this survey is by no means exhaustive, it seems clear that cytokines do have profound effects on the biophysical properties of neurons as well as gating ion channels, and hence synaptic transmission.

Cytokines can also produce changes in brain neurochemistry that may have electrophysiological outcomes. The best-characterized is the activity of cytokines on 5-HT. Serotonin turnover has been shown to be altered by administration of LPS in a number of animal models (Anisman, Merali, Poulter, and Hayley, 2005). In addition, cytokines may also alter the expression of 5-HT receptors. INF-α has been shown to reduce the expression of $5HT_{1A}$ receptors (Anisman, 2009). Serotonin activity in the brain is mediated by a number of receptors coupled to G proteins that activate various intracellular signaling cascades; only one 5-HT receptor is ion channel. However, many of these signaling cascades affect the electrophysiological properties of neurons directly and indirectly. Activation, of $5\text{-}HT_{1B}$ receptors leads to the inhibition of calcium channels activity in nerve terminal of the raphe nucleus neurons, resulting in a reduction of 5-HT release. Activation of $5\text{-}HT_{2A}$ receptors produces variable responses, depending on the region of the brain in which they are expressed. In piriform cortex, activation causes an increase in inhibitory activity on layer II pyramidal (excitatory) cells, while in the layer IV pyramidal neurons of the prefrontal cortex the activation induces increased excitatory synaptic transmission (Gellman and Aghajanian, 1994; Marek and Aghajanian, 1998). There also seem to be strong interactions between $5\text{-}HT_{2C}$ receptors and dopaminergic neurotransmission. For instance, in the ventral tegmental regions $5\text{-}HT_{2C}$ activation decreases DA release (Di, Di, Pierucci, and Esposito, 2008) owing to activation of local circuits (inhibitory interneurons) that regulate the activity of dopaminergic projection neurons from the VTA (Capuron and Miller, 2011). This list of activity is by no means exhaustive but indicates that alterations in brain monoamine signaling can have profound electrophysiological affects if its balance is altered.

Electrophysiology is a powerful technique that is often able to describe in great detail how brain behavior is altered at its most fundamental level. As mentioned earlier, one can measure the activity of small groups of neurons to the level of single-ion channel function. The choice of which level to use depends on the question that the experimenter would like to answer. Generally, the broader the question the "further away" one becomes from the need to do single-cell recordings. As with any technique that can provide accurate and insightful observations, electrophysiology is not easy and a good deal of training is required to become proficient and learn how to avoid the generation of meaningless artifacts. From a practical point of view, the equipment can be expensive – requiring significant resources and know-how to set up the infrastructure. Thus, most researchers who wish to follow this line of inquiry usually arrange to visit and train in a laboratory that is expert in these techniques. Hence, for the purposes of this review we will merely outline the basic considerations that must be taken into account in the use of various neuronal preparations – culture, brain slice, and *in vivo*. We then provide an overview of the ways these techniques have been used to study the electrophysiological activity of immune mediators in these various preparations.

Neuronal cell culture

Neuronal cell cultures are almost always derived from freshly dissociated embryonic brain tissue, typically from rodent brain. Although with some care one can record from them as soon as a few hours after their isolation, they are typically allowed to grow for at least 2 weeks before they are used for recordings. By far the most popular technique for doing electrophysiology on these cells is patch clamp recording. After two to three weeks, cells form synaptic connections and develop spontaneous activity that can be used to follow the activity of various agents by perfusing of the culture dish. Because the cells form a monolayer, the concentrations and access of drugs to the neurons are uniform and can be precisely and quickly controlled. In brain slice and *in vivo* electrophysiology the control of drug applications is often slow and/or uncertain. The ability to carry out detailed and accurate pharmacological investigation is one of the main advantages of neuronal cultures. The cells are also relatively easy to patch. It is also easier to do more complicated drug-delivery techniques, such as concentration jumps that can be as quick as 50–100 μs. Also, obtaining single-channel recordings is usually less difficult than getting similar recordings in brain slices. The main disadvantage is that the neural circuitry that develops is not the same as, or even close to, the circuits that develop in normal brain (although organotypic slice culture may circumvent some of these issues). Further, maturation of ion-channel expression may not be complete, so a mixture of embryonic and mature ion channels may be expressed, confounding interpretation of the results. Overall, the main advantages of studying cells in culture are the ability to precisely control the extracellular, and sometimes intracellular, milieu, and the relative ease of making patch recordings. This comes at the expense of the cells being in a non-physiological environment, having no coherent circuitry.

Brain slices

Brain slice recordings represent the next level of complexity, offering the advantage of keeping the neural circuitry relatively intact. There are several technical challenges that require complex measures to be taken to ensure that high quality (viable) tissue is obtained. The most difficult issues during all steps is maintaining a proper balance of oxygenation, pH, salt (osmolarity), and temperature. Keeping all these physiological parameters under control is critical if the tissue is to respond in a manner that reasonably reflects the underlying physiological processes. As the vast majority of brain slice recordings are made from rodents we will limit our description to this animal model.

The first choice that must be made when planning these kinds of experiments is the age of rodent to be used. Young animals (10–14 days old) are easier to use for a number of reasons. First, their size makes them relatively easier to handle; isolation of the brain from the skull is easier, owing to the thin cranial bones; and any hypoxia that may occur during the isolation of the brain seems to be less damaging in younger animals. Thus, the slices that are isolated recover more readily. The disadvantages are that one is not studying responses in a mature brain. Neural network connectivity is not the same as adult (there are in fact more synapses), myelination is incomplete, and neurotransmitter systems (glutamate and GABA for example) are in transition from the expression pattern seen in embryos to those expressed in the adult. Most pertinent here is that immune function may not be mature and so the responses that are obtained may only pertain to non-adult rodents, making the extrapolation to human even less certain. The alternative is the use of adult rodents. For this preparation the critical issue is preventing/controlling significant hypoxia from occurring, as the adult brain does not recover from long (> 5 minutes) periods of hypoxia. The advantage of using adult brains is that more slices can be prepared (the brain is bigger) and the neural circuitry is more stable (though still plastic). A further advantage is that experiments can be conducted with the rodent being treated over a period of time long enough to enable longitudinal studies.

In vivo recordings

The next level of complexity is recording from animals that have either chronic electrode implants or are acutely anesthetized and have electrodes implanted. In the first case the only possible type of recordings are extracellular. These are made either with electrodes that record the local field potential (the ensemble activity of a small group of cells) or electrodes that register action potentials from a single cell (unit recordings). In the second case, acute experiments are performed where a number of recording techniques are possible. These include patch clamp, intracellular, extracellular, and unit recordings. These recording techniques are sometimes combined. For example, combining an intracellular (single-cell) recording with an extracellular one can provide information on how a single neuron participates in the ensemble activity of a group of neurons. This combination of techniques has been very useful in assigning function to differing classes of interneurons (Klausberger and Somogyi, 2008; Klausberger *et al.*, 2005). The main advantage of *in vivo* recordings is that one is recording from an intact brain that has normal blood supply. The disadvantages are that these recordings do not usually provide detailed information of cellular activity (voltage clamp is very difficult or impossible), and drug concentrations are difficult to estimate as the entire brain cannot be uniformly dosed. In the case of acute recordings, where anesthesia must be used, there is the uncertainty arising from the fact that responses are being collected from a brain whose synaptic activity is greatly depressed. The responses may be muted or absent depending on the region of the brain being studied. In sum, *in vivo* recordings provide information on function from intact brain at the expense of losing some control over the accuracy of cellular and pharmacological measurements that may be pertinent.

What has electrophysiology told us about immune function and brain activity?

Electrophysiology has provided considerable knowledge on physiology and pharmacology of neuronal function. As mentioned earlier, there are number of techniques that have been used including extracellular, sharp electrode (intracellular) and patch clamp recording technique. There are three kinds of information that are gathered by these types of recordings: network, cellular, and single-channel behavior. Studies of the activity of cytokines have largely focused on cellular behavior, while the other types of behaviors have not been studied in any detail to date. Thus, we will concentrate on outlining the types of information that have been found, and what might be investigated in the future, with regard to cytokine modulation of neural function.

The brain operates by communicating with other regions by sending out synchronized volleys of activity (action potentials) from excitatory cells which project their axons to specific neuronal targets. This activity occurs at differing frequencies, ranging from low (0.5–2 Hz) to very high-frequency oscillations (200–400 Hz). For over 80 years it has been recognized that certain brain rhythms can be correlated to various behaviors. For example, sleep rhythms are associated with δ (2–4 Hz) oscillations, while γ (20–80 Hz) oscillations are associated with learning and/or the directing of attention to stimuli. The underlying cellular mechanisms of the ways that projection neurons' activities are synchronized have largely been elucidated by *in vitro* electrophysiology (Traub, Jefferys, J. and Whittington, 1999), although more recent work has used *in vivo* recordings (Klausberger and Somogyi, 2008). The analogy that has been used to describe this process is that the brain works like a badly driven car. The gas is always on and the car is controlled by applying the brakes. So, oscillations are created by inhibiting neurons that are constantly receiving excitatory input (which of course can vary in strength). However, the relationship between how interneurons control the differing oscillatory patterns is complicated by the recognition that interneurons are very diverse. For example, different types of inhibitory synaptic connections exist (Freund, 2003), with interneurons giving rise to connections that may either facilitate, run down, or be stable (Gupta, Wang, and Markram, 2000). Also, the phenotypes of both the interneuron and its target have a role in determining the type of synaptic connection. Thus, when these basic characteristics are coupled with the heterogeneous firing properties of the interneuron subtypes and the diversity of their anatomical connections (dendritic, axonal and/or somatic), an intriguing level of complexity is evident.

More recent *in vivo* studies (Klausberger, Roberts, and Somogyi, 2002; Klausberger *et al.*, 2005; Klausberger and Somogyi, 2008) have revealed that differing subtypes of interneurons play unique roles controlling brain oscillations. This has been termed as a "division of labour"; some interneurons participate in θ (3–6 Hz) oscillations, while other subtypes are more important for γ frequencies. For example, cholecystokinin (CCK) interneurons that target hippocampal dendrites fire during the rising phase of γ oscillations. This suggests that they are important in phasing the activity of the pyramidal cells. Other studies have shown oscillations in brain slices (Bartos *et al.*, 2002; Oren, Mann, Paulsen, and Hajos, 2006; Traub *et al.*, 1996) that suggest that perisomatic targeting interneurons, such as basket cells, have a predominant role in generating γ waves *in vitro* and *in vivo*. Importantly, evidence also suggests that interneuron plasticity can alter both the phase and frequency of the pattern generators (Soto-Trevino, Thoroughman, Marder, and Abbott, 2001).

How any of these synchronizing processes are affected by the immune system is almost completely unexplored. Nevertheless, several possibilities exist where one might hypothesize that brain rhythms may be altered by the immune system, since many cytokine effects on brain theoretically alter interneuron function. Perhaps the most obvious are those neurotransmitter systems that are known to alter interneuron excitability, such as 5-HT, CRF or GABA, which have been shown to be influenced by cytokines/or immune challenges. For example, acute and prolonged exposure to LPS alters 5-HT turnover, so it be might expected that normal brain rhythms may be affected. Further, LPS may stimulate the HPA axis to produce CRF which may heighten central stress responses (Black, 2002). CRF release from interneurons has been shown to increase GABA release on pyramidal neurons. In prefrontal cortex (PFC), 5-HT regulates GABAergic inhibitory transmission by enhancing the release and size of inhibitory postsynaptic current (IPSCs) (Tan, Zhong, and Yan, 2004). This enhancement desensitizes over a period of about 4 minutes. However, if the PFC slices were pre-exposed to CRF, the effect of 5-HT was prolonged, lasting 8–10 minutes. Interestingly, this enhancement of inhibition occurred on pyramidal neurons, which presumably would reduce the output of the PFC. Acute stress mimicked the effect of CRF and this was antagonized by the CRF antagonist α-helical $CRF_{9\text{-}4}$. The PFC and amygdala have strong reciprocal connections, and the anxiety response is due to alteration in the patterns of circuit behavior between these two brain regions. Importantly as the "inflammatory response" has many neurochemical similarities to the "stress response", causing the release of central neuropeptides like CRF, there is a strong suggestion that immune challenges can modify the activity of the neural circuits that mediate behavioral outcomes such as anxiety. However, the exact electrophysiological mechanism(s) by which cytokines and other neuropeptides may alter pattern generation is still largely unknown.

Another possible interaction between cytokines and brain function is in the development of epileptic seizures. Epilepsy can be conceptually thought of as the (inappropriate) hypersynchrony of the brain. This means that mechanisms that generate normal oscillatory behaviour have been augmented to the point that large regions of brain begin to synchronise to the point where normal behavior is disturbed. Seizures can also induce excitotoxicity and sudden death. How and why this synchrony arises has been the focus of intense studies that have implicated many mechanisms involving many electrophysiological phenomena (GABA and glutamate, for example) that will not be discussed here. However, a particularly intriguing recent development in the understanding and treatment of epilepsy is the idea that neuroinflammation may be involved in generating and perhaps exacerbating seizures. However, the question as to whether the antiflammatory/antiseizure actions are due to direct activity on neurons/glia or whether it is merely a secondary effect from reducing blood brain barrier permeability, which is increased by seizures, is debatable. Evidence for direct effects comes from a study of the antiseizure medication levetiracetam (LEV), which was shown to have anti-inflammatory activity (Stienen *et al.*, 2011). Specifically, LEV was shown to restore normal resting membrane potentials in astrocytes. This occurs via an interaction with both inward and outward rectifier currents. This restoration of the "normal state" promoted expression of transforming growth factor, TGFβ1. In addition, LEV and TGFβ1 facilitated the generation of astrocyte voltage-gated currents. The authors suggested that LEV likely reduces the spread of excitation within the astroglial functional syncytium that, in turn, stabilizes and normalizes neuronal–glial interactions. Other studies have implicated cytokine receptors in the modulation of neuronal activity in such a way that their activation would be predicted to be seizuregenic. In particular, CXCR4 receptor has been demonstrated to reduce glutamate receptor activity likely by a presynaptic mechanism that reduces glutamate release (Ragozzino, Renzi, Giovannelli, and Eusebi, 2002). By contrast, the coexpression of CXCR2 with glutamate receptor GluR1 in HEK-293 cells was shown to increase activity. The same study showed the amplitude of spontaneous excitatory postsynaptic currents (sEPSCs) was also increased in rat cerebellar granule cells (Lax *et al.*, 2002).

Patch clamp experiments performed on fetal mouse hypothalamic neurons in culture have shown that SDF-1α (10 nM) decreased the peak and rising slope of the action potentials and spike discharge frequency and was blocked by the CXCR4 antagonist AMD 3100 (1 μM). Interestingly this effect involved the depression of both voltage-dependent sodium and potassium currents (Guyon *et al.*, 2005). Whole-cell patch clamp recordings of hippocampal neurons in culture show that CX(3)CL1-induced depression of glutamate-receptor-mediated current (AMPA-current), is associated with adenosine receptor type activity. This appears to occur by another glial–neuronal interaction whereby CX(3)CL1 activity induces a significant release of adenosine from microglial cells which in turn modulates AMPA receptor activity (Lauro *et al.*, 2008). In summary, chemokines can modulate neuronal activity by a) altering the gating of voltage-dependent channels (sodium, potassium, and calcium); b) activation of the G-protein-activated inward rectifier potassium current, and c) augmenting GABA, glutamate, and DA release (Guyon *et al.*, 2009; Lauro *et al.*, 2008). As each of these processes have been shown to play important roles in the control of neuronal synchrony, the development of medications directed against these targets appears to be an important new direction in drug development.

Summary

It is clear that immune function alters brain neuronal processes and brain neurochemical functioning through numerous processes that can act acutely or for sustained periods. The findings described in this chapter reflect a good beginning to our understanding of how cytokines may cause changes in brain neurochemistry and electrophysiological responses. Questions that still need to be addressed include: How do the signaling cascades mediated by cytokine receptors activation interact with biochemical pathways that synthesize and break down neurotransmitters? How do the same receptors alter ion-channel function? How do alterations in ion-channel function created by cytokines have an impact on network behavior to create complex emotional states like depression? And, finally, How do all of these come together to affect normal and dysfunctional behavior?

Acknowledgments

Supported by the Canadian Institutes for Health Research (CIHR).

References

Anisman, H. (2009). Cascading effects of stressors and inflammatory immune system activation: implications for major depressive disorder. *Journal of Psychiatry and Neuroscience*, 34, 4–20.

Anisman, H., Kokkinidis, L., and Merali, Z. (1996). Interleukin-2 decreases accumbal dopamine efflux and responding for rewarding lateral hypothalamic stimulation. *Brain Research*, 731, 1–11.

Anisman, H., Merali, Z., Poulter, M.O., and Hayley, S. (2005). Cytokines as a precipitant of depressive illness: animal and human studies. *Current Pharmaceutical Design*, 11, 963–972.

Bartos, M., Vida, I., Frotscher, M., Meyer, A., Monyer, H., Geiger, J.R. et al. (2002). Fast synaptic inhibition promotes synchronized gamma oscillations in hippocampal interneuron networks. *Proceedings of the National Acadademy of Sciences of the USA*, 99, 13222–13227.

Black, P.H. (2002). Stress and the inflammatory response: a review of neurogenic inflammation. *Brain, Behavior, Immunity*, 16, 622–653.

Capuron, L. and Miller, A.H. (2011). Immune system to brain signaling: neuropsychopharmacological implications. *Pharmacology and Therapeutics*, 130, 226–238.

Cartier, L., Hartley, O., Dubois-Dauphin, M., and Krause, K.H. (2005). Chemokine receptors in the central nervous system: role in brain inflammation and neurodegenerative diseases. *Brain Research, Brain Research Reviews*, 48, 16–42.

Desson, S.E. and Ferguson, A.V. (2003). Interleukin 1beta modulates rat subfornical organ neurons as a result of activation of a non-selective cationic conductance. *Journal of Physiology*, 550, 113–122.

Di, G.G., Di, M., V, Pierucci, M., and Esposito, E. (2008). Serotonin–dopamine interaction: electrophysiological evidence. *Progress in Brain Research*, 172, 45–71.

Dunn, A.J. (1988). Systemic interleukin-1 administration stimulates hypothalamic norepinephrine metabolism paralleling the increased plasma corticosterone. *Life Sciences*, 43, 429–435.

Dunn, A.J. (1992). Endotoxin-induced activation of cerebral catecholamine and serotonin metabolism: comparison with interleukin-1. *Journal of Pharmacology and Experimental Therapeutics*, 261, 964–969.

Freund, T.F. (2003). Interneuron Diversity series: Rhythm and mood in perisomatic inhibition. *Trends in Neuroscience*, 26, 489–495.

Gellman, R.L. and Aghajanian, G.K. (1994). Serotonin2 receptor-mediated excitation of interneurons in piriform cortex: antagonism by atypical antipsychotic drugs. *Neuroscience*, 58, 515–525.

Gupta, A., Wang, Y., and Markram, H. (2000). Organizing principles for a diversity of GABAergic interneurons and synapses in the neocortex *Science*, 287, 273 278.

Guyon, A., Rovere, C., Cervantes, A., Allaeys, I., and Nahon, J.L. (2005). Stromal cell-derived factor-1alpha directly modulates voltage-dependent currents of the action potential in mammalian neuronal cells. *Journal of Neurochemistry*, 93, 963–973.

Guyon, A., Skrzydelski, D., De, G., I, Rovere, C., Conductier, G., Trocello, J.M. et al. (2009). Long term exposure to the chemokine CCL2 activates the nigrostriatal dopamine system: a novel mechanism for the control of dopamine release. *Neuroscience*, 162, 1072–1080.

Hellstrom, I.C., Danik, M., Luheshi, G.N., and Williams, S. (2005). Chronic LPS exposure produces changes in intrinsic membrane properties and a sustained IL-beta-dependent increase in GABAergic inhibition in hippocampal CA1 pyramidal neurons. *Hippocampus*, 15, 656–664.

Hori, T., Kiyohara, T., Nakashima, T., Mizuno, K., Muratani, H., and Katafuchi, T. (1992). Effects of temperature and neuroactive substances on hypothalamic neurones in vitro: possible implications for the induction of fever. *Physiological Research*, 41, 77–81.

Ikeda, H., Tsuda, M., Inoue, K., and Murase, K. (2007). Long-term potentiation of neuronal excitation by neuron–glia interactions in the rat spinal dorsal horn. *European Journal of Neuroscience*, 25, 1297–1306.

Kabiersch, A., del Rey, A., Honegger, C.G., and Besedovsky, H.O. (1988). Interleukin-1 induces changes in norepinephrine metabolism in the rat brain. *Brain, Behavior, Immunity*, 2, 267–274.

Kakizaki, Y., Watanobe, H., Kohsaka, A., and Suda, T. (1999). Temporal profiles of interleukin-1beta, interleukin-6, and tumor necrosis factor-alpha in the plasma and hypothalamic paraventricular nucleus after intravenous or intraperitoneal administration of lipopolysaccharide in the rat: estimation by push–pull perfusion. *Endocrine Journal*, 46, 487–496.

Kaur, D., Cruess, D.F., and Potter, W.Z. (1998). Effect of IL-1alpha on the release of norepinephrine in rat hypothalamus. *Journal of Neuroimmunology*, 90, 122–127.

Klausberger, T., Marton, L.F., O'Neill, J., Huck, J.H., Dalezios, Y., Fuentealba, P. et al. (2005). Complementary roles of cholecystokinin- and parvalbumin-expressing GABAergic neurons in hippocampal network oscillations. *Journal of Neuroscience*, 25, 9782–9793.

Klausberger, T., Roberts, J.D.B., and Somogyi, P. (2002). Cell type and input specific differences in the number and subtypes of synaptic $GABA_A$ receptors in the hippocampus. *Journal of Neuroscience*, 22, 2513–2521.

Klausberger, T. and Somogyi, P. (2008). Neuronal diversity and temporal dynamics: the unity of hippocampal circuit operations. *Science*, 321, 53–57.

Lacosta, S., Merali, Z., and Anisman, H. (1999a). Behavioral and neurochemical consequences of lipopolysaccharide in mice: anxiogenic-like effects. *Brain Research*, 818, 291–303.

Lacosta, S., Merali, Z., and Anisman, H. (1999b). Influence of acute and repeated interleukin-2 administration on spatial learning, locomotor activity, exploratory behaviors, and anxiety. *Behavioural Neuroscience*, 113, 1030–1041.

Lauro, C., Di, A.S., Cipriani, R., Sobrero, F., Antonilli, L., Brusadin, V. et al. (2008). Activity of adenosine receptors type 1 Is required for CX3CL1-mediated neuroprotection and neuromodulation in hippocampal neurons. *Journal of Immunology*, 180, 7590–7596.

Lax, P., Limatola, C., Fucile, S., Trettel, F., Di, B.S., Renzi, M. et al. (2002). Chemokine receptor CXCR2 regulates the functional properties of AMPA-type glutamate receptor GluR1 in HEK cells. *Journal of Neuroimmunology*, 129, 66–73.

Lukats, B., Egyed, R., Lenard, L., and Karadi, Z. (2005). Homeostatic alterations induced by interleukin-1beta microinjection into the orbitofrontal cortex in the rat. *Appetite*, 45, 137–147.

Marek, G.J. and Aghajanian, G.K. (1998). The electrophysiology of prefrontal serotonin systems: therapeutic implications for mood and psychosis. *Biological Psychiatry*, 44, 1118–1127.

Maurino, R., Machado, A., and Santiago, M. (2010). Effect of in vivo striatal perfusion of lipopolysaccharide on dopamine metabolites. *Neuroscience Letters*, 475, 121–123.

Merali, Z., Lacosta, S., and Anisman, H. (1997). Effects of interleukin-1beta and mild stress on alterations of norepinephrine, dopamine and serotonin neurotransmission: a regional microdialysis study. *Brain Research*, 761, 225–235.

MohanKumar, S.M. and MohanKumar, P.S. (2005). Systemic Interleukin-1beta stimulates the simultaneous release of norepinephrine in the paraventricular nucleus and the median eminence. *Brain Research Bulletin*, 65, 451–456.

Oren, I., Mann, E.O., Paulsen, O., and Hajos, N. (2006). Synaptic currents in anatomically identified CA3 neurons during hippocampal gamma oscillations in vitro. *Journal of Neuroscience*, 26, 9923–9934.

Pauli, S., Linthorst, A.C., and Reul, J.M. (1998). Tumour necrosis factor-alpha and interleukin-2 differentially affect hippocampal serotonergic neurotransmission, behavioural activity, body temperature and hypothalamic–pituitary–adrenocortical axis activity in the rat. *European Journal of Neuroscience*, 10, 868–878.

Pita, I., Jelaso, A.M., and Ide, C.F. (1999). IL-1beta increases intracellular calcium through an IL-1 type 1 receptor mediated mechanism in C6 astrocytic cells. *International Journal of Developmental Neuroscience*, 17, 813–820.

Puma, C., Danik, M., Quirion, R., Ramon, F., and Williams, S. (2001). The chemokine interleukin-8 acutely reduces Ca(2+) currents in identified cholinergic septal neurons expressing CXCR1 and CXCR2 receptor mRNAs. *Journal of Neurochemistry*, 78, 960–971.

Ragozzino, D., Renzi, M., Giovannelli, A., and Eusebi, F. (2002). Stimulation of chemokine CXC receptor 4 induces synaptic depression of evoked parallel fibers inputs onto Purkinje neurons in mouse cerebellum. *Journal of Neuroimmunology*, 127, 30–36.

Shintani, F., Kanba, S., Nakaki, T., Nibuya, M., Kinoshita, N., Suzuki, E. et al. (1993). Interleukin-1 beta augments release of norepinephrine, dopamine, and serotonin in the rat anterior hypothalamus. *Journal of Neuroscience*, 13, 3574–3581.

Slaney, T.R., Nie, J., Hershey, N.D., Thwar, P.K., Linderman, J., Burns, M.A. et al. (2011). Push–pull perfusion sampling with segmented flow for high temporal and spatial resolution in vivo chemical monitoring. *Analytical Chemistry*, 83, 5207–5213.

Smagin, G.N., Swiergiel, A.H., and Dunn, A.J. (1996). Peripheral administration of interleukin-1 increases extracellular concentrations of norepinephrine in rat hypothalamus: comparison with plasma corticosterone. *Psychoneuroendocrinology*, 21, 83–93.

Song, C., Merali, Z., and Anisman, H. (1999). Variations of nucleus accumbens dopamine and serotonin following systemic interleukin-1, interleukin-2 or interleukin-6 treatment. *Neuroscience*, 88, 823–836.

Soto-Trevino, C., Thoroughman, K.A., Marder, E., and Abbott, L.F. (2001). Activity-dependent modification of inhibitory synapses in models of rhythmic neural networks. *Nature Neuroscience*, 4, 297–303.

Stevenson, C.W. and Gratton, A. (2003). Basolateral amygdala modulation of the nucleus accumbens dopamine response to stress: role of the medial prefrontal cortex. *European Journal of Neuroscience*, 17, 1287–1295.

Stienen, M.N., Haghikia, A., Dambach, H., Thone, J., Wiemann, M., Gold, R. et al. (2011). Anti-inflammatory effects of the anticonvulsant drug levetiracetam on electrophysiological properties of astroglia are mediated via TGFbeta1 regulation. *British Journal of Pharmacology*, 162, 491–507.

Summy-Long, J.Y., Hu, S., Long, A., and Phillips, T.M. (2008). Interleukin-1beta release in the supraoptic nucleus area during osmotic stimulation requires neural function. *Journal of Neuroendocrinology*, 20, 1224–1232.

Tan, H., Zhong, P., and Yan, Z. (2004). Corticotropin-releasing factor and acute stress prolongs serotonergic regulation of GABA transmission in prefrontal cortical pyramidal neurons. *Journal of Neuroscience*, 24, 5000–5008.

Tancredi, V., D'antuono, M., Cafe, C., Giovedi, S., Bue, M.C., D'Arcangelo, G. et al. (2000). The inhibitory effects of interleukin-6 on synaptic plasticity in the rat hippocampus are associated with an inhibition of mitogen-activated protein kinase ERK. *Journal of Neurochemistry*, 75, 634–643.

Traub, R.D., Jefferys, J.G.R., and Whittington, M.A. (1999). *Fast Oscillations in Cortical Circuits.* Cambridge, MA: MIT Press.

Traub, R.D., Whittington, M.A., Colling, S.B., Buzsaki, G., and Jefferys, J.G. (1996). Analysis of gamma rhythms in the rat hippocampus in vitro and in vivo. *Journal of Physiology (London)*, 493, 471–484.

Vereker, E., Campbell, V., Roche, E., McEntee, E., and Lynch, M.A. (2000). Lipopolysaccharide inhibits long term potentiation in the rat dentate gyrus by activating caspase-1. *Journal of Biological Chemistry*, 275, 26252–26258.

Watanobe, H. and Takebe, K. (1993). Intrahypothalamic perfusion with interleukin-1-beta stimulates the local release of corticotropin-releasing hormone and arginine vasopressin and the plasma adrenocorticotropin in freely moving rats: a comparative perfusion of the paraventricular nucleus and the median eminence. *Neuroendocrinology*, 57, 593–599.

Watanobe, H. and Takebe, K. (1994). Effects of intravenous administration of interleukin-1-beta on the release of prostaglandin E2, corticotropin-releasing factor, and arginine vasopressin in several hypothalamic areas of freely moving rats: estimation by push–pull perfusion. *Neuroendocrinology*, 60, 8–15.

Zalcman, S., Green-Johnson, J.M., Murray, L., Nance, D.M., Dyck, D., Anisman, H. et al. (1994). Cytokine-specific central monoamine alterations induced by interleukin-1, -2 and -6. *Brain Research*, 643, 40–49.

4

Control and Contributions of the Blood–Brain Barriers to Cytokine Levels in the CNS

William A. Banks

Geriatrics Research Education and Clinical Center, Veterans Affairs, Puget Sound Health Care System and Division of Gerontology and Geriatric Medicine, Department of Internal Medicine, University of Washington School of Medicine, USA

Overview

The tenet of neuroimmunology is that the immune and central nervous systems communicate with one another. One of the main mechanisms of this communication is via humoral factors such as cytokines. Originally thought to be produced only by leukocytes, cytokines are now known to be secreted by a variety of other cells including those within the brain and those forming the blood–brain barriers (BBBs).

As currently elucidated, the BBBs are known to contribute to cytokine levels within the CNS through three major mechanisms: restrictive barrier function, transport function, and secretory function (Figure 4.1). Specific studies show that the immune–brain communications that result from these mechanisms mediate the influences of cytokines on cognition, temperature, neurodegeneration, pathogen penetration of the BBB, and, possibly, appetite. To further understand how these three mechanisms act and interact, some understanding of the BBB is needed.

The Blood–Brain Barrier

Evidence for a barrier separating the brain and blood was first gathered at the end of the nineteenth century (Davson and Segal, 1996a). Some dyes stained the brain, and bile acids caused seizures when injected directly into the brain but did not do so when injected peripherally. This and other work led to the concept that the capillary bed of the brain prevented by some means the unrestricted leakage of substances from blood into brain. Other work showed that the cerebrospinal fluid differed radically from plasma and lymph. This gave rise to the concept of a blood–CSF barrier (Davson and Segal, 1996b). In the late 1960s, electron microscopy revealed the anatomical basis for the barriers. Most capillary beds are quite leaky, producing an ultrafiltrate that nourishes the tissue bed. This leakage arises because of channels

The Wiley-Blackwell Handbook of Psychoneuroimmunology, First Edition. Edited by Alexander W. Kusnecov and Hymie Anisman.

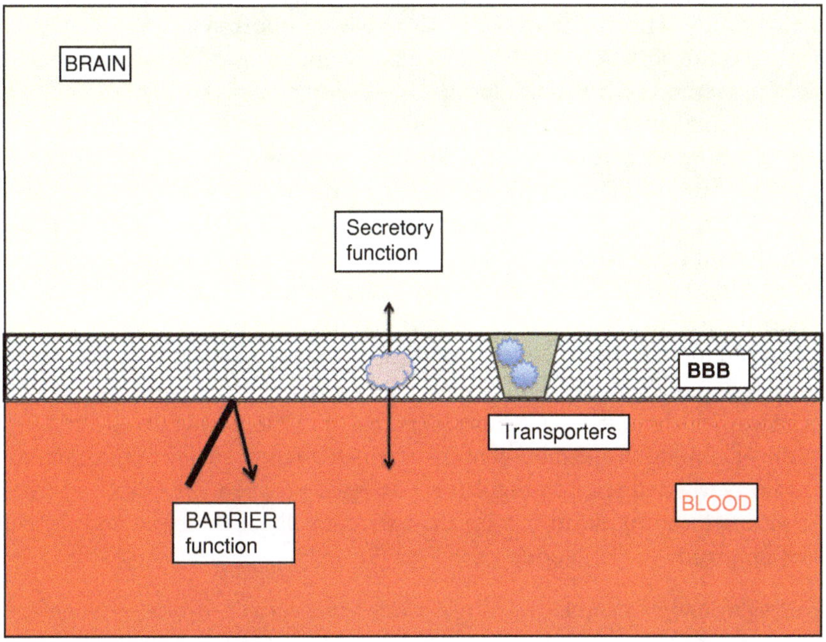

Figure 4.1 Three major characteristics of the blood–brain barriers that affect brain levels of cytokines. The physical aspects of the BBB prevent the unregulated leakage of cytokines into the brain. The cells comprising the blood–brain barrier secrete neuroimmune-active substances, including cytokines. Some cytokines are transported across the BBB by saturable systems.

that span the endothelial cell wall (fenestrae) and large vesicles that shuttle between blood and tissue (macropinocytosis), but brain endothelial cells are almost totally devoid of these. Furthermore, brain endothelial cells and the ependymal cells that define the choroid plexus are joined together by tight junctions that prevent intercellular leaks. As a result of nearly absent fenestrae, greatly reduced macropinocytosis, and tight intercellular junctions, the capillary bed of the brain does not leak.

Box 4.1 The Blood–Brain Barrier: A Brief History

The best-known of the late-nineteenth-century experiments that define the BBB were those of Paul Ehrlich. As a student, Ehrlich noted that some dyes injected into the body did not stain the brain. While others correctly interpreted these results as evidence for a barrier between the CNS and blood, Ehrlich contended that brain tissue was simply unable to bind these dyes. The existence and nature of the BBB was debated throughout the early and middle twentieth century, with some proposing that a virtual absence of interstitial space provided no room for dyes to be taken up. Not until electron microscopy experiments in the late 1960s was the ultrastructural basis of the BBB discovered. During this time, Hugh Davson and others continued to define the BBB in new terms. In addition to being a physical barrier, Davson and others noted that lipid-soluble substances could cross the BBB. To this day, most drugs used to treat CNS conditions are small, lipid-soluble drugs. The ability to study saturable transport systems was given a great boost with the introduction of the brain uptake index by Oldendorf in the 1970s. The graphical method (AKA multiple-time regression analysis) of Patlak, Blasberg, and Fenstermacher introduced in the early 1980s is critical to the study of molecules with slow rates of transport across the BBB, such as cytokines (Banks, Ortiz, Plotkin, and Kastin, 1991). Studies of the BBB as an enzymatic barrier were extended greatly in the 1980s, as a transporter of regulatory proteins in the 1990s, and as a secretor of immune-active substances in the early part of the twenty-first century, although the first studies in each of these fields date back some years before. The BBB has suffered greatly from premature reification: many outside the field assume that the incorporation of "barrier" within its name indicates that virtually nothing crosses it. The discoveries that immune cells, peptides, regulatory proteins, and antisense molecules can cross the BBB all contended with the untested assumptions that these substances could not cross the BBB. At the beginning of the third century in which it has been a field of study, the BBB is once again newly defined as a regulatory interface between the CNS and circulation that is in intimate communication with the adjacent cells of the brain and the cells and hormones circulating in the blood.

The barrier to leakage is both good news and bad news for the central nervous system. The need for such a barrier is likely twofold: 1) It is the first major defense for protecting the CNS from circulating substances that would be toxic to the neurons and other cells within the CNS. The evolutionary roots of the BBB run deep (Abbott, 2005). Essentially, any creature that has nerve-like tissue in contact with some type of circulating fluid has a barrier-like cell between the two. 2) Once encased in the skull, production of an ultrafiltrate would be problematic. This is because the amount of ultrafiltrate produced by a tissue bed can increase and decrease depending on osmotic and oncotic factors. Sudden increases in ultrafiltrate volume inside the rigid cranium would result in increased intracranial pressure. In the extreme case, these increased pressures force the brain downward, pressing the respiratory centers of the brain stem against the foramen magnum of the skull. This can result in respiratory arrest and death. Barrier function, therefore, helps to provide the CNS with a toxin-free environment and to control intracranial pressures.

The bad news is that the CNS is deprived of the production of a nourishing ultrafiltrate. Without an ultrafiltrate, there is no lymph produced to drain toxins from the tissue bed. The CNS has devised alternative ways to bring in nutrients and rid itself of toxins, and these alternatives involve the BBBs. A multitude of transporters exist at the capillary and choroid plexus barriers that supply the CNS with glucose, amino acids, vitamins, minerals, free fatty acids, and other needed substances. Efflux (brain-to-blood) transporters further block circulating toxins from entering the CNS and help to rid the CNS of toxins that have been produced locally. Metabolic free water produced by cells in the brain parenchyma, and CSF produced by the choroid plexus, flow through and around the brain to be reabsorbed at the arachnoid villi and by the primitive nasal lymphatics, thus producing a flow of fluid from the CNS to the blood.

Enzymatic activity at the BBBs provides a further level of barrier to some molecules, as exemplified by monoamines. Transporters deliver to the brain not only nutrients but also informational molecules including peptides and regulatory proteins. The endothelial and ependymal cells which form the BBB can also secrete substances into blood, brain interstitial fluid, or CSF.

Thus, the barrier function of the BBB is owed to morphological modifications (lack of fenestrae and macropinocytosis and presence of tight junctions), enzymatic activity, and efflux transporters. Additionally, through their enzymatic, transport, and secretory properties the BBBs have major roles in maintaining brain nutrition, homeostasis, and communication between the CNS and peripheral tissues (Neuwelt *et al.*, 2008). In short, the BBBs are not just barriers, but rather form a blood–brain interface endowed with numerous properties that first separate and then, in a highly regulated way, reconnect the CNS by way of the blood with the peripheral tissues (Figure 4.1).

The Blood–Brain Barrier and the Immune Privileged CNS

The CNS under healthy conditions was once thought to be separated from the immune system in an absolute sense. This separation was considered to be caused by a BBB that itself was absolute. Leukocytes, for example, were thought to enter the CNS only when there was an infection in the brain and only because the BBB had broken down. The flaw in this thinking was that although it appreciated that the BBB prevented the unregulated leakage of circulating substances into the brain, it failed to deal with the fact that simultaneously the BBB regulated entry.

The modern view has replaced an absolute immune privilege enforced by an absolute BBB with a relative, conditional, and contextual immune privilege regulated in part by a blood–brain regulatory interface. For example, leukocytes do not enter the CNS because the BBB is no longer intact and so unable to retain them in the circulation. Rather, communication between activated immune cells and brain endothelial cells orchestrate diapedesis, a complex cell-to-cell interaction in which leukocytes penetrate through brain endothelial cells (Engelhardt, 2008).

The BBBs are a major factor in controlling the entry of leukocytes into the CNS, and these leukocytes can then be a source of CNS cytokines. As such, leukocyte trafficking is one mechanism by which the BBB can be thought of as controlling CNS cytokine levels, albeit an indirect one. This review, however, will concentrate on the direct ways in which the BBB affects the levels of cytokines in the CNS: barrier function and the transport and secretion of cytokines and chemokines.

Restrictive barrier function

The first way that the BBB acts to control brain levels of cytokines is by its physical, restrictive barrier. This is not a barrier that only blocks cytokines or chemokines but is generalized to ions, small molecules, peptides, and other proteins. Small molecules and peptides can to varying extents overcome this barrier by melding with membranes that form the BBB and passing through by the mechanism of transmembrane diffusion. The ideal molecule for using this mechanism is small and lipid-soluble. The largest molecule shown to have some degree of penetration across the BBB is cytokine-induced neutrophil chemoattractant-1 (Pan and Kastin, 2001) at 7.8 kDa. However, increasing molecular weight generally penalizes penetration.

One cytokine for which there is virtually no penetration of the BBB is interleukin (IL)-2. Interestingly, a number of mechanisms combine to prevent IL-2 from crossing the BBB (Banks, Niehoff, and Zalcman, 2004). In the absence of a blood-to-brain transporter, the large size and low lipid-solubility of IL-2 would keep transmembrane penetration quite low. Another mechanism that prevents blood-borne IL-2 from accumulating in the CNS is a robust enzymatic barrier. Finally, IL-2 is transported out of the brain by a saturable efflux system. This makes IL-2 the only cytokine to date discovered to have its saturable transport system pointing in the brain-to-blood direction. The combination of a physical barrier, an enzymatic barrier, and a brain-to-blood transporter combine to prevent IL-2 from crossing the BBB.

Whether disruption can allow blood-borne cytokines significantly increased access to the CNS probably depends on the specific cytokine. Disruption can allow albumin, a molecule that at about 60 kDa is roughly four times larger than classic cytokines such as IL-1 or tumor necrosis factor α (TNF-α), to enter the brain in measurable amounts. IL-2, otherwise excluded from the CNS by multiple mechanisms, enters the CNS in measurable amounts when the BBB is disrupted by injecting sodium dodecylsulfate (Kobiler *et al.*, 1989). However, when transport systems dominate a substance's equilibrium between the CNS and blood, disruption has little effect. This has been illustrated both for a brain-to-blood efflux pump, in which case the efflux pump can easily handle the extra influx from a disrupted BBB, and for drug influx, in which case the normal rates of entry are so great that the amount contributed by disruption is negligible.

A special area of BBB–neuroimmune interactions resides at the circumventricular organs. (CVOs) (Banks, 2001). These are small areas of the brain (the median eminence, the subfornical organ, the neurohypophysis, the pineal gland, the area postrema, the organum vasculosum of the lamina terminalis, and the subcomissural organ) where their capillary beds do not form a BBB or a barrier less tight than in other regions of the brain. Circulating cytokines can enter these areas to interact directly with the cells of the CNS (Blatteis *et al.*, 1983). The CVOs are delineated from the rest of the CNS by a tanycytic layer, which, for all practical purposes, is another arm of the BBB in addition to the vascular and blood–CSF barriers (Rodriguez, Blazquez, and Guerra, 2010). All together, they comprise about 5% of the brain by weight. However, the CVOs are integrated with the rest of the CNS and both receive and send neuronal input.

Box 4.2 Circumventricular Organs: Another Kind of Blood–Brain Interface

The CVOs are areas of the brain in which the capillaries that course through them do not express the blood–brain barrier phenotype. These small areas tend to not be as leaky as peripheral tissues, but still considerably more leaky than CNS tissues. As a result, the cells within the CVO are in intimate contact with circulating substances. Neurons residing in the CVO project to areas far removed from the CVO and other neurons project nerve terminals to the CVO. As a result, the CVO can act as both an early-warning system for changes in the circulation and also communicate information gleaned from the circulation to areas deep within the brain. The CVOs have major influences on emesis (responding to toxins appearing in the blood), thirst and salt hunger, and appetite (the anorectic effects of amylin are largely mediated through a CVO). However, one way that the CVOs do not communicate intimately with the rest of the CNS is by unrestricted diffusion. Molecules entering a CVO are blocked from diffusing to non-CVO regions by a tanycytic barrier that delimits the CVO from other brain regions. Whether the tanycytic barrier, like the vascular and CSF barriers, contains transporters, enzymes, and secretory properties are important areas of investigation.

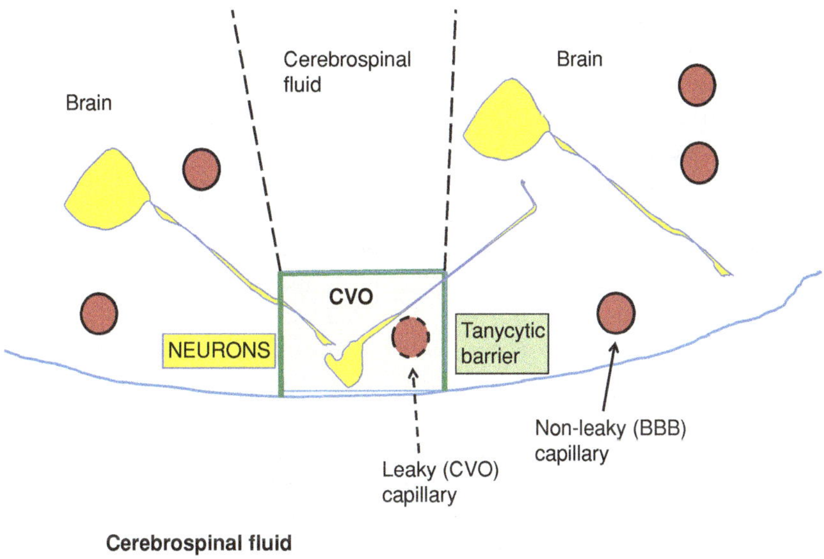

In summary, the barrier function of the BBB prevents the free leakage of blood-borne cytokines into the CNS. This, in turn, sets the stage for the BBB to contribute to cytokine levels in brain by two other mechanisms: the controlled blood-to-brain transport of cytokines, and secretion by the cells which form the BBB.

The transport of cytokines across the BBB

Numerous cytokines have been shown, by several labs, to cross the BBB. The first cytokines to be discovered to have blood-to-brain transport systems were the IL-1 molecules (α and β), IL-6, and TNF-α (Banks, Kastin, and Broadwell,1995). Three separate systems were shown to transport each of these three groups of cytokines. Many other cytokines and chemokines have been shown to cross the BBB, usually by way of a saturable transport system. To date, most transporters are unique for a given cytokine; that is, many cytokines are not sharing a small number of transporters. One exception to this rule is the IL-1 family in that IL-1α, IL-1β, and IL-1 receptor antagonist cross-inhibit each other's transport activity. This indicates that they are either transported by a single transporter or a family of transporters with overlapping affinity (Banks, Kastin, and Broadwell, 1995).

The nature of the transport protein is often not known. In some cases the transporter is the same protein that functions in other cells as the receptor. In other cases the transporter is a protein different from the receptor. For example, mice which do not express the epidermal growth factor (EGF) receptor still transport EGF across the BBB (Pan and Kastin, 1999).

Cytokine transporters as a rule have a heterogeneous distribution within the CNS. Furthermore, this distribution differs among cytokines. For example, the uptake of TNF-α by the hypothalamus is 10 times faster than its uptake by the parietal cortex. Uptake of IL-1 is fastest by the pons medulla, but two regions of the brain in the CD-1 mouse (a strain of the standard white lab mouse), the striatum and midbrain, do not take up IL-1. The SAMP8 mouse, a strain used as a model of Alzheimer's disease, also does not take up IL-1 at the hippocampus, thalamus, hypothalamus, and occipital cortex. Thus, cytokine transport across the BBB shows brain region differences, differences among cytokines, and differences among mouse strains.

Diseases alter the rate at which cytokines are transported across the BBB (Pan and Kastin, 2008). As mentioned about, the SAMP8 has a more limited regional distribution of IL-1 transport than the CD-1. Mice in which experimental allergic encephalitis, a model of multiple sclerosis, has been induced have a greatly increased transport rate of TNF that mirrors the onset and recovery of clinical disease. Spinal cord injury and other insults to the CNS result in altered transport of cytokines.

These variations in cytokine transport rates are assumed to be important in the neuroimmunology of cytokine actions. One example of this is work demonstrating that transport of IL-1 across the BBB produces CNS effects (Banks *et al.*, 2001). The area of the brain with the fastest transport rate for IL-1 is the posterior division of the septum (PDS). We have shown that cytokine injected into the blood stream crosses the BBB to act within the PDS to produce deficits in memory (Banks, Farr, La Scola, and Morley, 2001). This exogenous IL-1 also stimulates the release of endogenous IL-1 that further impairs memory. In these experiments, it was not determined whether the endogenous cytokine was released from peripheral or CNS sources. However, a similar pattern was found for the neurotoxic effects of TNF (Qin *et al.*, 2007). That paper showed that blood-borne TNF crossed the BBB to induce release of TNF from CNS sources, which in turn produced neurotoxic effects in dopamine cells of the substantia nigra.

The above work illustrates several important implications of cytokine transport across the BBB (Figure 4.2): 1) such transport participates in the neuroimmune axis (the IL-1 work illustrates its participation in a feature of sickness behavior); 2) transport can contribute to neurodegenerative processes (the TNF work illustrates how it could participate in Parkinson's disease); 3) it may be a general feature that cytokine crossing the BBB reinforces its level by stimulating further release from sources endogenous to the CNS. Thus, the relatively small amounts of cytokine crossing the BBB may be a signal that releases larger stores from within the CNS.

Secretion of immunoactive substances by the BBBs

An emerging area in BBB–neuroimmune relations is the study of immunoactive secretions by the cells that comprise the BBB. Cells that are secretory include the endothelial cells of the vascular BBB, the ependymal cells of the blood–CSF barrier, and the tanycytes of the tanycytic

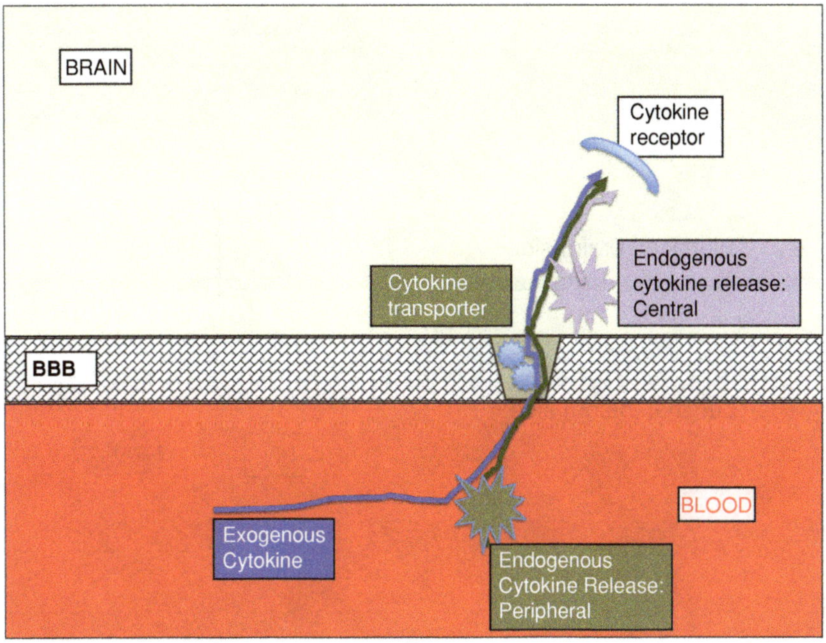

Figure 4.2 Schematic relations among BBB transporters and peripheral and central sources of cytokines. Exogenous cytokines can stimulate the release of endogenous cytokines in the periphery. Some exogenous and endogenous cytokines cross the BBB directly. Cytokines crossing the BBB can stimulate the release of cytokines from CNS sources. Cytokines from all these sources can act at CNS receptors.

CVO barriers. Immunoactive substances secreted include cytokines, chemokines, nitric oxide, and prostaglandins (Dorheim, Tracey, Pollock, and Grammas, 1994; Mcguire *et al.*, 2003; Reyes Fabry, and Coe, 1999). Some of these substances are constitutively secreted, and many are stimulated by lipopolysaccharide (LPS). Stimulants such as LPS can act at either the brain side or the blood side, and secretion likewise can be either into the CNS or into the peripheral side.

BBB cells are unique cells in the body in that while one cell membrane faces into the CNS, the other cell membrane interfaces with blood-borne products. As a result, BBB cells can receive information from one side, but secrete into the other (Figure 4.3). For example, HIV-1 interacting with the luminal side of the BBB can induce release of endothelin-1 from the abluminal side (Didier *et al.*, 2002); LPS applied to the brain side of monolayers of cultured brain endothelial cells induces release of LPS from the blood side. Thus, the cells of the BBB are able to relay signals from one side of the neuroimmune axis to the other, and so the BBB forms a unique aspect of CNS–peripheral tissue communication.

Secretions from the vascular BBB regulate the temperature effects of IL-1 and LPS, the transfer of HIV-1 across the BBB, and may influence appetite. IL-1 or LPS circulating in the blood stimulates cyclooxygenase-2 (COX-2) production in brain endothelial cells. These endothelial cells then secrete prostaglandin-E2 into brain interstitial fluid, which then induces fever (Cao, Watanabe, Yamagata, and Matsumura, 1997). LPS increases the rate at which HIV-1 as free virus crosses the vascular BBB. LPS induces brain endothelial cells to secrete

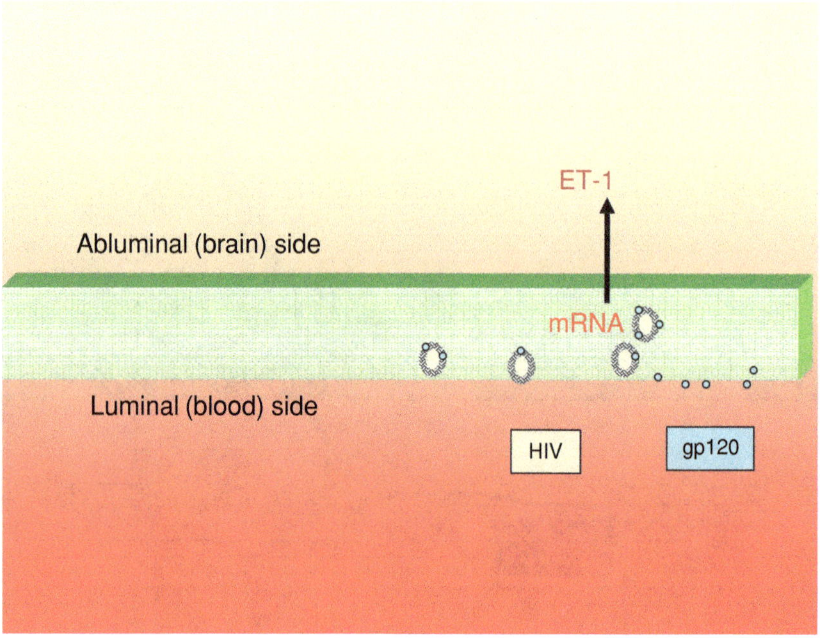

Figure 4.3 BBB secretions as an axis in neuroimmune communication. HIV-1 or its surface glycoprotein gp120 acts at the luminal surface of brain endothelial cells grown in a monolayer culture. BBB mRNA expression for endothelin-1 (ET-1) is then increased and subsequently the protein is secreted from the abluminal side. By receiving a proinflammatory stimulus from the blood and secreting neuroimmune substances into the brain, BBB secretions can relay information from the periphery into the CNS, forming a portion of the neuroimmune axis.

GM-CSF and IL-6 (unpublished data). GM-CSF and IL-6 then act in paracrine fashion at the luminal surface of the brain endothelial cells to induce the MAPK pathways which underlie the ability of HIV-1 to cross. BBB secretions may also modulate the effects of adiponectin on appetite regulation. Adiponectin crosses the BBB in very small amounts, less than the rate at which albumin crosses the BBB, but is able to influence feeding. Adiponectin also induces the release of IL-6 from the brain side of brain endothelial cells. However, adiponectin and IL-6 have the opposite effects on feeding, and so in this instance cytokine secretion may be acting as a counter-regulatory mechanism to the inducer.

Other mechanisms by which the BBB could control brain cytokines

The BBB has other mechanisms that would affect cytokine levels in the brain. However, these are indirect or are ultimately mediated through one of the mechanisms outlined above. For example, the BBB interacts with immune cells to control and regulate their trafficking through the CNS. This regulation not only affects the number of immune cells entering the CNS, but is also selective for type and activation status. By these processes, the BBB indirectly influences the contribution that CNS immune cells make to brain cytokine levels.

The BBB also influences the ability of drugs to enter the CNS (Greig *et al.*, 1995). Some of these, such as nonsteroidal anti-inflammatory drugs, in turn affect the ability of cells to secrete or respond to cytokines. Similarly, the BBB regulates brain levels of endogenous substances that influence neuroinflammatory status. An example of this is amyloid-β peptide. The BBB transports amyloid-β peptide both into and out of the CNS. Amyloid-β peptide, in turn, induces oxidative stress and neuroinflammation in the CNS.

Conclusions

The BBBs are involved in the regulation of brain cytokine levels through several mechanisms. The BBB first acts as a barrier to cytokines, preventing their unregulated leakage into the tissue bed of the CNS. The BBB then has several saturable transport systems that are highly selective for cytokines. Of those currently known, all but the one for IL-2 is directed in the blood-to-brain region. Finally, the cells which comprise the BBBs can themselves secrete cytokines directly into the CNS. Each of these mechanisms are themselves influenced, affected, and regulated by immune cells and immune-active substances.

References

Abbott, N.J. (2005). Dynamics of CNS barriers: evolution, differentiation, and modulation. *Cellular and Molecular Neurobiology*, 25, 5–23.

Banks, W.A. (2001). Cytokines, CVOs, and the blood–brain barrier. In R. Ader, D.L. Felten, and N. Cohen, (eds.) *Psychoneuroimmunology* (pp. 483–497). San Diego: Academic Press.

Banks, W.A., Farr, S.A., La Scola, M.E., and Morley, J.E. (2001). Intravenous human interleukin-1 alpha impairs memory processing in mice: Dependence on blood–brain barrier transport into posterior division of the septum. *Journal of Pharmacology and Experimental Therapeutics*, 299, 536–541.

Banks, W.A., Kastin, A.J. and Broadwell, R.D. (1995). Passage of cytokines across the blood–brain barrier. *Neuroimmunomodulation*, 2, 241–248.

Banks, W.A., Niehoff, M.L., and Zalcman, S. (2004). Permeability of the mouse blood–brain barrier to murine interleukin-2: Predominance of a saturable efflux system. *Brain,Behavior, and Immunity*, 18, 434–442.

Banks, W.A., Ortiz, L., Plotkin, S.R. and Kastin, A.J. (1991). Human interleukin (IL) 1 alpha, murine IL-1 alpha and murine IL-1 beta are transported from blood to brain in the mouse by a shared saturable mechanism. *Journal of Pharmacology and Experimental Therapeutics*, 259, 988–996.

Blatteis, C.M., Bealer, S.L., Hunter, W.S., Llanos, Q.J., Ahokas, R.A., and Mashburn, T.A., Jr. (1983). Suppression of fever after lesions of the anteroventral third ventricle in guinea pigs. *Brain Research Bulletin*, 11, 519–526.

Cao, C., Watanabe, Y., Yamagata, K., and Matsumura, K. (1997). Involvement of cyclooxygenase-2 in LPS-induced fever and regulation of its mRNA by LPS in the rat brain. *American Journal of Physiology*, 272, R1712–R1725.

Davson, H., and Segal, M.B. (1996a). *Physiology of the CSF and Blood–Brain Barriers*, Boca Raton: CRC Press.

Davson, H., and Segal, M.B. (1996b). The proteins and other macromolecules of the CSF. *Physiology of the CSF and the blood–brain barrier*. Boca Raton: CRC Press.

Didier, N., Banks, W.A., Creminon, C., Dereuddre-Bosquet, N., and Mabondzo, A. (2002). HIV-1-induced production of endothelin-1 in an in vitro model of the human blood–brain barrier. *Neuroreport*, 13, 1179–1183.

Dorheim, M.A., Tracey, W.R., Pollock, J.S., and Grammas, P. (1994). Nitric oxide synthase activity is elevated in brain microvessels in Alzheimer's disease. *Biochemical and Biophysical Research Communications*, 205, 659–665.

Engelhardt, B. (2008). The blood–central nervous system barriers actively control immune cell entry into the central nervous system. *Current Pharmaceutical Design*, 14, 1555–1565.

Greig, N.H., Brossi, A., Pei, X.F., Ingram, D.K., and Soncrant, T.T. (1995). Designing drugs for optimal nervous system activity. In J. Greenwood, D.J. Begley, and M.B. Segal, (eds.) *New Concepts of a Blood–Brain Barrier* (pp. 251–264). New York: Plenum Press.

Kobiler, D., Lustig, S., Gozes, Y., Ben Nathan, D., and Akov, Y. (1989). Sodium dodecylsulphate induces a breach in the blood–brain barrier and enables a West Nile virus variant to penetrate into mouse brain. *Brain Research*, 496, 314–316.

McGuire, T.R., Trickler, W.J., Hock, L., Vrana, A., Hoie, E.B., and Miller, D.W. (2003). Release of prostaglandin E-2 in bovine brain endothelial cells after exposure to three unique forms of the antifungal drug amphotericin-B: role of COX-2 in amphotericin-B induced fever. *Life Sciences*, 72, 2581–2590.

Neuwelt, E., Abbott, N.J., Abrey, L., Banks, W.A., Blakley, B., Davis, T., et al. (2008). Strategies to advance translational research into brain barriers. *Lancet Neurology*, 7, 84–96.

Pan, W., and Kastin, A.J. (1999). Entry of EGF into brain is rapid and saturable. *Peptides*, 20, 1091–1098.

Pan, W., and Kastin, A.J. (2001). Changing the chemokine gradient: CINC1 crosses the blood–brain barrier. *Journal of Neuroimmunology*, 115, 64–70.

Pan, W., and Kastin, A.J. (2008). Cytokine transport across the injured blood–spinal cord barrier. *Current Pharmaceutical Design*, 14, 1620–1624.

Qin, L., Wu, X., Block, M.L., Liu, Y., Breese, G.R., Hong, J.S. et al. (2007). Systemic LPS causes chronic neuroinflammation and progressive neurodegeneration. *Glia*, 55, 453–462.

Reyes, T.M., Fabry, Z., and Coe, C.L. (1999). Brain endothelial cell production of a neuroprotective cytokine, interleukin-6, in response to noxious stimuli. *Brain Research*, 851, 215–220.

Rodriguez, E.M., Blazquez, J.L., and Guerra, M. (2010). The design of barriers in the hypothalamus allows the median eminence and the arcuate nucleus to enjoy private milieus: the former opens to the portal blood and the latter to the cerebrospinal fluid. *Peptides*, 31, 757–76.

5

The Immune–Neuroendocrine Network in Health and Disease

Adriana del Rey and Hugo O. Besedovsky

Division of Immunophysiology, Institute of Physiology and Pathophysiology, Medical Faculty, Philipps University, Marburg, Germany

Introduction

The immune system contributes to the maintenance of the constancy of the molecular and cellular components of the organism, and adapts to changeable environmental and endogenous conditions. As with all physiological systems, the immune system is under neuroendocrine control and it interacts and works in a concerted action with other systems of the body. Indeed, immune cells possess receptors for most hormones, neurotransmitters, and neuropeptides, allowing them to mediate immunoregulatory signals. Conversely, products of immune cells can affect mechanisms that are directly or indirectly under the control of the brain. There is also evidence that mediators that were initially discovered in one system can also be produced by the other system. Although the immune system is permanently in operation, its level of activity increases when it is challenged by foreign or modified self-antigens, when there is tissue damage, or when it is exposed to agents that cause inflammation. Neuroendocrine responses, which vary according to the type of immune mechanism activated, are triggered when the immune response reaches certain intensity. In the following sections we refer to aspects related to immune–neuroendocrine interactions, such as their control and integration at brain levels and the pathological consequences of their disruption. To illustrate these aspects, we use examples that are mainly based on our own work.

Historical Perspective and Views: The Immune and Nervous System Talk to Each Other

More than 30 years ago, we approached the question of whether and, if so, how, the immune system can communicate with the nervous system and affect its functioning, and, in consequence, the neuroendocrine mechanisms known at that time to affect immune processes. Our strategy was to study possible changes in endocrine, autonomic, and brain activity that could be causally related to the immune response. Immunization with innocuous antigens was mandatory to exclude potential confounding factors, such as neural and endocrine responses caused by a disease itself, e.g. tissue damage, or the stress of feeling sick. This approach allowed us to

The Wiley-Blackwell Handbook of Psychoneuroimmunology, First Edition. Edited by Alexander W. Kusnecov and Hymie Anisman.

detect changes in the activity of the hypothalamic–pituitary–adrenal (HPA) and -thyroid axes, and in the activity of defined brain neurons triggered by the immune response itself. Later, we observed that neuroendocrine changes also occur during infectious, inflammatory, and autoimmune diseases, indicating that immune/inflammatory responses of sufficient magnitude are followed by neuroendocrine responses.

The next step was to identify which immune-derived messengers could convey afferent information to the brain. At a time when cytokines were not available in pure form, we tested whether conditioned medium from immune cells stimulated *in vitro* were capable of affecting neuroendocrine mechanisms when administered to a naïve host. These studies showed that products from activated immune cells can stimulate the HPA axis, affect the sympathetic nervous system (SNS), and alter catecholaminergic neurons in the brain. Other strategies were to study neuroendocrine responses following administration of sublethal doses of endotoxin to hosts depleted from macrophages (Derijk *et al.*, 1991), or injection to normal hosts of supernatants from Newcastle Disease virus-stimulated lymphocytes, in which IL-1 was neutralized. In both models, the stimulation of the HPA axis was abrogated or significantly diminished. It was later found that several immune-cell-derived products can, directly or indirectly, affect neural and endocrine mechanisms that are under brain control. (References documenting these aspects can be found in Besedovsky and del Rey, 1996 and 2007.)

From a physiological point of view, it was still necessary to show that the changes in the levels of hormones, neurotransmitters, and neuropeptides that are mediated by immune cell products have an immunoregulatory consequence and can influence the course of a disease. For example, it has been shown that an increase in corticosterone levels during the immune response to an antigen is necessary for the manifestation of antigenic competition. This phenomenon, in which injection of an antigen inhibits the immune response to an unrelated antigen administered sequentially, is abrogated when the increase in glucocorticoid levels induced by the first antigen is impeded by adrenalectomy. We interpreted these results as evidence that the HPA axis contributes to impose limits to the activation of the immune system. Today, there is multiple evidence of the immunoregulatory and pathophysiological relevance of the changes in endogenous neuroendocrine mediators induced by immune cell products.

In recent years we have returned to our original concept that immune–neuroendocrine feedback/forward responses and autonomic reflexes are the expression of a network of interactions between the immune, endocrine, and nervous systems (Besedovsky and Sorkin, 1977). Each of these systems operates as a network in and of itself, and we shall refer to them as "intrinsic networks." In the superimposed immune–neuroendocrine (INE) network, the intrinsic networks are connected with each other at multiple levels. Thus, a perturbation in one intrinsic network requires parallel readjustments in the others in order to assure changes towards a new level of stability. For example, stimulation of the immune network impacts on the endocrine system intrinsic network, which consequently changes its level of activity. In physiological terms, interactions between intrinsic networks result in changes leading to another state of equilibrium that enable better coping with the new condition. This concept, which has been called "allostasis" (adaptation through change), and which has a cost, has been related to the pernicious effects of chronic stress. However, in our view, when the perturbation occurs primarily at the level of the immune system, which in many cases implies a shift from health to disease, the situation is more complex. Neuroendocrine adjustments are not solely based on a passive transmission of perturbations in the immune network to the other intrinsic networks resulting in an adaptive redistribution of forces until a new equilibrium is established. In our view, this is an active, preprogrammed process. As we shall discuss, during diseases that trigger immune/inflammatory responses there is an active change not only in the levels of hormones or neurotransmitters, but also in the set-points that control and regulate neuroendocrine mechanisms. This resetting of set-points leads to the stabilization of neuroendocrine and metabolic variables around levels that are more adequate during disease than during health, and that, within strict limits, favor the operation of the immune system. However, when, for example, infectious diseases are prolonged, the new level of stability triggered by immune cell products can become deleterious, since it is established at the expense of other components of the network that are essential for life.

In the following sections we discuss some recent examples, mainly based on work in our own and associated laboratories, showing that immune cell products are part of a permanently operative INE network of signals during both health and disease. We shall provide evidence that the immune system can take the command of homeostasis during disease, an effect that is only adaptive to a certain extent. We shall also propose that some of the mediators of the immune system that are produced at the level of the CNS affect interactions between neural cells, contribute to brain physiology, and serve to integrate immune and psychosensorial signals under physiologic and pathologic conditions.

Cytokines Mediate a Resetting of the INE Network During Immune and Inflammatory Responses

While hormones, neurotransmitters, and neuropeptides can convey efferent regulatory signals to the immune system, mediators released by immune cells constitute the afferent input in this network. When the immune system becomes overactivated, a condition usually linked to disease, the impact of immune signals on the INE network increases and a new level of stability is reached. The response to dangerous conditions such as infections is very demanding in terms of energy (Kominsky, Campbell, and Colgan, 2010) and its duration is unpredictable. The evidence discussed below supports the existence of mechanisms that under disease conditions take command of homeostasis by fixing the stabilization of the network at a level that favors the immune system. Furthermore, there are indications that a neuronal–cytokine network also operates in the CNS. This central network can receive immune and neuronal inputs and can modulate relevant physiologic functions of the brain.

Cytokines can take command of homeostasis during disease

The concept of homeostasis, a term coined by W. Cannon, derives from observations by C. Bernard that although body temperature or the concentration of sugar in blood can be raised or lowered by a number of processes, the net outcome of these processes is that physiological parameters remain within certain limits. As mentioned, this concept evolved to account for more dynamic and adaptive views that emphasize the tendency of organisms to stabilize essential biological values at a given, well-adapted, level. Indeed, levels of a biological parameter that are optimal at different stages of life under health conditions may not be adequate during diseases that induce a change in the activity of the immune system. Under these conditions it is necessary to reset the control systems. There is evidence that such resetting is an active process mediated by immune cell products. The capacity of cytokines to reset thermoregulation is broadly accepted. We shall concentrate here on another aspect, namely the capacity of immune-derived cytokines to reset glucose homeostasis, a process that, according to our studies, is predominately mediated by IL-1 (for references see Besedovsky and del Rey, 2010; del Rey and Besedovsky, 1989; del Rey *et al.*, 2006b).

Glucose is the main fuel for immune cells, and the immune response is a process highly demanding in terms of energy (Kominsky, Campbell, and Colgan, 2010). Glucose uptake markedly increases in activated immune cells, which use predominantly the insulin-independent glucose transporter GLUT1. We have shown that exogenous and endogenous IL-1 can induce a prolonged hypoglycemia, a surprising effect considering the capacity of the cytokine to increase glucocorticoid levels. IL-1-induced hypoglycemia is long lasting and more prolonged than that caused by insulin (Figure 5.1A). On the other hand, there is evidence that, by acting in an autocrine/paracrine fashion, IL-1 can increase glucose uptake by several types of cells, including immune cells.

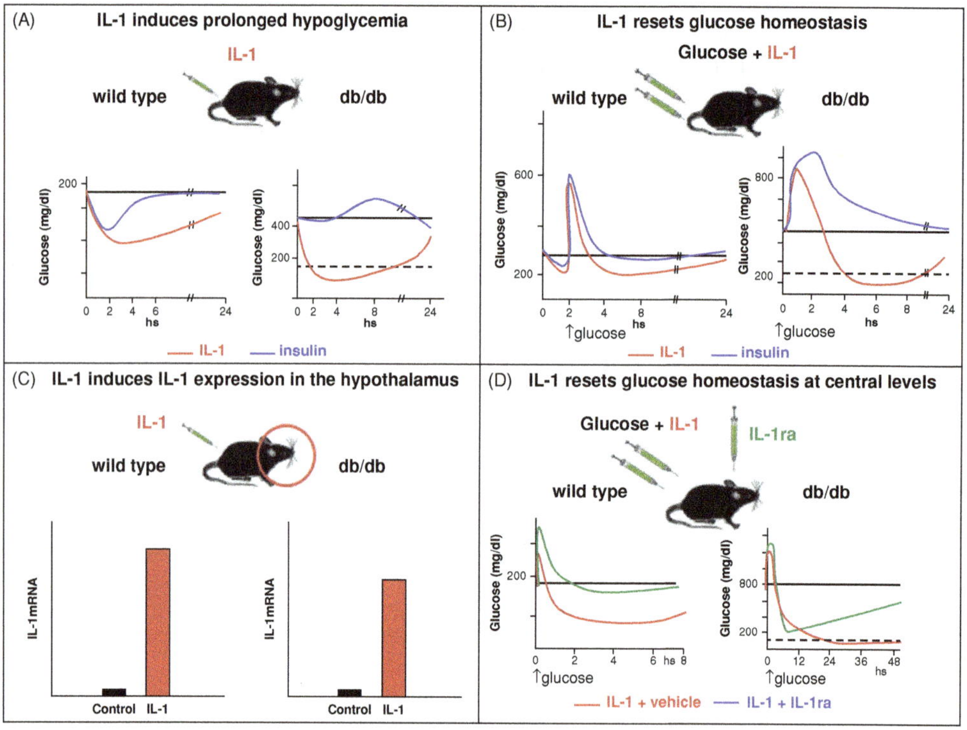

Figure 5.1 IL-1 resets glucose homeostasis. A) IL-1 induces a prolonged hypoglycemia in normal (wild type) and insulin-resistant, Type 2 diabetic (*db/db*) mice, as compared to insulin. B) Wild type mice received IL-1 or insulin at time 0 and a glucose load 2 hours later. IL-1-injected mice quickly returned to the hypoglycemic levels induced by IL-1. *Db/db* mice received IL-1 or insulin and a glucose load injected simultaneously. Diabetic mice not only returned quickly to their initial hyperglycemic values but also reached levels comparable to those of the normoglycemic wild type mice. C) Intraperitoneal injection of IL-1 induces IL-1 gene expression in the hypothalamus of normal and diabetic mice. D) Blockade of IL-1 receptors in the brain of normal and diabetic mice interferes with the effect of IL-1 on the host response to a glucose load. The horizontal gray bars in A, B and D indicate the range of the corresponding controls. The dotted gray line in the graphics showing the results in diabetic mice indicates the range of the normoglycemic animals. (The original data can be found in del Rey and Besedovsky, 1989, and del Rey *et al.*, 2006b).

The hypoglycemic effect of IL-1 is not mediated by insulin since it is also observed in insulin-resistant, Type 2 diabetic animals (Figure 5.1A), and is dissociable from pyrogenic, anorexic, and inflammatory effects of the cytokine. The dissociation of hypoglycemia from deleterious inflammatory effects of IL-1 is important because it has been shown that this cytokine is involved in the pathogenesis of Type 1 diabetes by affecting pancreatic β cells (for references see Besedovsky and del Rey, 2010).

During diseases that induce a strong activation of the immune system, such as infections, the priority is to provide energy, predominantly derived from glycolysis, to support immune cell activity. Indeed, the immune system is probably the only bodily system that requires cell proliferation and clonal expansion to fulfill its physiological functions. The amount of energy required for these processes is illustrated by the fact that during infective, inflammatory, and autoimmune diseases, secondary lymphoid organs grow (lymph node enlargement, splenomegaly), leading in some cases to a severalfold increase in mass compared to healthy individuals. At peripheral levels, the effect of IL-1 is mediated by increased glucose transport in GLUT1- and GLUT3-expressing tissues, including immune cells (Fox *et al.*, 2005).

While IL-3 and IL-7 contribute to provide energy for hematopoiesis and to quiescent immune cells respectively (Fox *et al.*, 2005), there is evidence that IL-1 can supply fuel support during immune responses, since it can induce glucose uptake in lymphoid tissue (Metzger *et al.*, 2004). Besides its pro-inflammatory and adjuvant actions, and its capacity to activate a cytokine network, IL-1 acts as a co-stimulatory signal for T cells, either directly or through interactions with other co-stimulatory molecules, such as B7/CD28, and is an inducer of IL-2 and IL-17 (Dinarello, 2009). Its capacity to induce glucose uptake suggests that IL-1 produced by antigen-presenting cells, and other cells, is a major candidate for increasing the supply of glucose to immune cells during immune and inflammatory responses (see references in Besedovsky and del Rey, 2010). Although insulin is an important growth factor for immune cells, the effect of IL-1 is largely independent from that of insulin. As mentioned, both molecules act via different glucose transporters, and the hypoglycemic effect of IL-1 is proportionally even more profound in insulin-resistant diabetic animals (del Rey and Besedovsky, 1989).

There is evidence derived from genetically manipulated mice to show the long lasting metabolic consequences of increased or reduced IL-1 signals. Long-lasting IL-1 overproduction in normal mice results in hypoglycemia, increased glucose utilization, and a lean phenotype (Metzger *et al.*, 2004), whereas IL-1 receptor type I knockout, or transgenic mice which overexpress IL-1 receptor antagonist (IL-1ra), develop Type 2 diabetes (Garcia *et al.*, 2006, Matsuki, Horai, Sudo, and Iwakura, 2003). However, in genetically predisposed individuals, the local inflammatory effect of IL-1 on pancreatic β cells can contribute to the pathogenesis of Type 1 diabetes (see references in Besedovsky and del Rey, 2010). A local ectopic over production of IL-1 in adipose tissue and pancreatic islets of animals subject to a high-fat diet also induces reduction of insulin signals (resistance and decreased production) and favors the development of Type 2 diabetes.

Considering that glucose homeostasis is tightly regulated by efficient counterregulatory mechanisms, the long lasting hypoglycemic effects of IL-1 are difficult to explain unless it is postulated that the cytokine could change the set-point of glucoregulation. We have explored this possibility and showed that a change in the set-point induced by IL-1 is clearly manifested during a glucose load. Normal and Type 2 diabetic animals treated with IL-1 and challenged with a glucose load not only show accelerated glucose clearance (probably due to a peripheral component) but return to the hypoglycemic values attained by injection of the cytokine (del

Rey *et al.*, 2006b) (Figure 5.1B). Administration of insulin at doses that induce a comparable hypoglycemia does not indicate any change in the glucoregulatory set-point, since animals return to the preset euglycemic values after the glucose load. As mentioned, IL-1 also dramatically reduces hyperglycemia in insulin-resistant diabetic mice such as *db/db* and *ob/ob* mice. This effect also involves a resetting of glucose homeostasis. In fact, *db/db* mice treated with IL-1 and receiving a glucose load, reach glucose values comparable to normal heterozygous litter-mates, levels that are maintained for at least 24 hours. Again, no comparable effects result from insulin administration (Figure 5.1B). Further evidence that IL-1 can change the set-point of glucoregulation is that the counterregulation to hypoglycemia seems to be inhibited by this cytokine. Although an early counterregulatory response, involving increased glucagon, catecholamine, and glucocorticoid secretion is observed after IL-1 administration, these changes are surprisingly short-lasting and disappear after 4 hours, about the time of maximal reduction in glucose blood levels induced by IL-1. In normal rats, IL-1-induced hypoglycemia is less marked, but it is paralleled by a clear compensatory decrease in insulin secretion (del Rey and Besedovsky, 1987). An initial hyperglycemia that can be followed by hypoglycemia is noticed in septic patients, in which different cytokines are overproduced, but there is an important increase in glucose consumption that is not mediated by insulin (McGuinness, 2005). In the following section, we provide more direct evidence that IL-1 changes the set-point of glucoregulation by acting at brain levels.

There is also evidence indicating that IL-1 can reset other homeostatic mechanisms, such the response of the HPA axis to stress (Tilders and Schmidt, 1998), and the response of cardiovascular centers to baroreceptor signals (Rogausch, Vo, del Rey, and Besedovsky, 2000). Taken together, it is becoming clear that under conditions in which the input of immune signals into the INE network is increased, there is a resetting of the activity of the network. This resetting is expected to be more adaptive than the previous equilibrium since it favors the activity of the immune system, for example during infectious diseases. However, if the resetting of the INE network induced by immune signals is prolonged, it can result, as we discuss below, in deleterious effects, since such resetting is done at the expense of other physiological mechanisms. This view is schematically represented in Figure 5.2, taking as an example the effects of IL-1 on glucose homeostasis.

The neuronal–cytokine network in the healthy brain

Several decades ago, it was discovered that cytokines can be produced in the brain during pathological conditions. It is now recognized that glial cells (microglia and astrocytes) and even some neurons can produce cytokines such as IL-1, TNF-α and IL-6. There is now evidence that these cytokines can also be produced in the "healthy" brain, and can be induced peripherally during an immune response, and centrally during increased neuronal activity at levels that can affect CNS functions.

Peripheral immune signals mediate cytokine production and action in the healthy brain More than 15 years ago, it was shown that acute stimulation of peripheral immune cells with LPS induces cytokine production in the hypothalamus (Laye, Parnet, Goujon, and Dantzer, 1994; van Dam, Brouns, Louisse, and Berkenbosch, 1992). We confirmed that even doses of the endotoxin that do not affect the blood–brain barrier induce cytokine production in different brain regions (Pitossi, del Rey, Kabiersch, and Besedovsky, 1997). More recently, we have also shown that during an adaptive immune response, IL-1 and IL-6 are produced in the brain (del

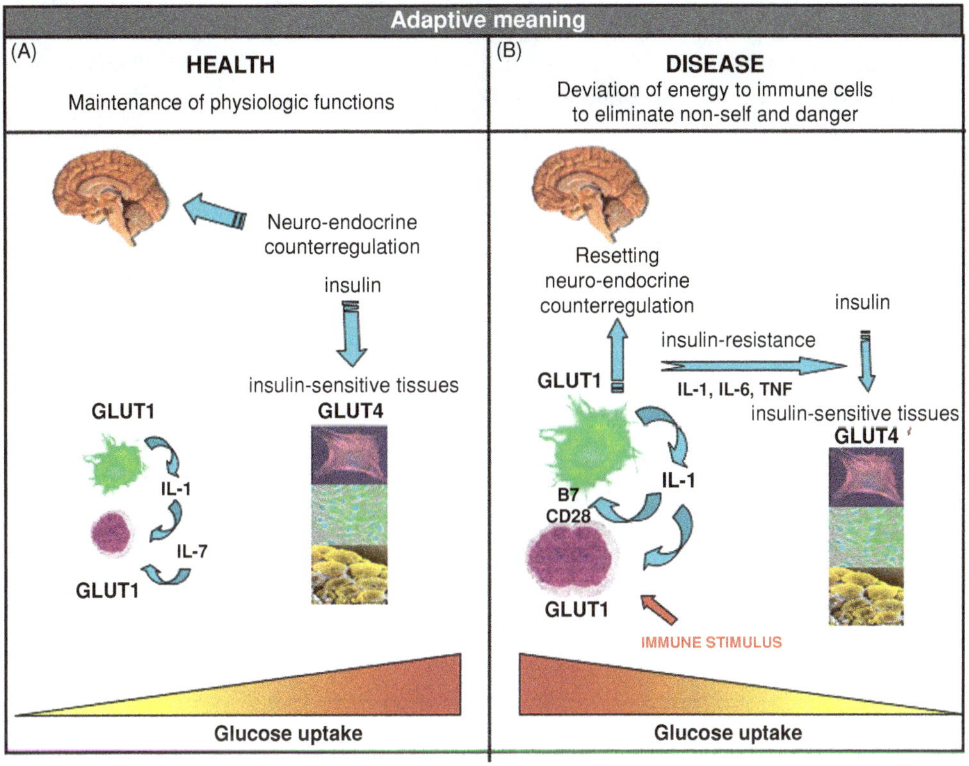

Figure 5.2 Cytokines can take command of homeostasis during disease. A) During health conditions and under basal activity of the immune system, glucose homeostasis is controlled by the classical interplay between insulin and neuroendocrine counterregulatory mechanisms. B) During diseases in which the immune system is overtly activated, IL-1 contributes to divert glucose to immune cells at the expenses of insulin-sensitive tissues. This cytokine can also mediate the resetting of the mechanisms that control glucose homeostasis at brain levels.

Rey *et al.*, 2008) and that chronic neuropathic pain results in the expression of these cytokines along the nociceptive pathway (del Rey *et al.*, 2011). Furthermore, we have shown that there is a type of "memory" that is evoked by a second inflammatory insult, as reflected by a different pattern of cytokine induction in the hypothalamus of animals previously exposed to another pro-inflammatory stimulus (del Rey *et al.*, 2009).

As discussed, IL-1 is capable of changing the set-point of glucoregulation by interfering with endocrine and autonomic counterregulatory mechanisms that are usually triggered during hypoglycemia. Furthermore, the long-lasting reduction in glucose blood levels induced by IL-1 does not trigger the expected compensatory increase in food intake, a behavioral response that occurs, for example, following insulin induced-hypoglycemia. Since neuroendocrine counterregulation and feeding behavior are under brain control, we have explored whether the described change in the set-point of glucoregulation is integrated at CNS levels. Different lines of evidence support this possibility: a) IL-1β gene expression is markedly increased in the hypothalamus of normal and diabetic mice that received IL-1β or LPS administered peripherally (Figure 5.1C); b) IL-1β mRNA transcripts in the hypothalamus negatively correlate with blood glucose levels in normal and diabetic mice treated with IL-1β; c) central administration of IL-1β reduces glucose levels; d) blockade of IL-1 receptors in the brain mediates a quick return to euglycemia after a glucose load in IL-1β-treated, normal and diabetic mice (Figure 5.1D). Taking this evidence together, the described results constitute the first evidence that an immune cell product can reset essential regulatory mechanism such as glucose homeostasis by acting at brain levels (del Rey *et al.*, 2006b).

Neuronal signals mediate cytokine production and action in the healthy brain As mentioned, immune signals can elicit physiologically significant cytokine production in the brain. As a counterpart to this finding, we have studied the converse situation, namely whether signals from activated neurons can also increase cytokine expression in the brain. For this purpose, we used as a model long-term potentiation (LTP) of synaptic activity in the hippocampus, a process characterized by a sustained enhancement in synaptic transmission and postsynaptic neuronal activity following a high-frequency stimulation of afferent fibers. LTP induction enables us to explore whether a long-lasting increase in the responsiveness of a defined population of neurons affects the production of a given cytokine, and whether, in turn, this cytokine can affect the activity of these neurons. A clear increase in IL-1β and IL-6 gene expression, triggered by glutamergic neurons via NMDA receptors, was observed in hippocampal slices and in freely moving rats during the course of LTP (Balschun *et al.*, 2004, Schneider *et al.*, 1998) (Figure 5.3A). More recently, we have detected that IL-1 receptor antagonist (IL-1ra) but not TNF-α, is induced during LTP in freely moving rats (del Rey *et al.*, 2013). These data constitute the

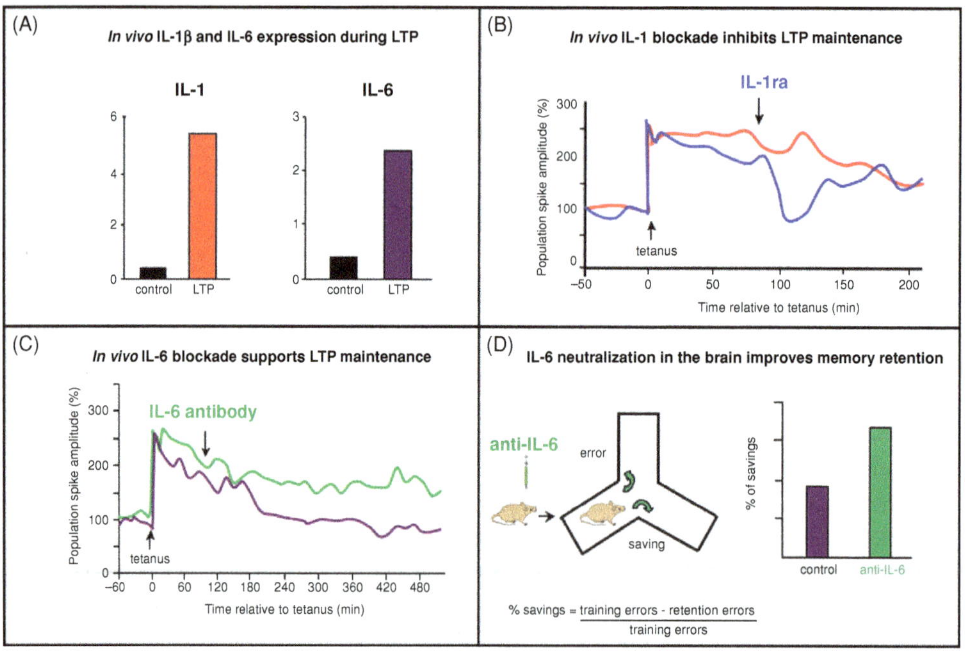

Figure 5.3 Neuronal signals mediate cytokine production and action in the healthy brain. A) IL-1 and IL-6 are expressed in the rat hippocampus during LTP. B) Blockade of IL-1 receptors by i.c.v. injection of IL-1ra inhibits LTP maintenance. C) Neutralization of IL-6 by i.c.v. injection of an IL-6 antibody supports LTP maintenance. D) IL-6 neutralization 90 minutes after the training session improves memory retention in a hippocampal dependent Y-maze spatial alternation task. (The original data can be found in Schneider *et al.*, 1998; and Balschun *et al.*, 2004).

first direct evidence that cytokine gene expression in the brain can be triggered by a presynaptic induced increase in the activity of a discrete population of neurons.

Using IL-1ra, the specific IL-1 receptor antagonist, we found that both *in vivo* and in hippocampal slices, blockade of IL-1 receptors results in inhibition of LTP maintenance (Schneider *et al.*, 1998) (Figure 5.3B). This effect is reversible and occurs only when the antagonist is administered after LTP is triggered, that is at a time when increased IL-1 levels are expected. Studies in Type 1 IL-1 receptor knockout mice, in which LTP cannot be induced, are in line with this finding (Avital *et al.*, 2003).

We have also found that, in contrast to the supportive effect of IL-1, IL-6 contributes to the extinction of a well-consolidated LTP (Balschun *et al.*, 2004) (Figure 5.3C). Collectively, these results strongly suggest that IL-1β and IL-6 control the maintenance of LTP in the brain, a process that is assigned a role in memory formation and in certain types of learning. Furthermore, these studies provide evidence for a physiological, neuromodulatory role for cytokines originally described as immune mediators.

It is necessary to distinguish between studies based on exogenous administration of cytokines and those that focus on the effects of cytokines endogenously produced by brain cells. There is a vast literature showing that exogenous administration *in vivo* and *in vitro* of cytokines can affect LTP induction and synaptic plasticity. Administration of IL-1, IL-2, IFN α and γ, TNF-α, IL-6, and IL-18 inhibits LTP (for references see Besedovsky and del Rey, 2011). These studies, although important from the pharmacological point of view, cannot reliably reveal the effect of cytokines endogenously produced in the brain. In fact, it should be considered that the maintenance of LTP is protein synthesis-dependent and involves the activation of genes in a given sequence and the release of their products in specific quantity.

As in the case of LTP, the effects of cytokine administration on learning, memory, and behavior in general have been extensively investigated (for references see Besedovsky and del Rey, 2011). Again, these pharmacological studies, although of unquestionable clinical relevance, may not reflect the effect of cytokines in the "normal" brain. Only possible physiological effects of endogenous cytokines on memory and learning are discussed below.

As mentioned above, a transient blockade of endogenous IL-1 results in inhibition of LTP maintenance. Considering that it is currently accepted that LTP underlies certain forms of memory, it was predicted that this process would be inhibited in animals in which IL-1 effects cannot be manifested. Several paradigms of memory function and hippocampal plasticity have been studied in IL-1 receptor type I knockout mice (Avital *et al.*, 2003; Yirmiya, Winocur, and Goshen, 2002). Compared to wild type controls, type 1 IL-1 receptor knockout mice display significantly longer latency to reach a hidden platform in the spatial version of the water maze test, and exhibit diminished contextual fear conditioning, but behave similarly to control animals in hippocampal-independent memory tasks. Blockade of IL-1 receptors in the brain of normal animals with IL-1ra administered in the brain and following a learning task (Morris water maze), causes memory impairment only in hippocampal-dependent tasks. IL-1ra causes memory impairment in the passive avoidance response, which also depends on hippocampal functions. Similar results were observed in transgenic mice overexpressing IL-1ra in the brain (for references see Besedovsky and del Rey, 2011). These results suggest that IL-1 signaling in the hippocampus plays a critical role in learning and memory processes (Avital *et al.*, 2003). The same authors have recently reported that enrichment can reverse the alterations in LTP and memory in mice with defective IL-1 signaling, indicating that genetically manipulated animals develop mechanisms that compensate to a certain extent the absence of effects of this cytokine (Goshen *et al.*, 2009).

As discussed above, IL-6 is produced during LTP, and neutralization of the cytokine after tetanization results in a clear prolongation of increased neuronal activity (Balschun *et al.*, 2004). This finding led us to study the role of IL-6 in memory consolidation, and we found that blockade of endogenous IL-6 after hippocampus-dependent spatial alternation learning results in a significant improvement of long-term memory (Balschun *et al.*, 2004) (Figure 5.3D). In agreement with this finding, IL-6 KO mice exhibit a facilitation of radial maze learning (Braida *et al.*, 2004).

In summary, cytokines are induced during increased neuronal activity and affect synaptic strength. The data reported constitute the first evidence that cytokines such as IL-1 and IL-6 are involved in this basic aspect of brain physiology. However, an uncontrolled overexpression of these cytokines during brain diseases results in cognitive deficits that include disturbances in synaptic strength and memory formation.

Taking the described results together with the previously reported evidence that cytokines such as IL-1 and IL-6 can be induced in the brain following stimulation of peripheral immune cells, it can be concluded that there are confluences and interactions between immune and neuronal signals at CNS levels.

Pathophysiological Consequences of Alterations in the INE Network

As in all processes based on the equilibrium between connections in a network of interactions, there could be conditions in which such links are disrupted or unbalanced. When alterations occur in the INE network, as in the example we discuss below, they can be non-adaptive and favor pathologies.

Disruption of immune–brain communication during autoimmune, lymphoproliferative, and inflammatory diseases

We shall discuss here examples in which the connection between sympathetic nerves and immune cells, one of the links of the INE network, is disrupted and can contribute to aggravate the course of autoimmune (AD), lymphoproliferative and inflammatory diseases. Compared to endocrine effects and sexual dimorphism, the relevance of the SNS in the pathogenesis of AD is more limited (for references see del Rey and Besedovsky, 2008).

It has been found that sympathetic activity is inhibited in experimentally induced autoimmune encephalomyelitis (EAE), the best-studied model of multiple sclerosis (MS), and that chemical sympathectomy augments the severity of the disease. In this model, as well as in MS patients, the predominant autoimmune effect is considered to be mediated by T_H1-related cellular responses. On the contrary, systemic lupus erythematosus (SLE) has been mainly associated with a T_H2 shift and increased humoral responses. SLE is a chronic, autoimmune lymphoproliferative disease characterized by exacerbations and remissions. We have used lpr/lpr mice, which develop a genetically determined autoimmune lymphoproliferative disease that shares several characteristics with SLE, to study the possible relevance of noradrenergic innervation for the development and expression of lymphoproliferative autoimmune diseases. Retrospectively, this animal model might also apply to the more recently described autoimmune lymphoproliferative syndrome (ALPS).

Mice homozygous for the autosomal recessive lpr gene lack functional Fas expression, and thus no Fas-dependent lymphoid cell apoptosis can occur. Massive lymphoproliferation and lymphadenopathy, splenomegaly, dysfunctions in B-cell functioning, increased immunoglobulin concentration, production of autoantibodies, expansion of double negative $B220^+CD3^+CD4^-CD8^-$ cells, and an altered T_H1/T_H2 cytokine balance are observed in these mice. All these defects are intrinsic to the immune system.

Since we have found that noradrenaline (NA), the main sympathetic neurotransmitter, can induce apoptosis in lymphoid cells in a Fas-independent manner, we studied whether this neurotransmitter could partially compensate for the lack of Fas-induced cell death in lpr/lpr mice. We have found that splenic NA concentration is increased in 1-week-old lpr/lpr mice when compared to age- and sex-matched normal litter-mates and to newborn lpr/lpr mice (del Rey *et al.*, 2006a), and this increase is still noticed until the 4th week of life in male lpr/lpr mice. This is interesting, since we have previously reported that NA concentration in the spleen of 1-week-old normal mice is actually decreased when compared to newborn mice, and this time coincides with the first detection of T-cells in this organ (Besedovsky *et al.*, 1987). Later in ontogeny, splenic sympathetic innervation is progressively lost in lpr/lpr mice, as reflected by a decreased NA concentration and a reduced density of noradrenergic nerve fibers in the spleen. These results are schematically represented in Figure 5.4.

The mechanism underlying these alterations in the spleen of lpr/lpr mice is not known but, in our view, it is related to increased immune activity, a phenomenon that we have denominated an immune–sympathetic reflex mechanism (del Rey *et al.*, 1981). This possibility is supported by our finding that the immune response to sheep erythrocytes results in decreased NA content and turnover rate in the spleen, and that the initial (hours) activation of the SNS during the immune response to the superantigen staphylococcal enterotoxin B is followed by a marked decreased in splenic NA concentration in the following days (del Rey, Kabiersch, Petzoldt, and Besedovsky, 2002). Also, the converse evidence, showing that reduced immune activity caused either by the lack of mature T-cells in athymic nude mice or by reduced antigenic challenge in germ-free rats results in increased sympathetic activity in lymphoid organs, agrees with this possibility (for references see del Rey and Besedovsky, 2008).

In young lpr/lpr mice and in the normal litter-mates of all ages studied, we found a positive correlation between IgM levels in blood and splenic NA concentration. However, a negative correlation between splenic NA concentration and the progression of the disease is established in adult lpr/lpr mice (del Rey *et al.*, 2006a). These results suggested that the loss of noradrenergic fibers might contribute to the development of the lymphoproliferative disease in lpr/lpr mice. In fact, advancing the loss of innervation that occurs spontaneously in adult lpr/lpr mice by sympathetic denervation at birth results in a marked increase in IgM plasma levels during adulthood when compared to non-treated lpr/lpr mice and denervated normal litter-mates. A significant portion of the autoantibodies found in lpr/lpr mice belongs to the IgG2a subclass, and IgG2a-producing B-cells in lpr/lpr mice are densely clustered in the T-cell-rich lymphatic sheath of the spleen, a location that coincides exactly with the richest area of splenic sympathetic innervation in normal mice. Neonatal sympathetic denervation also resulted in even higher concentrations of IgG2a in blood of adult lpr/lpr mice.

It is interesting to note that an increase in IgG2a production, which indicates T_H1 predominance, has been associated with acceleration of the lupus-like autoimmune syndrome. In fact, lymphadenopathy appeared earlier in denervated lpr/lpr mice and markedly accelerated the lethal course of the disease (for references see del Rey *et al.*, 2006a). These results provide clear evidence that noradrenergic nerves can affect the expression of the lupus-like autoimmune

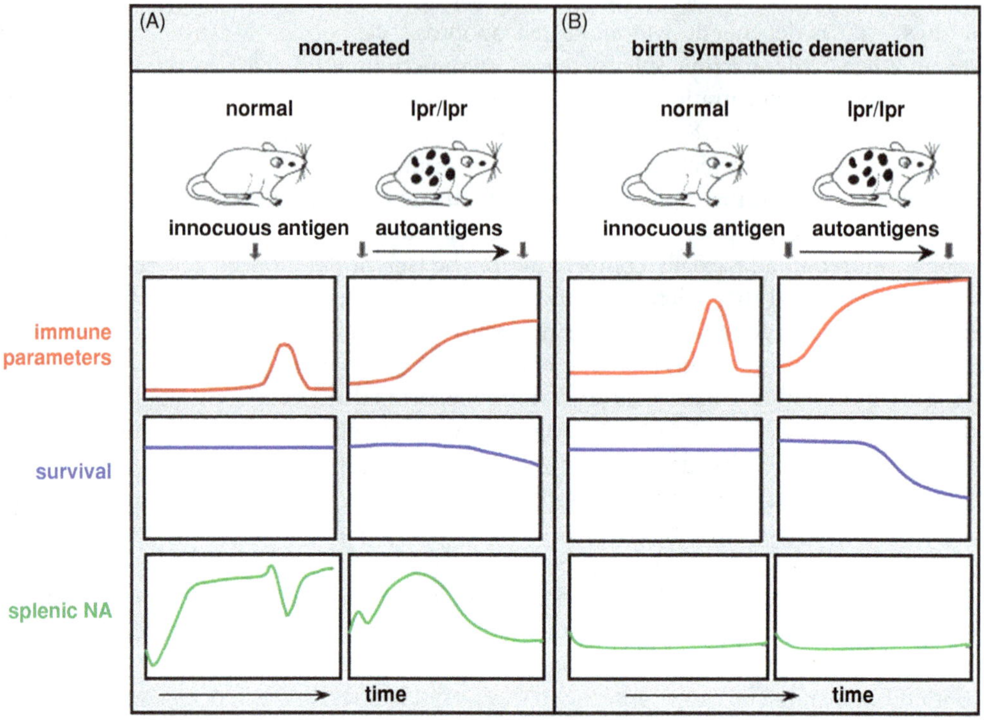

Figure 5.4 Disruption of immune-brain communication during autoimmune, lymphoproliferative diseases. A) Schematic representation of changes in immune parameters, survival and splenic NA concentration in normal mice that received an innocuous antigen at the time indicated by the gray arrow. The same parameters are depicted for lpr/lpr mice, in which the immune system is permanently activated by autoantigens (indicated by the two gray arrows). B) Normal and lpr/lpr mice were sympathetically denervated at birth. In normal mice, this treatment results in an increased immune response to an innocuous antigen, without affecting survival. In lpr/lpr mice, a comparable treatment markedly increases the autoimmune response and accelerates the lethal course of the lymphoproliferative disease. (The original data can be found in del Rey *et al.*, 2006a. The diagram has been modified from del Rey and Besedovsky, 2008 and reproduced by permission of S. Karger AG, Basel).

disease, and, to the best of our knowledge, they represent the first example that noradrenergic nerves contribute to control the expression of lymphoproliferative diseases. When this control system fails, as it occurs in lymphoid organs of adult lpr/lpr mice, the onset and lethal course of the disease are markedly accelerated. Although it is not known at present if alterations in the sympathetic innervation of lymphoid organs are observed in SLE patients, it has been shown that treatment with β-blockers can cause "drug-induced" lupus in humans, and that patients with SLE have a decreased density of β2-adrenergic receptors on peripheral $CD19^+$ cells (for references see del Rey *et al.*, 2006a).

Another example of disrupted sympathetic nerve–immune cell interactions derives from studies in rheumatoid arthritis (RA) (references related to this section can be found in del Rey *et al.*, 2008). The disease is characterized by synovitis, joint swelling, tenderness, and pain, morning stiffness, and limitation of joint mobility. TNF-α and IL-1β are particularly involved in the inflammatory and destructive process that can lead to cartilage and bone erosion and even to loss of function. Among other parameters, activated T-cells, macrophages, and plasma cells in the synovial membrane of the compromised joints, neutrophils in the synovial fluid, and increased expression of Toll-like receptors in the synovium, indicate the complex activation of the immune process during RA. We have hypothesized that alterations in immune–neuroendocrine interactions might also be involved in the pathology of this disease. To test this hypothesis, we have used a model of bovine type II collagen (CII)-induced arthritis in rats, and evaluated several neuro- and endocrine parameters at peripheral and central levels at different times after immunization. Besides the expected changes in the production of pro-inflammatory cytokines, we detected alterations in the functioning of the HPA axis, in adrenaline levels in plasma, and in the expression of IL-1β and IL-6 and in the content of NA in the hypothalamus.

The quantification of nerve fibers containing tyrosine hydroxylase (the rate-limiting enzyme in NA synthesis) in the joints of the arthritic rats showed that sympathetic innervation gradually disappears as the disease progresses. Similar observations have been also done in a model of arthritis in mice and in RA patients (for review see del Rey *et al.*, 2010). The results indicate that there is a disconnection between the immune system and the neuroendocrine responses expected to occur during the development of CII-induced arthritis. In the context discussed here, there is an interruption of the efferent sympathetic signals to the affected joints because nerve fibers are destroyed during the disease. There is also an uncoupled response of the SNS with both the HPA axis and hypothalamic noradrenergic neurons, and cytokine expression. Taken together, the results indicate that brain-integrated neuroendocrine responses mediated by the HPA axis and the SNS are disorganized and disrupted during the inflammatory/immune response that causes arthritis, even before symptoms of the disease are detected.

The changes and eventual interferences in the communication of the SNS and the immune system seem to be related to the level of activity of immune cells. Indeed, there is multiple evidence indicating that prolong and intense immune cell activity results in sympathetic denervation of lymphoid organs, and, conversely, a decreased activity of the immune system results in opposite effects. This evidence indicates the plasticity and vulnerability of the noradrenergic input to the INE network.

Deleterious Effects of the INE Network During Prolonged Infections: Pulmonary Tuberculosis as an Example

As mentioned, there is evidence that a causally related and biologically significant neuroendocrine response is triggered following the immune response linked to infections and other diseases that involve the activation of immune cells and inflammatory processes. With the aim of exploring whether such coupled immune and neuroendocrine responses also occur during human diseases, we have conducted translational studies taking human pulmonary tuberculosis (TB) as a model.

Mycobacterium tuberculosis is a major pathogen for humans. According to the 2010 WHO report, one-third of the world population is infected with this bacillus, and 5% of infected individuals develop TB. The clinical manifestations are greatly influenced by the immune response to *M. tuberculosis.* Indeed, a cellular immune response with polarization towards a pattern of T_H1 cytokines at early stages of the infection is sufficient to impede in most cases the overt expression of the disease since this pattern favors the development of delayed type hypersensitivity and macrophage activation. However, when the infected individual is unable to cope quickly enough with the bacillus, the tendency towards a T_H1 polarization is gradually lost, and the immune response becomes inadequate, contributing to the overexpression of the disease.

Neuroendocrine responses during chronic infections like lung tuberculosis are poorly characterized, or the studies performed were based on the evaluation of single hormonal systems. This is surprising considering that hormonal changes are likely to occur, since some of the cytokines produced during these diseases could affect endocrine mechanisms that, in turn, influence the course of infectious/inflammatory processes. We studied a wide range of pituitary, adrenal, gonadal, and thyroid hormones and adipokines in parallel to inflammatory and anti-inflammatory cytokines in the same patients with pulmonary TB (del Rey *et al.*, 2007; for a review see Bottasso, Bay, Besedovsky, and del Rey, 2009).

These studies were complemented with clinical, radiological, and body mass index (BMI) evaluations that allowed the classification of HIV-negative, newly diagnosed, untreated male patients as having mild, moderate, or advanced lung tuberculosis. Age- and sex-matched, healthy controls and household contacts (HHCs) were used for comparison. HHCs live together, and share socioeconomic conditions, with contagious TB patients but develop a subclinical and self-controlled process (latent tuberculosis).

Dehydroepiandrosterone (DHEA) and testosterone plasma concentrations were profoundly decreased and growth hormone levels markedly elevated in the patients, in parallel to increased concentration of thyroid hormones and to modestly increased levels of cortisol, estradiol, and prolactin. Leptin levels were clearly decreased but not other adipokines, and IFN-γ, IL-10, IL-6 and IL-18 levels were elevated in the patients. The magnitude of the alterations in practically all the endocrine parameters studied, as well as the decrease in the BMI, depended on the intensity of the disease. The endocrine profile of TB patients would favor a reduction of protective cell-mediated immunity and an exacerbation of inflammation, leading to perpetuation of the lung injury and to the hypercatabolic condition that characterizes this disease (Figure 5.5). Interestingly, HHCs, who, as mentioned, did not show overt symptoms of TB, had decreased DHEA levels. It is possible that a decrease in this powerful anti-inflammatory hormone, together with a well-balanced adaptive immune response, could favor the survival of *M. tuberculosis* in appropriated niches without causing further tissue injury.

We have also shown that, upon stimulation with antigens from the mycobacterium, peripheral blood mononuclear cells from the patients produce factors that can significantly inhibited DHEA secretion. We have recently found that TGF-β is among the factors that mediate this effect (D'Attilio *et al.*, 2012). These results support the hypothesis that at least some of the endocrine changes observed in the patients may be mediated by endogenous cytokines. Furthermore, the fact that non-symptomatic HHCs showed decreased levels of DHEA is a strong indication that this effect is also immune-mediated because it to be expected that they are also infected.

Appropriated multivariable discriminant analysis identified DHEA, C-reactive protein and BMI as the more significant variables to predict the characterization of the patients within the whole set of individuals studied (Santucci *et al.*, 2011). The implications of weight loss and the BMI in TB were recently discussed (for a review see Bottasso, Bay, Besedovsky, and del Rey, 2009).

DHEA is known to stimulate helper T-cell functions, facilitate T_H1 responses, and also exert potent anti-inflammatory effects. Our results are in line with data from patients with chronic disabling inflammatory diseases in which a prolonged immune aggression coexists with a deficient production of adrenal steroids. Decreased DHEA levels have also been found

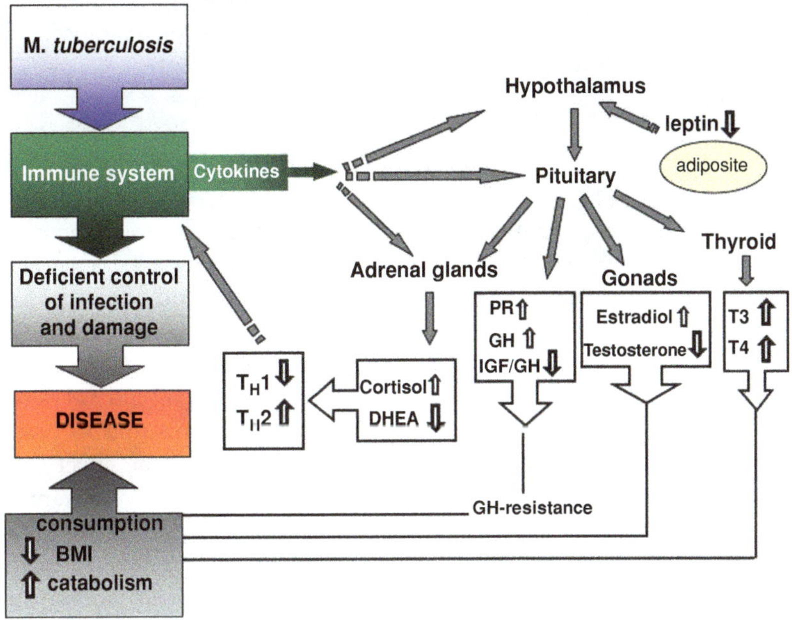

Figure 5.5 Deleterious effects of the INE network during pulmonary tuberculosis. The pattern of neuroendocrine responses in patients with tuberculosis favors a T_H2-type of immune response, which is inadequate to control the infection by the intracellular mycobacteria, and induces a hypercatabolic state that leads to "consumption." (The diagram has been modified from Bottasso, Bay, Besedovsky, and del Rey, 2009, and reproduced by permission of S. Karger AG, Basel).

in other infectious diseases of chronic nature, such as leishmaniasis and Chagas disease (for references see Bottasso, Bay, Besedovsky, and del Rey, 2009).

In summary, patients with established pulmonary TB develop an immune response that is not efficient in controlling the bacillus and the inflammatory process that results in lung injury. Parallel to this immune derangement, the patients develop a neuroendocrine and metabolic response that favors a catabolic condition that leads to cachexia. The fact that these processes are all related to the intensity of the disease would indicate that, without treatment, the patients would enter a state historically termed "consumption." The decreased BMI linked to the gravity of the disease can be taken as predictor of a lethal course. Several of the cytokines that are released during TB are known to stimulate the HPA axis, which should result in increase in powerful anti-inflammatory hormones such as cortisol and DHEA. However, the modest increase in cortisol and the markedly reduced DHEA levels observed in the plasma of TB patients already indicate a disruption in the INE network, most likely mediated by immune products. Furthermore, the lack of an increase in insulin-like growth factor in parallel to elevated levels of growth hormone is an indication that TB patients develop resistance to growth hormone, which has well recognized immune-stimulatory effects. Taking the evidence together, it appears that when the immune system cannot rapidly control the disease, the INE network becomes either uncoupled or disruptive. Such conditions indicate that, although initially adaptive, prolonged host neuroendocrine responses may lead to effects that are neither adequate to support the immune system nor to re-establish health. The lack of efficiency of host responses to long-lasting infections can be linked, as we have previously proposed taking a natural selection point of view, to an immune-mediated process of active negative selection based on the deletion of infected individuals who can propagate transmissible diseases (Besedovsky and del Rey, 1996).

Conclusions and Proposal

As mentioned, since the components of the INE network can reciprocally serve as regulatory signals, their final effects depend on their interactions at tissue or cellular target level. The signals conveyed by hormones, neurotransmitters, and neuropeptides could either be restricted to a particular target or exert more general effects. However, the production of neuroendocrine agents is directly or indirectly under brain control, a process that requires information from the periphery and the external world. In the other direction, peripheral sensorial nerves transmit afferent signals to the brain, and hormones send feedback information to particular CNS centers. In some cases, such feedback information is provided by the effect they cause, as for example, the effect of hormones and peripheral autonomic nerves on parameters such as glycemia or osmolarity. In other cases, peripheral information to the brain is based on the tissue-specific release of mediators. For example, leptin signals the brain about changes in adipose mass. However, in our view, it is still unknown how the brain monitors information about final effects on peripheral target cells exposed either simultaneously or sequentially to multiple signals. We have proposed that still undefined mediators that we have tentatively called retro-hormones or retro-transmitters serve to convey this information (Besedovsky and del Rey, 1996). In addition, to evaluate the overall effect of afferent signaling systems, it is necessary to consider their integration with inputs from sensorial structures and stimuli generated in the brain itself.

As mediators within the INE network, cytokines interact with neuroendocrine agents by a reciprocal modulation of the number and sensitivity of receptors, the induction of the same second messengers and other intracellular mediators that control gene transcription and posttranscriptional, secretory, and even epigenetic events. However, as we have discussed previously, immune cell products also send information to the brain. On these bases, we have defined the immune system as a sensorial organ that conveys information to the brain about changes in cellular and molecular components of the body, intrusion of pathogens and effects of different types of danger (Besedovsky *et al.*, 1983). Because such information becomes cognitive only during pathological conditions, it is not integrated in a given cortical area as the sensory and motor homunculus. Thus, we have proposed a kind of plastic sensorial immune homunculus located, but not topologically represented, in subcortical structures, the generation of which depends on the type of immune response in operation.

As discussed, there is also a network of interactions between cytokines and classical neural cell products that operate in the "healthy" brain. In our view, astrocytes, the most abundant cell type in the brain, play an important role in these interactions. These cells have been traditionally considered to be a type of helper cell, providing support to neurons by controlling local blood and fuel supply and by removing excessive quantities of neurotransmitters released at synaptic levels. At present, there is solid evidence that, in addition to these functions, astrocytes play an active role in brain functions linked to synaptic plasticity, and they have been proposed as the third component of a tripartite synapse (Allen and Barres, 2009).

The maintenance of LTP is a process that requires protein synthesis and the sequential activation of NF-κβ and other transcription factors that are affected by cytokines. Increased neuronal activity implies a big energetic cost, and the main source of energy is glycolysis, fuelled by glucose. Cytokines such as IL-1 may contribute to fuel supply to neural cells (for references Gavillet, Allaman, and Magistretti, 2008) because it can stimulate glucose uptake using predominantly GLUT1 in astrocytes. Since, as discussed above, IL-1 production is induced during LTP, we have proposed that this cytokine can enhance fuel supply to both astrocytes and neurons during a sustained increase in activity. Since astrocytes are considered the main suppliers of energy, acting directly or following the astrocyte–neuron lactate shuttle (Belanger, Allaman, and Magistretti, 2011), we have proposed that the stimulation of these cells by endogenously produced IL-1 would support the metabolic demands of the activated neurons that they contact (Besedovsky and del Rey, 2011).

In addition to the capacity of astrocytes to affect synaptic plasticity and brain functions, they have all the necessary machinery to be involved in immune processes in the brain. For example, they can process antigens, act as antigen-presenting cells and be affected, in a paracrine or autocrine fashion, by cytokines (Farina *et al.*, 2007). Thus, astrocytes have two "faces": on one hand they exchange signals with neurons; on the other they can detect and react to peripheral and central immune signals. Based on these properties, astrocytes can be considered as neuroimmune cells, and cytokines such IL-1 and IL-6 as mediators of their dual functions. Indeed, these cytokines are released by astrocytes, on which they exert biologically relevant effects both during increased synaptic plasticity, e.g. during LTP, and following stimulation of peripheral immune cells.

The concept of tripartite synapses has emerged in recent years. This considers astrocytes which surround neurons as a third synaptic component that not only influence neuronal metabolism but also affect synaptic strength, and several brain functions, such as memory consolidation.The facts that IL-1 and IL-6 are induced in the brain during increased neuronal activity, and that these cytokines can influence both neurons and astrocytes, strongly suggests that they function as mediators within the tripartite synapse. Since the production of IL-1, IL-6 and other cytokines can also be induced in the brain upon activation of peripheral immune cells, tripartite synapses would constitute an interface between the immune system and the central nervous system. The fact that astrocyte processes are part of the blood–brain-barrier and can be affected by peripheral signals also contributes to the establishment of such an interface. Furthermore, afferent nerve fibers also convey information from the immune system to the brain and, by acting on defined neurons, they can also have an input on tripartite synapses.

Under basal conditions, the release of low amounts of cytokines by brain cells could be one of the various inputs that modulate the activity of neurons involved in the regulation of adaptive functions integrated at the level of the hypothalamus and the limbic system. Under conditions during which the activity of the immune system changes, peripheral cytokines and other mediators would trigger the initial steps of neuroendocrine responses that occur as consequence of immune cell stimulation. The rapid neuroendocrine response observed when certain cytokines are administered peripherally may indicate that this initial step does not involve the synthesis de novo of cytokines in the brain. However, peripheral immune mediators and neurons and glial cells activated during this initial step would trigger increased expression of cytokines in the brain. This confluence of signals may contribute to determine a defined pattern of central cytokine expression during an immune response. This pattern may differ in relation to the type of immune response that is elicited and on the neurosensorial inputs on the neurons that receive immune signals. Thus, the final immune, neuromodulatory, and adaptive outcome will be the result of the balance between different convergent inputs on the affected set of neural cells.

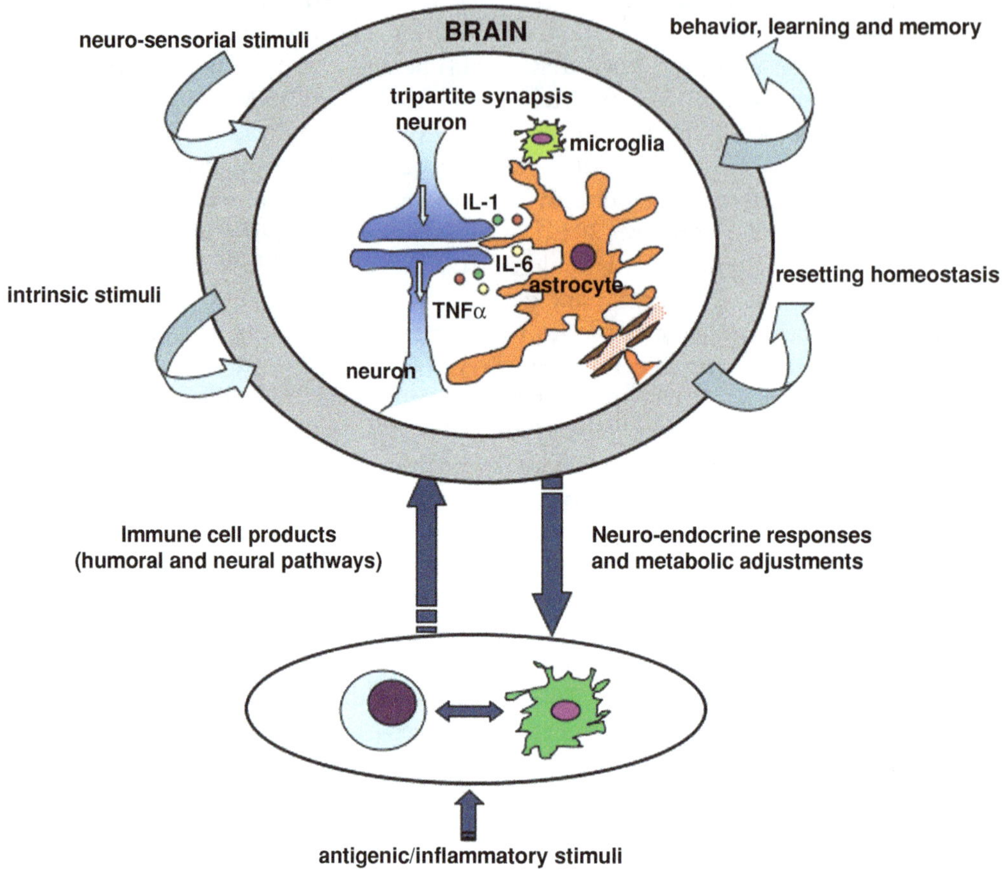

Figure 5.6 Tripartite synapses subject to cytokine inputs act as a relay system in immune-brain connectivity. A tripartite synapse surrounded by brain-borne cytokines, different neural and immune inputs generated inside and outside the brain, and the neuroendocrine and behavioral responses that can be elicited are schematically represented in the figure. It is not well understood at present how the cellular and molecular mechanisms involved in immune–brain communication are integrated at CNS levels. We propose that tripartite synapses, composed by neurons and astrocytes, could serve as a relay system in this process. Besides their relevant function in synaptic plasticity and in the control of neuronal metabolism, astrocytes are also part of the brain immune system. Cytokines such as IL-1 and IL-6, which are known to affect the three components of tripartite synapses, are overexpressed during potentiation of synaptic activity. These cytokines can modulate LTP maintenance, a process that underlies physiological brain functions such as learning and memory. In addition, some cytokines are produced in the brain during increased peripheral immune cell activity. Thus, besides receiving neural inputs derived from sensorial or intrinsic brain signals, certain tripartite synapses can also be affected by immune signals. The final effect mediated by these tripartite synapses on neurons involved in different brain functions would therefore depend on the relative "weight" of the confluent neural- and immune-derived signals. Acting as a relay system, defined tripartite synapses could differentially modulate neuroendocrine and metabolic adjustments that are behaviorally and immunologically relevant.

On these bases, we postulate that tripartite synapses posses the cellular and molecular components to function as a "relay system" capable of receiving and integrating peripheral immune signals with central neural signals. Considering that these signals can induce either synergistic or antagonist effects, the integration of their effects would result in neuroendocrine and behavioral responses with different outcomes. Thus, this integrative relay system is expected to be relevant in determining to what extent neuroendocrine and metabolic mechanisms under brain control can contribute to maintain health, and also influence the course and consequences of a disease (Figure 5.6).

We have discussed examples based mainly on our own results, indicating that there is a constantly operative INE network that can be exposed to multiple inputs and respond with adaptive adjustments when the outcome is well-balanced. As proposed here, such balance is modulated at brain levels by a superimposed intrinsic brain network, whose key components are tripartite synapses that might integrate immune and neurosensorial signals. In our view, disruption of this integrative process contributes not only to peripheral but also to central diseases. We are far from understanding the molecular and cellular bases of these superimposed and interactive networks and from unraveling which are the hierarchical components that predominate to maintain and reestablish health at different stages of life. At this point, we have only delineated superimposed networks that involve the main regulatory signaling systems, and we dimly perceive its enormous complexity.

Acknowledgements

This work was supported by the Deutsche Forschungsgemeinschaft (DFG RE 1451/3-1).

References

Allen, N. J. and Barres, B. A. (2009). Neuroscience: Glia – more than just brain glue. *Nature*, 457, 675–677.

Avital, A., Goshen, I., Kamsler, A., Segal, M., Iverfeldt, K., Richter-Levin, G. and Yirmiya, R. (2003). Impaired Interleukin-1 signaling is associated with deficits in hippocampal memory processes and neural plasticity. *Hippocampus*, 13, 826–834.

Balschun, D., Wetzel, W., del Rey, A., Pitossi, F., Schneider, H., Zuschratter, W. and Besedovsky, H. O. (2004). Interleukin-6: A cytokine to forget. *FASEB Journal*, 18, 1788–1790.

Belanger, M., Allaman, I. and Magistretti, P. J. (2011). Brain energy metabolism: Focus on astrocyte–neuron metabolic cooperation. *Cell Metabolism*, 14, 724–738.

Besedovsky, H., del Rey, A., Sorkin, E., Da Prada, M., Burri, R. and Honegger, C. (1983). The immune response evokes changes in brain noradrenergic neurons. *Science*, 221, 564–566.

Besedovsky, H. and Sorkin, E. (1977). Network of immune–neuroendocrine interactions. *Clinical and Experimental Immunology*, 27, 1–12.

Besedovsky, H. O. and del Rey, A. (1996). Immune–neuroendocrine interactions: Facts and hypotheses. *Endocrine Reviews*, 17, 64–102.

Besedovsky, H. O. and Del Rey, A. (2007). Physiology of psychoneuroimmunology: A personal view. *Brain, Behavior, Immunity*, 21, 34–44.

Besedovsky, H. O. and Del Rey, A. (2010). Interleukin-1 resets glucose homeostasis at central and peripheral levels: Relevance for immunoregulation. *Neuroimmunomodulation*, 17, 139–141.

Besedovsky, H. O. and del Rey, A. (2011). Central and peripheral cytokines mediate immune–brain connectivity. *Neurochemical Research*, 36, 1–6.

Besedovsky, H. O., del Rey, A., Sorkin, E., Burri, R., Honegger, C. G., Schlumpf, M. and Lichtensteiger, W. (1987). T lymphocytes affect the development of sympathetic innervation of mouse spleen. *Brain, Behavior, Immunity*, 1, 185–193.

Bottasso, O., Bay, M. L., Besedovsky, H. and del Rey, A. (2009). Immunoendocrine alterations during human tuberculosis as an integrated view of disease pathology. *Neuroimmunomodulation*, 16, 68–77.

Braida, D., Sacerdote, P., Panerai, A. E., Bianchi, M., Aloisi, A. M., Iosue, S. and Sala, M. (2004). Cognitive function in young and adult IL (Interleukin)-6 deficient mice. *Behavioural Brain Research*, 153, 423–249.

D'Attilio, L., Bozza, V. V., Santucci, N., Bongiovanni, B., Dídoli, G., Radcliffe, S., Besedovsky, H., del Rey, A., Bottasso, O. and Bay, M. L. (2012). TGF-β neutralization abrogates the inhibited DHEA production mediated by factors released from M. tuberculosis-stimulated PBMC. *Annals of the New York Academy of Sciences*, 1262, 1–9.

del Rey, A., Balschun, D., Wetzel, W., Randolf, A. and Besedovsky, H. O. (2013). A cytokine network involving brain-borne IL-1β, IL-1ra, IL-18, IL-6, and TNF-α operates during long-term potentiation and learning. *Brain, Behavior, Immunity* pii: S0889-1591(13)00201-8. doi: 10.1016/j.bbi.2013.05.011. [Epub ahead of print]

del Rey, A. and Besedovsky, H. (1987). Interleukin 1 Affects glucose homeostasis. *American Journal of Physiology*, 253, R794–798.

del Rey, A. and Besedovsky, H. (1989). Antidiabetic effects of Interleukin 1. *Proceedings of the National Academy of Sciences of the USA*, 86, 5943–5947.

del Rey, A. and Besedovsky, H. O. (2008). Sympathetic nervous system–immune interactions in autoimmune lymphoproliferative diseases. *Neuroimmunomodulation*, 15, 29–36.

del Rey, A., Besedovsky, H. O., Sorkin, E., Da Prada, M. and Arrenbrecht, S. (1981). Immunoregulation mediated by the sympathetic nervous system, II. *Cellular Immunology*, 63, 329–334.

del Rey, A., Kabiersch, A., Petzoldt, S. and Besedovsky, H. O. (2002). Involvement of noradrenergic nerves in the activation and clonal deletion of T cells stimulated by superantigen in vivo. *Journal of Neuroimmunology*, 127, 44–53.

del Rey, A., Randolf, A., Wildmann, J., Besedovsky, H. O. and Jessop, D. S. (2009). Re-exposure to endotoxin induces differential cytokine gene expression in the rat hypothalamus and spleen. *Brain, Behavior, Immunity*, 23, 776–783.

del Rey, A., Roggero, E., Kabiersch, A., Schafer, M. and Besedovsky, H. O. (2006a). The role of noradrenergic nerves in the development of the lymphoproliferative disease in fas-deficient, lpr/lpr mice. *Journal of Immunology*, 176, 7079–7086.

del Rey, A., Roggero, E., Randolf, A., Mahuad, C., Mccann, S., Rettori, V. and Besedovsky, H. O. (2006b). IL-1 resets glucose homeostasis at central levels. *Proceedings of the National Academy of Sciences of the USA*,103, 16039–16044.

del Rey, A., Wolff, C., Wildmann, J., Randolf, A., Hahnel, A., Besedovsky, H. O. and Straub, R. H. (2008). Disrupted brain–immune system – joint communication during experimental arthritis. *Arthritis and Rheumatism*, 58, 3090–3099.

del Rey, A., Wolff, C., Wildmann, J., Randolf, A., Straub, R. H. and Besedovsky, H. O. (2010). When immune–neuroendocrine interactions are disrupted: Experimentally induced arthritis as an example. *Neuroimmunomodulation*, 17, 165–168.

del Rey, A., Yau, H. J., Randolf, A., Centeno, M. V., Wildmann, J., Martina, M., Besedovsky, H. O. and Apkarian, A. V. (2011). Chronic neuropathic pain-like behavior correlates with IL-1beta expression and disrupts cytokine interactions in the hippocampus. *Pain*, 152, 2827–2835.

del Rey, A. D., Mahuad, C. V., Bozza, V. V., Bogue, C., Farroni, M. A., Bay, M. L., Bottasso, O. A. and Besedovsky, H. O. (2007). Endocrine and cytokine responses in humans with pulmonary tuberculosis. *Brain, Behavior, Immunity*, 21, 171–179.

Derijk, R., Van Rooijen, N., Tilders, F. J., Besedovsky, H. O., del Rey, A. and Berkenbosch, F. (1991). Selective depletion of macrophages prevents pituitary–adrenal activation in response to subpyrogenic, but not too pyrogenic, doses of bacterial endotoxin in rats. *Endocrinology*, 129, 330–338.

Dinarello, C. A. (2009). Immunological And inflammatory functions of the Interleukin-1 family. *Annual Reviews in Immunology*, 27, 519–550.

Farina, C., Aloisi, F. and Meinl, E. (2007). astrocytes are active players in cerebral innate immunity. *Trends in Immunology*, 28, 138–145.

Fox, C. J., Hammerman, P. S. and Thompson, C. B. (2005). Fuel feeds function: Energy metabolism and the T-cell response. *Nature Reviews Immunology*, 5, 844–852.

Garcia, M. C., Wernstedt, I., Berndtsson, A., Enge, M., Bell, M., Hultgren, O., Horn, M., Ahren, B., Enerback, S., Ohlsson, C., Wallenius, V. and Jansson, J. O. (2006). Mature-onset obesity in Interleukin-1 receptor I knockout mice. *Diabetes*, 55, 1205–1213.

Gavillet, M., Allaman, I. and Magistretti, P. J. (2008). Modulation of astrocytic metabolic phenotype by proinflammatory cytokines. *Glia*, 56, 975–989.

Goshen, I., Avital, A., Kreisel, T., Licht, T., Segal, M. and Yirmiya, R. (2009). Environmental Enrichment restores memory functioning in mice with impaired IL-1 signaling via reinstatement of long-term potentiation and spine size enlargement. *Journal of Neuroscience*, 29, 3395–3403.

Kominsky, D. J., Campbell, E. L. and Colgan, S. P. (2010). Metabolic shifts in immunity and inflammation. *Journal Of Immunology*, 184, 4062–4068.

Laye, S., Parnet, P., Goujon, E. and Dantzer, R. (1994). Peripheral administration of lipopolysaccharide induces the expression of cytokine transcripts in the brain and pituitary of mice. *Brain Research, Molecular Brain Research*, 27, 157–162.

Matsuki, T., Horai, R., Sudo, K. and Iwakura, Y. (2003). IL-1 plays an important role in lipid metabolism by regulating insulin levels under physiological conditions. *Journal of Experimental Medicine*, 198, 877–888.

Mcguinness, O. P. (2005). Defective glucose homeostasis during infection. *Annual Review of Nutrition*, 25, 9–35.

Metzger, S., Nusair, S., Planer, D., Barash, V., Pappo, O., Shilyansky, J. and Chajek-Shaul, T. (2004). Inhibition of hepatic gluconeogenesis and enhanced glucose uptake contribute to the development of hypoglycemia in mice bearing Interleukin-1beta-secreting tumor. *Endocrinology*, 145, 5150–5156.

Pitossi, F., del Rey, A., Kabiersch, A. and Besedovsky, H. (1997). Induction of cytokine transcripts in the central nervous system and pituitary following peripheral administration of endotoxin to mice. *Journal of Neuroscience Research*, 48, 287–298.

Rogausch, H., Vo, N. T., del Rey, A. and Besedovsky, H. O. (2000). Increased sensitivity of the baroreceptor reflex after bacterial endotoxin. *Annals of the New York Academy of Sciences*, 917, 165–168.

Santucci, N., D'attilio, L., Kovalevski, L., Bozza, V., Besedovsky, H., del Rey, A., Bay, M. L. and Bottasso, O. (2011). A multifaceted analysis of immune–endocrine–metabolic alterations in patients with pulmonary tuberculosis. *PLOS One*, 6, E26363.

Schneider, H., Pitossi, F., Balschun, D., Wagner, A., del Rey, A. and Besedovsky, H. O. (1998). A neuromodulatory role of Interleukin-1beta in the hippocampus. *Proceedings of the National Academy of Sciences of the USA*, 95, 7778–7783.

Tilders, F. J. and Schmidt, E. D. (1998). Interleukin-1-induced plasticity of hypothalamic CRH neurons and long-term stress hyperresponsiveness. *Annals of the New York Academy of Sciences*, 840, 65–73.

Van Dam, A. M., Brouns, M., Louisse, S. and Berkenbosch, F. (1992). Appearance of Interleukin-1 in macrophages and in ramified microglia in the brain of endotoxin-treated rats: A pathway for the induction of non-specific symptoms of sickness? *Brain Research*, 588, 291–296.

Yirmiya, R., Winocur, G. and Goshen, I. (2002). Brain Interleukin-1 is involved in spatial memory and passive avoidance conditioning. *Neurobiology of Learning and Memory*, 78, 379–389.

6

Neural Functions of Hematopoietic-derived Cells

Noël C. Derecki and Jonathan Kipnis

Center for Brain Immunology and Glia (BIG), Department of Neuroscience, University of Virginia, Charlottesville, VA, USA

Introduction

The immune system and the central nervous system (CNS) are more alike than different. Both systems, and the cells within them, learn constantly from experience – although both systems are also "hard wired" to some degree. Both communicate discreet parcels of information over tiny distances by means of synapses, and over vast distances via intricate chemical signaling networks. More broadly, of course, both systems are utterly critical to an organism's survival. This last point may be the most critical to the seemingly paradoxical relationship between the immune and central nervous systems, for extraordinarily, each is widely believed to live out its days in enforced isolation from the other. This systemic segregation, known as "immune privilege," has long been believed to be near-absolute. It is only recently – within the last couple of decades – that an empirically based challenge has been mounted against this particularly resilient bit of scientific dogma.

Ground-breaking progress – en route to a far more nuanced understanding of the role of the immune system in the CNS – was first made in the 1990s, when Irun Cohen published a series of works espousing entirely radical ideas regarding *autoimmunity*, or immune reaction against the "self" (Cohen, 1992a, b). Namely, Cohen questioned the well-entrenched notion that autoimmunity was a wholly unwanted situation. Instead, he suggested that auto-antigen recognition was part of the indispensable foundation of a smoothly functioning and indeed, intelligent immune system. He writes, "Autoimmunity is not merely a burden and an opportunity, it is a necessity" (Cohen, 1992a). The first experimental evidence to support these ideas came from the Schwartz group, suggesting a beneficial role for the immune system in CNS pathology. These data overarchingly demonstrated that a well-controlled amplification of the autoimmune response could be correlated with improved neuronal survival in models of acute CNS injury (Moalem *et al.*, 1999; Schwartz, Moalem, Leibowitz-Amit, and Cohen, 1999) and chronic neurodegenerative conditions (Kipnis and Schwartz, 2002; Hofstetter *et al.*, 2003). These findings were not, of course, greeted by universal acceptance – quite the contrary, in fact. This was to be expected, however, since the preponderance of evidence gathered until then unequivocally implicated the vagaries of the immune system as a major contributor to secondary neuronal degeneration following CNS injury, and to neuroinflammation and

The Wiley-Blackwell Handbook of Psychoneuroimmunology, First Edition. Edited by Alexander W. Kusnecov and Hymie Anisman.

destructive demyelination. History was more or less clearly on the side of the conservative scientific establishment as well, since anatomical dogma from the time of Ehrlich (1885), Lewandowski (1900), and Goldmann (1900) had dictated that the so-called "blood–brain barrier" was virtually unbreachable by the immune system, except in cases that concerned detrimental pathological outcomes. Thus, the idea that the immune system could be beneficial in cases of disease (or perhaps even more radically, be *necessary* to healthy and normal CNS function) was practically heresy to most immunologists and neuroscientists alike. Nevertheless, the floodgates of inquiry had opened, and hot on the heels of these seminal papers on immune system benefit in CNS injury came similarly innovative findings that implicated T lymphocytes as critical to normal learning and memory (Ziv *et al.*, 2006; Brynskikh. Warren, Zhu, and Kipnis, 2008), and thus, the function of the healthy CNS (Kipnis, Cohen, Cardon, and Schwartz, 2004).

The Blood–Brain Barrier, Past to Present

The brain, in terms of its relationship with the rest of the body, is a peculiar organ, indeed. Comprising roughly two percent of the weight of the human body, the brain nevertheless consumes approximately 20% of the body's energy, gobbling up oxygen and glucose as quickly as they can be supplied to it. Yet this same organ, which in terms of energy and metabolic exchange is analogous to an eight-lane highway, becomes an all-but-impassably-narrow road when the transfer of most other molecules (and cells) from the circulation are concerned. This eccentric nature of the brain to hoard and exchange certain blood-borne substances, yet eschew the transport of others, is largely attributed to a structure – or series of structures – known as the blood–brain barrier (BBB).

Fundamental insights into the nature of this assembly of structures emerged from a series of experiments performed around the turn of the century. In 1885, German bacteriologist Paul Ehrlich, who was injecting redox-sensitive "intravital" dyes into the circulatory system to label structures adjacent to capillaries, stumbled upon a surprising – and given the aim of his experiment, probably annoying – phenomenon. While his aniline dyes stained most internal organs thoroughly, he noted that the brains of the animals he had injected remained oddly untouched. Frustrated, he repeated his experiment, but with the same strange results. Ehrlich initially concluded (albeit incorrectly) that the brain tissue *itself* was resistant to his dyes (Ehrlich, 1885). It was not until a few years later that one of Ehrlich's students, Ernst Goldmann, attempted the reverse experiment, injecting similar dyes into the cerebrospinal fluid (CSF). Goldmann got the reverse result, with the brain staining gloriously and the external organs not at all (Goldmann, 1900). Together, these data suggested to them that some sort of biological "membrane" existed that separated the blood and brain, and that it was generally impermeable in either direction. Surprisingly, this initial notion of imperviousness, concomitant with a notion of complete "immune privilege" for the CNS, has remained almost unchanged for over a century – at least in the collective consciousness of most of biology. It should be stressed that the dogma persists even today.

It was not until the mid-1960s that a more explicitly detailed picture of the BBB was revealed by electron microscopy (Karnovsky, 1967). The inner workings of transport and adhesion were subsequently shown using molecular and biochemical techniques (Persidsky, Ramirez, Haorah, and Kanmogne, 2006). Along these lines, it has now been elucidated that several mechanisms are key to the proper function of the BBB. These can be roughly divided into three groups: acellular barriers, cellular checkpoints, and molecular transport mechanisms.

Two major cellular barriers stand guard between the CNS parenchyma and the circulation. The first of these is a network of tight junctions; the second is the astrocytic endfeet of the glia limitans. Tight junctions, or zonula occludens, serve mainly to stitch together the capillary endothelium, but are also found in epithelial cells in the choroid plexus. These specialized connections rely upon several molecules, namely occludins, claudins, junctional adhesion molecules, or "JAMs," (Guo *et al.*, 1998; Martin-Padura *et al.*, 1998; Abbott, Ronnback, and Hansson, 2006) and the eponymous zonula occludins, including ZO-1, ZO-2, and ZO-3 (Stevenson *et al.*, 1986; Ando-Akatsuka *et al.*, 1999; Itoh, Morita, and Tsukita, 1999a; Itoh *et al.*, 1999b). Anchoring all of these within the cytoplasm is actin.

While the multiplicity of molecular strategies that endothelial cells use to form tight junctions speaks well to the powerful structural integrity of the barrier formed, it also suggests that many avenues remain open to the endothelium in terms of a subtle regulation of barrier permeability, rather than the "all or none" situation which is normally imputed to the BBB. Furthermore, the situation does not seem to be one of "belt and suspenders," since changes to any piece of the above molecular puzzle yield a surprising increase in the permeability of tight junctions (Carvey, Hendey, and Monahan, 2009), though no single change yields total breach of the barrier. Indeed, a large number of immune effectors – both blood-borne and brain-derived, are able to exert changes in permeability at the level of the tight junction. The principal group is that of the pro-inflammatory cytokines, including interleukin (IL)-6, and, in particular, tumor necrosis factor (TNF); the latter has recently been shown to act from either side of the tight junction to increase the "leakiness" of the normally tight seal (Fletcher *et al.*, 2009). Notably, the finding that inflammatory signaling across the BBB is bidirectional (Zhao, Kalvass, and Pollock, 2009) suggests that peripheral changes in the circulation are not alone in being able to modify the properties of the BBB, but that parenchymal changes may also be important. One possible implication is that CNS microglia and astrocytes, by selectively weakening the BBB through TNF production, are encouraging the infiltration of the peripheral immune system into the brain; certainly, this would be a reversal of the dogma that the immune system is not "wanted" in the CNS. Equally worthy of note is the possibility that the BBB may be far more than a static barrier, and in fact could be a key point of, or perhaps even an initiator of, communication between the periphery and the parenchyma.

The second cellular barrier, this time on the parenchymal side, is provided by the endfeet of astroglia that surround the endothelium (with basement membrane in-between) to form the abluminal part of the glia limitans. (Iadecola and Nedergaard, 2007). Asserting that astrocytes are everywhere the BBB is would not be overstating the point, for astrocytes ensheath the majority of the capillary endothelium in the CNS. Microglia must also be mentioned, however, for though they are in the minority, these macrophages of the brain also intercalate periodically within the glia limitans (Hanisch and Kettenmann, 2007) and may comprise up to 25% of it. While there is ample evidence (Janzer and Raff, 1987; Goldstein, 1988; Rubin and Staddon, 1999) that astrocytes actively signal to endothelial cells in orchestrating the formation of the BBB, the possibility of additional players, for example pericytes (Krueger and Bechmann, 2010; Guillemin and Brew, 2004), is likely. Conclusive proof of the primary role of astrocytes, in terms of the identification of specific secreted-protein mediators, has remained elusive. Whether astrocytes are the conductors, or merely players, however, does not change the fact that they are integral to BBB function.

Structurally, astrocytes are interconnected by gap junctions and adherens junctions. The former can be harnessed in the service of signaling, while the latter are wholly structural. In contrast to endothelial cells, however, astrocytes are physically separated by 20–30 nm gaps through which horseradish peroxidase is able to easily diffuse (Brightman and Reese, 1969), suggesting that astrocytes do not function to the same degree as the endothelium as a mechanical barrier, at least in terms of passive molecular transmission. In conjunction with the abluminal basal lamina, however, astrocytes still present a formidable obstacle, when necessary, to potential invading cells, macromolecules, and larger pathogens.

In post-capillary venules, three basement membranes (in addition to the two basement membranes associated with the endothelial and astroglial layers, a third layer called the tunica media, or smooth muscle layer, is associated with its own basement membrane) stand between the blood and brain; in capillaries there are two. In large part, they are more specifically "foundational" in structure than the two previously discussed cellular barriers. These basement membranes are largely acellular, consisting of a matrix of proteins like elastin, glycoproteins such as laminin, fibrillin, fibronectin, and dystroglycan, and collagen bundles, as well as smaller interlinking proteins (Karnovsky, 1968). These membranes are dense, and surround the capillary endothelium and astrocytic endfeet to the point of engulfment; yet they are not so dense as to preclude the diffusion of macromolecules, and thus cannot be considered an impenetrable barrier. Interestingly, the composition of the glial membrane and the postcapillary membrane degrade differentially, suggesting that certain mediators are more important for parenchymal infiltration by immune cells than for post-extravasation, since the glial membrane is far more subject to MMPs. Apart from this, however, it does not seem that the basement membranes are able to signal, per se, and are a relatively static barrier when left unperturbed.

The choroid plexus

The choroid plexus is anatomically located within the lateral ventricles of the brain, and extends from the ventricle walls to fill much of the ventricular space. Its nominal function is the secretion of cerebrospinal fluid (CSF). CSF bathes the inner surfaces of the brain within the ventricles, and the outer aspects of the brain and spinal cord as it flows within the subarachnoid space between the arachnoid mater and pia mater, the innermost layers of the meninges (Kivisakk *et al.*, 2003; Ransohoff, Kivisakk, and Kidd, 2003). The capillaries within the choroid plexus tissue are fenestrated (Dziegielewska, Habgood, and Saunders, 2001; Dziegielewska and Saunders, 2002), and thus differ substantially from the intraparenchymal capillaries and postcapillary venules described above. However, the choroid plexus is not considered to be "leaky," since tight junctions do exist between the cuboidal epithelial cells that surround the capillaries (Engelhardt, 2006). These tight junctions function to exclude blood proteins from the CSF, and thus constitute a structure similar to the BBB, known as the blood–CSF barrier.

The circumventricular organs (CVO)

In addition to areas within the meninges, ventricular margins, and the choroid plexus, the peripheral circulation and the CNS interact at key points known as the circumventricular organs (CVO) (Nadjar *et al.*, 2005; Quan and Banks, 2007). These comprise a collection of brain structures that, given their unique lack of BBB protection, constantly sample the circulation. It might logically follow that CVO should be uniquely situated to communicate with circulating factors, including immune-derived cytokines. In fact, it has been shown that IL-1β does enter the CVO via the circulation, and is able to propagate molecular cascades within the brain parenchyma itself (Dantzer *et al.*, 2008). Of interest are experiments demonstrating parenchymal IL1-β release in the area postrema (a CVO located in the medulla) in response to peripheral administration of the bacterial endotoxin lipopolysaccharide (LPS) (Marvel *et al.*, 2004).

Transport Systems

Reese and Karnovsky, who performed seminal electron microscopy work elucidating the ultrastructure of the BBB, remarked on the relative lack of visible transporters (Reese and Karnovsky, 1967). This is indeed the case, in comparison to vasculature within non-CNS tissues. Nevertheless, transport does indeed occur. Much of the transport into and out of the CNS across the BBB follows the canonical paradigm seen in other organs, i.e. nutrients, water, and glucose comprising the bulk of influx, with metabolites and toxins moving in the other direction back into the circulation. Specific molecular mechanisms have been identified that are key to understanding the ability of molecules to traffic between the CNS and circulation and vice-versa. These include transporters for ions (potassium, sodium, chloride, and others), peptides and growth factors (e.g. vasoactive intestinal peptide, insulin-like growth factor), neurotransmitters (e.g. glutamate, glycine), and cytokines (e.g. IL-6, IL-1β, and TNF).

To gain insight into the vicissitudes of transport within the BBB, it is perhaps useful to understand that not all players, or indeed all surfaces (luminal and abluminal) are identical in their properties; direction of transport makes a difference (Carvey, Hendey, and Monahan, 2009). Blood-to-brain transport is largely dependent on luminal receptors first, but it is critical that abluminal transport mechanisms function properly as well, in order for the utility of BBB transport to be complete (Abbott, Ronnback, and Hansson, 2006). While this may seem irrelevant, the implications are actually rather interesting when one considers that inflammation on the CNS side or on the blood side of the BBB could affect normal ion transport in very different ways. While circulating pro-inflammatory cytokines might have certain effects on their own when transported into the brain rather than generated within the brain by glia. For instance, anorexia and cachexia are common side-effects of peripheral inflammation (Yeh, Blackwood, and Schuster, 2008), yet are seldom seen as a direct result of CNS neuroinflammation without peripheral cytokine increases (Burgess *et al.*, 1998).

Consider also the importance of ions like potassium and sodium to basic neuronal function: if potassium transporters, which are highly enriched on the endfeet of astrocytes, are somehow compromised at the level of the BBB, consequences for neurons that depend upon low levels of potassium in the extracellular space could be profoundly affected. Clearly, this could have implications in pathologies like epilepsy, for instance, which has been linked to innate immune inflammation in numerous studies (Vezzani and Granata, 2005). Perhaps even more intriguing is the reverse possibility, which is that seizures promote inflammation in order to harness the immune system as a postseizure tissue clearance and rebuilding mechanism. In fact, immune-related glia-derived cytokines have been recently shown to be powerful mediators of synaptic plasticity in the form of long-term potentiation (LTP), long-term depression (LTD), and synaptic scaling (Kelly *et al.*, 2001; Beattie *et al.*, 2002; Ross, Allan, Rothwell, and Verkhratsky, 2003; Maher, Nolan,and Lynch, 2005; Stellwagen and Malenka, 2006).

The implications of directionality in BBB transport

To fully appreciate the possibilities for peripheral immune cells to exert biologically significant effects on brain parenchyma, it is helpful to understand the blood–brain barrier in terms of its selectivity on both a cellular and molecular scale. It is also important to understand that the BBB differs in its properties depending upon anatomical location. Thus, immune effects across the BBB may be expected to be differential depending upon locational permeability, and proximity to particular structures. It becomes clear that frank parenchymal infiltration is not necessary, as in the case of stroke or multiple sclerosis, for the immune system to impact neuronal function, as well as for the brain to affect the circulation. The BBB is commonly misunderstood as a monolithic "wall" between immune system and brain. In truth, it is actually far more subtly constructed. The BBB is dynamic, well-regulated, and allows for novel possibilities to be contemplated in terms of manipulation at the level of the peripheral immune system that can impact CNS function. In fairness, it should also be noted that a formidable barrier truly does exist between the two systems, in terms of the blockage of immune cell entry into the brain parenchyma under homeostatic conditions. However, the inferences that have been drawn from the existence of the BBB are highly questionable. The notion that the immune system is "bad" for the healthy CNS, and that it must be kept out at all costs, is simplistic at best, and potentially dangerous at worst, as in the rationale of broad-blanket immune suppression as an effective therapy for CNS pathology.

Immune Privilege Revisited

The blood–brain barrier is not alone in being somewhat overestimated. The "immune privilege" of the brain is also often thought to mean that the immune system simply "ignores" the brain except in situations of pathological disturbance. This interpretation is somewhat extreme. More accurately, the CNS would be considered privileged because the brain parenchyma itself lacks canonical antigen presentation by dendritic cells (DC) (Galea, Bechmann, and Perry, 2007). DC, which are professional antigen presenting cells (APC) would conceivably function in a nonprivileged scenario by presenting CNS antigen directly to T-cells within brain parenchyma. To date, conclusive evidence of such activity in healthy brain has not been presented, but a case has been made by some (Engelhardt and Ransohoff, 2005). In classic experiments, it was demonstrated that foreign tissue, when grafted into the brain parenchyma, could persist for a significant period of time without immune rejection (Medawar, 1948). Interestingly, though, rejection of the foreign tissue was shown to occur quickly if the same tissue were subsequently grafted into a location in the periphery. Taken together, these results suggested that immune surveillance was in fact occurring within the brain, but that the CNS lacked a lymphoid center in which to mount a response via the traditional route of antigen presentation by APC. Cserr was the first to identify the deep cervical lymph nodes as the likely draining lymph nodes for the CNS (Cserr, Harling-Berg, and Knopf, 1992; Cserr and Knopf, 1992), and this seminal work has since been built upon. Recent experiments have shown that T-lymphocytes migrate from the CNS through the cribroid plate, then the nasal mucosa, to reach their final destination in the cervical nodes (Goldmann *et al.*, 2006). Another common misconception is that the healthy CNS contains a paucity of immune cells. In fact, immune cells are found there in exceedingly large numbers. These include the resident immune cells of the brain, microglia, and the plentiful myeloid cells and lymphocytes found in the adjacent tissues and spaces – perivascular, meningeal, and ventricular – of the CNS.

Peripheral immune cells – not just in the periphery

Classical leukocytes, commonly thought of as being restricted to the periphery, have also been found to be surprisingly populous in the areas surrounding the internal and external surfaces of the brain. For example, as many as 175 to 500,000 leukocytes by some estimations (Kivisakk *et al.*, 2003), are present in the CSF of the normal, non-inflamed human CNS. $CD11b^+$ myeloid-derived cells, including macrophages and $CD11b^+/CD11c^+$ DC, are also found in the meninges in large numbers (McMenamin, 1999; McMenamin *et al.*, 2003), as are B-lymphocytes (Kerschensteiner *et al.*, 1999; Anthony, Crawford, and Bell, 2003). It should be stressed, however, that the above cells are rarely found within the parenchymal tissue itself under normal circumstances, but rather in the CSF, the perivascular spaces, the meningeal tissues, and the meningeal spaces.

Although the deep cervical lymph nodes, as noted earlier, are likely a primary center for CNS-related APC/T-cell interaction, it is quite clear that viable APC also exist within the CNS milieu. For example, in addition to the plentiful DC and macrophages found in meningeal tissue, a small population of DC have also been identified in the CSF (Engelhardt and Ransohoff, 2005). $CD11b^+$ perivascular cells may also be a source of antigen presentation in lieu of the classical scenario presented by the lymph nodes (Gregerson, Sam and McPherson, 2004) and have even been demonstrated to be able to fulfill this function *in vivo* (Hickey and Kimura, 1988). Along these lines, epitope spreading (the development of an immune response to molecular epitopes distinct from the original disease propagating antigen) in MS has been demonstrated to occur within the CNS, rather than in the periphery or cervical nodes, thus implicating local antigen presentation (McMahon *et al.*, 2005).

CNS immune traffic – molecular interactions

What is known about immune traffic across the BBB is largely centered on interactions between cell adhesion molecules (CAMs) and their binding partners, with these interactions being mediated by local chemokine expression. This complicated process can be broken down cleanly into six discrete steps (Man, Ubogu, and Ransohoff, 2007), each mediated by a specific set of necessary players (Butcher *et al.*, 1999).

The first step in a leukocyte's journey across the BBB into the CNS – or into most tissues, for that matter – is necessarily to slow down and begin to leave the circulation. Key to this initial step, called tethering and rolling, is the action of selectins and their respective glycosylated ligands (Lee and Benveniste, 1999). Selectins comprise a family of transmembrane glycoproteins, and are expressed both on endothelial cells and on leukocytes (Haverslag, Pasterkamp, and Hoefer, 2008). Three selectin family members, namely P-, E-, and L-selectin, are expressed moderately on the luminal aspect of the endothelial cells that line both capillaries and post-capillary venules, and are heavily represented within the pial microvessels that crisscross the innermost layer of the meninges (Engelhardt, 2008). A notable exception to this general rule is P-selectin, which is not expressed in parenchymal microvessels (Barkalow *et al.*, 1996).

As the rolling leukocyte is slowed down and proceeds along the luminal surface of the endothelium, it is able to sample vessel walls for the presence of chemokines, a sizable cohort of which (summarized in Man, Ubogu, and Ransohoff, 2007) may function in the second step, which is the activation of heterodimeric integrins on the leukocyte. Once activated, the integrin heterodimer will transition from a low- to a high-affinity/avidity state (Engelhardt and

Ransohoff, 2005), and can bind to either VCAM (vascular cell adhesion molecule)-1 or ICAM (intercellular adhesion molecule)-1, which are expressed on endothelial surfaces. Evidence to support these integrin/CAM interactions is based primarily on studies of cellular infiltration of the CNS during the induction of experimental autoimmune encephalitis (EAE, a model for multiple sclerosis) in rodents. Evidence from these numerous studies, taken together, suggests that the α4β1 integrin heterodimer, very late antigen (VLA)-4, pairs specifically with VCAM-1, and that LFA-1 binds to ICAM-1. In support of the importance of the former interaction, a monoclonal antibody to VLA-4, (Natalizumab), has been shown to be efficacious in the treatment of MS in humans (Miller *et al.*, 2003), and strikingly reduces T-cell infiltration of lesions in the CNS (Yednock *et al.*, 1992; Piraino *et al.*, 2005).

Binding of these co-receptor pairs brings the leukocyte to a full stop, which is the third step, known as adhesion. It is important to point out here that steps 1 through 3 are generally applicable to all situations of endothelial crossing by leukocytes, including the situation of transcellular, or "through cells" transmigration, which does not necessitate the uncoupling of endothelial tight junctions. Steps 4 through 6 that follow are specific to paracellular, or "between cells" extravasation.

The leukocyte, having now completely left the circulation, may crawl (locomotion, the fourth step) along the endothelial wall in search of an intercellular tight junction. Upon locating a tight junction, the leukocyte is likely guided by the presence of chemokines produced at the abluminal aspect of the endothelial wall. CCL19, CCL21, and CCL22 have been implicated by some as being critical in EAE-associated infiltration (Columba-Cabezas *et al.*, 2002, 2003), but experimental proof of this particular interaction in healthy tissue is still lacking to date.

The immune cell will then extend a process into the junction, following the chemokine gradient (process extension, the fifth step). Following process extension, molecules primarily involved in the formation of the tight endothelial junctions, such as the junctional adhesion molecule JAM-1, can now bind to leukocyte-expressed integrins, such as leukocyte function associated molecule (LFA)-1 (Del Maschio *et al.*, 1999), and thus mediate extravasation of the immune cell into the perivascular space (the sixth and final step).

Immune cell crossing at the choroid plexus is necessarily different from crossing at the capillary or venule. The capillaries within the choroid plexus tissue are fenestrated, and thus do not present the same obstacles to potential transmigration by leukocytes. Choroidal capillaries also present a different landscape in terms of selectin expression, with P-selectin believed to be critical (Engelhardt and Ransohoff, 2005), since antibodies to P-selectin drastically limit T-cell numbers in the meninges and choroid plexus, (Carrithers, Vintin, Kang, and Janeway, 2000) though this is somewhat surprising, since IHC does not reveal expression in this area (Engelhardt, Vestweber, Hallman, and Schultz, 1997, but also see Kivisakk *et al.*, 2003); it is surmised that levels below detection, or antibodies with poor specificity are responsible for this apparent paradox. Selectin expression (including E-selectin and L-selectin) in the choroid plexus area in general, in fact, is controversial. This is due not only to the paucity of conclusive IHC results, but also to a seeming disparity between selectin-mediated mechanisms in humans and mice – at least as they are examined in EAE studies. What is known is that selectins, especially P-selectin, are key to the tethering and rolling of leukocytes in the choroid plexus venules, and that CAMs, including ICAM-1 and mucosal vascular addressin cell adhesion molecule (MadCAM)-1, are involved in transepithelial migration, similar to the transendothelial migration in parenchymal venules mediated by ICAM-1 and VCAM-1. Interestingly, abluminal expression of ICAM-1 and MadCAM-1 has also been noted in choroid plexus (Steffen *et al.*, 1996), perhaps indicating a reverse pathway from CSF back into blood.

It becomes clear that the immune privilege of the CNS is considerably less extreme than originally thought. Such a realization must prompt a modification in the way we consider the resolution of CNS injury, the etiology of inflammation-associated CNS pathology, and of psychiatric disorders that may be affected (or caused) by the workings of the immune system. We must even necessarily amend our considerations of the ramifications of CNS immunity on the modulation of neural function in support of higher thought processes such as learning, memory, and cognition.

Immune system–CNS Crosstalk

While the manifestation of pathology in any part of the body may ultimately be disruptive to the function of the entire organism, it is almost always the rule – rather than the exception – when disease or injury strikes the CNS. Without the brain, brainstem, and spinal cord, the rest of the body will simply cease to live at all. Thus, it is imperative that the CNS be protected, even at great cost, from injury or infection. Yet, the same argument in terms of importance to the whole can be made for the immune system. Indeed, without a proper defense against the furious onslaught of fungi, viruses, bacteria, and parasites that seek to propagate themselves at the cost of their host, higher organisms (as we know them), humans included, would likely have vanished from the earth long ago. Given that the CNS and the immune system are each so integral to the maintenance and proliferation of our species, it might rationally be supposed that they work together in ways that are mutually beneficial. Surprisingly, though, as we have seen in the case of the way the BBB and immune privilege are viewed, the assumption that the two systems must remain separate except at peril to the whole is far more commonly accepted than the reverse. Yet, as Abraham Lincoln famously wrote, "A house divided upon itself cannot stand." Recent data show that there is, in fact, an elegant interplay requiring communication and cooperation between the CNS and the immune system.

CNS–immune communication: Direct, bidirectional, and necessary

The immune system enjoys a great deal of independence in its workings. A dendritic cell or macrophage will present antigen as readily in a Petri dish as it will in the body (Lanzavecchia and Watts, 1994). It will not, however, do much else in the absence of the ever-changing plethora of signaling, cues, and cofactors to be found in the body. Thus, neither immune cells nor the immune system are entirely autonomous. As it happens, the CNS, a central regulator of most systems in the body, is able to exert a measure of control over the immune system. A case in point of CNS–immune influence can be clearly seen in the immune stress response, in which glucocorticoid (GC) synthesis via the hypothalamic–pituitary–adrenal (HPA) axis is responsible for widespread changes in the immune system.

Chronic, acute, and injury-induced stress Chronic stress has been shown to affect immune function in primarily suppressive ways. Classic experiments showing thymic involution (Selye, 1936) and the apoptosis of lymphocytes resulting from increased GC levels provide striking evidence of stress-induced immune suppression on both the anatomical and cellular level (Selye and Horava, 1953; Tarcic, Ovadia, Weiss, and Weidenfeld, 1998) More recently, the expression of canonical immune-derived pro-inflammatory cytokines such as IL1-β and TNF have also been shown to be severely suppressed by chronic GC exposure (De Bosscher, Vanden Beghe, and Haegeman, 2003). Synthetic formulations of GC molecules, like dexamethazone, are widely used by the medical community in immunosuppressive regimens (Lowenberg, Stahn, Hommes, and Buttgereit, 2008). For these reasons, the GC-mediated effects of stress are assumed to be generally immunosuppressive; yet, it is critically important that such an oversimplification not be applied to all stressors or GC-mediated processes. When the effects of acute stress are compared to those mediated by chronic stress, for instance, it becomes clear that bidirectional modulation is indeed the rule rather than the exception.

Acute stress, in fact, has been shown to upregulate expression of MHC-II on both peripheral myeloid cells and CNS microglia (Frank *et al.*, 2007), and stimulate proliferation of natural killer cells (Schedlowski *et al.*, 1996), thus preparing the body for an imminent immune response. GC also prevent apoptosis of neutrophils, the first-line granulocyte responders of the cellular immune compartment (Cox, 1995; Liles, Dale, and Klebanoff, 1995). Importantly, this effect does not generalize to all to granulocytes; an opposite effect is seen upon GC exposure in the other two granulocyte populations, eosinophils and basophils (Schleimer and Bochner, 1994; Yoshimura *et al.*, 2001) indicating that the prevention of neutrophil apoptosis is not simply an unintended epiphenomenon of GC influence. In sum, the above findings suggest a "priming" effect on the immune system of stress-induced acute GC release. This priming effect is demonstrated elegantly by Johnson and coworkers, who showed that an acute stressor in mice, in the form of inescapable tail shock given 24 hours before the introduction of LPS, significantly increases the level of pro-inflammatory cytokine release as measured in both plasma and in brain (Johnson *et al.*, 2002).

The Immune System in Response to Neuroinflammation and Neurodegeneration

It is remarkable that the immune system is seen as a beneficial entity in most of the body, and critical to the healing process – yet the reverse is perceived in terms of immune presence in the CNS. Much of this difference can likely be attributed to data that highlights the destructive role of pro-inflammatory cytokines (Druzhyna, Musiyenko, Wilson, and LeDoux, 2005; Frank-Cannon, Alto, McAlpine, and Tansey, 2009), superoxide radicals, like inducible nitric oxide synthase (iNOS) (Bagasra *et al.*, 1995) and prostaglandin synthases like cyclooxygenase (COX)-1 and -2 (Nogawa, Zhang, Ross, and Iadecola, 1997; Iadecola and Alexander, 2001). There is much controversy that persists, however, and a significant number of groups also report that the above mediators play roles in resolution of inflammation or neuroprotection (Iadecola, 1997; Nawashiro, Tasaki, Ruetzler, and Hallenbeck, 1997; Lawrence, Gilroy, Colville-Nash, and Willoughby, 2001), and healthy brain function (Kaufmann *et al.*, 1996; Stellwagen and Malenka, 2006). Clearly, there are two sides to the coin, and indeed, evidence suggests that timing and internal feedback mechanisms might be a key factor in determining the beneficial or pathological effects of these mediators (Shaked *et al.*, 2004; Serhan and Savill, 2005).

Further skewing the perception towards the viewpoint that immune activity is generally harmful in the CNS, is the interpretation of the activation status of innate immune cells such as microglia and macrophages. Activated microglia have primarily been assumed to be tissue-destructive (Block, Zecca, and Hong, 2007) but this idea has been challenged lately by data that suggest a more complex heterogeneity in microglial function (Hanisch and Kettenmann,

2007). Recent studies implicate microglia (Persson, Brantefjord, Hansson, and Ronnback, 2005; Butovsky *et al.*, 2006), as well as blood-borne myeloid cells (Shechter *et al.*, 2009) in neuroprotective roles. Thus, the presence and identification of cell phenotype – namely pro-inflammatory (M1) or anti-inflammatory/suppressive (M2) myeloid cells (Mantovani, Sica, and Locati, 2005) and microglia (Michelucci *et al.*, 2009; Ransohoff and Perry, 2009) – has become increasingly important to our understanding of CNS immunity. The realization that innate immune cell phenotype in the CNS is plastic, rapid and completely reversible (Appel, Beers, and Henkel, 2009) may be key to understanding specifically when inflammation should be blocked, and when it should actually be encouraged. Similarly, it bears mentioning that innate cell phenotype is critical in dictating the attraction and phenotype of adaptive immune cells like T-cells, which have recently been shown to play unanticipated beneficial roles in CNS pathologies.

T-cells in the resolution of acute CNS injury

The phenomenon of autoimmune T-cell activity, in particular, is most often viewed as an example of an immune system "run amok," and perhaps for good reason; this destructive paradigm is demonstrated convincingly by CNS viral diseases like progressive multifocal leukoencephalopathy (PML), and autoinflammatory pathologies like MS. Along these lines, the adaptive immune system has customarily been seen as a significant detrimental factor in the phenomenon of secondary neuronal degeneration that follows the primary insult of CNS injuries (Aarli, 1983; Zamvil *et al.*, 1985). Thus, when it was revealed that autoimmune T-cells were actually associated with protection from secondary neuronal degeneration following CNS axotomy (Moalem *et al.*, 1999) the response from the scientific community was far from uniformly accepting or supportive. Yet, this discovery was not an anomalous finding. Rather, it proved seminal to a series of related findings from unrelated investigators that autoreactive T-cells were indeed crucial to neuronal recovery post-insult (Yoles *et al.*, 2001). Jones and coworkers showed that severe combined immunodeficient (SCID) mice, lacking both T-cells and B-cells, were significantly impaired in recovery of function after facial nerve transection, as compared to wild type controls with a full immune cell complement (Serpe *et al.*, 2002). It was subsequently shown by the same group that stimulation by CNS autoantigen was required by the $CD4^+$ T-cells responsible for nerve repair (Serpe, Coers, Sanders, and Jones, 2003; Byram *et al.*, 2004) implicating autoimmune mechanisms as key to recovery of facial nerve function.

T-cells in the resolution of chronic CNS neurodegeneration

Evidence that T-cells are important in modulating the resolution of CNS neurodegeneration comes from other pathologies as well. An interesting example is that of amyotrophic lateral sclerosis (ALS). ALS is an adult-onset disorder that selectively targets upper and lower motor neurons for destruction, resulting in muscle weakness, spasticity, and ultimately, death (Boillee, Van de Velde, and Cleveland, 2006). Human ALS pathology can be recapitulated in mouse via a mutant form of the superoxide dismutase (mSOD1) gene (Gurney *et al.*, 1994). Neuroinflammation is a hallmark of ALS, and it has been thought that lymphocyte infiltration seen in ALS lesions was evidence of immune-mediated destruction of neurons (Engelhardt, Tajti, and Appel, 1993), and initiated by T-cells. To better understand the contribution of T-cells to neurodegeneration seen in ALS, Appel and coworkers bred mSOD1 mice also lacking functional T-cells. When they examined these mice, the unexpected result was that disease progression in animals lacking T-cells was accelerated rather than slowed, thus indicating that T-cells were playing a beneficial role (Chiu *et al.*, 2008). This discovery was supported by a subsequent finding demonstrating a beneficial effect of adoptively transferred T-cell subsets in mSOD1 mutants. Specifically, both $CD4^+$ T_{reg} and effector T (T_{eff}) (activated T-cells produced during the proliferative burst T-cells undergo after being primed by antigen) were sufficient to extend lifespan and reduce severity of disease in mSOD1 mice (Banerjee *et al.*, 2008). T_{eff} that had been isolated from other disease-bearing mSOD1 mice – thus T-cells specific for CNS autoantigen – conferred greater benefit than T-cells isolated from wild type mice. Interestingly, T_{reg} conferred neuroprotection late in disease progression, but not early, suggesting that immune suppression was only beneficial in the final stages of disease, when innate cells would be likely to switch the phenotype of T_{eff} cells from anti-inflammatory (T_H2) to pro-inflammatory (T_H1) phenotype. This last finding is perhaps particularly important, since it again elucidates the importance of timing in terms of the adaptive immune response, which will be crucial in designing appropriate therapies for neuroinflammatory disorders.

Complementary to the above studies, it is certainly worthy of note that there is little difference, if any, in terms of levels of circulating T-cells in healthy individuals compared to those suffering from autoimmune disease (Lohse *et al.*, 1996; Kipnis *et al.*, 2006). Autoimmunity is also evolutionarily conserved, and autoantigens can be well-categorized molecularly – even across species (Cohen, 1992a). Thus, it is reasonable to assume that well-controlled autoantigen recognition and reactivity would be part and parcel of a healthy immune system, rather than an aberration. Indeed, as will be detailed in the section to follow, the beneficial aspects of T-cells reactive to self antigen are not limited to cases of frank injury to the CNS, or to pathologies involving – and long thought to be caused by – neuroinflammation. In fact, it has been recently shown that T-cells are also important to the healthy function of the brain, and even perform in support of higher cognitive functions such as learning and memory.

The Immune System and Higher Brain Function

Since it was shown – roughly a decade ago – that a well-controlled autoreactive T-cell response after CNS injury reduces post-traumatic loss of neurons (Moalem *et al.*, 1999), a startling range of pathologies have been demonstrated to be to amenable to amelioration by the very same cells that were once thought to be anathema to CNS health. Nevertheless, a situation involving acute injury or pathological inflammation is still quite different from the day-to-day assembly and maintenance of the complex neural circuits that underlie higher brain functions such as learning and memory.

To begin with, there is a striking difference in scale between neural pathology and neural homeostasis in terms of their ability to attract the immune system. A CNS injury, by its very nature, is an acute situation, and would be likely to draw the prompt and targeted attention of the immune system, vis-à-vis the release of "danger" signals, in the form of dense chemokine and neurotransmitter gradients. Present also would be vast amounts of CNS autoantigen, composed of cellular and molecular debris. In such a case, the immune system might become activated and migrate into CNS tissue. In frank neuroinflammatory disease, the situation is analogous, demanding a heightened and targeted response to pathology. In contrast, a biologically significant immune presence affecting healthy CNS function would necessitate similar mechanisms, but on a scale much harder to detect, and constrained within the bounds of normal homeostatic levels of molecular mediators. Furthermore, the neural substrates of learning and memory are comparatively diffuse, thus shrouding the location of the target of action by the immune system, were it to be involved. Finally, there would be the question of access, given the higher threshold for CNS entrance than periphery for the immune system.

Thus, the finding that immunodeficient SCID mice were markedly impaired in tests of learning and memory such as the Morris water maze (MWM) (Kipnis *et al.*, 2004), Barnes maze, and radial arm maze (Brynskikh, Warren, Zhu, and Kipnis, 2008), while not unexpected, was indeed tantalizing, given the stark differences between CNS pathology and healthy function. Importantly, analogous learning deficiencies were shown in other immunodeficient strains, including athymic nude mice lacking T-cells, and recombinase activation gene (RAG) mutants, lacking mature T- and B-cells. Also striking was the corollary result that injection of T-cell-deficient mice with splenocytes from wild type counterparts improved their performance on learning and memory tasks to a level similar to that of wild type (Kipnis *et al.*, 2004). Importantly, the ability of simple passive transfer of splenocytes to rescue the phenotype of adult SCID mice in the MWM implied that the effects of immunodeficiency were not merely a developmental aberration.

Phenomenologically, it was clear that immune deficiency could negatively impact brain function, but many questions remained: What was the subgroup of splenocytes that were important – were they the same autoimmune T-cells that were found to be beneficial in CNS pathology? Where, indeed, were these cells promulgating their effects – in the periphery, or within the CNS? If they were in the CNS, then were they interacting directly with brain parenchyma or did they require local intermediaries? Was there a particular molecular factor produced by these cells that was crucial to brain function? Answers to some of these questions have been provided by subsequent research, and the others are being intensively studied, including by our lab.

Autoimmune T-cells in learning and memory

Clues to the identity of the immune cells important to learning and memory were provided when T_{MBP} transgenic mice (engineered to express only a T-cell receptor specific for an epitope of the myelin basic protein (MBP) self-antigen), and T_{ova} transgenic mice, (engineered to express only a T-cell receptor specific for an irrelevant antigen, ovalbumin) were compared to wild type mice in the MWM. Wild type mice showed significantly better performance than T_{ova}, and T_{MBP} showed significantly better performance than wild type, indicating that T-cells directed toward CNS antigen provided superior support to learning and memory function or were sufficient to support normal function. Presence of T-cells per se, as in the case of T_{ova} mice, was not sufficient to support normal cognitive function, and thus antigen is likely required. When hippocampi from these mice were examined, the same pattern was evident in that T_{ova} mice showed impaired levels of neurogenesis as compared to both wild type and T_{MBP} mice (Ziv *et al.*, 2006). These results, in sum, showed that T-cells, and CNS antigen-specific T-cells in particular, were key players in the support of the normal renewal of cells in the hippocampus. It was further shown that T-cells were essential for cognitive improvement, because transfusion of T-cell-depleted splenocytes to SCID mice did not provide enhancement in cognitive function (Brynskikh, Warren, Zhu, and Kipnis, 2008). $CD4^+$, but not $CD8^+$ T-cells were recently shown to mediate the effect on cognition (Wolf *et al.*, 2009) in experiments that deleted these specific subsets.

While the above experiments demonstrated clear "phenomenological" evidence that immune cells (and specifically $CD4^+$ T-lymphocytes) were key players in the support of learning and memory, many questions remained. First, where were T-cells acting – in the periphery, in the parenchyma of the brain, or somewhere in-between? Were all T-cells important to the phenomenon, or was a particular subset critical, i.e. memory T-cells, naïve T-cells, pro- or anti-inflammatory T-cells? Did T-cells produce molecular messengers that served to activate downstream cells? Were APC important intermediaries, or were T-cells acting directly on brain parenchymal cells, i.e. neurons and glia?

IL-4 and cognition: The importance of meningeal immunity

Our recent findings indicate that the immune system benefits the brain function through the meningeal spaces. Meninges and choroid plexus consists of a large numbers of cells therein positive for CD11b, a myeloid cell marker, and MHC-II – indicating that meningeal T-cells were likely in dialogue with these local antigen presenting cells; this scenario would be a prerequisite for dynamic T-cell regulation right "next door" rather than directly within the brain. Thus, we considered fully the possibility that T-cells were important regulators of the meningeal immune milieu, and that these ventricular and exterior CNS structures might offer more than just protection from physical insult.

To better understand the function of these meningeal T-cells, we considered methods of restricting their entrance, but keeping them in the periphery. By using an antibody to VLA-4, a molecule critical for T-cell diapedesis (Yednock *et al.*, 1992; Baron *et al.*, 1993), and thus preventing the access of T-cells to the meningeal areas, we found that we could detrimentally affect CNS function. The impaired learning phenotype of these otherwise wild type animals with normal immune systems – except for the fact that levels of meningeal T-cells were drastically reduced – was reminiscent of constitutively T-cell deficient animals. Importantly, this suggested that meningeal immune cells had a specific and critical job to do in support of normal brain activity, and that they needed to act locally to be effective. Of significance, we found that when we blocked T-cell entrance into the meninges, the level of pro-inflammatory cytokines expressed by meningeal myeloid cells increased substantially. Given that T-cells are assumed to be "bad actors" when found close to the brain, as is shown in mouse models of CNS inflammatory diseases, our results went directly against the dogmatic assumption that removing T-cells from the CNS regions would lower inflammation. Therefore, the meningeal areas emerged as a key location from which T-cells could augment – or inhibit – higher brain function by upregulating or downregulating the expression of pro- and anti-inflammatory factors by resident myeloid cells, plentiful in the meningeal areas. These findings gave important anatomical context to much previous data implicating pro-inflammatory cytokines as being unfavorable to healthy cognitive function. It had previously been suggested that circulating pro-inflammatory cytokines could act detrimentally on the CNS (Hasegawa *et al.*, 2000; Chen *et al.*, 2007; McAfoose and Baune, 2009), but before our work, a paucity of data reflected a local contribution of the meninges to higher brain function.

When we examined T-cells found within the meninges, and compared mice that had undergone MWM training with naïve animals, it became apparent that trained mice not only had increased levels of T-cells in these areas, but that these T-cells, after training, expressed high levels of IL-4. Based on this striking observation, we compared wild type and $IL4^{-/-}$ mice in the MWM, and demonstrated that the latter group was severely learning impaired (Derecki *et al.*, 2010). This indicated a key role for IL-4 in spatial learning and memory. In fact, there was tangential support for this, from recent work showing IL-4 to be beneficial in a mouse model of Alzheimer's disease (Cao *et al.*, 2009). What was novel and unexpected, however, was the fact that it had never been previously considered that IL-4 secreted by circulating immune cells would conceivably have significant effects on normal, healthy brain function.

Following this, we performed irradiation and bone marrow transfer experiments with IL-$4^{-/-}$ mice and wild type mice and demonstrated that we could impair the performance of wild type animals or improve the performance of knockout animals in the Morris water maze following replacement of the immune system of each with that of the other. These experiments demonstrated the immune system specificity of the IL-4 source (Derecki *et al.*, 2010).

Finally, we examined the possibility that neurotrophins might be regulated by IL-4, and thus provide one link between IL-4 and learning. We showed that IL-4 robustly increased brain-derived neurotrophic factor (BDNF) production by primary astrocytes, that IL-4 was able to block BDNF downregulation by pro-inflammatory cytokines, and that interestingly, $IL4^{-/-}$ mice showed no BDNF increase in the hippocampus after MWM training; this phenomenon in wild type mice has been well-demonstrated by other groups as being concomitant with learning in hippocampally-based assays including MWM and foot shock avoidance (Kesslak *et al.*, 1998; Hall, Thomas, and Everitt, 2000).

Of no small consequence, these experiments were done in adult animals. This fact suggested that the immune system could be harnessed to *acutely* modify brain function. In terms of therapeutic potential, this is important, since it opens the door to direct treatment of pathology, rather than simply prophylactic treatment. We showed that immune factors, more than being important during brain development (Huh *et al.*, 2000; Stevens *et al.*, 2007) were also critical in adulthood, and were dynamic players in day-to-day "real-time" CNS function.

Thus, this work was the first to demonstrate a specific molecular mechanism that might begin to explain the striking phenomenon that adaptive immune-deficient mice were severely impaired in assays of spatial learning and memory, and the corollary finding that passive transfer of wild type T-cells could dramatically improve function in these mice. More specifically, our data implicated an immune molecule, IL-4, which could feasibly work in two very different ways to modulate CNS function. First, IL-4 is a prototypical anti-inflammatory cytokine; thus, IL-4 can directly dictate the fate of downstream myeloid cells to a similarly anti-inflammatory "M2" phenotype, centrally important for healing, tissue growth and repair. Second, by identifying a specific peripheral cytokine involved in controlling the production of a critical CNS parenchymal neurotrophic factor, BDNF, we reasoned that we might be able to harness this previously uncharacterized mechanism to skew glial phenotype to a pro-neuronal state in pathological situations.

Meningeal myeloid cells as key players in cognitive disorders

While T-cells are extraordinarily versatile and powerful cells, they carry with them the risk, when used in clinical therapies, of touching off catastrophic autoimmune disease. Thus, we wanted to examine whether meningeal myeloid cells, which we had shown were pushed to an M2 anti-inflammatory phenotype by T-cell-derived IL-4, could impart similar effects within the context of learning and memory as T-cells.

We chose adaptive immune-deficient SCID mice for our experiments, since they are impaired in learning and memory (Kipnis *et al.*, 2004), and display a pro-inflammatory meningeal myeloid skew (Derecki, Quinnies, and Kipnis, 2011). Mice were injected i.v. with syngeneic bone-marrow-derived myeloid cells skewed ex-vivo to either pro-(with rIFN-γ) or anti-inflammatory fate (with rIL-4) and then assayed in the MWM. SCID mice injected with M2 macrophages performed significantly better than M1-injected or control animals. When we examined meningeal immunity in these mice, we confirmed that the injected M2 cells were sufficient to push already-resident meningeal myeloid cells to an anti-inflammatory phenotype, producing increased levels of IL-10 and decreased levels of tissue-destructive TNF (Derecki, Quinnies, and Kipnis, 2011).

These results suggest that M2 cells could contribute directly (in a T-cell-independent manner) to cognitive function, and might be developed in the future as an eminently feasible therapeutic approach for cognitive conditions associated with T-cell malfunction. This was the first demonstration of the ability of myeloid cells to improve cognitive function. This is extremely important because HIV-dementia, immunosuppressive chemotherapy regimens, allotransplantation, allograft, and age-related dementia are several conditions that are associated with cognitive impairment and are also pathologies that might preclude the use of T-cells as a practical therapy. Theoretically, however, macrophages from such a patient could easily be expanded ex vivo, skewed to an anti-inflammatory phenotype, then re-injected with minimal risk of autoimmune disease. M2 cells might even shift T-cell immunity towards an anti-inflammatory TH2 phenotype, leading to a self-propagating beneficial response. These results were obtained in a model lacking T-cells altogether, thus models more analogous to human conditions, such as wild type mice treated with chemotherapeutic agents need to be explored.

Summary Conclusions

Our grasp of the workings of the blood–brain barrier and of CNS immune privilege has undergone a veritable sea change in recent years. Far from being impassable bulwarks separating body from brain, the BBB and immune privilege have been newly recharacterized as integral parts of an elegant and complex neuroimmune network. Moreover, it has now been demonstrated that the brain is far from impenetrable to immune cells and their molecular mediators. In this way, the BBB can be thought of as a *facilitator* of communication rather than an impediment to it. Thus, a plethora of unanticipated factors, long considered to be germane only to the hematopoietic and immune systems, will need be taken into account when considering both day-to-day function and pathological dysfunction of the CNS. Accordingly, our understanding of the term "neuroimmunology," and what it encompasses, has necessarily also changed. Once concerned exclusively with a small cohort of pathological conditions involving clear *attack* of the CNS by the immune system, neuroimmunologists are now beginning to uncover *healthy physiological interactions* between the two systems that have implications far beyond the setting of frank pathology. Immune mediators have lately been shown to dictate CNS processes as fundamental as neuronal guidance, as subtle as synaptic refinement and maintenance, and as complex as learning, memory, and higher cognitive function. Even within the realm of disease, the purview of the neuroimmunologist is now considerably extended beyond "core" neuroinflammatory disorders such as MS. Pathologies like Parkinson's, Alzheimer's, and Huntington's disease have all been demonstrated to feature immune dysregulation as contributing factors, and the list is ever-growing. Psychiatric disorders, including major depression, bipolar disorder, and schizophrenia, all of which have previously been attributed to CNS-exclusive dysfunction, have recently been suggested to have strong immune links.

Thus, it is not surprising that much attention is now also being paid to the possible role of the immune system in what is perhaps the newest frontier of all in neuroimmunology: immune regulation of higher brain functions, including learning and memory. There is general agreement by now that a fair number of immune molecules are necessary for normal development and functioning of the brain. It has yet to be established, however, whether the role of peripheral immune cells is restricted to maintenance of CNS homeostasis or whether the immune system is directly involved in brain function. Thus, for example, in the case of cognitive function, it is not yet known whether the immune system participates actively in learning and memory processes, or simply helps the brain to cope with the stress associated with learning, and thus allows the learning process to be more efficient. Nevertheless, as clearly demonstrated by findings summarized here, we can no longer ignore immune malfunction as a potentially contributory or even causative factor in the etiology of neurodevelopmental, cognitive, and psychiatric dysfunction, and as a possible critical supporting factor in healthy cognitive function.

Along these lines, it can be argued that healthy brain function depends upon the ability of the immune system to successfully regulate the production of "proneuronal" factors. These include the secretion of growth factors, like BDNF and IGF-1, the preservation of homeostatic balance between pro- and anti-inflammatory cytokines within the CNS milieu, and the proper maintenance of the CNS cellular environment by appropriate clearance of cellular detritus and toxic compounds, such that normal neuronal development may occur. Thus, we propose that impaired brain function and CNS pathology may be amenable to amelioration by manipulation of either or both meningeal and parenchymal immunity.

References

Aarli, J.A. (1983). The immune system and the nervous system. *Journal of Neurology*, 229, 137–154.

Abbott, N.J., Ronnback, L., and Hansson, E. (2006). Astrocyte–endothelial interactions at the blood–brain barrier. *Nature Reviews in Neuroscience*, 7, 41–53.

Ando-Akatsuka, Y., Yonemura, S., Itoh, M., Furuse, M., and Tsukita, S. (1999). Differential behavior of E-cadherin and occludin in their colocalization with ZO-1 during the establishment of epithelial cell polarity. *Journal of Cell Physiology*, 179, 115–125.

Anthony, I.C., Crawford, D.H., and Bell, J.E. (2003). B lymphocytes in the normal brain: contrasts with HIV-associated lymphoid infiltrates and lymphomas. *Brain*, 126, 1058–1067.

Appel, S.H., Beers, D.R., and Henkel, J.S. (2009). T cell–microglial dialogue in Parkinson's disease and amyotrophic lateral sclerosis: are we listening? *Trends in Immunology*, 31, 7–17.

Bagasra, O., Michaels, F.H., Zheng, Y.M., Bobroski, L.E., Spitsin, S.V., Fu, Z.F. et al. (1995). Activation of the inducible form of nitric oxide synthase in the brains of patients with multiple sclerosis. *Proceedings of the National Academy of Sciences of the USA*, 92, 12041–12045.

Banerjee, R., Mosley, R.L., Reynolds, A.D., Dhar, A., Jackson-Lewis, V., Gordon, P.H. et al. (2008). Adaptive immune neuroprotection in G93A-SOD1 amyotrophic lateral sclerosis mice. *PLoS ONE* 3:e2740.

Barkalow, F.J., Goodman, M.J., Gerritsen, M.E., and Mayadas, T.N. (1996). Brain endothelium lack one of two pathways of P-selectin-mediated neutrophil adhesion. *Blood*, 88, 4585–4593.

Baron, J.L., Madri, J.A., Ruddle, N.H., Hashim, G., and Janeway, C.A., Jr. (1993). Surface expression of alpha 4 integrin by CD4 T cells is required for their entry into brain parenchyma. *Journal of Experimental Medicine*, 177, 57–68.

Beattie, E.C., Stellwagen, D., Morishita, W., Bresnahan, J.C., Ha, B.K., Von Zastrow, M., et al. (2002). Control of synaptic strength by glial TNFalpha. *Science*, 295, 2282–2285.

Block, M.L., Zecca, L., and Hong, J.S. (2007). Microglia-mediated neurotoxicity: uncovering the molecular mechanisms. *Nature Reviews in Neuroscience*, 8, 57–69.

Boillee, S., Vande Velde, C., and Cleveland, D.W. (2006). ALS: a disease of motor neurons and their nonneuronal neighbors. *Neuron*, 52, 39–59.

Brightman, M.W. and Reese, T.S. (1969). Junctions between intimately apposed cell membranes in the vertebrate brain. *Journal of Cell Biology*, 40, 648–677.

Brynskikh, A., Warren, T., Zhu, J., and Kipnis, J. (2008). Adaptive immunity affects learning behavior in mice. *Brain, Behavior, Immunity*, 22, 861–869.

Burgess,W., Gheusi, G., Yao, J., Johnson, R.W., Dantzer, R., and Kelley, K.W. (1998). Interleukin-1beta-converting enzyme-deficient mice resist central but not systemic endotoxin-induced anorexia. *American Journal of Physiology*, 274, R1829–1833.

Butcher, E.C., Williams, M., Youngman, K., Rott, L., and Briskin, M. (1999). Lymphocyte trafficking and regional immunity. *Advances in Immunology*, 72, 209–253.

Butovsky, O., Landa, G., Kunis, G., Ziv, Y., Avidan, H., Greenberg, N.S. et al. (2006). Induction and blockage of oligodendrogenesis by differently activated microglia in an animal model of multiple sclerosis. *Journal of Clinical Investigation*, 116, 905–915.

Byram, S.C., Carson, M.J., DeBoy, C.A., Serpe, C.J., Sanders, V.M., and Jones, K.J. (2004). CD4-positive T cell-mediated neuroprotection requires dual compartment antigen presentation. *Journal of Neuroscience*, 24, 4333–4339.

Cao, C., Arendash, G.W., Dickson, A., Mamcarz, M.B., Lin, X., and Ethell, D.W. (2009). Beta-specific Th2 cells provide cognitive and pathological benefits to Alzheimer's mice without infiltrating the CNS. *Neurobiology of Disease*, 34, 63–70.

Carrithers, M.D., Visintin, I., Kang, S.J., and Janeway, C.A., Jr. (2000). Differential adhesion molecule requirements for immune surveillance and inflammatory recruitment. *Brain*, 123 (Pt 6), 1092–1101.

Carvey, P.M., Hendey, B., and Monahan, A.J. (2009). The blood–brain barrier in neurodegenerative disease: a rhetorical perspective. *Journal of Neurochemistry*, 111, 291–314.

Chen, J., Buchanan, J.B., Sparkman, N.L., Godbout, J.P., Freund, G.G., and Johnson, R.W. (2007). Neuroinflammation and disruption in working memory in aged mice after acute stimulation of the peripheral innate immune system. *Brain, Behavior, Immunity*, 22, 301–311.

Chiu, I.M., Chen, A., Zheng, Y., Kosaras, B., Tsiftsoglou, S.A., Vartanian, T.K. et al. (2008). T lymphocytes potentiate endogenous neuroprotective inflammation in a mouse model of ALS. *Proceedings of the National Academy of Sciences of the USA*, 105, 17913–17918.

Cohen, I.R. (1992a). The cognitive paradigm and the immunological homunculus. *Immunology Today*, 13, 490–494.

Cohen, I.R. (1992b). The cognitive principle challenges clonal selection. *Immunology Today*, 13, 441–444.

Columba-Cabezas, S., Serafini, B., Ambrosini, E., and Aloisi, F. (2003). Lymphoid chemokines CCL19 and CCL21 are expressed in the central nervous system during experimental autoimmune encephalomyelitis: implications for the maintenance of chronic neuroinflammation. *Brain Pathology*, 13, 38–51.

Columba-Cabezas, S., Serafini, B., Ambrosini, E., Sanchez, M., Penna, G., Adorini, L., and Aloisi, F. (2002). Induction of macrophage-derived chemokine/CCL22 expression in experimental autoimmune encephalomyelitis and cultured microglia: implications for disease regulation. *Journal of Neuroimmunology*, 130, 10–21.

Cox, G. (1995). Glucocorticoid treatment inhibits apoptosis in human neutrophils. Separation of survival and activation outcomes. *Journal of Immunology*, 154, 4719–4725.

Cserr, H.F. and Knopf, P.M. (1992). Cervical lymphatics, the blood–brain barrier and the immunoreactivity of the brain: a new view. *Immunology Today*, 13, 507–512.

Cserr, H.F., Harling-Berg, C.J., and Knopf, P.M. (1992). Drainage of brain extracellular fluid into blood and deep cervical lymph and its immunological significance. *Brain Pathology*, 2, 269–276.

Dantzer, R., O'Connor, J.C., Freund, G.G., Johnson, R.W., and Kelley, K.W. (2008). From inflammation to sickness and depression: when the immune system subjugates the brain. *Nature Reviews in Neuroscience*, 9, 46–56.

De Bosscher, K., Vanden Berghe, W., and Haegeman, G. (2003). The interplay between the glucocorticoid receptor and nuclear factor-kappaB or activator protein-1: molecular mechanisms for gene repression. *Endocrine Reviews*, 24, 488–522.

Del Maschio, A., De Luigi, A., Martin-Padura, I., Brockhaus, M., Bartfai, T., Fruscella, P. et al. (1999). Leukocyte recruitment in the cerebrospinal fluid of mice with experimental meningitis is inhibited by an antibody to junctional adhesion molecule (JAM). *Journal of Experimental Medicine*, 190, 1351–1356.

Derecki, N.C., Quinnies, K.M., and Kipnis, J. (2011). Alternatively activated myeloid (M2). cells enhance cognitive function in immune compromised mice. *Brain, Behavior, Immunity*, 25, 379–385.

Derecki, N.C., Cardani, A.N., Yang, C.H., Quinnies, K.M., Crihfield, A., Lynch, K.R., and Kipnis, J. (2010). Regulation of learning and memory by meningeal immunity: a key role for IL-4. *Journal of Experimental Medicine*, 207, 1067–1080.

Druzhyna, N.M., Musiyenko, S.I., Wilson, G.L., and LeDoux, S.P. (2005). Cytokines induce nitric oxide-mediated mtDNA damage and apoptosis in oligodendrocytes. Protective role of targeting 8-oxoguanine glycosylase to mitochondria. *Journal of Bioligical Chemistry*, 280, 21673–21679.

Dziegielewska, K.M. and Saunders, N.R. (2002). The ins and outs of brain–barrier mechanisms. *Trends in Neuroscience*, 25, 69–71.

Dziegielewska, K.M., Ek, J., Habgood, M.D., and Saunders, N.R. (2001). Development of the choroid plexus. *Microscopy Research and Technique*, 52, 5–20.

Ehrlich, P. (1885). *Das Sauerstoff-Bedürfnis des Organismus. Eine farbenanalytische Studie.* [On the oxygen consumption of the body. A study using intravital dyes.]. Verlag von August Hirschwald, Berlin.

Engelhardt, B. (2006). Molecular mechanisms involved in T cell migration across the blood–brain barrier. *Journal of Neural Transmission*, 113, 477–485.

Engelhardt, B. (2008). Immune cell entry into the central nervous system: involvement of adhesion molecules and chemokines. *Journal of Neurological Science*, 274, 23–26.

Engelhardt, B. and Ransohoff, R.M. (2005). The ins and outs of T-lymphocyte trafficking to the CNS: anatomical sites and molecular mechanisms. *Trends in Immunology*, 26, 485–495.

Engelhardt, B., Vestweber, D., Hallmann, R., and Schulz, M. (1997). E- and P-selectin are not involved in the recruitment of inflammatory cells across the blood–brain barrier in experimental autoimmune encephalomyelitis. *Blood*, 90, 4459–4472.

Engelhardt, J.I., Tajti, J., and Appel, S.H. (1993). Lymphocytic infiltrates in the spinal cord in amyotrophic lateral sclerosis. *Archives of Neurology*, 50, 30–36.

Fletcher, N.F., Bexiga, M.G., Brayden, D.J., Brankin, B., Willett, B.J., Hosie, M.J. et al. (2009). Lymphocyte migration through the blood–brain barrier (BBB) in feline immunodeficiency virus infection is significantly influenced by the pre-existence of virus and tumour necrosis factor (TNF).–alpha within the central nervous system (CNS): studies using an in vitro feline BBB model. *Neuropathology and Applied Neurobiology*, 35, 592–602.

Frank, M.G., Baratta, M.V., Sprunger, D.B., Watkins, L.R., and Maier, S.F. (2007). Microglia serve as a neuroimmune substrate for stress-induced potentiation of CNS pro-inflammatory cytokine responses. *Brain, Behavior, Immunity*, 21, 47–59.

Frank-Cannon, T.C., Alto, L.T., McAlpine, F.E., and Tansey, M.G. (2009). Does neuroinflammation fan the flame in neurodegenerative diseases? *Molecular Neurodegeneration*, 4, 47.

Galea, I., Bechmann, I., and Perry, V.H. (2007). What is immune privilege (not)? *Trends in Immunology*, 28, 12–18.

Goldmann, E. (1900). Vitalfärbungen am Zentralnervensystem. Beitrag zur Physio-Pathologie des Plexus Choroideus und der Hirnhäute. [Intravital labelling of the central nervous system. A study on the pathophysiology of the choroid plexus and the meninges.] *Abhandlungen der königlich preußischen Akademie der Wissenschaften, Physikalisch-Mathematische Classe 1* (1913), 1–64.

Goldmann, J., Kwidzinski, E., Brandt, C., Mahlo, J., Richter, D., and Bechmann, I. (2006). T cells traffic from brain to cervical lymph nodes via the cribroid plate and the nasal mucosa. *Journal of Leukocyte Biology*, 80, 797–801.

Goldstein, G.W. (1988). Endothelial cell–astrocyte interactions. A cellular model of the blood–brain barrier. *Annals of the New York Academy of Sciences*, 529, 31–39.

Gregerson, D.S., Sam, T.N., and McPherson, S.W. (2004). The antigen-presenting activity of fresh, adult parenchymal microglia and perivascular cells from retina. *Journal of Immunology*, 172, 6587–6597.

Guillemin, G.J. and Brew, B.J. (2004). Microglia, macrophages, perivascular macrophages, and pericytes: a review of function and identification. *Journal of Leukocyte Biology*, 75, 388–397.

Guo, C., Zheng, C., Martin-Padura, I., Bian, Z.C., and Guan, J.L. (1998). Differential stimulation of proline-rich tyrosine kinase 2 and mitogen-activated protein kinase by sphingosine 1-phosphate. *European Journal of Biochemistry*, 257, 403–408.

Gurney, M.E., Pu, H., Chiu, A.Y., Dal Canto, M.C., Polchow, C.Y., Alexander, D.D. et al. (1994). Motor neuron degeneration in mice that express a human Cu,Zn superoxide dismutase mutation. *Science*, 264, 1772–1775.

Hall, J., Thomas, K.L. and Everitt, B.J. (2000). Rapid and selective induction of BDNF expression in the hippocampus during contextual learning. *Nature Neuroscience*, 3, 533–535.

Hanisch, U.K. and Kettenmann, H. (2007). Microglia: active sensor and versatile effector cells in the normal and pathologic brain. *Nature Neuroscience*, 10, 1387–1394.

Hasegawa, Y., Sawada, M., Ozaki, N., Inagaki, T., and Suzumura, A. (2000). Increased soluble tumor necrosis factor receptor levels in the serum of elderly people. *Gerontology*, 46, 185–188.

Haverslag, R., Pasterkamp, G., and Hoefer, I.E. (2008). Targeting adhesion molecules in cardiovascular disorders. *Cardiovascular and Haematological Disorders – Drug Targets*, 8, 252–260.

Hickey, W.F. and Kimura, H. (1988). Perivascular microglial cells of the CNS are bone marrow-derived and present antigen in vivo. *Science*, 239, 290–292.

Hofstetter, H.H., Sewell, D.L., Liu, F., Sandor, M., Forsthuber, T., Lehmann, P.V., and Fabry, Z. (2003). Autoreactive T cells promote post-traumatic healing in the central nervous system. *Journal of Neuroimmunology*, 134, 25–34.

Huh, G.S., Boulanger, L.M., Du, H., Riquelme, P.A., Brotz, T.M., and Shatz, C.J. (2000). Functional requirement for class I MHC in CNS development and plasticity. *Science*, 290, 2155–2159.

Iadecola, C. (1997). Bright and dark sides of nitric oxide in ischemic brain injury. *Trends in Neuroscience*, 20, 132–139.

Iadecola, C. and Alexander, M. (2001). Cerebral ischemia and inflammation. *Current Opinion in Neurology*, 14, 89–94.

Iadecola, C. and Nedergaard, M. (2007). Glial regulation of the cerebral microvasculature. *Nature Neuroscience*, 10, 1369–1376.

Itoh, M., Morita, K., and Tsukita, S. (1999a). Characterization of ZO-2 as a MAGUK family member associated with tight as well as adherens junctions with a binding affinity to occludin and alpha catenin. *Journal of Biological Chemistry*, 274, 5981–5986.

Itoh, M., Furuse, M., Morita, K., Kubota, K., Saitou, M., and Tsukita, S. (1999b). Direct binding of three tight junction-associated MAGUKs, ZO-1, ZO-2, and ZO-3, with the COOH termini of claudins. *Journal of Cell Biology*, 147, 1351–1363.

Janzer, R.C. and Raff, M.C. (1987). Astrocytes induce blood–brain barrier properties in endothelial cells. *Nature*, 325, 253–257.

Johnson, J.D., O'Connor, K.A., Deak, T., Stark, M., Watkins, L.R., and Maier, S.F. (2002). Prior stressor exposure sensitizes LPS-induced cytokine production. *Brain, Behavior, Immunity*, 16, 461–476.

Karnovsky, M.J. (1967). The ultrastructural basis of capillary permeability studied with peroxidase as a tracer. *Journal of Cell Biology*, 35, 213–236.

Karnovsky, M.J. (1968). The Ultrastructural Basis of Transcapillary Exchanges. *Journal of General Physiology*, 52, 64–95.

Kaufmann, W.E., Worley, P.F., Pegg, J., Bremer, M., and Isakson, P. (1996). COX-2, a synaptically induced enzyme, is expressed by excitatory neurons at postsynaptic sites in rat cerebral cortex. *Proceedings of the National Academy of Sciences of the USA*, 93, 2317–2321.

Kelly, A., Lynch, A., Vereker, E., Nolan, Y., Queenan, P., Whittaker, E. et al. (2001). The anti-inflammatory cytokine, interleukin (IL).-10, blocks the inhibitory effect of IL-1 beta on long term potentiation. A role for JNK. *Journal of Biological Chemistry*, 276, 45564–45572.

Kerschensteiner, M., Gallmeier, E., Behrens, L., Leal, V.V., Misgeld, T., Klinkert, W.E. et al. (1999). Activated human T cells, B cells, and monocytes produce brain-derived neurotrophic factor in vitro and in inflammatory brain lesions: a neuroprotective role of inflammation? *Journal of Experimental Medicine*, 189, 865–870.

Kesslak, J.P., So, V., Choi, J., Cotman, C.W., and Gomez-Pinilla, F. (1998). Learning upregulates brain-derived neurotrophic factor messenger ribonucleic acid: a mechanism to facilitate encoding and circuit maintenance? *Behavioral Neuroscience*, 112, 1012–1019.

Kipnis, J. and Schwartz, M. (2002). Dual action of glatiramer acetate (Cop-1). in the treatment of CNS autoimmune and neurodegenerative disorders. *Trends in Molecular Medicine*, 8, 319–323.

Kipnis, J., Cardon, M., Strous, R.D., and Schwartz, M (2006). Loss of autoimmune T cells correlates with brain diseases: possible implications for schizophrenia? *Trends in Molecular Medicine*, 12, 107–112.

Kipnis, J, Cohen, H, Cardon, M, Ziv, Y, and Schwartz, M. (2004). T cell deficiency leads to cognitive dysfunction: implications for therapeutic vaccination for schizophrenia and other psychiatric conditions. *Proceedings of the National Academy of Sciences of the USA*, 101, 8180–8185.

Kivisakk, P., Mahad, D.J., Callahan, M.K., Trebst, C., Tucky, B., Wei, T. et al. (2003). Human cerebrospinal fluid central memory CD4+ T cells: evidence for trafficking through choroid plexus and meninges via P-selectin. *Proceedings of the National Academy of Sciences of the USA*, 100, 8389–8394.

Krueger, M. and Bechmann, I. (2010). CNS pericytes: concepts, misconceptions, and a way out. *Glia*, 58, 1–10.

Lanzavecchia, A. and Watts, C. (1994). Peptide partners call the tune. *Nature*, 371, 198–199.

Lawrence, T., Gilroy, D.W., Colville-Nash, P.R., and Willoughby, D.A. (2001). Possible new role for NF-kappaB in the resolution of inflammation. *Nature Medicine*, 7, 1291–1297.

Lee, S.J. and Benveniste, E.N. (1999). Adhesion molecule expression and regulation on cells of the central nervous system. *Journal of Neuroimmunology*, 98, 77–88.

Lewandowski; M. (1900). Zur Lehre von der Cerebrospinalflüssigkeit. [On the cerebrospinal fluid.] *Z. Klein Forsch.*, 40, 480–494

Liles, W.C., Dale, D.C., and Klebanoff, S.J. (1995). Glucocorticoids inhibit apoptosis of human neutrophils. *Blood*, 86, 3181–3188.

Lohse, A.W., Dinkelmann, M., Kimmig, M., Herkel, J., and Meyer zum Buschenfelde, K.H. (1996). Estimation of the frequency of self-reactive T cells in health and inflammatory diseases by limiting dilution analysis and single cell cloning. *Journal of Autoimmunity*, 9, 667–675.

Lowenberg, M., Stahn, C., Hommes, D.W., and Buttgereit, F. (2008). Novel insights into mechanisms of glucocorticoid action and the development of new glucocorticoid receptor ligands. *Steroids*, 73, 1025–1029.

Maher, F.O., Nolan, Y., and Lynch, M.A. (2005). Downregulation of IL-4-induced signalling in hippocampus contributes to deficits in LTP in the aged rat. *Neurobiology of Aging*, 26, 717–728.

Man, S., Ubogu, E.E., and Ransohoff, R.M. (2007). Inflammatory cell migration into the central nervous system: a few new twists on an old tale. *Brain Pathology*, 17, 243–250.

Mantovani, A., Sica, A., and Locati, M. (2005). Macrophage polarization comes of age. *Immunity*, 23, 344–346.

Martin-Padura, I., Lostaglio, S., Schneemann, M., Williams, L., Romano, M., Fruscella, P. et al. (1998). Junctional adhesion molecule, a novel member of the immunoglobulin superfamily that distributes at intercellular junctions and modulates monocyte transmigration. *Journal of Cell Biology*, 142, 117–127.

Marvel, F.A., Chen, C.C., Badr, N., Gaykema, R.P., and Goehler, L.E. (2004). Reversible inactivation of the dorsal vagal complex blocks lipopolysaccharide-induced social withdrawal and c-Fos expression in central autonomic nuclei. *Brain, Behavior, Immunity*, 18, 123–134.

McAfoose, J. and Baune, B.T. (2009). Evidence for a cytokine model of cognitive function. *Neuroscience and Biobehavioral Reviews*, 33, 355–366.

McMahon, E.J., Bailey, S.L., Castenada, C.V., Waldner, H., and Miller, S.D. (2005). Epitope spreading initiates in the CNS in two mouse models of multiple sclerosis. *Nature Medicine*, 11, 335–339.

McMenamin, P.G. (1999). Distribution and phenotype of dendritic cells and resident tissue macrophages in the dura mater, leptomeninges, and choroid plexus of the rat brain as demonstrated in wholemount preparations. *Journal of Comparative Neurology*, 405, 553–562.

McMenamin, P.G., Wealthall, R.J., Deverall, M., Cooper, S.J., and Griffin, B. (2003). Macrophages and dendritic cells in the rat meninges and choroid plexus: three-dimensional localisation by environmental scanning electron microscopy and confocal microscopy. *Cell Tissue Research*, 313, 259–269.

Medawar, P.B. (1948). Immunity to homologous grafted skin; the fate of skin homografts transplanted to the brain, to subcutaneous tissue, and to the anterior chamber of the eye. *British Journal of Experimental Pathology*, 29, 58–69.

Michelucci, A., Heurtaux, T., Grandbarbe, L., Morga, E., and Heuschling, P. (2009). Characterization of the microglial phenotype under specific pro-inflammatory and anti-inflammatory conditions: Effects of oligomeric and fibrillar amyloid-beta. *Journal of Neuroimmunology*, 210, 3–12.

Miller, D.H., Khan, O.A., Sheremata, W.A., Blumhardt, L.D., Rice, G.P., Libonati, M.A. et al. (2003). A controlled trial of natalizumab for relapsing multiple sclerosis. *New England Journal of Medicine*, 348, 15–23.

Moalem, G., Leibowitz-Amit, R., Yoles, E., Mor, F., Cohen, I.R., and Schwartz, M. (1999). Autoimmune T cells protect neurons from secondary degeneration after central nervous system axotomy. *Nature Medicine*, 5, 49–55.

Nadjar, A., Combe, C., Busquet, P., Dantzer, R., and Parnet, P. (2005). Signaling pathways of interleukin-1 actions in the brain: anatomical distribution of phospho-ERK1/2 in the brain of rat treated systemically with interleukin-1beta. *Neuroscience*, 134, 921–932.

Nawashiro, H., Tasaki, K., Ruetzler, C.A., and Hallenbeck, J.M. (1997). TNF-alpha pretreatment induces protective effects against focal cerebral ischemia in mice. *Journal of Cerebral Blood Flow and Metabolism*, 17, 483–490.

Nogawa, S., Zhang, F., Ross, M.E., and Iadecola, C. (1997). Cyclo-oxygenase-2 gene expression in neurons contributes to ischemic brain damage. *Journal of Neuroscience*, 17, 2746–2755.

Persidsky, Y., Ramirez, S.H., Haorah, J., and Kanmogne, G.D. (2006). Blood–brain barrier: structural components and function under physiologic and pathologic conditions. *Journal of Neuroimmune Pharmacology*, 1, 223–236.

Persson, M., Brantefjord, M., Hansson, E., and Ronnback, L. (2005). Lipopolysaccharide increases microglial GLT-1 expression and glutamate uptake capacity in vitro by a mechanism dependent on TNF-alpha. *Glia*, 51, 111–120.

Piraino, P.S., Yednock, T.A., Freedman, S.B., Messersmith, E.K., Pleiss, M.A., and Karlik, S.J. (2005). Suppression of acute experimental allergic encephalomyelitis with a small molecule inhibitor of alpha4 integrin. *Multiple Sclerosis*, 11, 683–690.

Quan, N., and Banks, W.A. (2007). Brain–immune communication pathways. *Brain, Behavior, Immunity*, 21, 727–735.

Ransohoff, R.M., and Perry, V.H. (2009). Microglial physiology: unique stimuli, specialized responses. *Annual Reviews in Immunology*, 27, 119–145.

Ransohoff, R.M., Kivisakk, P., and Kidd, G. (2003). Three or more routes for leukocyte migration into the central nervous system. *Nature Reviews in Immunology*, 3, 569–581.

Reese, T.S. and Karnovsky, M.J. (1967). Fine-structural localization of a blood–brain barrier to exogenous peroxidase. *Journal of Cell Biology*, 34, 207–217.

Ross, F.M., Allan, S.M, Rothwell, N.J., and Verkhratsky, A. (2003). A dual role for interleukin-1 in LTP in mouse hippocampal slices. *Journal of Neuroimmunology*, 144, 61–67.

Rubin, L.L. and Staddon, J.M. (1999). The cell biology of the blood–brain barrier. *Annual Reviews in Neuroscience*, 22, 11–28.

Schedlowski, M., Hosch, W., Oberbeck, R., Benschop, R.J., Jacobs, R., Raab, H.R., and Schmidt, R.E. (1996). Catecholamines modulate human NK cell circulation and function via spleen-independent beta 2-adrenergic mechanisms. *Journal of Immunology*, 156, 93–99.

Schleimer, R.P. and Bochner, B.S. (1994). The effects of glucocorticoids on human eosinophils. *Journal of Allergy and Clinical Immunology*, 94, 1202–1213.

Schwartz, M., Moalem, G., Leibowitz-Amit, R., and Cohen, I.R. (1999). Innate and adaptive immune responses can be beneficial for CNS repair. *Trends in Neuroscience*, 22, 295–299.

Selye, H. (1936). A syndrome produced by diverse nocuous agents. 1936. *Journal of Neuropsychiatry and Clinical Neuroscience*, 10, 230–231.

Selye, H. and Horava, A. (1953). Stress Research. *Science*, 117, 509.

Serhan, C.N. and Savill, J. (2005). Resolution of inflammation: the beginning programs the end. *Nature Immunology*, 6, 1191–1197.

Serpe, C.J., Coers, S., Sanders, V.M. and Jones, K.J. (2003). CD4+ T, but not CD8+ or B, lymphocytes mediate facial motoneuron survival after facial nerve transection. *Brain, Behavior, Immunity*, 17, 393–402.

Serpe, C.J., Tetzlaff, J.E., Coers, S., Sanders, V.M., and Jones, K.J. (2002). Functional recovery after facial nerve crush is delayed in severe combined immunodeficient mice. *Brain, Behavior, Immunity*, 16, 808–812.

Shaked, I., Porat, Z., Gersner, R., Kipnis, J., and Schwartz, M. (2004). Early activation of microglia as antigen-presenting cells correlates with T cell-mediated protection and repair of the injured central nervous system. *Journal of Neuroimmunology*, 146, 84–93.

Shechter, R., London, A., Varol, C., Raposo, C., Cusimano, M., Yovel, G. et al. (2009). Infiltrating blood-derived macrophages are vital cells playing an anti-inflammatory role in recovery from spinal cord injury in mice. *PLoS Med* 6:e1000113.

Steffen, B.J., Breier, G., Butcher, E.C., Schulz, M., and Engelhardt, B. (1996). ICAM-1, VCAM-1, and MAdCAM-1 are expressed on choroid plexus epithelium but not endothelium and mediate binding of lymphocytes in vitro. *American Journal of Pathology*, 148, 1819–1838.

Stellwagen, D. and Malenka, R.C. (2006). Synaptic scaling mediated by glial TNF-alpha. *Nature*, 440, 1054–1059.

Stevens, B., Allen, N.J., Vazquez, L.E., Howell, G.R., Christopherson, K.S., Nouri, N. et al. (2007). The classical complement cascade mediates CNS synapse elimination. *Cell*, 131, 1164–1178.

Stevenson, B.R., Siliciano, J.D., Mooseker, M.S., and Goodenough, D.A. (1986). Identification of ZO-1: a high molecular weight polypeptide associated with the tight junction (zonula occludens). in a variety of epithelia. *Journal of Cell Biology*, 103, 755–766.

Tarcic, N., Ovadia, H., Weiss, D.W., and Weidenfeld, J. (1998). Restraint stress-induced thymic involution and cell apoptosis are dependent on endogenous glucocorticoids. *Journal of Neuroimmunology*, 82, 40–46.

Vezzani, A. and Granata, T. (2005). Brain inflammation in epilepsy: experimental and clinical evidence. *Epilepsia*, 46, 1724–1743.

Wolf, S.A., Steiner, B., Akpinarli, A., Kammertoens, T., Nassenstein, C., Braun, A. et al. (2009). CD4-positive T lymphocytes provide a neuroimmunological link in the control of adult hippocampal neurogenesis. *Journal of Immunology*, 182, 3979–3984.

Yednock, T.A., Cannon, C., Fritz, L.C., Sanchez-Madrid, F., Steinman, L., and Karin, N. (1992). Prevention of experimental autoimmune encephalomyelitis by antibodies against alpha 4 beta 1 integrin. *Nature*, 356, 63–66.

Yeh, S.S., Blackwood, K., and Schuster, M.W. (2008). The cytokine basis of cachexia and its treatment: are they ready for prime time? *Journal of the American Medical Directors Association*, 9, 219–236.

Yoles, E., Hauben, E., Palgi, O., Agranov, E., Gothilf, A., Cohen, A. et al. (2001). Protective autoimmunity is a physiological response to CNS trauma. *Journal of Neuroscience*, 21, 3740–3748.

Yoshimura, C., Miyamasu, M., Nagase, H., Iikura, M., Yamaguchi, M., and Kawanami, O. (2001). Glucocorticoids induce basophil apoptosis. *Journal of Allergy and Clinical Immunology*, 108, 215–220.

Zamvil, S., Nelson, P., Trotter, J., Mitchel, I.D., Knobler, R., Fritz, R., and Steinman, L. (1985). T-cell clones specific for myelin basic protein induce chronic relapsing paralysis and demyelination. *Nature*, 317, 355–358.

Zhao, R., Kalvass, J.C., and Pollack, G.M. (2009). Assessment of blood–brain barrier permeability using the in situ mouse brain perfusion technique. *Pharmaceutical Research*, 26, 1657–1664.

Ziv, Y., Ron, N., Butovsky, O., Landa, G., Sudai, E., Greenberg, N. et al. (2006). Immune cells contribute to the maintenance of neurogenesis and spatial learning abilities in adulthood. *Nature Neuroscience*, 9, 268–275.

7

Immunoregulatory Neuropeptides

Doina Ganea and Mario Skarica

Temple University School of Medicine, Philadelphia, PA, USA

Bidirectional Communication between the CNS and the Immune System

The bidirectional connection between the central nervous system (CNS) and the peripheral immune system includes the transmission of both ascending and descending information. Immune signals from the periphery travel to the CNS through several venues, 1) afferent nerves such as the vagus and trigeminal nerves directly activated by peripheral cytokines; 2) macrophages and dendritic cells in the circumventricular organs responding to incoming peripheral inflammatory signals by producing cytokines; 3) specific cytokine transporters at the brain-blood-barrier (BBB); and 4) cytokine activation of vascular brain endothelial cells resulting in local production of lipid mediators such as PGE2 (reviewed in Dantzer *et al.*, 2008; Tracey, 2010). In addition, CNS resident glial cells, including microglia and astrocytes, respond to signals provided by various ascending pathways by producing inflammatory mediators which serve as ligands for receptors expressed on neuronal and non-neuronal cells in the CNS parenchyma.

Interneuronal relays in the CNS spread and amplify the signals received from the periphery and initiate efferent CNS→peripheral immune system responses, which are mostly anti-inflammatory in nature. These include: 1) the hypothalamic–pituitary–adrenal (HPA) axis; 2. the so-called "cholinergic anti-inflammatory pathway"; and 3) the release of neurotransmitters and neuropeptides from the sympathetic and parasympathetic innervations of lymphoid organs. Activation of the HPA axis results in the release of glucocorticoids (GC) which suppress transcription of pro-inflammatory genes through various signaling pathways, including binding of activated GC receptors to glucocorticoid-response element (GRE) sites, sequestration of the nuclear coactivators CBP and p300, and de novo synthesis of the NF-κB inhibitor IκBα (reviewed in Rivest, 2009). The vagus, which mediates transmission of ascending information, is also involved in the rapid implementation of the anti-inflammatory action of the cholinergic pathway, by suppressing the innate immune response of monocytes and macrophages. The cholinergic anti-inflammatory pathway is mediated through acetylcholine→nicotinic α7-AChR interactions and results primarily in the suppression of TNF-α production (reviewed in Tracey, 2010). Finally, autonomic efferent nerves that innervate primary and secondary lymphoid organs release neurotransmitters (NT) and neuropeptides (NP) in the vicinity of immune cells. Norepinephrine (NE), the NT released by the sympathetic innervations, inhibits

The Wiley-Blackwell Handbook of Psychoneuroimmunology, First Edition. Edited by Alexander W. Kusnecov and Hymie Anisman.

T-cell proliferation and differentiation into T_H1 cells, and chemical sympathectomy exacerbates experimental autoimmune encephalomyelitis (EAE), a T_H1-type autoimmune disease (reviewed in Bellinger *et al.*, 2008). The immunoregulatory effects of neuroendocrine hormones and of neurotransmitters are discussed in detail in other chapters of this book.

Here we review the immunomodulatory role of neuropeptides, focusing on immune sources and targets, receptors and major signaling pathways, *in vivo* effects in models of inflammatory and autoimmune diseases, and future perspectives for clinical use. The emphasis is on vasoactive intestinal peptide (VIP), one of the best studied anti-inflammatory NP, with pleiotropic effects in both innate and adaptive immunity, and a member of the ancient antimicrobial peptide family.

Innate and Adaptive Immune Responses

To eliminate invading pathogens, the immune system mounts two different but interconnected responses, innate and adaptive immunity, which differ in terms of several important characteristics (Table 7.1).

The innate immune response includes the release of antimicrobial peptides, one of the ancient forms of defense against pathogens, and pathogen destruction by innate immune cells through phagocytosis, release of oxygen and nitrogen radicals, and production of proinflammatory cytokines and chemokines following recognition of foreign molecular patterns shared by groups of pathogens. The innate immune response occurs early (minutes to hours) after pathogen entry, and does not result in immunological memory. The major cell types involved in innate immunity are neutrophils (NΦ), macrophages (MΦ) and dendritic cells (DC) in the periphery, and microglia (MG) in the CNS. However, non-classical immune cells such as skin epithelial cells and Paneth cells in the intestine, which are major producers of antimicrobial peptides, also play an important role in innate immunity. Among neuroimmunomodulators, neuropeptides are the only ones reported to have direct antimicrobial activity (Table 7.2). In addition, various

Table 7.1 Innate and Adaptive Immune Response

Immune response	*Innate*	*Adaptive*
Timing	Immediate/early (min to hours)	Late (days)
Specificity	Low for antimicrobial peptide release (recognizes pathogens in general) Intermediate for MΦ, NΦ, DC activation (recognize groups of pathogens through TLRs, NLRs, RLHs)	High for B- and $T_{\alpha\beta}$-cells (recognize specific antigenic epitopes)
Memory	No	Yes
Cells	Classical immune: MΦ, NΦ, DC, MG Non-immune: epithelial cells, Paneth cells	B- and T-lymphocytes
Molecules	Antimicrobial peptides Complement Cytokines (TNF-α, IL-1β, IL-6, IL-10) and chemokines Oxygen and nitrogen radicals	Antibodies T-cell cytokines (IFNγ, IL-2, IL-4, IL-5, IL-17, etc) Perforin and granzymes

DC, dendritic cells; MΦ, macrophages; MG, microglia; NΦ, neutrophils; NLRs, Nucleotide-binding and Oligomerization Domain (NOD)-like receptors; RLHs, Retinoic acid inducible gene-I (RIG-I)-like helicases; TLRs, Toll-like receptors.

Table 7.2 Immunoregulatory Neuropeptides

NP	*Immune source*	*Signaling*	*Receptors on immune cells*	*Immune functions*	*Therapeutic effect*	*Reviewed in*
Adrenomedullin (AM)	MΦ, Mo	cAMP/PKA	CRLR/RAMP2-3 MF, Mo, DC	↓ Inflammatory cytokines and chemokines, T_H1 differentiation ↑ T_{reg}, Antimicrobial	Sepsis IBD EAE	Delgado and Ganea, 2008; Wiesner and Vilcinskas, 2010; Zudaire, Portal-Nunez, and Cuttitta, 2006
Corticostatin (CST)	MΦ, Mo, T-cells	cAMP/PKA	SST1-5 MΦ, Mo, DC, T-cells	↓ Inflammatory cytokines and chemokines, T_H1 differentiation, COX2 ↑ T_{reg}, Antimicrobial (defensin H)	Sepsis RA IBD	Brogden, Guthmiller, Salzet, and Zasloff, 2005; Dello Russo, Lisi, Navarra, and Tringali, 2009; Gonzalez-Rey, Ganea, and Delgado, 2010
Ghrelin (GHR)	MΦ, Mo	AMP-activated protein kinase (AMPK)	GHSR MΦ, Mo, DC, T-cells	↓ Inflammatory cytokines and chemokines, T_H1 differentiation ↑ T_{reg}	Sepsis EAE IBD RA	Delgado and Ganea, 2008; Taub, 2008
α-melanocyte stimulating hormone (α-MSH)	MΦ	cAMP MAPK	MC-1R, -3R, -5R MΦ, NΦ, T- and B-cells, mast cells	↓ Inflammatory cytokines, Cell migration, Adhesion molecules, COX 2, Apoptosis ↑ T_{reg}, Antimicrobial	Contact dermatitis EAE Ocular inflammation, allergic airway inflammation RA Septic shock Peritoneal sepsis DSS-Colitis	Brzoska, Luger, Maaser, Abels, and Bohm, 2008; Catania *et al.*, 2006; Luger, Scholzen, Brzoska, and Bohm, 2003; Taylor, 2007

Neuropeptide Y (NPY)	?		?	Y1 MΦ, DC, T- and B-cells	↓ ↑	Bimodal: On T-cells T_H1 On MΦ and DC TNF, IL-12 Phagocytosis Activation of allogeneic T-cells	EAE DSS-colitis	Wheway, Herzog, and Mackay, 2007
Opioids (enkephalins, endorphins, dynorphins)	Leukocytes		cAMP	OP1, OP3 MΦ, Mo, lymphocyte	↓ ↓	Phagocytosis Inflammatory cytokines, NO NK cells T_H1, IFNγ	Sepsis	Odunayo, Dodam, Kerl, and DeClue, 2010
Pituitary adenylate cyclase activating polypeptide (PACAP)	?	↓	cAMP, PKA,PI3K NF κβ MAPK	MΦ, Mo, DC, T- and B-cells	↓ ↑	Inflammatory cytokines and chemokines T_H1 differentiation T_{reg}, T_H2	Sepsis IBD RA EAE Type I diabetes	Delgado and Ganea, 2008; Gonzalez-Rey *et al.*, 2010
Substance P (SP)	MΦ, Mo, T- and B-cells	↑	NF-κβ PLC, Ca^{2+}	NK1R DC, MΦ, Mo, T- and B-cells	↑	Inflammatory cytokines and chemokines	Promotes neuroinflammation Therapeutic effects of SP antagonists in EAE	Douglas and Leeman, 2011
Urocortin (UCT)	MΦ, Mo, T- and B-cells, mast cells		CREB	CRFR2 MΦ, Mo, DC, T-cells	↓ ↑	Inflammatory cytokines and chemokines T_H1 differentiation T_{reg}	Sepsis IBD RA EAE Uveoretinitis	Delgado and Ganea, 2008; Gravanis and Margioris, 2005; Snoek, Borensztajn, van den Wijngaard, and de Jonge, 2010
Vasoactive intestinal peptide (VIP)	T_H2 cells, mast cells	↓	cAMP/PKA NFkB, MAPK JAK1/STAT1	MΦ, Mo, DC, T-and B-cells	↓ ↑	Inflammatory cytokines and chemokines T_H1 differentiation T_{reg}, T_H2 Antimicrobial	Sepsis IBD RA EAE Type I diabetes Parkinson's disease Brain injury	Delgado and Ganea, 2008; Gonzalez-Rey *et al.*, 2010

DC, dendritic cell; DSS, dextran sodium sulfate; EAE, experimental autoimmune encephalomyelitis; IBD, inflammatory bowel disease; MΦ, macrophage; Mo, monocyte, NΦ, neutrophil; NP, neuropeptide; RA, rheumatoid arthritis; T_{reg}, regulatory T-cells.

NPs were reported to modulate innate immune responses by affecting phagocytosis, release of oxygen and nitrogen radicals, and especially the production of pro- and anti-inflammatory cytokines and chemokines by activated MΦ, MG and DC (Table 7.2).

In addition to their immediate function in killing pathogens, MΦ, MG and especially DC have the capacity to process antigen, and initiate an adaptive immune response through stimulatory and costimulatory contacts with naïve T-cells bearing the appropriate T-cell receptor (TCR). In contrast to the innate response, the adaptive immune response which involves B- and $T_{\alpha\beta}$-lymphocytes evolved later, and is characterized by a high degree of specificity, i.e. receptors specific for a unique antigenic epitope, a lag period of days instead of minutes or hours, and the capacity to develop immunological memory, reacting stronger and faster to subsequent exposures to the same pathogen (Table 7.1). More recently, B- and T-cells of an intermediary type, including B_1 cells and $T_{\gamma\delta}$, have been reported to function more like innate immune cells, suggesting a stepwise evolution rather than a sudden change in the development of adaptive immunity.

Although the immune response is required for the successful elimination of pathogens, an uncontrolled inflammatory response can lead to tissue damage, organ failure, and death. Therefore, endogenous anti-inflammatory factors such as glucocorticoids, lipid mediators, anti-inflammatory cytokines, and neuropeptides play an important role in the successful resolution of the acute inflammatory response and the prevention of the development of chronic inflammation.

Immunomodulatory Neuropeptides

The growing field of immunoregulatory neuropeptides includes mostly anti-inflammatory agents, with the exception of substance P (SP) which stimulates the immune response, and of neuropeptide Y (NPY) which inhibits proinflammatory T-cell differentiation while stimulating innate immune cells such as macrophages (MΦ) and dendritic cells (DC) (Table 7.2).

Neurons are the classical neuropeptide (NP) source. NPs are synthesized as pro-NP precursors that are packaged and processed to mature NPs within secretory granules, axonal transported to nerve terminals and released into the extracellular space following depolarization and Ca^{2+} influx. The close association of peptidergic nerve terminals with lymphocytes and macrophages within various lymphoid organs has been previously reported (reviewed in Stevens-Felten and Bellinger, 1997). In addition to nerve terminals, immune cells themselves have been shown to express various NP genes and function as NP sources (Table 7.2). The detailed processing and secretion of NPs from immune cells requires further investigation. Also, whether both neuronal and immune NPs have the same biological effects remains to be determined. A recent report using bone-marrow chimeras to distinguish between the contribution of neuronal and hematopoietic VIP suggests that T-cell derived VIP plays the essential role in the effects on anti-viral immunity (Li *et al.*, 2011). However, this might be a reflection of an autocrine effect, with anti-viral T-cells being the source of immune VIP.

Pro-inflammatory Neuropeptides

The vast majority of immunoregulatory NPs are anti-inflammatory in nature (Table 7.2). At the present time, only two NPs, substance P (SP) and neuropeptide Y (NPY), function at least partially as immunostimulators. SP, a member of the tachykinin family, is a sensory neurotransmitter which plays a major role in neurogenic inflammation (reviewed in Douglas and Leeman, 2011). In addition to the central and peripheral nervous system, SP is expressed in most immune cells and can function as an autocrine or paracrine immunoregulator for cells expressing NK1R. In contrast to other NPs, signaling through NK1R activates NF-κB, the major transcription factor for pro-inflammatory cytokine and chemokine gene expression. In addition, SP signaling in immune cells also includes activation of phospholipase C (PLC), production of IP3, and Ca^{2+} influx. As a result, SP initiates or enhances expression and production of pro-inflammatory MΦ-, DC- and T-cell-derived cytokines such as TNFα, IL-1β, IL-6, IL-2 and IFNγ, and promotes T_H1 pro-inflammatory responses. *In vivo*, SP was reported to have a positive or negative effect in various types of viral infections, to maintain neuroinflammation in EAE, and to facilitate granuloma formation in models of schistosomiasis (Douglas and Leeman, 2011).

NPY, a NP localized in the sympathetic innervation, has been initially described as a suppressor of T_H1 differentiation, with beneficial effects in T_H1-type autoimmune diseases such as EAE and RA (Bedoui *et al.*, 2004). However, more recent studies revealed opposite effects in DSS-colitis and led to a detailed analysis of NPY effects on T-cells and antigen-presenting cells (APC) using Y1R-deficient mice. The results confirmed that NPY has a suppressive effect on T_H1 function, but has the opposite effect on APC, enhancing their capacity to stimulate naïve T-cells and therefore promote T-cell differentiation (Wheway, Herzog, and Mackay, 2007). This classifies NPY as a bimodal immune regulator, which on one hand promotes T-cell differentiation, and on the other hand inhibits the function of already differentiated T_H1 cells. An important aspect that has not been investigated yet, is the effect of NPY on the differentiation and function of T_H17, effector T-cells recently identified as major players in autoimmune diseases.

Anti-inflammatory Neuropeptides

The majority of the NPs listed in Table 7.2 are anti-inflammatory in nature. Although they belong to different structural families and act on different receptors, the anti-inflammatory NPs share a number of similarities: production by both neurons and immune cells, and binding to G-protein-coupled receptors that induce cAMP. Based on extensive existing literature, we selected VIP as the prototype for anti-inflammatory NPs, and therefore the remainder of this chapter is focused on aspects of VIP biology directly related to its immunoregulatory role. If the reader is interested, further information on VIP, its receptors and detailed actions on cell functions can be found in the review by Delgado and Ganea (2011).

Endogenous VIP: sources and immunoregulatory role

As with most NPs, two different sources of VIP have been described in lymphoid organs, *i.e.* the local innervations and the immune cells. VIPergic nerve fibers were identified in lymphoid organs, and immune cells, especially $CD4^+$ T_H2 and $CD8^+$ T2 cells were shown to express VIP mRNA, to process preproVIP, and to secrete the mature peptide.

The role of endogenous immune VIP as an immunoregulatory factor is supported by *in vitro* and *in vivo* data. As expected from the anti-inflammatory role of exogenous VIP, VIP-deficient mice are more susceptible to LPS-induced septic shock and more prone to develop bronchial asthma with high numbers of infiltrating immune cells and high levels of pro-inflammatory cytokines (Hamidi *et al.*, 2006). In a different context, VIP-deficient mice showed improved survival after viral infections associated with increased numbers of activated anti-viral cytotoxic T-cells (Li *et al.*, 2011). The biological significance of endogenous immune VIP, produced and secreted by T-cells, has also been addressed. *In vitro* experiments analyzing T_H1/T_H2 differentiation in purified T-cell cultures established that T-cell-derived VIP affected T-cell differentiation favoring the development of T_H2 at the expense of T_H1 cells (J. Voice *et al.*, 2004). A similar conclusion was reached *in vivo*, where increased anti-viral immunity was observed in wild-type (wt) radiation chimeras engrafted with VIP-KO hematopoietic cells. Since neuronal VIP production was not affected in the bone-marrow chimeras, the increased anti-viral response was attributed to the lack of VIP production by hematopoietic cells (Li *et al.*, 2011).

VIP receptors in immune cells

To date, three types of VIP/PACAP receptors have been cloned and classified as VPAC1, VPAC2 and PAC1. VPAC1 and 2 bind VIP with equal affinity ($K_d \approx 1$ nM) and activate primarily the adenylate cyclase pathway. PAC1 has low affinity for VIP ($K_d > 500$ nM) and activates both adenylate cyclase and phospholipase C. The pleiotropic effects of VIP are mediated through receptors which are widely distributed in CNS and peripheral tissues. In immune cells, VPAC1 is constitutively expressed in lymphocytes, macrophages, monocytes, dendritic cells, microglia and mast cells, and VPAC2, expressed at low levels in naïve or resting cells, is induced following stimulation (reviewed in Delgado, Pozo, and Ganea, 2004). PAC1 is expressed only in cells of the macrophage/monocyte lineage. Defects in the VIP receptor/signaling system might be a predisposing factor in the development of autoimmune diseases, since immune cells of patients with autoimmune/inflammatory diseases such as ankylosing spondylitis, rheumatoid arthritis and osteoarthritis express lower VPAC1 levels and respond poorly to VIP, and MS patients exhibit decreased VPAC2 expression in T_H1 cells.

Effects of VIP on Innate Immune Cells

Effects on cytokine/chemokine production

Although activated innate immune cells are essential for the elimination of pathogens, sustained release of pro-inflammatory factors is detrimental, causing tissue and organ damage. The resolution of acute inflammation is an active process which requires the participation of anti-inflammatory agents including NPs. All anti-inflammatory NPs presently identified suppress pro-inflammatory cytokine and chemokine production from innate immune cells (Table 7.2). VIP was shown to inhibit the production of TNF-α, IL-6, IL-12, to reduce iNOS and COX2 expression, and to stimulate the production of the anti-inflammatory cytokine IL-10 in LPS-stimulated MΦ and MG (Figure 7.1) (reviewed in Delgado, Pozo, and Ganea, 2004). Recent reports indicate that VIP also downregulates MΦ-derived high mobility group box-1 (HMGB1), a late-occurring cytokine involved in lethal endotoxemia and sepsis, suppresses the inflammatory response of MG exposed to beta-amyloid fibrils, and prevents *in vivo* neurodegeneration and MG activation in models of neuroinflammation.

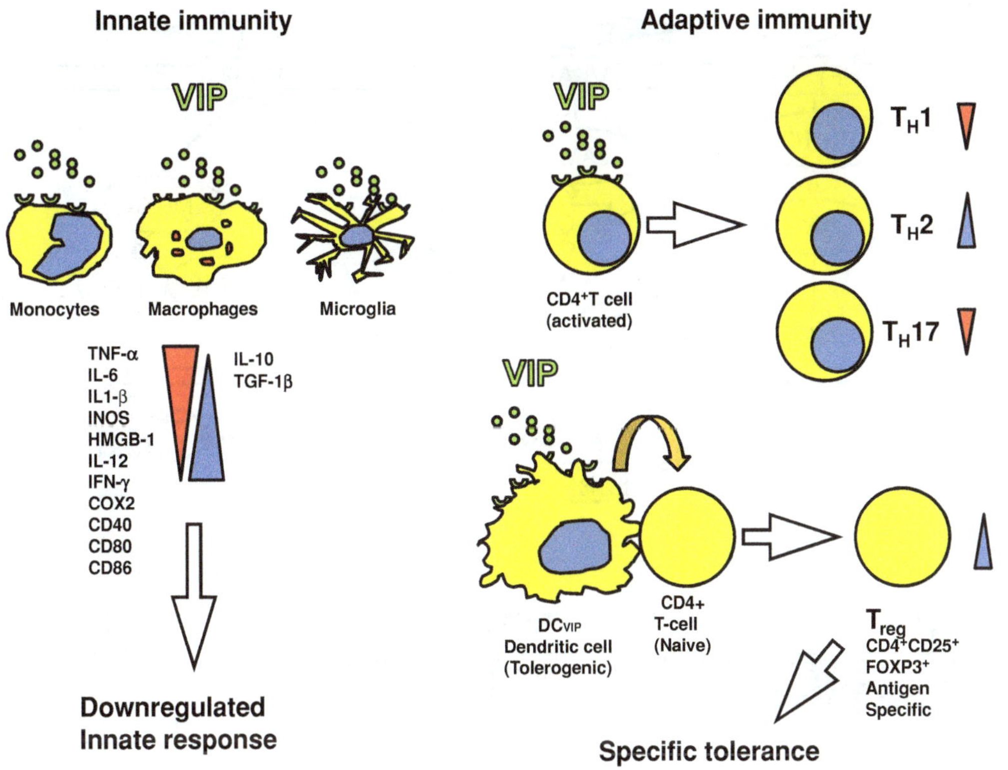

Figure 7.1 Effects of VIP on innate and adaptive immunity. Innate Immunity: VIP signals primarily through VPAC1 in monocytes, macrophages and microglia suppressing the pro-inflammatory response and upregulating the expression of anti-inflammatory cytokines. Adaptive Immunity: VIP affects $CD4^+$ T-cells differentiation by suppressing T_H1 and T_H17 (*in vivo*), and upregulating T_H2 differentiation. The direct effects on T-cells are mediated primarily through VPAC2. VIP induces antigen-specific $CD4^+CD25^+Foxp3^+$ T_{reg} through the generation of tolerogenic dendritic cells.

Accumulation of immune cells at the inflammatory site is mediated primarily through chemokines. *In vitro*, VIP inhibited the expression of proinflammatory chemokines in mouse MΦ and MG, and in human peripheral blood monocytes. *In vivo*, VIP reduced neutrophil, macrophage, and lymphocyte recruitment to the peritoneal cavity in a model of acute peritonitis.

Signaling pathways

VIP affects the expression of pro-inflammatory factors in activated MΦ and MG by regulating the expression and/or transactivating activity of the transcription factors (TF) AP-1, NF-κB, CREB, and IRF-1 (Figure 7.2) (reviewed in Delgado, Pozo, and Ganea, 2004). NF-κB is an ubiquitous TF involved in the expression of pro-inflammatory genes, and its inhibition explains the wide range of cytokines and chemokines negatively affected by VIP. The inhibitory effect of VIP on NF-κB is mediated through both cAMP-dependent and cAMP-independent signaling pathways. The cAMP-independent pathway stabilizes IκB by inhibiting IKK, and maintains

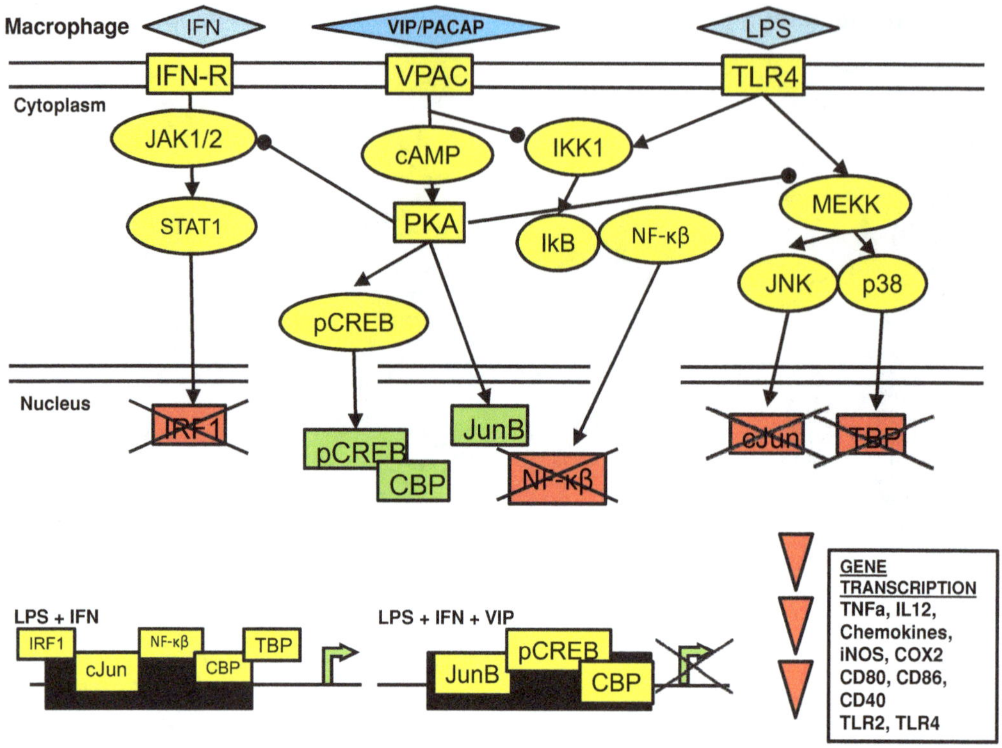

Figure 7.2 Signaling pathways involved in the effects of VIP on activated macrophages. In response to ligands such as VIP or PACAP, VPAC receptors signal through cAMP-dependent and cAMP-independent pathways. The cAMP-dependent pathway activates PKA resulting in CREB phosphorylation, Jun B expression, as well as inhibition of JNK/p38 kinases, and of the JAK1/2-STAT1 pathway. This results in increased pCREB and JunB nuclear translocation, and in the suppression of c-Jun, TATA-box binding protein (TBP) and IRF1. The cAMP-independent pathway inhibits IKK1, stabilizing IκB and maintaining cytoplasmic IκB /NF-κB complexes. As a result, NF-κB nuclear translocation is reduced. In addition, nuclear pCREB sequesters the coactivator CBP, which becomes unavailable to form transcriptionally active NF-κB/CBP complexes. The replacement of c-Jun with JunB in AP-1 complexes reduces their transcriptional activity. Transcription of proinflammatory genes is also reduced through the inhibition of IRF-1 synthesis and of TBP phosphorylation and DNA binding.

the p65/p50/IκB complex in the cytoplasm. The cAMP-dependent pathway phosphorylates CREB, leading to its nuclear translocation and subsequent binding to and sequestration of the co-activator CBP, which is thus prevented from binding to nuclear p65/p50 NF-κB. As a result, the transcriptional activity of NF-κB is severely impaired. The cAMP-dependent pathway also mediates changes in the TNFα promoter CRE-binding complex, reducing c-Jun and increasing CREB, and reduces IRF-1 binding to iNOS and IL-12p40 promoters by inhibiting JAK1/STAT1 phosphorylation. In addition, the cAMP-dependent pathway inhibits the MEKK1/MEK4/JNK pathway, resulting in reduced c-Jun phosphorylation and induces JunB synthesis, replacing c-Jun with JunB in AP-1 complexes with subsequent reduction in AP-1 binding to the TNFα promoter. Moreover, by inhibiting the MEKK1/MEK3/6/p38 pathway, VIP reduces the phosphorylation of TBP resulting in a reduced recruitment of RNA polymerase II.

Effects of VIP in Adaptive Immunity

Effects on T-cell activation and proliferation

VIP affects adaptive immunity by inhibiting T-cell activation and proliferation, switching the T_H1/T_H2 balance in favor of the anti-inflammatory T_H2 subset, and inducing regulatory T-cells (T_{reg}) (Figure 7.1). The inhibition of T-cell activation is mediated indirectly through the inhibition of expression of CD80 and CD86 costimulatory molecules in DC, and directly through the induction of the cell cycle arrest molecule $p27^{kip1}$ in T-cells. In addition, VIP also directly inhibits T-cell derived IL-2 production, further reducing the proliferation of activated T-cells (reviewed in Delgado, Pozo, and Ganea, 2004).

VIP promotes T_H2 differentiation

Activated $CD4^+$ T-cells differentiate into several subsets of effector cells, i.e. T_H1, T_H2, and the recently described T_H17. Both T_H1 and T_H17 cells are pro-inflammatory, active participants in acute and chronic inflammation, as well as in a number of autoimmune diseases. In contrast, T_H2 cells, although major players in allergic reactions and asthma, are considered anti-inflammatory owing to their inhibitory effect on T_H1/T_H17 differentiation. As with many of the anti-inflammatory NPs (Table 7.2), VIP inhibits T_H1 and favors T_H2 differentiation (Figure 7.1). Transgenic mice overexpressing VPAC2 in CD4 T-cells develop prevalent T_H2 immunity, whereas the T_H1 response prevails in VPAC2-deficient mice (Goetzl *et al.*, 2001; J. K. Voice *et al.*, 2001). A number of non-excluding mechanisms contribute to the VIP-induced T_H2 bias (Figure 7.3). IL-12 signaling is required for T_H1 differentiation and c-Maf and JunB are TF required for T_H2 differentiation. VIP affects T_H1/T_H2 generation indirectly by inhibiting IL-12 production in activated APCs, and directly, by blocking IL-12 signaling and by inducing c-Maf and JunB in T-cells. VIP also supports T_H2 survival *in vivo* and *in vitro*. T_H2 cells express higher levels of VIP receptors which mediate the inhibitory effect of VIP on the expression of FasL and granzyme B, molecules involved in the apoptosis of activated effector CD4 T-cells (Sharma, Delgado, and Ganea, 2006).

Does VIP affect T_H17 differentiation?

The recently discovered T_H17 cells play a major role in autoimmunity, dominating the inflammatory response in rheumatoid arthritis (RA), multiple sclerosis (MS), psoriasis, and Crohn's disease. The effect of VIP on T_H17 differentiation and function is controversial. *In vivo* studies using models of type I diabetes and RA suggest an inhibitory VIP effect on T_H17 differentiation or function (Deng *et al.*, 2010; Jimeno *et al.*, 2010). In contrast, *in vitro* studies showed that VIP and TGF-β induced similar numbers of T_H17 as the classical IL-6 plus TGF-β combination (Yadav, Rosenbaum, and Goetzl, 2008). The fact that VIP appears to replace IL-6, a major pathogen-induced cytokine, raises the interesting possibility that VIP might contribute to the maintenance of homeostatic levels of T_H17.

VIP induces T_{reg}

Both natural and inducible regulatory T-cells (T_{reg}) play an essential role in maintaining tolerance and preventing immune attacks against self-antigens. Deficiencies in T_{reg} were reported

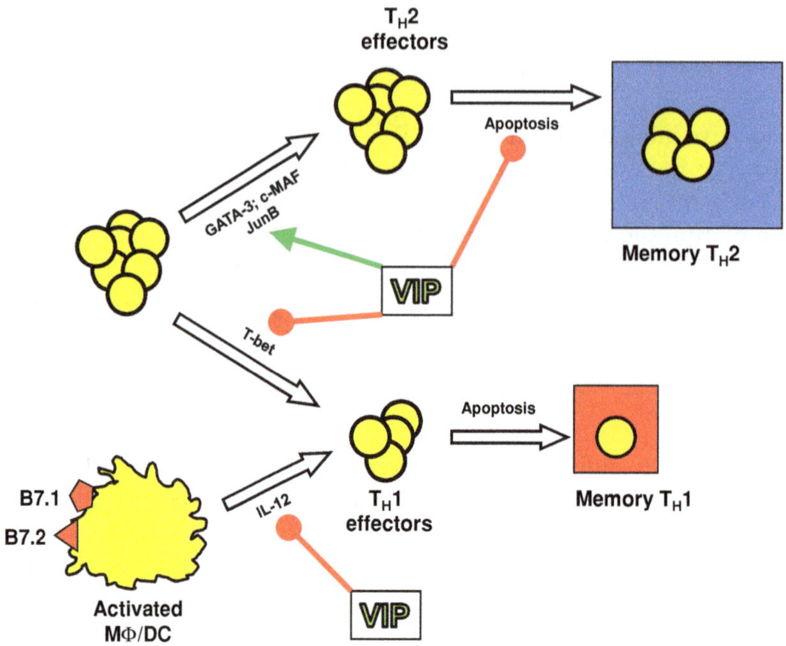

Figure 7.3 VIP promotes TH2 differentiation. VIP reduces T_H1 and promotes T_H2 differentiation through several direct and indirect molecular mechanisms. VIP reduces T-bet expression in activated $CD4^+$ T-cells and inhibits macrophage/DC/microglia IL-12 production, suppressing T_H1 differentiation directly and indirectly. On the other hand, VIP upregulates c-Maf and Jun B expression in activated T-cells and inhibits activation-induced cell death in T_H2, but not T_H1 effectors, promoting T_H2 differentiation.

in human autoimmune diseases, and were documented in experimental autoimmune models. The majority of the anti-inflammatory NPs have been reported to induce T_{reg}. The major advantage of inducing antigen-specific T_{reg} resides in their specificity and long-term survival.

Recent studies showed that VIP induces T_{reg} through the generation of tolerogenic DC (tDC). tDC play an important role in maintaining tolerance by inducing antigen-specific regulatory T-cells (iT_{reg}), and are of major therapeutic interest since they can be induced with biological and pharmacological agents and manipulated to present specific autoantigens. Together with galectin 1, vitamin D3, IL-10 and TNFα, VIP belongs to the group of biological agents that induce tDC (Maldonado and von Andrian, 2010). Exposure to VIP during differentiation of bone marrow- or monocyte-derived DC leads to the development of tolerogenic DC_{VIP} which induce IL-10-producing $CD4^+Foxp3^+$ T_{reg} (Figure 7.1). The DC_{VIP}-induced T_{reg} inhibit the proliferation of antigen-specific T-cells and transfer tolerance to naïve recipients (reviewed in Gonzalez-Rey *et al.*, 2010).

VIP administration has been reported to induce T_{reg} *in vivo*. Inoculation of VIP together with a low dose of antigen resulted in the expansion of $CD4^+CD25^+Foxp3^+$ T_{reg}, which inhibited the proliferation of antigen-specific T-cells, transferred suppression, and inhibited T_H1 responses *in vivo* (Delgado *et al.*, 2005). VIP administration in collagen-induced arthritis, murine type I diabetes and EAE resulted in the generation of T_{reg} usually associated with a decrease in T_H17 (Chen *et al.*, 2008; Delgado *et al.*, 2005; Deng *et al.*, 2010; Fernandez-Martin, Gonzalez-Rey, Chorny, Ganea, and Delgado, 2006; Fernandez-Martin, Gonzalez-Rey, Chorny, Martin et al., 2006; Jimeno *et al.*, 2010). Upon transfer to mice with established disease, T_{reg} from VIP-treated arthritic mice suppressed and ameliorated disease progression (Gonzalez-Rey, Fernandez-Martin, Chorny, and Delgado, 2006). Along the same lines, *in vivo* delivery of a VIP-expressing lentiviral vector to arthritic mice at different phases of the disease resulted in significant disease amelioration concomitant with a reduction of the inflammatory and autoimmune process and the induction of $CD4^+CD25^+Foxp3^+$ T_{reg} in the draining lymph nodes (Delgado *et al.*, 2008). In humans, the use of nebulized VIP in patients with sarcoidosis also resulted in increased numbers of $CD4^+Foxp3^+CD25^+$ T_{reg} in the bronchoalveolar lavage (Prasse *et al.*, 2010).

NPs as Natural Antimicrobial Peptides

Recently, a new and somewhat surprising biological role for NPs emerged, as members of the natural antimicrobial peptide family. Several studies identified SP, NPY, AM, α-MSH, proenkephalin A, ghrelin and VIP as natural antimicrobial peptides against both Gram-positive and Gram-negative bacteria and fungi (reviewed in Brogden, Guthmiller, Salzet, and Zasloff, 2005). NPs resemble natural antimicrobial peptides in terms of small size and cationic amphipathic secondary structure, which allows NP insertion into and destabilization of bacterial or fungal cell membranes. In addition, VIP was also reported to cause cell death of the parasite *Trypanosoma brucei* through autophagy following VIP endocytosis by the parasite (reviewed in Gonzalez-Rey *et al.*, 2010). The recently described antimicrobial role of VIP provides an explanation for the previously described secretion of the VIP fragments $VIP_{6–28}$ and $VIP_{10–28}$ by neutrophils and mast cells. Although these fragments fail to signal through VIP receptors, they exhibit antimicrobial activities (Delgado *et al.*, 2009; El Karim, Linden, Orr, and Lundy, 2008).

NP: Therapeutic Perspective

Most, if not all, anti-inflammatory NPs have the advantage of targeting a wide range of immune cells, affecting both innate and adaptive immune responses. Another advantage resides in the large number of pro-inflammatory cytokines and chemokines affected through the inhibition of ubiquitous TFs such as AP-1 and NF-κB. Therefore, NPs are potentially among the most efficient modifiers of the immune response. Indeed, adrenomedullin, corticostatin, ghrelin, α-MSH, urocortin and VIP are therapeutic in models of inflammatory diseases such as septic shock (Table 7.2), primarily through the suppression of pro-inflammatory cytokine expression in innate immune cells. In addition, the downregulation of the high-mobility group box-1 (HMGB1), an essential cytokine in lethal endotoxemia and sepsis, by VIP, ghrelin and urocortin contributes to the protective role of these NPs, and is a good predictor for their potential therapeutic effect in human septic shock and in hemorrhagic shock and reperfusion injury. Inflammatory responses of microglia occur in various CNS conditions. VIP and ghrelin suppressed microglia inflammatory responses induced by beta-amyloid fibrils and the neurotoxin MPTP, and were protective in murine models of Parkinson's disease (reviewed in Gonzalez-Rey *et al.*, 2010). This raises the possibility of using NPs in the treatment of Alzheimer and Parkinson's disease.

Autoimmune diseases such as MS, RA, and Crohn's disease exhibit both an inflammatory innate immune response and a pro-inflammatory T_H1/T_H17 component. Anti-inflammatory NPs suppress T_H1 differentiation. Although a decrease in T_H17 was reported following VIP therapy in a model of type I diabetes (Jimeno *et al.*, 2010), the effects of NPs on T_H17 differentiation or function remain to be established. In agreement with the observed suppression of T_H1 cells, adrenomedullin, corticostatin, ghrelin, α-MSH, urocortin and, particularly, VIP showed efficacy in EAE (model for MS), collagen-induced arthritis (model for RA) and hapten (TNBS)-induced colitis (model for Crohn's disease). In EAE, VIP treatment resulted in fewer CNS infiltrating immune cells, a reduction in encephalitogenic T-cells with a concomitant increase in T_{reg}, and reduced microglia activation (Fernandez-Martin, Gonzalez-Rey, Chorny, Ganea *et al.*, 2006; Gonzalez-Rey, Fernandez-Martin, Chorny, Martin *et al.*, 2006). The induction of T_{reg} by NPs such as VIP, α-MSH, urocortin, corticostatin and adenomedullin represents one of the most important findings in recent years (reviewed in Gonzalez-Rey *et al.*, 2010). T_{reg} play an essential role in maintaining tolerance in the periphery by suppressing the proliferation and function of effector T-cells, and therefore their induction represents a tempting therapeutic target for the treatment of autoimmune diseases.

Taking into account the multiple cellular and molecular targets of NPs, direct NP administration in inflammatory/autoimmune disorders is a reasonable therapeutic approach. There are, however, serious issues related to NP stability and possible side-effects on organs other than the immune system. Natural NPs are small, hydrophilic molecules, highly susceptible to rapid *in vivo* clearance and degradation by peptidases. They also affect various tissues, primarily the vascular and GI tract. Therefore, therapeutic use of NPs requires improved methods of delivery to target tissues combined with protection against degradation. Several options are currently considered, including stable NP derivatives generated through amino acid substitutions, formulations based on liposomes or nanoparticles, combined treatment with peptidase inhibitors, or serum NP-binding proteins. Some of these approaches have been already tested. For example, stable VIP derivatives showed efficacy as inhalable formulations in an asthma/COPD model, VIP-containing liposomes were used in a model of autoimmune uveoretinits, and silver-protected VIP nanoparticles were shown to inhibit *in vitro* microglia activation (reviewed in Gonzalez-Rey *et al.*, 2010). Clinical trials using VIP inhalations in chronic sarcoidosis and idiopathic pulmonary arterial hypertension are in progress and have shown efficacy (Leuchte *et al.*, 2008; Prasse *et al.*, 2010).

Cell-based therapies represent a viable alternative to the use of natural or modified peptides such as VIP. As described previously, murine bone marrow- and human monocyte-derived DC generated in the presence of VIP (DC_{VIP}) developed into tolerogenic DC capable of inducing T_{reg} specific for the antigen loaded on DC_{VIP}. The potential use of DC_{VIP} in cellular therapy is aimed at the *in vivo* generation of Ag-specific T_{reg}. Cellular therapy with DC_{VIP} was tested in models of inflammatory/autoimmune diseases. In collagen-induced arthritis (CIA), DC_{VIP} pulsed with collagen II were administered to mice with established disease and shown to stop disease progression, reduce the proliferation of antigen-specific T-cells, and induce T_{reg}. Similar results were obtained in EAE and TNBS-induced colitis (Chorny *et al.*, 2005; Gonzalez-Rey and Delgado, 2006). A similar cell-based therapy could be developed in humans by generating DC_{VIP} *in vitro* from blood monocytes, loading them with specific antigens and reinjecting them into the patients. The *in vivo* generation of antigen-specific, long-lived T_{reg} represents an enormous advantage. The challenge is the identification of specific antigens or antigenic epitopes characteristic for various autoimmune conditions.

Cell-based therapy could also offer a good alternative in terms of targeted NP delivery. Antigen-specific T-cells transduced with adeno-associated viral (AAV) vectors expressing α-MSH were used to deliver the NP at the inflammation site in EAE models (Han *et al.*, 2007). We developed a lentiviral VIP expressing vector which was used to transduce differentiating DC (lentiVIP-DC). The tolerogenic, IL-10 producing lentiVIP-DC serves a double purpose, i.e. local delivery of VIP at the inflammation site to suppress innate immune responses and induction of T_{reg} specific for antigens acquired at the inflammation site. LentiVIP-DC proved to be therapeutic in both EAE and sepsis models (Toscano *et al.*, 2010). See Box 7.1, Lentivirus.

Box 7.1 Lentivirus

Lentiviruses belong to the Retroviridae family. Lentiviruses can deliver a significant amount of genetic information into the host cell and replicate in dividing and non-dividing cells. HIV, SIV, and FIV are all examples of lentiviruses. Lentiviral vectors are primarily used as a research tool used to introduce a new genes into cells or to block the expression of a specific gene using RNA interference technology.

Conclusions

The central nervous system and the immune system communicate bidirectionally through a common array of molecules and receptors, including neurotransmitters, neuropeptides, cytokines, and chemokines. Neuropeptides present in both the sympathetic and parasympathetic innervation are released within the lymphoid organs in the vicinity of immune cells. In addition, immune cells themselves express and release neuropeptides. Whether neuronal and immune-derived neuropeptides are interchangeable in terms of function remains to be determined. Immune cells express G-protein coupled neuropeptide receptors which initiate cell signaling upon ligand binding. Most immunoregulatory neuropeptides, with the exception of substance P and possibly neuropeptide Y, function as endogenous anti-inflammatory factors and play an important role in resolution of inflammation and return to homeostasis following an immune response. Specific immunoregulatory functions shared by anti-inflammatory neuropeptides include: 1) "deactivation" of innate immune cells such as macrophages and microglia; 2) reduction in the capacity of dendritic cells to present antigen and stimulate naïve T-cells; 3) inhibition of T_H1 and possibly T_H17 differentiation, while promoting T_H2 and T_{reg} development. These shared properties characterize anti-inflammatory neuropeptides as potent immunoregulators which affect both innate and adaptive immunity. Most interestingly, both pro- and anti-inflammatory neuropeptides act as natural antimicrobial agents and share structural similarities with defensins and cathelicidins. This suggests that the primeval role of neuropeptides could have been as antimicrobial peptides and explains their presence in primitive organisms and the fact that they are highly conserved across species.

References

Bedoui, S., Miyake, S., Straub, R. H., von Horsten, S., and Yamamura, T. (2004). More sympathy for autoimmunity with neuropeptide Y? *Trends in Immunology*, 25(10), 508–512.

Bellinger, D. L., Millar, B. A., Perez, S., Carter, J., Wood, C., ThyagaRajan, S., et al. (2008). Sympathetic modulation of immunity: relevance to disease. *Cellular Immunology*, 252(1-2), 27–56.

Brogden, K. A., Guthmiller, J. M., Salzet, M., and Zasloff, M. (2005). The nervous system and innate immunity: the neuropeptide connection. *Nature Immunology*, 6(6), 558–564.

Brzoska, T., Luger, T. A., Maaser, C., Abels, C., and Bohm, M. (2008). Alpha-melanocyte-stimulating hormone and related tripeptides: biochemistry, antiinflammatory and protective effects in vitro and in vivo, and future perspectives for the treatment of immune-mediated inflammatory diseases. *Endocrine Reviews*, 29(5), 581–602.

Catania, A., Colombo, G., Rossi, C., Carlin, A., Sordi, A., Lonati, C., et al. (2006). Antimicrobial properties of alpha-MSH and related synthetic melanocortins. *Scientific World Journal*, 6, 1241–1246.

Chen, G., Hao, J., Xi, Y., Wang, W., Wang, Z., Li, N., et al. (2008). The therapeutic effect of vasoactive intestinal peptide on experimental arthritis is associated with CD4+CD25+ T regulatory cells. *Scandinavian Journal of Immunology*, 68(6), 572–578.

Chorny, A., Gonzalez-Rey, E., Fernandez-Martin, A., Pozo, D., Ganea, D., and Delgado, M. (2005). Vasoactive intestinal peptide induces regulatory dendritic cells with therapeutic effects on autoimmune disorders. *Proceedings of the National Academy of Sciences of the USA*, 102(38), 13562–13567.

Dantzer, R., O'Connor, J. C., Freund, G. G., Johnson, R. W., and Kelley, K. W. (2008). From inflammation to sickness and depression: when the immune system subjugates the brain. *Nature Reviews Neuroscience*, 9(1), 46–56.

Delgado, M., Anderson, P., Garcia-Salcedo, J. A., Caro, M., and Gonzalez-Rey, E. (2009). Neuropeptides kill African trypanosomes by targeting intracellular compartments and inducing autophagic-like cell death. *Cell Death and Differentiation*, 16(3), 406–416.

Delgado, M., Chorny, A., Gonzalez-Rey, E., and Ganea, D. (2005). Vasoactive intestinal peptide generates CD4+CD25+ regulatory T cells in vivo. *Journal of Leukocyte Biology*, 78(6), 1327–1338.

Delgado, M., and Ganea, D. (2008). Anti-inflammatory neuropeptides: a new class of endogenous immunoregulatory agents. *Brain, Behavior, Immunity*, 22(8), 1146–1151.

Delgado, M. and Ganea, D. (2011). Vasoactive intestinal peptide: a neuropeptide with pleiotropic immune functions. *Amino Acids. 2011 Dec 3.* DOI: 10.1007/s00726-011-1184-8

Delgado, M., Pozo, D., and Ganea, D. (2004). The significance of vasoactive intestinal peptide in immunomodulation. *Pharmacological Reviews*, 56(2), 249–290.

Delgado, M., Toscano, M. G., Benabdellah, K., Cobo, M., O'Valle, F., Gonzalez-Rey, E., et al. (2008). In vivo delivery of lentiviral vectors expressing vasoactive intestinal peptide complementary DNA as gene therapy for collagen-induced arthritis. *Arthritis & Rheumatism*, 58(4), 1026–1037.

Dello Russo, C., Lisi, L., Navarra, P., and Tringali, G. (2009). Diverging effects of cortistatin and somatostatin on the production and release of prostanoids from rat cortical microglia and astrocytes. *J Neuroimmunology*, 213(1-2), 78–83.

Deng, S., Xi, Y., Wang, H., Hao, J., Niu, X., Li, W., et al. (2010). Regulatory effect of vasoactive intestinal peptide on the balance of Treg and Th17 in collagen-induced arthritis. *Cellular Immunology*, 265(2), 105–110.

Douglas, S. D., and Leeman, S. E. (2011). Neurokinin-1 receptor: functional significance in the immune system in reference to selected infections and inflammation. *Annals of the New York Academy of Sciences*, 1217, 83–95.

El Karim, I. A., Linden, G. J., Orr, D. F., and Lundy, F. T. (2008). Antimicrobial activity of neuropeptides against a range of micro-organisms from skin, oral, respiratory and gastrointestinal tract sites. *J Neuroimmunology*, 200(1-2), 11–16.

Fernandez-Martin, A., Gonzalez-Rey, E., Chorny, A., Ganea, D., and Delgado, M. (2006). Vasoactive intestinal peptide induces regulatory T cells during experimental autoimmune encephalomyelitis. *European Journal of Immunology*, 36(2), 318–326.

Fernandez-Martin, A., Gonzalez-Rey, E., Chorny, A., Martin, J., Pozo, D., Ganea, D., et al. (2006). VIP prevents experimental multiple sclerosis by downregulating both inflammatory and autoimmune components of the disease. *Annals of the New York Academy of Sciences*, 1070, 276–281.

Goetzl, E. J., Voice, J. K., Shen, S., Dorsam, G., Kong, Y., West, K. M., et al. (2001). Enhanced delayed-type hypersensitivity and diminished immediate-type hypersensitivity in mice lacking the inducible VPAC(2) receptor for vasoactive intestinal peptide. *Proceedings of the National Academy of Sciences of the USA*, 98(24), 13854–13859.

Gonzalez-Rey, E. and Delgado, M. (2006). Therapeutic treatment of experimental colitis with regulatory dendritic cells generated with vasoactive intestinal peptide. *Gastroenterology*, 131(6), 1799–1811.

Gonzalez-Rey, E., Fernandez-Martin, A., Chorny, A., and Delgado, M. (2006). Vasoactive intestinal peptide induces CD4+,CD25+ T regulatory cells with therapeutic effect in collagen-induced arthritis. *Arthritis & Rheumatism*, 54(3), 864–876.

Gonzalez-Rey, E., Fernandez-Martin, A., Chorny, A., Martin, J., Pozo, D., Ganea, D., et al. (2006). Therapeutic effect of vasoactive intestinal peptide on experimental autoimmune encephalomyelitis: down-regulation of inflammatory and autoimmune responses. *American Journal of Pathology*, 168(4), 1179–1188.

Gonzalez-Rey, E., Ganea, D., and Delgado, M. (2010). Neuropeptides: keeping the balance between pathogen immunity and immune tolerance. *Current Opinion in Pharmacology*, 10(4), 473–481.

Gravanis, A. and Margioris, A. N. (2005). The corticotropin-releasing factor (CRF) family of neuropeptides in inflammation: potential therapeutic applications. *Current Medicinal Chemistry*, 12(13), 1503–1512.

Hamidi, S. A., Szema, A. M., Lyubsky, S., Dickman, K. G., Degene, A., Mathew, S. M., et al. (2006). Clues to VIP function from knockout mice. *Annals of the New York Academy of Sciences*, 1070, 5–9.

Han, D., Tian, Y., Zhang, M., Zhou, Z., and Lu, J. (2007). Prevention and treatment of experimental autoimmune encephalomyelitis with recombinant adeno-associated virus-mediated alpha-melanocyte-stimulating hormone-transduced PLP139-151-specific T cells. *Gene Therapy*, 14(5), 383–395.

Jimeno, R., Gomariz, R. P., Gutierrez-Canas, I., Martinez, C., Juarranz, Y., and Leceta, J. (2010). New insights into the role of VIP on the ratio of T-cell subsets during the development of autoimmune diabetes. *Immunology & Cell Biology*, 88(7), 734–745.

Leuchte, H. H., Baezner, C., Baumgartner, R. A., Bevec, D., Bacher, G., Neurohr, C., et al. (2008). Inhalation of vasoactive intestinal peptide in pulmonary hypertension. *European Respiratory Journal*, 32(5), 1289–1294.

Li, J. M., Southerland, L., Hossain, M. S., Giver, C. R., Wang, Y., Darlak, K., et al. (2011). Absence of vasoactive intestinal peptide expression in hematopoietic cells enhances Th1 polarization and antiviral immunity in mice. *Journal of Immunology*, 187(2), 1057–1065.

Luger, T. A., Scholzen, T. E., Brzoska, T., and Bohm, M. (2003). New insights into the functions of alpha-MSH and related peptides in the immune system. *Annals of the New York Academy of Sciences*, 994, 133–140.

Maldonado, R. A. and von Andrian, U. H. (2010). How tolerogenic dendritic cells induce regulatory T cells. *Advances in Immunology*, 108, 111–165.

Odunayo, A., Dodam, J. R., Kerl, M. E., and DeClue, A. E. (2010). Immunomodulatory effects of opioids. *J Journal of Veterinary Emergency and Critical Care (San Antonio)*, 20(4), 376–385.

Prasse, A., Zissel, G., Lutzen, N., Schupp, J., Schmiedlin, R., Gonzalez-Rey, E., et al. (2010). Inhaled vasoactive intestinal peptide exerts immunoregulatory effects in sarcoidosis. *American Journal of Respiratory and Critical Care Medicine*, 182(4), 540–548.

Rivest, S. (2009). Regulation of innate immune responses in the brain. *Nature Reviews Immunology*, 9(6), 429–439.

Sharma, V., Delgado, M., and Ganea, D. (2006). Granzyme B, a new player in activation-induced cell death, is down-regulated by vasoactive intestinal peptide in Th2 but not Th1 effectors. *Journal of Immunology*, 176(1), 97–110.

Snoek, S. A., Borensztajn, K. S., van den Wijngaard, R. M., and de Jonge, W. J. (2010). Neuropeptide receptors in intestinal disease: physiology and therapeutic potential. *Current Pharmaceutical Design*, 16(9), 1091–1105.

Stevens-Felten, S. Y. and Bellinger, D. L. (1997). Noradrenergic and peptidergic innervation of lymphoid organs. *Chemical Immunology*, 69, 99–131.

Taub, D. D. (2008). Novel connections between the neuroendocrine and immune systems: the ghrelin immunoregulatory network. *Vitamins & Hormones*, 77, 325–346.

Taylor, A. W. (2007). Ocular immunosuppressive microenvironment. *Chemical Immunology & Allergy*, 92, 71–85.

Toscano, M. G., Delgado, M., Kong, W., Martin, F., Skarica, M., and Ganea, D. (2010). Dendritic cells transduced with lentiviral vectors expressing VIP differentiate into VIP-secreting tolerogenic-like DCs. *Molecular Therapy*, 18(5), 1035–1045.

Tracey, K. J. (2010). Understanding immunity requires more than immunology. *Nature Immunology*, 11(7), 561–564.

Voice, J., Donnelly, S., Dorsam, G., Dolganov, G., Paul, S., and Goetzl, E. J. (2004). c-Maf and JunB mediation of Th2 differentiation induced by the type 2 G protein-coupled receptor (VPAC2) for vasoactive intestinal peptide. *Journal of Immunology*, 172(12), 7289–7296.

Voice, J. K., Dorsam, G., Lee, H., Kong, Y., and Goetzl, E. J. (2001). Allergic diathesis in transgenic mice with constitutive T cell expression of inducible vasoactive intestinal peptide receptor. *FASEB Journal*, 15(13), 2489–2496.

Wheway, J., Herzog, H., and Mackay, F. (2007). NPY and receptors in immune and inflammatory diseases. *Current Topics in Medicinal Chemistry*, 7(17), 1743–1752.

Wiesner, J. and Vilcinskas, A. (2010). Antimicrobial peptides: the ancient arm of the human immune system. *Virulence*, 1(5), 440–464.

Yadav, M., Rosenbaum, J., and Goetzl, E. J. (2008). Cutting edge: vasoactive intestinal peptide (VIP) induces differentiation of Th17 cells with a distinctive cytokine profile. *Journal of Immunology*, 180(5), 2772–2776.

Zudaire, E., Portal-Nunez, S., and Cuttitta, F. (2006). The central role of adrenomedullin in host defense. *Journal of Leukocyte Biology*, 80(2), 237–244.

8

Regulation of Immune Cell Activity by Norepinephrine and β2-Adrenergic Receptor Engagement

Caroline J. Padro,[1,2] Jaclyn W. McAlees,[1,2] and Virginia M. Sanders[1]

[1]*Department of Molecular Virology, Immunology, and Medical Genetics, Ohio State University, Columbus, OH, USA*
[2]*Integrated Biomedical Science Graduate Program*

Introduction

Until relatively recently, the nervous and immune systems were thought to be separate entities that did not interact, but the discoveries described below were among the first to establish that there is a strong neuro–immune interaction that is important for maintaining homeostasis and defense against pathogens. In 1975, Ader and Cohen showed that an immune response could be classically conditioned, suggesting for the first time that behavior influenced immunity (Ader and Cohen, 1975). This finding also suggested that such an association between the brain and the immune system might have biological relevance for the cause and treatment of disease. A few years later, using the administration of pharmacologic adrenergic inhibitors *in vivo*, Besedovsky and del Rey showed that the peripheral sympathetic nervous system, which synthesizes and releases the catecholamine norepinephrine, was responsible for causing modest adjustments to the magnitude of an immune reaction that was activated by an antigen (Besedovsky *et al.*, 1979). This finding indicated a possible mechanism by which behavior might influence the level of immunity, as was noted in the conditioning experiments by Ader and Cohen. In an attempt to establish the mechanism by which sympathetic regulation of immune activity was initiated centrally, Besedovsky and del Rey also showed that a soluble product of antigen-activated immune cells was responsible for inducing a decrease in central hypothalamic neuronal activity, which released the negative control on sympathetic nervous system output to the periphery (Besedovsky *et al.*, 1983). This finding suggested that the immune system produced mediators that communicated with central mechanisms to activate the peripheral SNS, providing a mechanism to explain the antigen-induced increase in norephinephrine release within lymphoid organs and subsequent immune modulation. Around the same time, Felten and his colleagues provided an anatomical basis for these findings by showing that every

The Wiley-Blackwell Handbook of Psychoneuroimmunology, First Edition. Edited by Alexander W. Kusnecov and Hymie Anisman.

lymphoid organ was innervated with sympathetic nerve fibers, and that their nerve terminals were located within the parenchyma, which is where immune cells reside (Williams and Felten, 1981; Williams *et al.*, 1981). In addition, radioligand binding analysis and pharmacological data confirmed that adrenergic receptors were expressed on immune cells and were responsible for mediating the norephinephrine-induced changes in immune cell activity and function (Sanders Kasprowicz, Kohm, and Swanson, 2001). These and other findings collected from five decades of research have been reviewed extensively (Kohm and Sanders, 2001; Nance and Sanders, 2007) and have set the stage for the establishment of an entirely new direction of neuroimmunological studies, the study of neuroimmunomodulation. Today, the goal of pharmacological studies in this area is to identify which of the various molecular pathways and signaling intermediates activated by adrenergic receptor engagement on immune cells are specifically linked to the changes induced in immune cell activity and effector function.

Innervation of Lymphoid Tissue, Release of Norepinephrine, and Adrenergic Receptor Expression

Neuroanatomical and neurochemical data have confirmed a structural basis for the communication between the nervous and immune systems, showing that the sympathetic nervous system provides the primary pathway for direct neural modulation of immune cell activity (Nance and Sanders, 2007). Sympathetic nerve activity is typically associated with the fight or flight response by regulation of the cardiovascular and respiratory systems in response to a perceived threat. In addition, norephinephrine is considered a factor that aids in the maintenance of immune system function in response to the threat of antigen (Nance and Sanders, 2007). In order for the rest of the immune system to become activated via the nervous system during the fight against an antigen, innate immune cells must release cytokines after their initial encounter with the antigen. These cytokines bind to their cognate receptors and stimulate central nervous system neurons that are connected to the sympathetic nerve pathway via peripheral nerves with efferent activity, crossing of the cytokines of the blood–brain barrier via specific cytokine transporters, or via immune cells crossing the blood–brain barrier in times of altered blood–brain barrier permeability (Kohm and Sanders, 2001). Sympathetic neurotransmission from the CNS to the periphery occurs via projections from the paraventricular nucleus of the hypothalamus, rostral ventrolateral medulla, ventromedial medulla, and caudal raphe nucleus (Sawchenko and Swanson, 1982). Axons of the hypothalamic neurons project to the spinal cord and synapse on postganglionic sympathetic neurons located in the sympathetic chain ganglia along the spinal column, and the celiac, superior mesenteric, and inferior mesenteric ganglia located in the abdominal cavity. The axons of the postganglionic neurons then follow the vasculature to innervate target organs, including all primary (thymus and bone marrow) and secondary (spleen and lymph node) lymphoid organs (Elenkov, Wilder, Chrousos, and Vizi, 2000; Kohm and Sanders, 2001) (illustrated in Figure 8.1). Therefore, an anatomical basis for neurotransmission was established that resulted in the release of norephinephrine from granules from sympathetic nerve terminals upon sympathetic nerve activation.

As the neuronal pathways were documented to establish the connection from the CNS to lymphoid organs, further studies were performed to determine how sympathetic neurotransmission affected immune cell function in tissues previously thought to be excluded from sympathetic nerve activity. Electron-microscopic studies of the splenic white pulp showed that

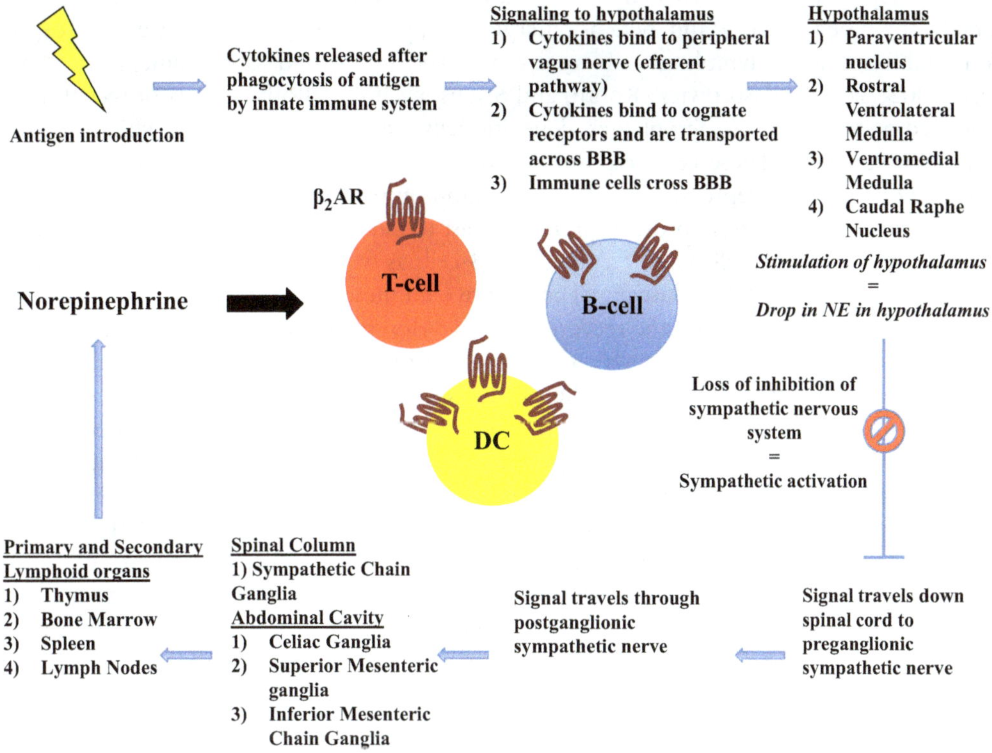

Figure 8.1 Anatomical basis for neurotransmission via the sympathetic pathway upon antigen exposure. Antigen introduction via injury allows for the release of inflammatory cytokines by innate immune cells upon phagocytosis of antigen at the site of injury. Cytokines stimulate the hypothalamus using three different pathways: 1) binding to cognate receptors on peripheral nerves and sending an efferent signal to the hypothalamus; 2) binding to cognate receptors and transport across the blood–brain barrier (BBB); 3) immune cell permeation of the BBB which is often compromised due to infection. Stimulation of the hypothalamus inhibits norepinephrine (NE) release and leads to a loss of inhibition of preganglionic sympathetic neurons within the hypothalamus. Preganglionic sympathetic neurons synapse on postganglionic sympathetic neurons at the level of the spinal cord and into the abdominal cavity. The sympathetic ganglia, celiac ganglia, superior mesenteric ganglia, and inferior mesenteric chain ganglia follow the vasculature and innervate the primary and secondary lymphoid organs: thymus, bone marrow, spleen, and lymph nodes. It is at these junctures where NE is released in the proximity of B-cells, T-cells, and dendritic cells (DC) that express the β_2AR. This is the mechanism by which immune homeostasis is maintained. However, there are other types of pharmacological agonists that bypass the sympathetic innervation pathway and target the β_2AR directly as a result of drug therapy for certain clinical conditions, such as in allergic asthma and heart dysfunction.

sympathetic nerve terminals are in close proximity to T-cells, interdigitating dendritic cells, and B-cells (Felten and Olschowka, 1987) and that norephinephrine is released within 8–18 hours of antigen administration to mice (Kohm, Tang, Sanders, and Jones, 2000). Flierl *et al.* (2007) have shown that, in addition to sympathetic nerve terminals, phagocytes release norepinephrine and express the enzymes for norepinephrine synthesis and degradation, providing an autocrine mechanism by which norepinephrine can be released within the immediate vicinity of the immune cells to affect their function.

Norepinephrine binds to two families of adrenergic receptors expressed on immune cells, namely the alpha- (αAR) and beta-adrenergic receptor (βAR), so the pattern of expression established which lymphoid cells were more likely to respond to norepinephrine (Kavelaars, 2002; Sanders Kasprowicz, Kohm, and Swanson, 2001). Both families of receptors are expressed on monocytes/macrophages, dendritic cells (DC), and neutrophils, which are called innate immune cells. These cells respond quickly and are able to recognize pathogens using antigen-non-specific receptors, e.g., pattern-recognition receptors, but are unable to develop memory to ensure long-term protection. In contrast to innate immune cells, adaptive immune cells, i.e., the $CD4^+$ T-cell, $CD8^+$ T-cell, and B-cell, as well as the innate natural killer cell (NKC), express the β_2AR exclusively. The adaptive immune cells react slowly to a pathogen using high-affinity antigen-specific receptors and develop memory to provide long-term protection. The dichotomy in adrenergic receptor expression by these immune cells is interesting, given that adaptive immune cells and the innate NKC develop from lymphoid precursors in the bone marrow, as opposed to all other innate immune cells that develop from myeloid precursors. The level of adrenergic receptor expression varies among the different immune cell types and is regulated by a variety of factors, including the activation state of the cell, cytokines, and neurotransmitters (Sanders, Kasprowicz, Kohm, and Swanson, 2001). Findings also suggest that the timing of receptor expression may play an important role in mediating neurotransmitter regulation of immune cells (Nance and Sanders, 2007). For example, naïve $CD4^+$ T-cells express the β_2AR, but upon differentiation, the T_H2 cell loses expression of the β_2AR, whereas the T_H1 cell retains expression of the β_2AR (Sanders, Kasprowicz, Kohm, and Swanson, 2001). Expression of the β_2AR was regulated by epigenetic histone methylation patterns within the β_2AR promoter (McAlees *et al.*, 2011). Thus, immune cells express an adrenergic receptor that binds to the NE released from nerve terminals residing within lymphoid tissue and/or the immune cell itself.

Activation of Molecular Pathways and Signaling Intermediates

Before discussing the functional effects that are induced by β_2AR engagement of an immune cell, we will first discuss the molecular pathways and signaling intermediates that are activated by β_2AR engagement. We think it is essential for researchers in this field to understand the complexity of this receptor and to understand that all effects induced by β_2AR engagement are not necessarily mediated by the activation of one given molecular pathway. As will be discussed below, a number of surprising findings emphasize the need to understand all of the potential adrenergic receptor molecular pathways and signaling intermediates activated by β_2AR engagement so that we can develop rational, therapeutic approaches for immune-related diseases.

Adrenergic receptors are seven-transmembrane spanning receptors that associate with heterotrimeric GTP-binding proteins (G-proteins) and are, therefore, known as G-protein coupled receptors (GPCRs). Early mechanistic studies of the β_2AR focused on the study of $G\alpha_s$ activation and subsequent elevation in cAMP, which was thought at the time to be the exclusive signaling intermediate activated by this receptor. (For a comprehensive review of the findings from early studies of cAMP-mediated effects in immune cells, see Kohm and Sanders, 2001.) More recent studies, as summarized in Figure 8.2, have revealed that the β_2AR is able to associate with either the G-protein $G\alpha_s$ or $G\alpha_i$, each of which activates a distinct molecular pathway within an immune cell to differentially regulate its function (Zamah, Delahunty, Luttrell, and Lefkowitz, 2002). Lefkowitz and his colleagues discovered that the β_2AR also associates with

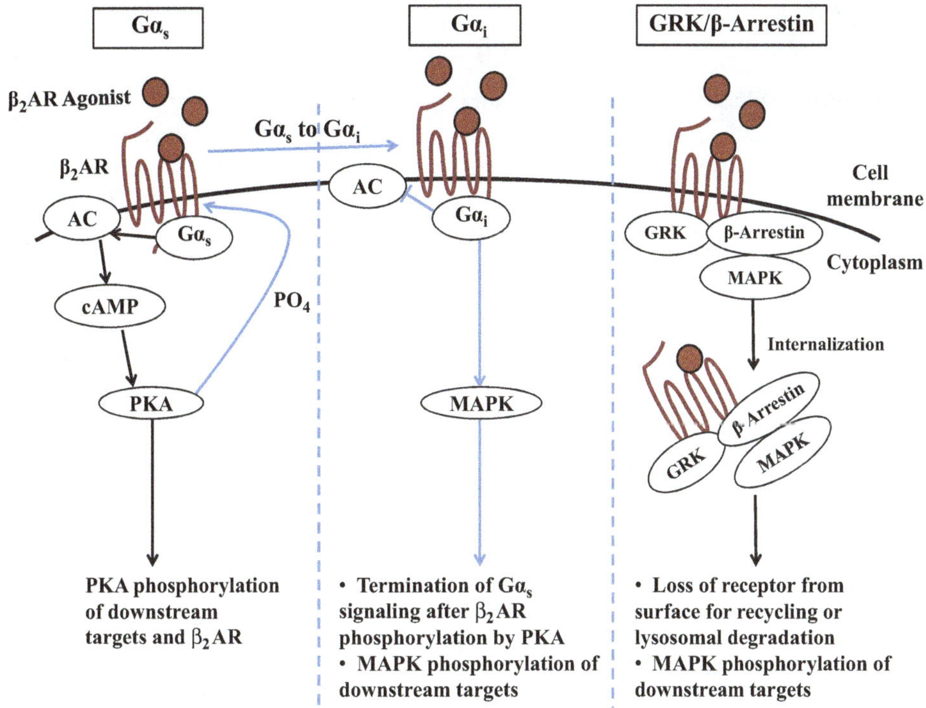

Figure 8.2 Molecular pathways activated intracellularly by β_2AR engagement on an immune cell. The sympathetic neurotransmitter, norepinephrine (NE), binds to the β_2AR. Ligand binding to the receptor will induce receptor binding to a heterotrimeric G-protein complex comprised of the Gα-protein and the β and γ subunits. GDP will be released from the Gα-protein and replaced by GTP, leading to activation and separation of the heterotrimeric G-protein complex to $G\alpha_s$ and βγ, after which the following events occur: 1) Gαs activates the enzyme adenylate cyclase to subsequently raise the level of cAMP. cAMP activates PKA, a kinase that phosphorylates multiple substrates. PKA also phosphorylates the intracellular tail of the β_2AR to cause a $G\alpha_s$-to-$G\alpha_i$ switch and, subsequently, activates a negative-feedback pathway through $G\alpha_i$; 2) Activation of $G\alpha_i$ halts β_2AR binding to $G\alpha_s$ and inhibits the $G\alpha_s$ signaling pathway. β_2AR binding to $G\alpha_i$ also leads to activation of molecules of the MAPK family of proteins; and 3) Ligand binding to the β_2AR activates a G-protein-independent molecular pathway, GRK/β-arrestin2. Receptor stimulation recruits GRK, which binds to and phosphorylates specific sites on the β_2AR to create a binding site for β-arrestin2. This complex will internalize the receptor and inhibit all G-protein-mediated signaling. β-arrestin2 can then serve as a scaffolding protein to bind and activate molecules of the MAPK family of proteins. All three pathways lead to phosphorylation of targeted transcription factors that will induce changes in gene expression and immune cell effector function.

G-protein-coupled receptor kinases (GRKs) and β-arrestins that activate signaling pathways independently of Gα-proteins (Shenoy and Lefkowitz, 2003). Activation of each of these signaling intermediates requires ligand binding to the receptor. This requirement is one reason why early studies using cAMP analogs, which bypass Gα-proteins and/or β-arrestin activation, may be misleading. For this reason, current research needs to be aimed toward understanding which molecular pathways and signaling intermediates are activated by adrenergic receptor stimulation on an immune cell to mediate transcriptional, genetic, and functional changes that develop hours-to-days after receptor stimulation.

Gα_s signaling in B-cells mediates the NE/β_2AR-induced change in the antibody response

Classically, agonist binding to the β_2AR on an intact cell induces coupling to the Gα_s subunit that activates the enzyme adenylate cyclase to cause a rapid transient increase in cAMP levels. cAMP subsequently activates cAMP-dependent protein kinase A (PKA), which mediates phosphorylation of either the transcription factor CREB or the phosphatase hematopoietic protein tyrosine phosphatase (HePTP) that is involved in the regulation of ERK1/2 and p38 mitogen-activated protein kinase (MAPK). These two PKA-induced molecular pathways, CREB vs HePTP, appear to differentially regulate the level of IL-4-dependent IgG$_1$ and IgE antibody produced by B-cells, respectively. Specifically, while the β_2AR-induced increase in PKA activation regulates the level produced of both IgG$_1$ and IgE, the PKA-induced increase in CREB activation regulates IgG$_1$ alone and the PKA-induced increase in HePTP and p38MAPK activation regulates IgE alone (Figure 8.3) (Pongratz et al., 2006). For IgG$_1$,

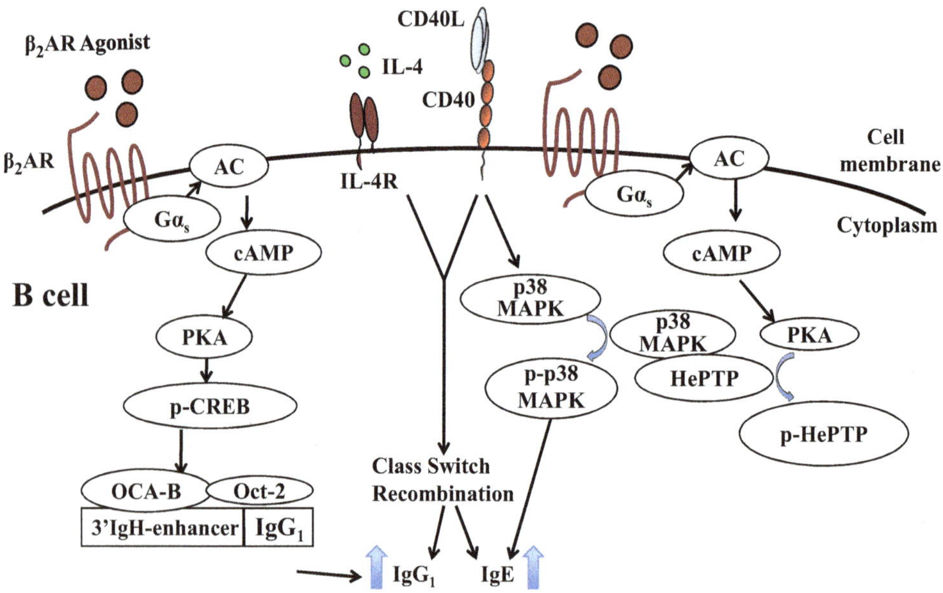

Figure 8.3 β_2AR stimulation increases IgE and IgG1 production by primed B-cells using two distinct pathways. Stimulation of the β_2AR on a CD40L/IL-4 primed B-cell works through two separate pathways to increase production of IgE and IgG1 without affecting class switch recombination. The increase in IgG$_1$ production is mediated by the molecular pathway that includes Gα_s activation of adenylyl cyclase, cAMP, and PKA. PKA phosphorylates CREB, which allows for OCA-B production. OCA-B binds OCT-2 to create a heterodimer that binds to the 3′IgH-enhancer, which promotes an increase in the rate of IgG1 transcription. For IgE, Gα_s activation allows for the activation of adenylyl cyclase, cAMP, and PKA. However, the molecular pathway differs from above in that PKA phosphorylates hematopoietic protein tyrosine phosphatase (HePTP) that is bound to p38 MAPK (p38 MAPK-HePTP), releasing p38 to be phosphorylated by the MAPK pathway that was activated by the engagement of CD40. The phosphorylated p38 MAPK is now responsible for mediating the increase in IgE, involving other signaling intermediates such as CD23 and ADAM10. The existence of two unique molecular pathways involving unique signaling intermediates provides an opportunity to therapeutically target the level of production of either IgE or IgG1 in an isotype-specific manner.

PKA-phosphorylated CREB translocates to the nucleus to transcribe the transcriptional co-activator OCA-B, which heterodimerizes with the transcription factor Oct-2, to regulate the rate of mature IgG_1 transcription (Podojil and Sanders, 2005). For IgE, PKA phosphorylates HePTP, which is bound to p38 MAPK. Phosphorylation of HePTP allows for a conformational change to occur so that p38 MAPK is released from HePTP, making it free to be phosphorylated by the MAP kinase pathway (McAlees and Sanders, 2009). This increase in p38 MAPK phosphorylation allows for gene transcription of downstream targets. Blockade of this pathway using pharmacological inhibitors affects IgE production and the IgE regulator, CD23 (Pongratz *et al.*, 2006). Thus, this is one example of how PKA activation by $G\alpha_s$ can activate two different substrates that each go on to selectively regulate the level of two different antibody isotypes produced by the B-cell, emphasizing the need to understand such differences when attempting to develop selective therapeutic interventions.

Regulator of G protein Signaling (RGS) proteins also affect β_2AR-mediated downstream transcription of CREB-responsive genes. In particular, RGS13 has been found to be especially prevalent in germinal center B-cells and can decrease the affinity of phosphorylated CREB (p-CREB) for p300 and CBP by translocating to the nucleus and binding to p-CREB. RGS13, therefore, decreases transcription of p-CREB target genes such as OCA-B and thereby may regulate the level of IgG1 enhancement induced by β_2AR engagement on a B-cell (Druey, 2009). In addition, the Epac group of proteins is activated by cAMP. cAMP has the same affinity for Epac as PKA. Epac proteins have been found in mature B-cells and are activated by B-Cell Receptor engagement. Downstream effectors include ERK1/2 and NF-κB (Figure 8.4) (Grandoch, Roscioni and Schmidt, 2010). As the cAMP-Epac signaling pathway is a recently discovered alternative to the classical cAMP-PKA pathway, further studies will be needed to determine their relevance in the β_2AR-$G\alpha_s$-stimulated effects on B-cells.

Taken together, these data indicate that $G\alpha_s$ activates more signaling intermediates than just cAMP and PKA, and that these additional signaling intermediates are associated with molecular pathways that exhibit specificity for the regulation of a particular immune cell effector function.

$G\alpha_i$ signaling in macrophages mediates the NE/β_2AR-induced change in cytokine production

Activation of PKA not only mediates $G\alpha_s$ activation of specific molecular pathways, but also mediates the switch from the β_2AR-induced activation of $G\alpha_s$ to the activation of $G\alpha_i$. Following $G\alpha_s$-mediated activation of cAMP and PKA, the active PKA phosphorylates the intracellular tail of the β_2AR to induce a negative feedback mechanism that switches β_2AR binding with $G\alpha_s$ to binding with $G\alpha_i$, effectively halting $G\alpha_s$ activity (Zamah, Delahunty, Luttrell, and Lefkowitz 2002). The switch from $G\alpha_s$ to $G\alpha_i$ is reported to differentially regulate MAPK-dependent cytokine production by macrophages, depending on the stimuli used for cell activation. β_2AR stimulation decreases the level of TNF-α and IL-12 production by LPS-activated macrophages via $G\alpha_s$ regulation of MAPKs, but increases the production of these cytokines in PMA-stimulated macrophages via $G\alpha_i$ regulation of MAPKs (Magocsi *et al.*, 2007; Szelenyi *et al.*, 2006). Interestingly, in the absence of any macrophage activating signals, β_2AR stimulation alone is reported to induce the production of the pro-inflammatory cytokines IL-6 and IL-1β via $G\alpha_i$ activation (Tan *et al.*, 2007). Taken together, these findings reveal that while $G\alpha_i$ activation depends on and inhibits $G\alpha_s$ activation, each signaling intermediate activates a distinct molecular pathway to differentially regulate an immune cell that is in any state of activation.

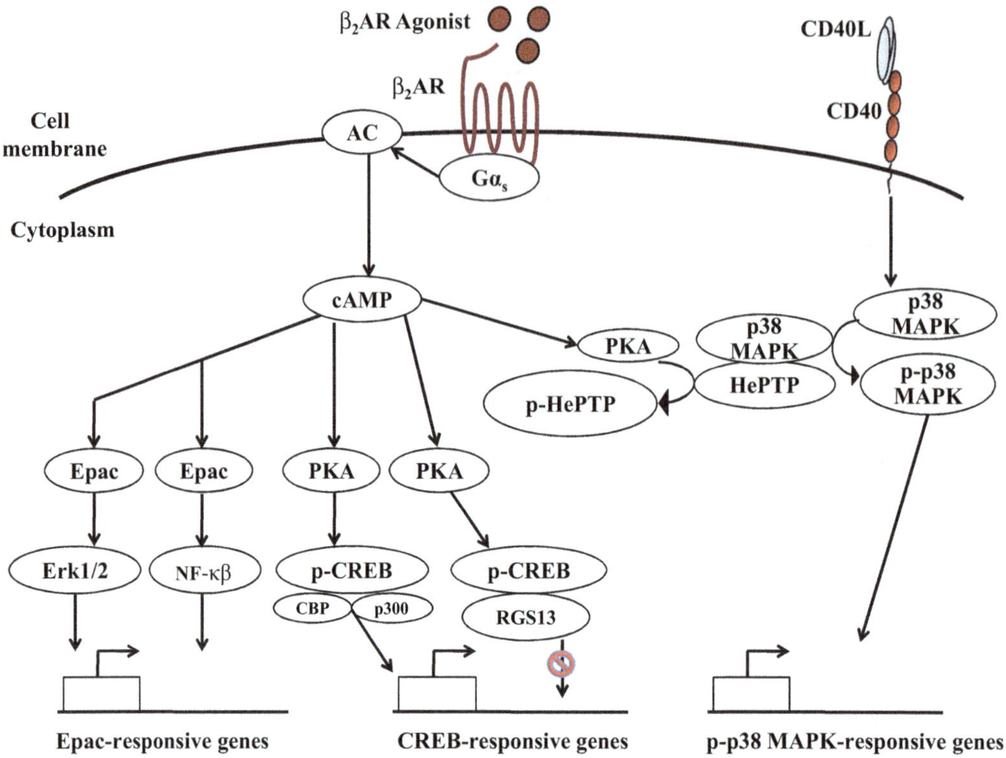

Figure 8.4 Signaling pathways activated by $G\alpha_s$ upon β_2AR stimulation. Several pathways are activated by $G\alpha_s$ and result in the activation of various transcriptional targets that will dictate the activated cellular response. The classical $G\alpha_s$ pathway results in adenylyl cyclase and cAMP activation. cAMP phosphorylates Epac and PKA, having the same affinity for both targets. Downstream targets of Epac include Erk1/2 and NF-κβ, while targets for PKA include CREB and HePTP. Phosphorylated CREB binds p300 and CREB Binding Protein (CBP) to form a complex that serves as a transcription factor for CREB-responsive genes. CREB also binds to Regulator of G Protein Signaling 13 (RGS13), which prevents p300 and CBP binding and, therefore, represses transcription of CREB-responsive genes. When PKA phosphorylates HePTP, p38 MAPK is released and phosphorylated by the CD40-activated MAPK cascade, allowing for transcription of phosphorylated p38 MAPK-responsive-genes. Ultimately, the engagement of one receptor, the β_2AR, can potentially result in the modulation of five different functional responses, and such possibilities need to be considered when studying any immune outcome of β_2AR-mediated signaling.

GRK/β-arrestin signaling is independent of PKA activation, but mediates a change in inflammatory response and immune cell migration

One of the most striking discoveries in the last few decades has been that engagement of the β_2AR also activates a G-protein-*independent* signaling cascade. Upon ligand binding to the β_2AR, a conformational change exposes several amino acid sites on the intracellular portion of the receptor that are specifically phosphorylated by a G-protein-coupled receptor kinase (GRK) (DeWire, Ahn, Lefkowitz, and Shenoy, 2007). Phosphorylation of the β_2AR at GRK-specific sites creates a binding site for β-arrestin, which is a molecule that mediates internalization and desensitization of the β_2AR to terminate all Gα-protein-mediated signaling events (DeWire, Ahn, Lefkowitz, and Shenoy, 2007). More recently, it was discovered that β-arrestins also serve as scaffolding proteins that bind and activate signaling intermediates such as ERK1/2 or c-Jun N-terminal kinase of the MAPK family (reviewed extensively in DeWire, Ahn, Lefkowitz, and Shenoy, 2007). Some data indicate that GRK/β-arrestins may play a role in regulating inflammatory responses and immune cell migration. For example, β-arrestin2-deficient mice have a normal antigen-specific IgE and IgG_1 response (McAlees and Sanders, 2009) but upon induction of allergic asthma, these mice show a decrease in lymphocyte and eosinophil infiltration into the lungs, a decreased level of the cytokines IL-4, IL-13, and IL-5 in the lung, and do not develop the signature lung inflammation that characterizes allergic asthma (Walker *et al.*, 2003). These findings suggest that β_2AR stimulation on an immune cell also activates the G-protein-independent molecular pathway, involving GRK and β-arrestins, to regulate inflammatory activity and migration of immune cells to an area of inflammation. Thus, studies involving β_2AR stimulation must rule out all other G-protein-dependent and -independent pathways before concluding that their effects are due to the classical Gas-cAMP-PKA-CREB signaling pathway.

General considerations about the temporal relationship among multiple β_2AR-activated molecular pathways

It is important to note that both G-protein- and GRK/β-arrestin-mediated activation of a molecular pathway requires ligand binding to the β_2AR (DeWire *et al.*, 2007). In addition, $G\alpha_i$ activation requires not only ligand binding to the receptor, but also $G\alpha_s$-induced activation of PKA, which subsequently induces the switch to $G\alpha_i$ activation by the receptor (Zamah *et al.*, 2002). While GRK/β-arrestin activation is independent of Gα-protein activity, the activation of Gα-mediated molecular pathways occurs prior to the activation of GRK/β-arrestin-mediated molecular pathways (DeWire *et al.*, 2007), suggesting that activation of these molecular pathways and signaling intermediates is temporally isolated. However, the $G\alpha_s$ pathway can diverge to include transcriptional regulation of downstream targets by p-CREB, HePTP-associated p38 MAPK, RGS13, and Epac. Therefore, $G\alpha_s$, $G\alpha_i$, and GRK/β-arrestins may all be activated upon norepinephrine binding to the β_2AR to create a complicated network of temporally isolated molecular pathways. Epigenetically speaking, genes that are downstream of these pathways ultimately depend on chromatin accessibility, which determines not only which genes are transcribed after norepinephrine binding to the β_2AR, but also the temporal nature of this response.

Clinical Implications

Norepinephrine-mediated regulation of immune cell activity is a mechanism by which homeostasis can be maintained. Therefore, disruption of the communication between norepinephrine and an immune cell, be it at the level of neurotransmitter release, receptor expression, or signaling intermediates available for activation, may have health and disease implications, particularly if a normal level of immune cell activity is either depressed or elevated.

IgE and allergic asthma

IgE plays a role in the clearance of allergens by activating the release of histamine that mediates many of the symptoms associated with an allergic response, such as watery eyes and cough, which help to eliminate the allergen from the system. Slight increases in the levels of IgE appear to correlate with the development of a more severe allergic asthma response to allergen (Oettgen and Geha, 1999). Paradoxically, the most effective treatments for the bronchoconstriction triggered by an allergic asthma attack involve the use of β_2AR agonists. Stimulation of the β_2AR on smooth muscle cells allows for bronchodilation, which allows normal air passage through the lungs. However, aside from the effect on bronchial smooth muscle cells, the effect of β_2AR engagement on immune cells located in the lung are unknown. For example, it is possible that the administration of a β_2AR agonist during an asthma attack may exacerbate the intensity of future allergic asthma attacks by increasing the level of IgE produced by the B-cells over time. This may have considerable physiological relevance since the half-life of a β_2AR agonist is considerably longer than norepinephrine, which is released when antigen enters the system in an effort to maintain homeostasis and, therefore, may exert effects on immune cells that influence the lung microenvironment for a longer period of time than that associated with the early allergic response alone.

Equally unknown is how Long-Acting Beta Agonist (LABA) therapy, by itself or coupled with glucocorticoid treatment, affects the level of IgE production. LABA monotherapy is associated with an increased risk of asthma-related death and has been given a black box warning by the FDA. Therefore, most maintenance therapy to prevent allergic asthma attacks by LABA includes glucocorticoid treatment. LABAs are named due to their ability to insert themselves into the membrane adjacent to the receptor they stimulate and, as a consequence, persist in the body longer and engage the β_2AR longer (Walker *et al.*, 2011). While LABAs stimulate the classical $G\alpha_s$ pathway, they have also been found to mediate their effects via the beta arrestin pathway (Qian *et al.*, 2011). It remains to be determined how LABA monotherapy and co-therapy with glucocorticoids affects the different signaling pathways of B-cells, as well as how this change affects the level of IgE production (Figure 8.5). In addition, the upregulation of β_2AR expression upon GC exposure (Hadcock and Malbon, 1988), which could potentially exacerbate the β_2AR-induced effect on the level of IgE produced. Given the evidence indicating that increased stimulation of a greater number of β_2ARs may occur when using this combination therapy, it is possible that co-therapy will worsen allergic asthma by steadily increasing IgE production over the long term. Investigations are currently under way on the use of inverse agonists, which are used to stabilize activity of the β_2AR, for the prevention of inflammation and allergic asthma attacks, suggesting that engagement of the β_2AR might play some role in allergic asthma development. Inverse agonists of the β_2AR carry with them the initial risk of causing an increase in bronchoconstriction. However, initial clinical trials showed that the benefit of chronic inverse agonist therapy far outweighs this risk by reducing methacholine responsiveness while still allowing the use of SABA for bronchorelaxation (Walker *et al.*, 2011). Currently, β_2AR agonist therapy, even with the drawbacks discussed above, is the most effective therapy for treating asthma attacks and should not be abandoned until an equally effective therapy or interventional approach is developed that concurrently maintains the bronchodilating effect of the β_2AR agonist, without exacerbating asthma symptoms resulting from β_2AR effects on immune cells. Thus, the possibility exists that treatment with a β_2AR agonist may worsen allergic asthma by increasing IgE and, therefore, illustrates the need for more focused studies to

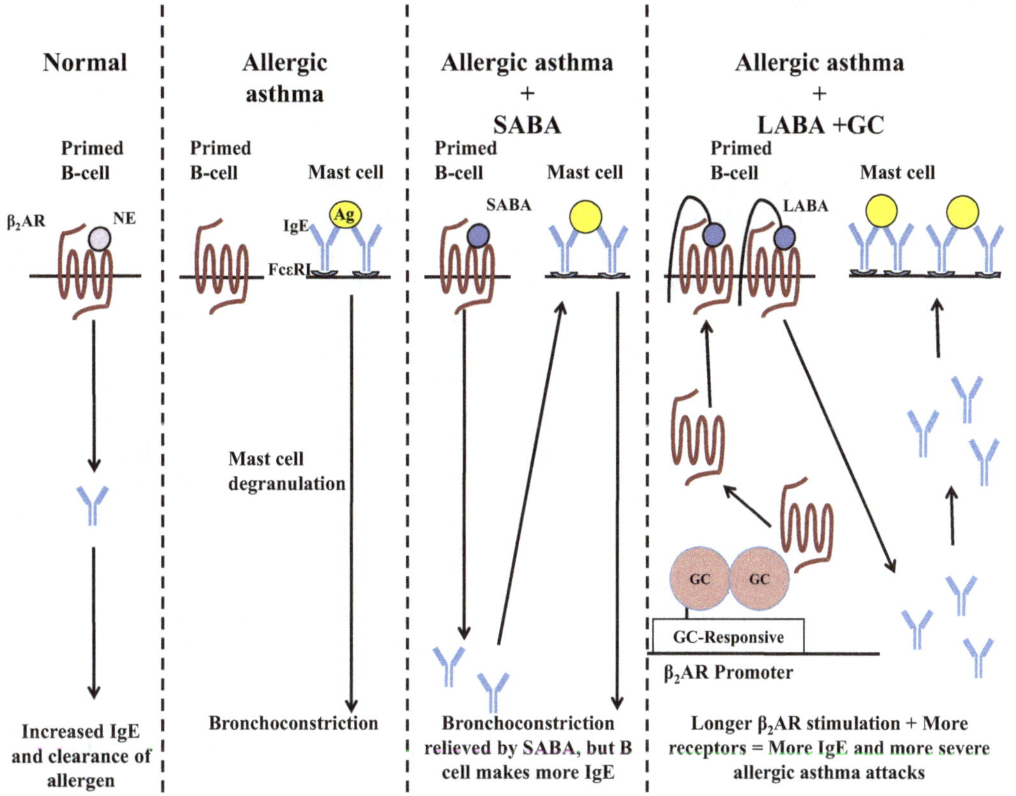

Figure 8.5 β_2AR stimulation and allergic asthma outcomes. The paradox of allergic asthma is that treatment with lifesaving β_2AR agonists may actually worsen attacks in the long run by inadvertently increasing the level of IgE, the mediator of allergic asthma, that is produced over time. In a normal situation when the host encounters allergen (Ag), β_2AR stimulation by NE increases the level of IgE produced, which will help to clear the allergen via the release of histamine and other inflammatory mediators. In the case of allergic asthma, Ag crosslinks specific IgE attached to high-affinity IgE receptors (FcεRI) and leads to mast cell degranulation. The mediators released by degranulation of a mast cell, such as histamine and inflammatory mediators, cause bronchoconstriction. Short Acting β_2AR Agonists (SABA) stimulate the β_2AR on smooth muscle cells surrounding the bronchioles to relieve the constriction and promote bronchodilation. An unintended consequence may be that IgE production is increased upon β_2AR stimulation by SABA on the primed B-cells in the lung or in other lymphoid organs. Of higher concern is the long-acting β_2AR agonist (LABA) that is administered with glucocorticoid therapy. LABAs remain in the body longer by inserting into the membrane adjacent to the β_2AR to which they bind. In addition, glucorticoids (GC) increase the number of β_2ARs expressed through a mechanism that involves the glucocorticoid-responsive element in the promoter for the β_2AR gene. When using this therapy, prolonged stimulation of more β_2ARs may intensify asthma symptoms that become refractory to therapy due to the unintended upregulation in the level of IgE production induced by the greater number of β_2ARs, which may worsen the severity of allergic asthma over the long term.

find therapeutic targets that are just as effective in providing asthma relief as those targeted by a β_2AR agonist.

Antibody production and immunity

Other aspects of immunity can also be affected by β_2AR engagement on immune cells. For example, β_2AR engagement on a B-cell increases the production of IgG_1, which is important for the clearance of bacterial pathogens such as Streptococcus pneumonia (Fine *et al.*, 1988) and plays a role in the development of autoimmune diseases such as lupus (Elenkov *et al.*, 2000; Kohm and Sanders, 2001). Also, β_2AR engagement on a T_H1 cell may change cell-migration patterns that affect the development of multiple sclerosis, an inflammatory disease of the central nervous system that is mediated by migration of T-cells into the brain and spinal cord, where they promote an inflammatory response (Elenkov *et al.*, 2000; Kohm and Sanders, 2001). In addition, β_2AR engagement on a macrophage may affect the production of cytokines that are important for the regulation of an innate immune response, as well as for the activation of the adaptive immune response to a pathogen. For example, a low level of pro-inflammatory cytokine production by macrophages leads to insufficient clearance of a pathogen, while an inability to control the level of pro-inflammatory cytokine production leads to sepsis, a potentially life-threatening condition (Mosser, 2003). Such β_2AR-induced effects on immune cell function might result directly from a β_2AR-induced effect on endogenous immune cell function, or indirectly from a β_2AR-induced change in either the level of norepinephrine released peripherally that could be affected by some exogenous factor that is known to regulate immune cell function such as stress or depression (Glaser and Kiecolt-Glaser, 2005), the level of lymphoid tissue innervation that might be affected by a disease process or aging (Elenkov *et al.*, 2000; Kohm and Sanders, 2001), and/or the level of adrenergic receptor expression on immune cells that might be affected by cytokines, drugs, or a disease process (Nance and Sanders, 2007). Therefore, it is important to understand how norepinephrine affects immune cell effector function so that we can not only better pinpoint where any changes might occur in neuro-to-immune communication, but also better identify pharmacological targets that might be able to modulate the finely tuned balance between the maintenance of health and the development of disease.

Conclusions

Recent data have greatly improved our understanding of the mechanisms by which the sympathetic nervous system regulates the immune system to maintain immune homeostasis. However, much more research is needed to determine the specific molecular pathways and signaling intermediates that are activated in an immune cell by either norepinephrine or a β_2AR pharmacologic agonist to mediate this regulation. When studying the mechanisms by which norepinephrine regulates immune cell activity, it is important to consider that while changes in signaling intermediates are detected seconds to minutes after β_2AR stimulation, many of the transcriptional, genetic, and functional changes occur from hours to days later. The time lag between the activation of early signaling intermediates by β_2AR engagement on an immune cell and the change induced in an end-point effector function confounds the interpretation of many study results and creates an air of skepticism about conclusions drawn on the mechanism by which norepinephrine modulates immune cell activity. However, this skepticism is dwindling as more molecular data are collected.

The work conducted recently in the B-cell provides an example of how an immediate β_2AR-mediated change in the activation of signaling intermediates has been linked directly to the cascade of molecular changes in B-cell activity that occur over a period of days. Importantly, the association between β_2AR-mediated early changes in cellular activity and those changes occurring days later were made possible through the use of gene-deficient mice, selective pharmacologic antagonists, enzyme inhibitors, and sensitive molecular techniques. When a B-cell is exposed to antigen and a β_2AR agonist concurrently, an increase in cAMP (Kohm, Mozaffarian and Sanders, 2002) as well as an increase in PKA and p38 MAPK activation (Pongratz *et al.*, 2006), are measured within minutes as compared to B-cells exposed to antigen alone. After approximately 16 hours, the B-cell surface molecule CD86 becomes expressed on the B-cell surface to a level higher after the β_2AR is engaged on B-cells (Kohm *et al.*, 2002). Two days later, the transcriptional co-activator OCA-B is maximally increased via the β_2AR-induced signaling pathway, while the transcription factor that binds to OCA-B, Oct-2, is increased when the CD86 molecule, which is increased in expression after β_2AR engagement, is engaged. Subsequently, both OCA-B and Oct-2 bind to specific gene sequences within the 3′-IgH enhancer that control the rate at which antibody genes will be transcribed (Podojil, Kin and Sanders, 2004). And finally, the increase in IgG_1 production is measurable on days 4-6 (Kasprowicz *et al.*, 2000). Therefore, when studying the responsiveness of immune cells to norepinephrine exposure, the classic idea of millisecond functional responsiveness needs to be changed now that we can link the cascade of intracellular events induced by norepinephrine that modulate the level of normal immune cell activity.

The goal of neuro-to-immune studies should be to design experiments that will provide results that will promote a better understanding of which molecular pathways and signaling intermediates are activated by β_2AR engagement by norepinephrine and, more importantly, how these pathways and intermediates are associated with changes in an immune cell effector function. Such results will help greatly to allow for the identification of novel pharmacological targets for the treatment of deficient or exacerbated immune responses that may be precipitated by a dysregulation in some component associated with sympathetic regulation of immune cell activity.

References

Ader, R. and Cohen, N. (1975). Behaviorally conditioned immunosuppression. *Psychosomatic Medicine*, 37, 333–340.

Besedovsky, H., del Rey, A., Sorkin, E., Da Prada, M., Burri, R., and Honegger, C. (1983). The immune response evokes changes in brain noradrenergic neurons. *Science*, 221, 564–566.

Besedovsky, H.O., del Rey, A., Sorkin, E., Da Prada, M., and Keller, H.H. (1979). Immunoregulation mediated by the sympathetic nervous system. *Cellular Immunology*, 48, 346–355.

DeWire, S.M., Ahn, S., Lefkowitz, R.J., and Shenoy, S.K. (2007). Beta-arrestins and cell signaling. *Annual Review of Physiology*, 69, 483–510.

Druey, K.M. (2009). Regulation of G-protein-coupled signaling pathways in allergic inflammation. *Immunologic Research*, 43, 62–76.

Elenkov, I.J., Wilder, R.L., Chrousos, G.P., and Vizi, E.S. (2000). The sympathetic nerve – an integrative interface between two supersystems: the brain and the immune system. *Pharmacological Reviews*, 52, 595–638.

Felten, S.Y. and Olschowka, J. (1987). Noradrenergic sympathetic innervation of the spleen: II. Tyrosine hydroxylase (TH)-positive nerve terminals form synaptic-like contacts on lymphocytes in the splenic white pulp. *Journal of Neuroscience Research*, 18, 37–48.

Fine, D.P., Kirk, J.L., Schiffman, G., Schweinle, J.E., and Guckian, J.C. (1988). Analysis of humoral and phagocytic defenses against *Streptococcus pneumoniae* serotypes 1 and 3. *Journal of Laboratory and Clinical Medicine*, 112, 487–497.

Flierl, M.A., Rittirsch, D., Nadeau, B.A., Chen, A.J., Sarma, J.V., Zetoune, F.S., McGuire, S.R., List, R.P., Day, D.E., Hoesel, L.M., Gao, H., Van Rooijen, N., Huber-Lang, M.S., Neubig, R.R., and Ward, P.A. (2007). Phagocyte-derived catecholamines enhance acute inflammatory injury. *Nature*, 449, 721–725.

Glaser, R. and Kiecolt-Glaser, J.K. (2005). Stress-induced immune dysfunction: implications for health. *Nature Reviews Immunology*, 5, 243–251.

Grandoch, M., Roscioni, S.S. and Schmidt, M. (2010). The role of Epac proteins, novel cAMP mediators, in the regulation of immune, lung and neuronal function. *British Journal of Pharmacology*, 159, 265–284.

Hadcock, J.R. and Malbon, C.C. (1988). Regulation of beta-adrenergic receptors by "permissive" hormones: glucocorticoids increase steady-state levels of receptor mRNA. *Proceedings of the National Academy of Sciences of the USA*, 85, 8415–8419.

Kasprowicz, D.J., Kohm, A.P., Berton, M.T., Chruscinski, A.J., Sharpe, A. and Sanders, V.M. (2000). Stimulation of the B cell receptor, CD86 (B7-2), and the beta 2-adrenergic receptor intrinsically modulates the level of IgG1 and IgE produced per B cell. *Journal of Immunology*, 165, 680–690.

Kavelaars, A. (2002). Regulated expression of alpha-1 adrenergic receptors in the immune system. *Brain, Behavior, Immunity*, 16, 799–807.

Kohm, A.P., Mozaffarian, A. and Sanders, V.M. (2002). B cell receptor- and beta 2-adrenergic receptor-induced regulation of B7-2 (CD86) expression in B cells. *Journal of Immunology*, 168, 6314–6322.

Kohm, A.P. and Sanders, V.M. (2001). Norepinephrine and beta 2-adrenergic receptor stimulation regulate CD4+T and B lymphocyte function in vitro and in vivo. *Pharmacological Reviews*, 53, 487–525.

Kohm, A.P., Tang, Y., Sanders, V.M., and Jones, S.B. (2000). Activation of antigen-specific CD4+ Th2 cells and B cells in vivo increases norepinephrine release in the spleen and bone marrow. *Journal of Immunology*, 165, 725–733.

Magocsi, M., Vizi, E.S., Selmeczy, Z., Brozik, A. and Szelenyi, J. (2007). Multiple G-protein-coupling specificity of beta-adrenoceptor in macrophages. *Immunology*, 122, 503–513.

McAlees, J.W. and Sanders, V.M. (2009). Hematopoietic protein tyrosine phosphatase mediates beta2-adrenergic receptor-induced regulation of p38 mitogen-activated protein kinase in B lymphocytes. *Molecular and Cellular Biology*, 29, 675–686.

McAlees, J.W., Smith, L.T., Erbe, R.S., Jarjoura, D., Ponzio, N.M. and Sanders, V.M. (2011). Epigenetic regulation of beta2-adrenergic receptor expression in T(H)1 and T(H)2 cells. *Brain, Behavior, Immunity*, 25, 408–415.

Mosser, D.M. (2003). The many faces of macrophage activation. *Journal of Leukocyte Biology*, 73, 209–212.

Nance, D.M. and Sanders, V.M. (2007). Autonomic innervation and regulation of the immune system (1987-2007). *Brain, Behavior, Immunity*, 21, 736–745.

Oettgen, H.C. and Geha, R.S. (1999). IgE in asthma and atopy: cellular and molecular connections. *Journal of Clinical Investigation*, 104, 829–835.

Podojil, J.R., Kin, N.W., and Sanders, V.M. (2004). CD86 and beta2-adrenergic receptor signaling pathways, respectively, increase Oct-2 and OCA-B Expression and binding to the 3′-IgH enhancer in B cells. *Journal of Biological Chemistry*, 279, 23394–23404.

Podojil, J.R. and Sanders, V.M. (2005). CD86 and beta2-adrenergic receptor stimulation regulate B-cell activity cooperatively. *Trends in Immunology*, 26, 180–185.

Pongratz, G., McAlees, J.W., Conrad, D.H., Erbe, R.S., Haas, K.M. and Sanders, V.M. (2006). The Level of IgE Produced by a B Cell Is Regulated by Norepinephrine in a p38 MAPK- and CD23-Dependent Manner. *Journal of Immunology*, 177, 2926–2938.

Qian, L., Wu, H.M., Chen, S.H., Zhang, D., Ali, S.F., Peterson, L., Wilson, B., Lu, R.B., Hong, J.S., and Flood, P.M. (2011). Beta2-adrenergic receptor activation prevents rodent dopaminergic neurotoxicity by inhibiting microglia via a novel signaling pathway. *Journal of Immunology*, 186, 4443–4454.

Sanders, V.M., Kasprowicz, D.J., Kohm, A.P., and Swanson, M.A. (2001). Neurotransmitter receptors on lymphocytes and other lymphoid cells. In R. Ader, D. Felten, and N. Cohen. (Eds.), *Psychoneuroimmunology* (pp. 161–196). San Diego, CA: Academic Press.

Sawchenko, P.E. and Swanson, L.W. (1982). The organization of noradrenergic pathways from the brainstem to the paraventricular and supraoptic nuclei in the rat. *Brain Research*, 257, 275–325.

Shenoy, S.K. and Lefkowitz, R.J. (2003). Multifaceted roles of beta-arrestins in the regulation of seven-membrane-spanning receptor trafficking and signalling. *Biochemical Journal*, 375, 503–515.

Szelenyi, J., Selmeczy, Z., Brozik, A., Medgyesi, D., and Magocsi, M. (2006). Dual beta adrenergic modulation in the immune system: stimulus-dependent effect of isoproterenol on MAPK activation and inflammatory mediator production in macrophages. *Neurochemistry International*, 49, 94–103.

Tan, K.S., Nackley, A.G., Satterfield, K., Maixner, W., Diatchenko, L., and Flood, P.M. (2007). Beta2 adrenergic receptor activation stimulates pro-inflammatory cytokine production in macrophages via PKA- and NF-kappaB-independent mechanisms. *Cellular Signalling*, 19, 251–260.

Walker, J.K., Fong, A.M., Lawson, B.L., Savov, J.D., Patel, D.D., Schwartz, D.A., and Lefkowitz, R.J. (2003). Beta-arrestin-2 regulates the development of allergic asthma. *Journal of Clinical Investigation*, 112, 566–574.

Walker, J.K., Penn, R.B., Hanania, N.A., Dickey, B.F., and Bond, R.A. (2011). New perspectives regarding beta(2) -adrenoceptor ligands in the treatment of asthma. *British Journal of Pharmacology*, 163, 18–28.

Williams, J.M. and Felten, D.L. (1981). Sympathetic innervation of murine thymus and spleen: a comparative histofluorescence study. *Anatomical Record*, 199, 531–542.

Williams, J.M., Peterson, R.G., Shea, P.A., Schmedtje, J.F., Bauer, D.C., and Felten, D.L. (1981). Sympathetic innervation of murine thymus and spleen: evidence for a functional link between the nervous and immune systems. *Brain Research Bulletin*, 6, 83–94.

Zamah, A.M., Delahunty, M., Luttrell, L.M., and Lefkowitz, R.J. (2002). Protein kinase A-mediated phosphorylation of the beta 2-adrenergic receptor regulates its coupling to Gs and Gi. Demonstration in a reconstituted system. *Journal of Biological Chemistry*, 277, 31249–31256.

9

Immune-to-Brain Communication in Pain

Historical Perspectives, New Directions

Peter M. Grace,[1,2] Linda R. Watkins,[2] and Mark R. Hutchinson[2,3]

[1] *Discipline of Pharmacology, School of Medical Sciences, University of Adelaide, Adelaide, South Australia*

[2] *Department of Psychology and the Center for Neuroscience, University of Colorado at Boulder, Boulder, CO, USA*

[3] *Discipline of Physiology, School of Medical Sciences, University of Adelaide, Adelaide, South Australia*

Introduction

The origins of pain research can be traced back to the scientist and philosopher, Rene Descartes, whose *Treatise of Man* was published in 1664. Descartes' specificity theory dominated the study and treatment of pain for the next 330 years. Ronald Melzack and Patrick Wall strongly disputed Descartes' idea that pain is transmitted from the skin to the brain via a single, specific pathway, as it implies that simply cutting this pathway will extinguish all pain. Many clinical cases demonstrate that this is not the case, but that damage to nerves can often result in exacerbation of painful symptoms, leading to unremitting pain. Thus, in 1965, Melzack and Wall published the gate control theory, which rejuvenated the study of pain; first initiating renewed investigation into the complex hard-wiring of the pain processing system, and, secondly, its plasticity. These insights have led to a consensus view that chronic pain is not simply the persistence of acute pain (See Box 9.1), but a disease in its own right.

Damage to the peripheral or central nervous system may result from traumatic injury, surgical intervention, disease such as diabetes, or infection, and leads to an acute phase response, which is characterized by "nociceptive pain," inflammation, and restriction of normal function. Such pain serves an important role in alerting the individual to danger and protecting against tissue damage, which is illustrated by a hereditary disorder that results in failed embryonic nociceptor survival, due to trkA receptor mutations. These patients lack pain sensitivity, so that they burn and chew their tongues and lips without detecting damage, lose the tips of their fingers due to irreparable injury, and damage their joints.

Usually, following an acute phase, there is a recovery period of diminishing inflammation, reduced pain, healing of the injury and a return to normal function. However, in about 10% of

The Wiley-Blackwell Handbook of Psychoneuroimmunology, First Edition. Edited by Alexander W. Kusnecov and Hymie Anisman.

Box 9.1 Pain: acute vs chronic

Acute pain	*Chronic pain*
Typically lasts < 3 months	Typically lasts > 3 months
Directly results from surgery or trauma	Not directly related to tissue damage
Adaptive: useful to signal damage or danger	Maladaptive: serves no useful purpose
Resolves as injury heals	May persists in the absence of tissue damage
Simple presentation	Complex presentation: often accompanied by psychological features such as anxiety, depression and/or altered sleep patterns

the general population, pain persists despite injury healing, resulting in a state of chronic neuropathic pain. Symptoms of neuropathic pain are often severely debilitating, such as spontaneous pain and dysaesthesia, and the exaggerated pain states of allodynia and hyperalgesia.

Pathological Pain Processing: A Neuronal Perspective

Research of recent years has shown pain is not modality-specific, but rather that pain processing is an integrated matrix that occurs at the peripheral, spinal, and supraspinal sites. Before the immune contribution to neuropathic pain can be appreciated, this neuronal pain-processing matrix will be briefly described, and the neuronal adaptations that contribute to pain pathology will be summarized (see the following reviews for greater depth: Woolf and Ma, 2007; Costigan, Scholz, and Woolf, 2009). Such an overview of these neuronal systems is vital to understanding where and how the immune system can modulate pain processing.

The peripheral nociceptive pathway

Fibers that innervate regions of the head and body arise from cell bodies in the trigeminal and dorsal root ganglia (DRG) respectively. These fibers are called nociceptors, a term coined by Sherrington (1906) over a century ago to describe the nerves responsible for detecting noxious stimuli. The nociceptor has four major functional components: 1) the peripheral terminal, which transduces external stimuli and initiates action potentials; 2) the axon, which conducts the action potentials; 3) the cell body, which controls the identity and integrity of the neuron in the DRG; 4) the central terminal, which forms the presynaptic element of the first synapse in the sensory pathway in the central nervous system (CNS; Figure 9.1). Peripheral fibers that transmit pain messages can be categorized into two main groups anatomically and functionally: Aα- and Aβ-nociceptors are large-diameter, myelinated fibers, detecting innocuous stimuli, but do not contribute to pain; Aδ-fibers are medium-diameter, thinly myelinated, rapidly conducting fibers; C-fibers are small-diameter, unmyelinated slow-conducting fibers. Nociceptors express many ion channels that detect noxious stimuli which lead to the generation of an action potential upon activation.

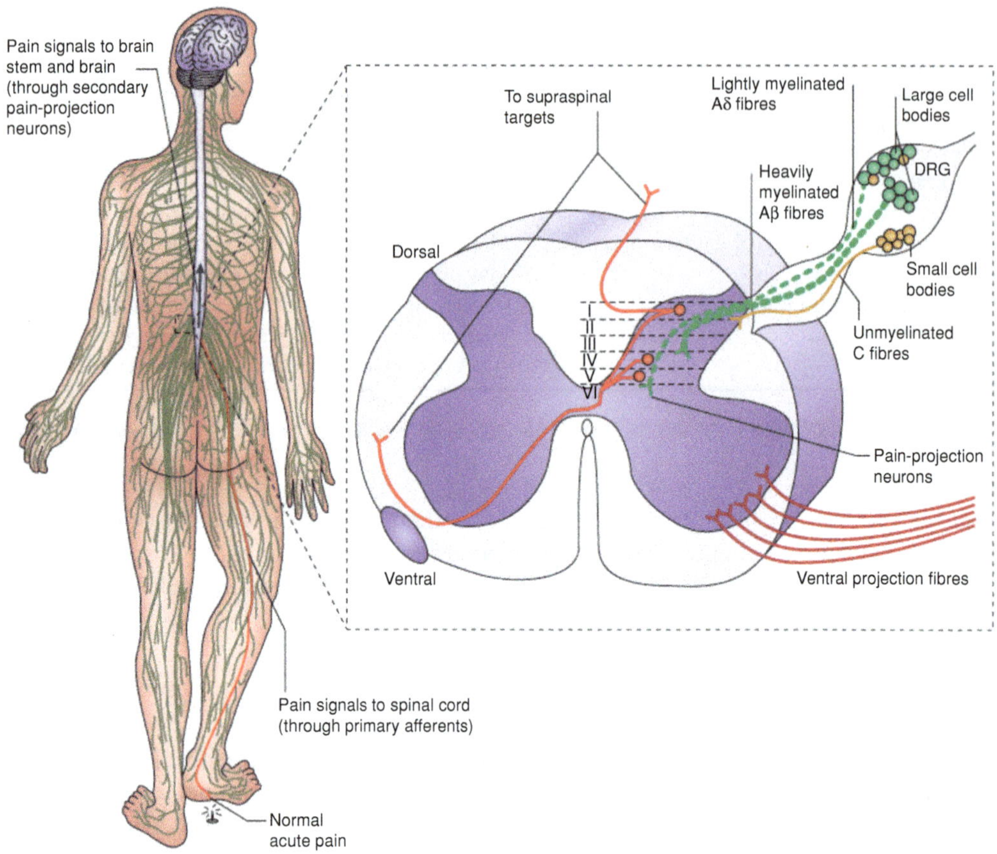

Figure 9.1 Nociception. Normal pain signalling in the body is transmitted to the spinal cord dorsal horn through nociceptors. Nociceptive pain, such as a pinprick to the foot, leads to the release of pain transmitters from primary afferent terminals that project onto pain-projection neurons primarily to laminae I, IV and V in the spinal cord dorsal horns. It is notable that Aβ-, Aδ- and C-fibers additionally project to laminae II–VI to a much lesser extent, but can alter pain-projection neuron activity. However, when tissue injury and skin inflammation ensue, chronic inflammatory signals are released from surrounding cells at the peripheral nerve terminal and lead to the sensitization of the nociceptors. Such factors include, but are not limited to, adenosine and its related mono- or polyphosphorylated compounds (AMP, ADP and ATP), bradykinin, glutamate, histamine, IL-1, IL-6, nerve growth factor, platelet-activating factor, prostaglandin E2, protons, serotonin, substance P, and TNF-α. Nociceptive signalling from the dorsal root ganglia (DRG) is then relayed to the dorsal spinal cord, brain stem and brain, where the experience of pain occurs. The inset shows a cross-section of spinal cord, including the spinal cord dorsal horn and the DRG. The DRG contain pseudounipolar sensory neurons – so called because they give rise to a single axon that bifurcates, with one part projecting to the periphery and the other projecting to the dorsal horn of the spinal cord. The cell bodies of nociceptive neurons in the DRG are broadly classified into large and small types. Immunohistochemical staining studies have shown that slow-conducting C- and Aδ-fibers have small cell bodies, whereas faster-conducting Aβ-fibers tend to have larger cell bodies. Reprinted by permission from Macmillan Publishers Ltd: *Nature Reviews Neuroscience* (Milligan and Watkins, 2009), © 2009.

The central nociceptive pathway

The nociceptors synapse in the dorsal horn of the spinal cord, which is organized into different laminae, extending from the superficial (lamina I) to the deep dorsal horn (lamina VI). Most nociceptive Aδ- and C-fibers terminate superficially in laminae I–II, with a smaller number reaching deeper laminae, whereas Aβ-fibers predominantly innervate laminae III–VI (Figure 9.1).

The nociceptors (first-order neurons) synapse with interneurons and second-order neurons, which signal between each other via many neurotransmitters and neuromodulators, including the excitatory glutamate, substance P, calcitonin gene related peptide (CGRP), and the inhibitory γ-aminobutyric acid (GABA), 5-hydroxytryptamine (5-HT; Figure 9.2A). The superficial laminae of the spinal dorsal horn are critical, as this region represents the junction of primary afferents, second-order ascending projections and third-order descending neurons, which modulate the ascending projection signals.

The main ascending projection is to the thalamus, via the spinothalamic tract. From the thalamus, neurons project to the somatosensory primary (S1) and secondary (S2) areas, the cingulate, insula, the prefrontal cortex and cerebellum. This network of brain structures is referred to as the "pain matrix" and encodes for the multidimensional pain experience. This experience includes the sensory–discriminative component, that is the perception or mapping of the intensity, location, duration, temporal pattern, and quality of noxious stimuli, encoded by the cortical regions. The sensory–discriminative component is likely an adaptive measure in triggering evasive action to a threatening noxious stimulus; the affective–emotional component, that is the relationship between pain and mood, attention, coping tolerance, and rationalization, encoded by the limbic system; and the cognitive component, that is the cognitive impairment, the inability to think clearly and make advantageous decisions, one of the consequences of persistent pain but for which the underlying neural mechanisms are not well understood. A neural circuit that involves prefrontal cortical areas and the amygdala appears to be of critical importance for cognitive functions such as decision-making.

The mammalian CNS has several well-defined, supraspinally organized, descending pathways. These pathways form a network of neural systems that modulate the ascending transmission of nociceptive information, with the best-described being the brainstem control of information at the level of the dorsal horn. Several supraspinal sites are known to contribute to the descending modulation of nociception, either by a direct projection of neurons to the spinal cord, or indirectly by projections to the spinal cord via other brainstem regions. These include the periaqueductal grey (PAG), locus coeruleus, and the rostral ventromedial medulla (RVM), which subsequently modulate nociception in the dorsal horn. These regions perform antinociceptive roles but can also perform facilitatory roles.

Pathological pain processing

The advent of a number of animal models of neuropathic pain conditions has facilitated understanding of the mechanisms involved when chronic neuropathic pain ensues. It is now known that many neuroplastic changes differentiate pathological and normal pain processing, including dynamic modifications at the peripheral terminus, in terms of increased ion channel density and reduced activation thresholds; at the DRG, in terms of increased Na^+ channel clustering leading to spontaneous activity of damaged nerves and cross-excitation to undamaged fibers; at the dorsal horn of the spinal cord, in terms of hypofunctioning inhibitory GABAergic and glycinergic neurons, increased synaptic strength and subthreshold activation of ascending

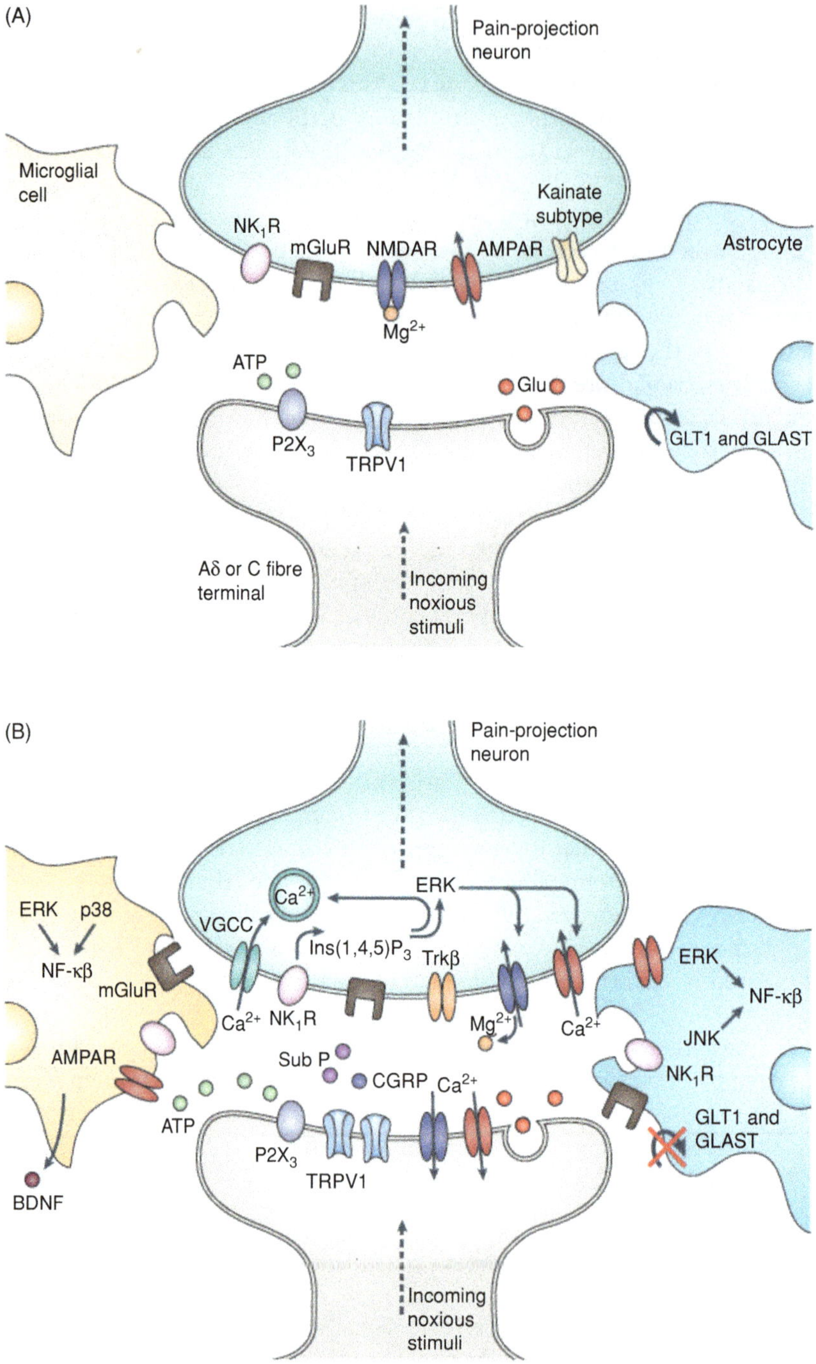

Figure 9.2 Molecules involved in pain processing. A) Under healthy circumstances, low-frequency activation of Aδ- and C-fiber nociceptors by mild noxious stimuli leads to glutamate (Glu) release from the central presynaptic afferent nerve terminals in the spinal cord dorsal horn. Short-term activation of AMPA (α-amino-3-hydroxy- 5-methyl-4-isoxazole proprionic acid) and kainate subtypes of ionotropic glutamate receptors ensues. Although also present, the NMDA (N-methyl-d-aspartate) ionotropic glutamate receptor subtype (NMDAR) remains silent because it is plugged by Mg^{2+}. This signalling to dorsal horn pain-projection neurons provides information about the time of onset, duration and intensity of noxious

second-order neurons, and recruitment of Aβ-fibers (central sensitization: see Box 9.2 and Figure 9.2B). Descending pathways from brainstem regions then modulate the integrated signal at the dorsal horn in either an inhibitory or facilitatory fashion. It is not clear what drives the transition from acute to chronic pain, especially as these changes to the pain-processing system have no adaptive benefits for the sufferer.

Box 9.2 Central Sensitization

Several mechanisms that bring about central sensitization have been described, since Woolf's first description (Woolf, 1983). The best-characterized involves a change in the function of neuronal NMDA receptors in the spinal cord dorsal horn. Activation of sensory neurons by painful stimuli leads to the release of transmitters (for example, substance P and excitatory amino acids) that bind to and activate pain-projection neurons in the spinal cord. During conditions that produce strong and/or persistent nociceptive stimulation, sufficient amounts of substance P and glutamate are released to sustain the depolarization of the spinal cord neurons. When this happens, Mg^{2+} that is normally present in the NMDA channel is removed, allowing Ca^{2+} to flow into the cell and facilitate signal transmission. The influx of Ca^{2+} causes the production and release of nitric oxide by Ca^{2+}-activated neuronal nitric oxide synthase and of prostaglandins by cyclooxygenase enzymes. These molecules both enhance the excitability of spinal cord neurons in response to incoming pain signals and cause an exaggerated release of neurotransmitters from sensory neuron presynaptic terminals to the spinal cord. Together, these downstream effects of NMDA activation result in the amplification of pain messages being relayed to higher brain centers.

Figure 9.2 (*continued*) stimuli from the periphery. Both astrocytes and microglia remain unchanged by these synaptic events. B) After repetitive synaptic communication, which can occur after a short barrage of nociceptive afferent input, there is an increase in the responsiveness of dorsal horn pain-projection neurons to subsequent stimuli (known as central sensitization) (see Box 9.2). A co-release of glutamate and neurotransmitters such as substance P (sub P) and calcitonin gene-related peptide (CGRP) mediates NMDAR activation, leading to voltage-gated Ca^{2+} currents (VGCCs). In addition, inositol-1,4,5-trisphosphate (Ins(1,4,5)P3) signaling and mitogen-activated protein kinases, such as extracellular signal-regulated kinase (ERK), p38, and c-Jun N-terminal kinase (JNK), are activated. In neurons, ERK can further sensitize excited AMPA receptors (AMPARs) and NMDARs. Activation of purinoreceptors ($P2X_3$) by ATP, activation of sub-P receptors (the neurokinin 1 receptor (NK1R)), activation of metabotropic glutamate receptors (mGluR), and release of brain-derived neurotrophic factor (BDNF) all contribute to enhanced nociceptive transmission. Astrocytes and microglia express various neurotransmitter receptors and are activated by glutamate, ATP and sub-P. At synapses the glutamate transporters, glutamate transporter 1 (GLT1) and glutamate–aspartate transporter (GLAST), which are crucial for clearing synaptic glutamate, become dysregulated after prolonged exposure to high levels of synaptic glutamate. Ongoing excitation can induce ERK, p38 and JNK activation in microglia and astrocytes. Each of these kinases can activate the transcription factor nuclear factor-κB (NF-κB), which induces the synthesis of inflammatory factors. Upregulation of the V1 transient receptor potential channel (TRPV1) after inflammation further contributes to the sensitization to noxious signals. During this time, normally non-nociceptive Aβ-fibers can also activate pain-projection neurons. Reprinted by permission from Macmillan Publishers Ltd: *Nature Reviews Neuroscience* (Milligan and Watkins, 2009), © 2009.

The Immune Contribution to Pathological Pain Processing

In the early 1990s, evidence was accumulating to support a hypothesis that pain signaling could not be solely explained by neuronal signaling. Around the same time that Watkins, Maier and colleagues (1994) were exploring the pro-nociceptive mechanisms of the classical sickness response, Garrison and colleagues (1991) reported that peripheral nerve damage, which created exaggerated nociception, also activated spinal cord glia (see Box 9.3 and Box 9.4). Furthermore, the N-methyl-D-aspartate (NMDA) antagonist MK801, which blocks neuropathy-induced allodynia and hyperalgesia, also blocked glial activation (Garrison, Dougherty and Carlton, 1994). These studies established that glial activation, at minimum, correlated with neuropathy-induced allodynia and hyperalgesia as well as their pharmacological resolution.

Box 9.3 Glia

Glia are the most abundant cell type in the CNS, outnumbering neurons ten to one. Microglia (~10%) and astrocytes (~50%), the two predominant glial cell types, are immunocompetent, that is, they are capable of recognizing and responding to traditional immune signals. Originally considered as merely structural support to neurons, glia are increasingly being recognized by the scientific and medical communities as more than just mere neuronal "housekeepers." It is now clear that astrocytes play a pivotal role in maintaining CNS homeostasis, with microglia constantly surveying the CNS microenvironment for damage or danger. Glia are recognized to contribute substantially to a diverse range of CNS pathologies. Owing to the sentinel role of microglia, they respond quickly producing large quantities of proinflammatory cytokines, followed soon after by astrocyte activation and upregulation of cell specific activation markers.

The potential implications of the studies by Garrison and colleagues were enormous. If glial activation was indeed a causal, rather than correlated, factor in the development of allodynia and hyperalgesia, it would be a complete paradigm shift from the classical view that exaggerated pain states are created and maintained solely by neurons. This, of course, raised the questions as to whether glia are necessary or sufficient for allodynia and hyperalgesia. Whilst every model that induced allodynia and/or hyperalgesia was associated with glial activation, these questions proved difficult to address, given the limited pharmacological tools available, and the further limited knowledge of how glia might alter nociception.

The question of whether glia are necessary for allodynia and hyperalgesia addresses whether exaggerated nociceptive responses will occur in the presence of neurons, but absence of glia. Two drugs have been employed to disrupt the function of glia: fluorocitrate, which selectively disrupts the Krebs energy cycle of glia by inhibiting the glia-specific enzyme aconitase; and minocycline, which disrupts the activation of microglia and is generally considered to be devoid of direct effect on neurons or astrocytes, although exceptions are now known. Both interventions have been very effective in blocking a wide range of models of allodynia/hyperalgesia,

Box 9.4 Glial activation

Activation is a fundamentally different phenomenon in neurons compared with that in glia. The term "activation" refers to an enhanced ability of a cell to perform a function beyond that present in a basal state. For neurons, activation is unidimensional, as it mainly relates to the production of action potentials. By contrast, activation of glia is multidimensional, because glia perform numerous functions. So there are many different activational states, with various components expressed with different time-courses and intensities that are dependent on the stimulus that triggers activation. For example, activated glia may have a pro-inflammatory (M1) or anti-inflammatory (M2) phenotype, although it should be noted that these are considered to be the extremes of a continuum.

Astrocyte activation occurs in response to CNS trauma, ischemia, tumors, neurodegeneration, and the presence of immunogenic components of viruses and bacteria. Activation is morphologically characterized by hypertrophy and increased production of intermediate filaments (glial fibrillary acidic protein (GFAP), vimentin and/or nestin), and functionally by increased production of a variety of pro-inflammatory substances. Notably, functional changes and morphological changes are not time-locked, so functional changes can be detected in the absence of increased intermediate filaments, and vice versa.

Microglial activation occurs in response to the same range of stimuli that activate astrocytes. It is a graded phenomenon, characterized by a specific morphology (retracted processes and hypertrophy; amoeboid morphology under strongly pathological circumstances), proliferation, increased expression of one or more cell- surface markers or receptors (such as the complement 3 receptor associated with adhesion, migration and phagocytosis, and scavenger receptors associated with phagocytosis), and/or changes in functional activities (migration to areas of damage, phagocytosis, production/release of pro-inflammatory substances). Notably, the changes in receptors, cell-surface markers and/or the production of pro-inflammatory substances can occur in the absence of morphological changes, proliferation or phagocytosis. So, as is the case for astrocyte activation, microglial activation is a multi-dimensional process. The manner in which activation is expressed is dependent on the type and intensity of the inductive stimulus, and different patterns and time-courses of responses can occur.

but two interesting findings are worth noting. Firstly, fluorocitrate, by inhibiting both astrocyte and microglial activation, appears to produce a more profound blockade of exaggerated nociception than minocycline, which targets microglia alone. Second, minocycline is far more effective in blocking, rather than reversing, exaggerated nociception (Raghavendra, Tanga, and DeLeo, 2003), suggesting that the most important role of microglia might be involvement in the initial induction of exaggerated responses to noxious stimuli. The temporal activation patterns of microglia and astrocytes following nerve injury (Tanga, Raghavendra, and DeLeo, 2004) supports the idea that microglial activation in turn leads to astrocyte activation that maintains the facilitation of nociception.

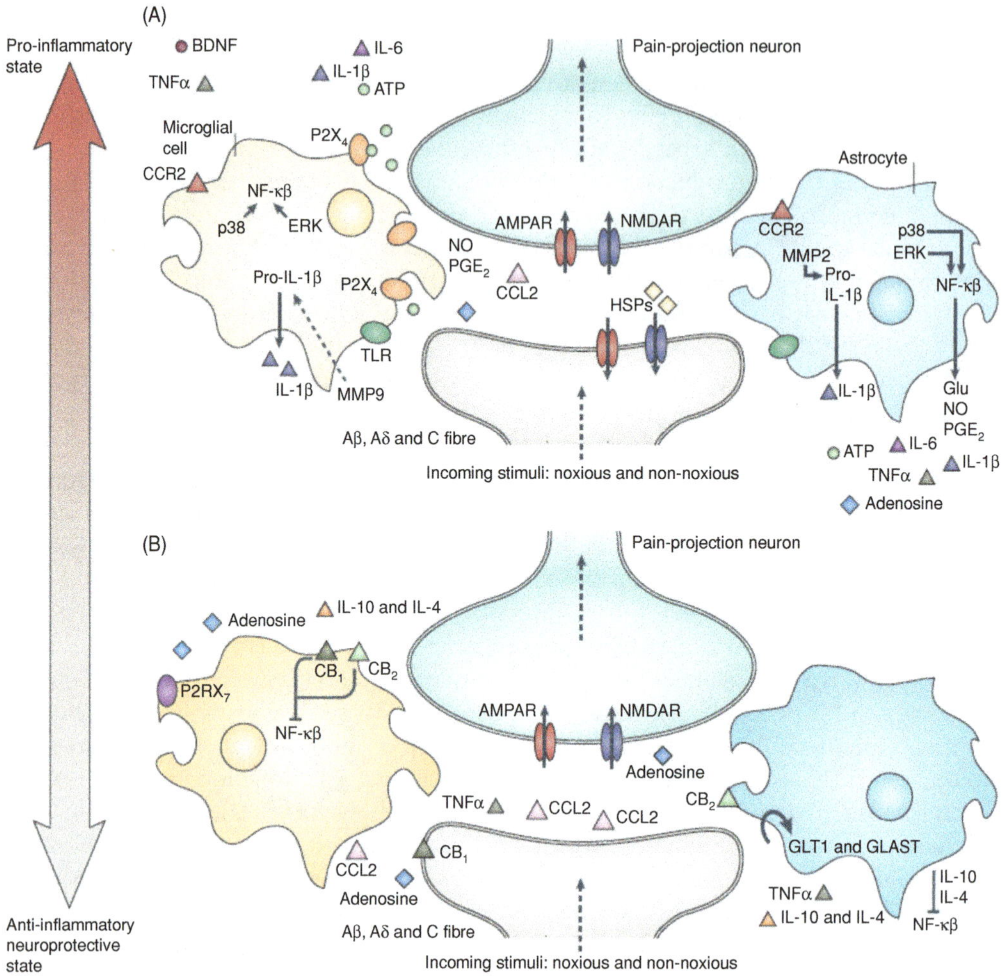

Figure 9.3 Glia activation: from pro-inflammatory to anti-inflammatory states. A) Pro-inflammatory roles for glia. If a noxious input persists, such as during chronic inflammation or nerve damage, sustained central sensitization leads to transcriptional changes in dorsal horn neurons that alter these neurons' function for prolonged periods. Astrocytes respond to this ongoing synaptic activity by mobilizing internal Ca^{2+}, leading to the release of glutamate (Glu), ATP that binds to $P2X_4$, tumor-necrosis factor-α (TNF-α), interleukin 1β (IL-1β), IL-6, nitric oxide (NO) and prostaglandin E2 (PGE2). Activated microglia are also a source of all of these pro-inflammatory factors. Matrix metalloproteinase 9 (MMP9) induces pro-IL-1β cleavage and microglial activation, whereas MMP2 induces pro-IL-1β cleavage and maintains astrocyte activation. The activation of p38 mitogen-activated protein kinase (p38 MAPK) is induced in both microglia and astrocytes on IL-1β signalling. Astrocytes and microglia express the chemokine receptors CX_3CR1 (not shown) and CCR2 and become activated when the respective chemokines bind. After nerve damage, heat-shock proteins (HSPs) are released and can bind to Toll-like receptors (TLRs) expressed on both astrocytes and microglia, leading to the further activation of these cell types. B) Activated glia can also be neuroprotective, as they release anti-inflammatory cytokines such as IL-10 and IL-4 and express cannabinoid receptors (CB1 and CB2) that have been shown to exert anti-inflammatory functions and to inhibit microglial toxicity by suppressing chemotactic responses and MAPK signal transduction, with consequent pro-inflammatory cytokine inhibition. The glutamate transporters,

A strategy to test whether glial activation is sufficient to induce allodynia/hyperalgesia was dependent on identifying ways to selectively activate these cells. Although studies of brain glial cultures have identified neurotransmitters that can activate glia (Araque, Parpura, Sanzgiri, and Haydon, 1999), that information was of little use, as there is marked heterogeneity in both receptor expression and response properties of glia isolated from various CNS regions, and even between spinal regions. Furthermore, the prospect of studying the effects of neurotransmitters on glia *in vivo* was confounded by the fact that they would also activate spinal neurons. Demonstration of a causal role for glia in generating nociceptive hypersensitivity rested upon the fact that glia are immunocompetent cell types, expressing receptors for, and being activated by, viruses and bacteria. Key studies showed that injection of the immunogenic portions of bacteria and viruses over spinal cord resulted in glial activation *and* exaggerated pain responses (Meller *et al.*, 1994; Milligan *et al.*, 2001). More recent approaches have delivered activated glia over the spinal cords of naïve rodents, resulting in exaggerated pain responses (e.g. Tsuda *et al.*, 2003). Glial activation, therefore, is causal to the allodynia and hyperalgesia observed in these studies, as the pain changes were blocked by disruption of glial function.

How do Glia Become Activated Following Nerve Injury?

Whilst glial activation could be demonstrated experimentally, the manner in which glia are activated following nerve injury was still unresolved. Apart from activation by the neurotransmitters and neuromodulators released from the presynaptic terminals of nociceptive primary afferents (e.g., glutamate, substance P: Milligan and Watkins, 2009), much of glial activation can be understood from their immunocompetent status (Figure 9.3A). The consequences of such activation will be discussed in more detail below.

Glial activation: Toll-like receptors

As the primary immunocompetent cells of the CNS, glia have the ability to mount an innate response against potential pathogens by detecting pathogen-associated molecular patterns (PAMPs) and danger-associated molecular patterns (DAMPs). These patterns are recognized by membrane bound toll-like receptors (TLRs; Box 9.5), allowing glia to become activated

Figure 9.3 (*continued*) glutamate transporter 1 (GLT1) and glutamate–aspartate transporter (GLAST), can resume normal glutamate clearance. Activation of microglial P2RX7 purinoreceptors by ATP leads to TNF-α release that protects neurons from glutamate-induced toxicity. Activated astrocytes reduce the spread of tissue degeneration after direct injury through the controlled removal of dying neurons and tissue debris, another neuroprotective effect. In quiescent cells (not shown), nuclear factor-κB (NF-κB) is sequestered in the cytosol by inhibitor of κB (IκB), which binds to specific regions on NF-κB and thereby prevents exposure of the nuclear-localization signal. On stimulation with pro-inflammatory cytokines, IκB proteins are phosphorylated, leading to their ubiquitin-dependent degradation. As a consequence, NF-κB translocates to the nucleus and binds to elements in the promoters of target genes, leading to activation of pro-inflammatory cytokine genes. Reprinted by permission from Macmillan Publishers Ltd: *Nature Reviews Neuroscience* (Milligan and Watkins, 2009), © 2009.

Box 9.5 Toll-like receptors

Toll like receptors (TLRs) are a family of ~13 single transmembrane receptors that recognize a diverse range of moieties or "patterns" on exogenous (e.g., lipopolysaccharide (LPS) of Gram-negative bacteria) and endogenous (e.g., heat-shock proteins and cell membrane components released from stressed/damaged cells) substances that are considered to be danger signals and hence warrant activation of the innate immune system to defend the host. The cell types that express TLRs, the molecules that activate them, and the products released as a consequence have recently been reviewed (Nicotra, Loram, Watkins, and Hutchinson, 2012). TLR4 has been extensively characterized, as it is the TLR that recognizes endotoxin (LPS). Binding of agonists to TLR4 and its accessory molecules, such as MD2 and CD14, activates similar downstream intracellular signalling pathways to those previously documented for IL-1β binding to its cognate receptor, resulting in a powerful pro-inflammatory signal. Indeed, the striking similarity of these pathways is reflected by it being called the TLR4/IL-1 signaling cascade. TLRs signal through two adaptor proteins; MyD88 and TRIF, which engage phosphorylation of kinases such as ERK, JNK and p38. Parallel activation of IP3/Akt signaling, together with the previously outlined kinase activation, culminates in pro-inflammatory transcription and eventual translation. The system is under negative regulation by several mechanisms, such as that by the newly discovered TIR8 pathway. Within the CNS, microglia and some astrocytes, but not neurons, express TLR4 basally.

Box 9.6 Opioid-induced glial activation

Studies of opioid–glial interactions have revealed that glia become progressively more proinflammatory upon repeated morphine exposure and this pro-inflammation, in turn, modulates the wanted and unwanted actions of morphine (Hutchinson *et al.*, 2011). This discovery was first made during studies of the analgesic effect of morphine in spinal cord, which showed that morphine caused gradual pro-inflammatory activation of spinal cord glia, evident by upregulation of both cell-type specific glial activation markers and neuroexcitatory glial products (e.g. pro-inflammatory cytokines and chemokines such as IL-1β). Importantly, this opioid-induced pro-inflammation had a behavioral consequence: the progressive loss of analgesia upon repeated morphine administrations (analgesic tolerance) was attenuated if either morphine-induced glial activation was inhibited or the actions of spinal glial proinflammatory cytokines were blocked (Hutchinson *et al.*, 2011). Opioid-induced proinflammatory spinal glial activation amplifies nociceptive transmission, opposing opioid analgesia. These data highlight the behavioral and, hence, the clinical importance of these non-neuronal actions of opioids.

The mechanism(s) by which opioids cause pro-inflammatory glial activation were unknown until quite recently. We have found that opioid-induced pro-inflammatory glial activation is not mediated by the classical opioid receptors, as it is non-stereoselective. Rather, *in vitro* and *in vivo* studies have demonstrated that opioid- and opioid metabolite-induced proinflammatory glial activation is mediated by TLR4, but in a rank order of potency totally dissimilar to μ-opioid receptor binding. These discoveries were complemented by the parallel discovery that the classical neuronal opioid receptor inactive (+)-isomers of the antagonists naloxone and naltrexone act as TLR4 signaling inhibitors. While highlighting the deleterious consequences for opioid analgesia, these discoveries also point towards novel ways of improving the therapeutic efficacy and reducing the adverse effect profile of opioids (Hutchinson *et al.*, 2011).

and mount an immune response. TLRs detect host DNA, RNA, heat-shock proteins, and cell membrane components that are released by cell stress and damage, such as nerve injury. Whilst TLR-mediated glial activation was implicated when the immunogenic portions of bacteria and viruses were injected over the spinal cord (Meller *et al.*, 1994, Milligan *et al.*, 2001), Tanga and colleagues (2004) showed a correlation between increased spinal microglial TLR4 activation with the onset of behavioral hypersensitivity. Tanga and colleagues (2005) subsequently showed that *TLR4* knockout (KO) mice had significantly attenuated behavioral hypersensitivity, decreased expression of microglial activation markers and proinflammatory cytokines following nerve injury. To date, TLR2, 3 and 4 have all been causally linked to neuropathy induced behavioral hypersensitivity (Kim *et al.*, 2007; Tanga, Nutile-McMenemy, and DeLeo, 2005). Furthermore, opioids have been demonstrated to activate glia via TLRs, with dramatic consequences for analgesia (Box 9.6).

Glial activation: cytokines and chemokines

Glia not only secrete proinflammatory cytokines in response to activation, but are also activated by them, expressing the cognate receptors. In addition, a range of chemokines (*chemo*tactic cyto*kines*) activate glia. CCL2 (monocyte chemotactic protein-1) has been especially well characterized, and constitutes a putative neuron-to-glia activation signal. CCL2 delivered over the spinal cord of uninjured rodents not only induces hyperalgesia, but also microglial activation. If the experiment is repeated, or a peripheral nerve injured, in *CCR2* genetic knockout mice, then microglial activation and nociceptive hypersensitivity is attenuated (Abbadie *et al.*, 2009). In response to nerve injury, CCL2 is upregulated in the DRG and spinal dorsal horn, and transported to the dorsal horn, where it is released in response to neuronal impulses, such as nociceptive signals. CCL2 signals via its upregulated cognate receptor on the membrane of microglia. Given that CCL2 upregulation in the spinal cord closely precedes microglial activation, CCL2 secretion by primary afferents appears to be an initiating microglial activation signal (Abbadie *et al.*, 2009).

Fractalkine (CX_3CL1) is another well-characterized chemokine, and is also posited as a neuron–glia activation signal, mediating neuropathic-like pain. Fractalkine is known to bind to only one receptor, CX_3CR1 (which binds only fractalkine), and is expressed by spinal cord neurons. CX_3CR1 is expressed mostly on microglia, and the injection of fractalkine over the spinal cord has been shown to activate microglia (Milligan and Watkins, 2009). Peripheral nerve injury or neuronal excitation in the spinal cord triggers matrix metalloproteinase (MMP)-induced cleavage of fractalkine and an increase in the expression of CX_3CR1 in microglia in pain-relevant areas. Activated microglia in the dorsal horn also express the lysosomal cysteine protease cathepsin S, an enzyme that may induce fractalkine cleavage during neuropathic pain states. Fractalkine and CX_3CR1 expression in astrocytes have also been found to increase during ongoing nociceptive hypersensitivity, suggesting that CX_3CR1 activation might be important for the chronic stages of neuropathic pain, as astrocyte activation is strongly implicated in ongoing pain changes (Abbadie *et al.*, 2009).

Glial activation: ATP

There is evidence that ATP signaling activates microglia via the $P2X_4$ and $P2X_7$ receptors, contributing to nociceptive hypersensitivity. Strong support comes from a study where microglia were activated by ATP ex vivo and then injected over the spinal cord of uninjured rats, inducing nociceptive hypersensitivity (Tsuda *et al.*, 2003). It was further shown that blockade of $P2X_4$ or $P2X_7$ receptors attenuates exaggerated pain responses induced by nerve injury. The source of ATP is unknown, but may be actively released from injured dorsal horn neurons, or may increase as primary afferent neurons degenerate.

Glial activation: signal transduction and transcription factors

Mitogen-activated protein kinases (MAPKs) are important for signal transduction in glial and neuronal cells. The MAPK family consists of three major members: extracellular signal-regulated kinases (ERK), p38, and c-Jun N-terminal kinase (JNK), although very little is known about JNK. Activation (phosphorylation) of MAPKs in both microglia and astrocytes leads to activation of signal transduction factors, such as NF-κB, resulting in transcription of a wide array of inflammatory genes (including those that encode tumor necrosis factor (TNF)α, interleukin (IL)1β and IL-6) and chemokines (such as CCL2), in addition to nitric oxide (NO) and prostaglandins.

Phosphorylated ERK was initially identified all over the spinal cord following nerve injury, but because these cells did not look like neurons, they were ignored. However, shortly afterwards, a number of studies began to report ERK activation in spinal microglia and astrocytes after nerve injury, with the temporal pattern supporting the conclusions drawn above, that microglial activation in turn leads to astrocyte activation. After nerve injury, ERK is essential for intracellular signaling in glial cells that lead to the production of pro-inflammatory/pro-nociceptive mediators.

Other studies have shown that neuropathic pain signaling also requires the activation of microglial p38 MAPK. p38 MAPK is involved in Ca^{2+}-sensitive intracellular signaling cascades that lead to the production of pro-inflammatory cytokines. It has been speculated that activation of $P2X_4$ increases intracellular Ca^{2+} and activates p38 MAPK. Further studies show that TNF-α and MMPs trigger microglial p38 MAPK activation in the spinal dorsal horn following peripheral nerve injury. MMP9-induced cytokine induction leads to p38

MAPK activation in microglia during the onset and early stages of neuropathic pain, whereas MMP2-induced cytokine induction leads to astrocyte activation during the ongoing and later stages of neuropathic pain.

What are the Consequences of Glial Activation for Pathological Pain Processing?

Neither astrocytes nor microglia can synaptically relay information about pain from the spinal cord to the brain, because they do not have axons. Rather, activated glia exert their influence on pain processing through release of neurotrophins and cytokines (predominantly TNF-α, IL-1β and IL-6), which amplify neuronal excitation and pain signaling. It should be noted that cytokines have been the focus of the majority of research, but that glia also release other substances that modulate pain signaling (e.g. ATP, NO, reactive oxygen species, prostaglandins, glutamate). The majority of research has focused on the pain-enhancing effects of cytokines in the spinal dorsal horn, where they are capable of acting directly on cytokine receptors expressed by neurons and other glia. The injection of exogenous proinflammatory cytokines over the spinal cord enhances nociception, and electrophysiological studies document rapid enhancement of neuronal excitability in response to noxious stimuli following injection of proinflammatory cytokines to the region (Milligan and Watkins, 2009). Conversely, the blockade of proinflammatory cytokine function, using either IL-1β receptor antagonist (IL-1ra), soluble TNF receptors, or anti-IL-6-neutralizing antibodies, reverses exaggerated nociception in virtually all models of neuropathic pain. The fact that established hyperalgesia and allodynia can be reversed by proinflammatory cytokine receptor antagonists supports the conclusion that cytokines are key contributors to the maintenance and induction of enhanced nociceptive states (Milligan and Watkins, 2009).

Aside from direct neuronal activation, proinflammatory cytokines alter synaptic transmission in dorsal horn neurons. TNF-α and IL-1β increase neuronal excitability and synaptic strength by increasing the expression, frequency (perhaps via enhanced glutamate release), and amplitude of NMDA and 2-amino-3-(5-methyl-3-oxo-1,2-oxazol-4-yl) propanoic acid (AMPA) receptor spontaneous excitatory currents in postsynaptic neurons, as well as the ensuing production of prostaglandins and nitric oxide. IL-1β, released by activated glia, increases NMDA receptor subunit phosphorylation, resulting in activation of the intracellular signaling cascade. Such phosphorylation is prevented by the application of fluorocitrate or IL-1ra to abolish glial signaling via IL-1β (Guo *et al.*, 2007).

Chronic astrocyte activation after nerve injury has been shown to disrupt synaptic homeostasis, being associated with extracellular-signal-regulated kinase (ERK) activation, and subsequent downregulation of the excitatory amino acid transporters, glutamate aspartate transporter (GLAST; EAAT1) and glutamate transporter-1 (GLT-1; EAAT2). These transporters normally function to clear glutamate from the synaptic cleft, where it is metabolized to glutamine via the enzyme glutamine synthetase, and shuttled back to the neuron for reconversion to glutamate. Dysfunction of these transporters can produce marked changes in spinal processing, as inhibition causes an elevation in extracellular glutamate concentrations and results in spontaneous nociceptive hypersensitivity.

Proinflammatory cytokines also facilitate disinhibition, decreasing the frequency and amplitude of spontaneous inhibitory postsynaptic GABA- and glycine- induced currents.

Groundbreaking work by Coull and colleagues (2005) has shown that ATP-stimulated microglia release brain-derived neurotrophic factor, which causes a depolarization shift in the pain-projection neurons that inverts the polarity of currents activated by the inhibitory neurotransmitter GABA in spinal lamina neurons.

Peripheral Immune Contributions to Pathological Pain Processing

A contribution of peripheral immune cells to mechanisms of nociceptive hypersensitivity was recently highlighted in our laboratory (Grace *et al.*, 2011), where we found that splenocytes from "high pain" donor rats (four sciatic nerve ligatures, demonstrating robust allodynia) adoptively transferred to "low pain" recipients (one sciatic nerve ligature, demonstrating mild allodynia prior to adoptive transfer) resulted in potentiated allodynia. The effect was abolished, however, if uninjured recipients were instead used, demonstrating that peripheral immune cells amplify existing nociceptive signals, but are incapable of initiating allodynia in their own right.

In response to peripheral nerve injury, an innate immune response ensues, with activation of the complement cascade, mast cell degranulation, and macrophage and neutrophil invasion at the site of injury and in the affected DRG. This gives way to an adaptive immune response, with the recruitment of T-cells, which may interact with activated Schwann cells, the glial cells of the peripheral nervous system. Schwann cells undergo dramatic phenotypic modulation, regaining capacity to proliferate, migrate, and interact with the immune system in T-cell mediated immune responses by expressing major histocompatibility complex (MHC) class II molecules. Throughout this process, vascular endothelial cells, originally considered to be passive lining cells, play an active role in the process of leukocyte recruitment and transendothelial migration into the affected tissue. In a similar fashion to that described above, cytokines and other inflammatory mediators are released by immune cells and act directly on nociceptors, as well as via indirect induction of agents, such as prostaglandins. In addition, there is evidence that DRG-infiltrating immune cells contribute to spontaneous activity of injured neurons. Representing more than a decade of research, this area has recently been thoroughly reviewed (Austin and Moalem-Taylor, 2010).

The CNS is no longer considered to be an entirely immune-privileged organ, especially following peripheral nerve injury. Such an injury alters immune privilege (blood–spinal cord barrier permeability; recruitment of antigen-presenting cells; a supportive CNS microenvironment) to allow T-cell and probably macrophage infiltration into the CNS (Grace, Rolan, and Hutchinson, 2011). Once in the CNS, T-cells secrete proinflammatory cytokines and likely interact with activated microglia to facilitate cytokine release from these cell types directly (Figure 9.4). Furthermore, converging lines of evidence suggest that T-cells may contribute to the maintenance of exaggerated pain states through glial interactions (Grace, Rolan, and Hutchinson, 2011). Studies in T-cell-deficient rodents have demonstrated that nerve-injury induces, but does not maintain allodynia/hyperalgesia (Grace, Rolan, and Hutchinson, 2011). This pattern is supported by microglial activation marker expression, but not astrocyte activation marker expression following peripheral nerve injury (Cao and DeLeo, 2008), suggesting that infiltrating T-cells may be critical mediators in the transition from microglial to astrocytic mediated pain, and therefore the transition of acute to chronic pain.

Therefore, peripheral immune cells represent yet another layer of complexity to immune modulation of nociceptive hypersensitivity arising from nerve injury. Peripheral immune cells

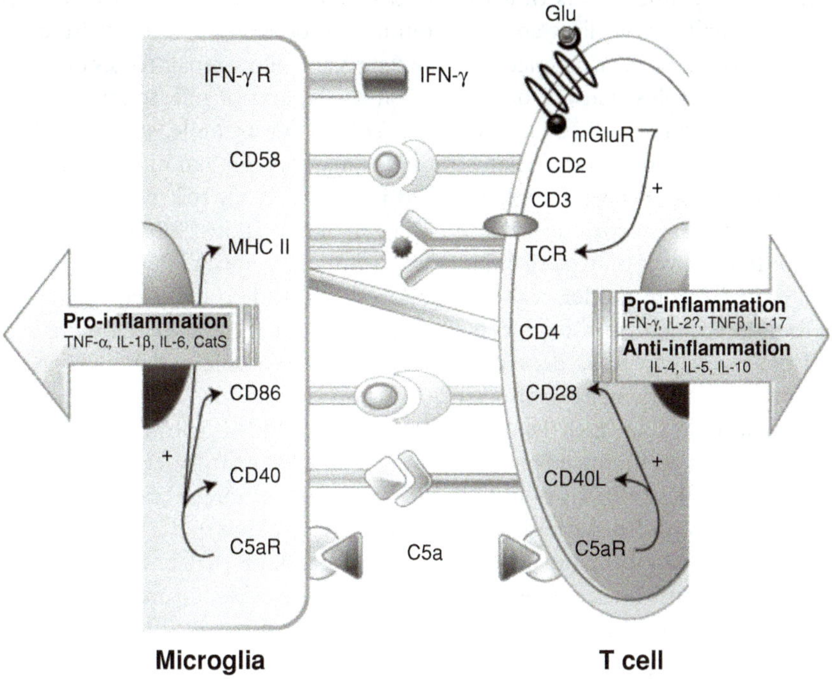

Figure 9.4 The CNS immunological synapse in neuropathic pain. The antigen-presenting cells of the CNS, microglia, present antigen via the major histocompatibility complex (MHC) class II. The antigen is recognized via the T-cell receptor (TCR)–CD3 complex and the co-receptor CD4 (signal 1). This is interaction is assisted and stabilized by adhesion molecules, such as CD2, which attach the microglial ligand LFA-3/CD58. Following the activation signal received via the TCR–CD3 complex, the signal is verified by co-stimulatory molecules, of which CD40 and CD86 have been identified in neuropathic pain (signal 2). Constitutive or inducible T-cell metabotropic glutamate receptors (mGluRs) and microglial and T-cell complement component 5a receptors (C5aR) may respectively direct an immune response against local antigens and enhance expression of MHC class II and co-stimulatory molecules. The result of this interaction is secretion of pro-inflammatory or anti-inflammatory products by both cell types depending on the helper T-cell subset (T_H1 vs T_H2 vs T_H17). CatS, cathepsin S; Glu, glutamate; IFN, interferon; IL, interleukin; TNF, tumour necrosis factor.Reprinted from *Brain, Behavior, and Immunity*, Vol. 25, Grace, P.M., Rolan, P.E., and Hutchinson, M.R., Peripheral immune contributions to the maintenance of central glial activation underlying neuropathic pain, pages 1322–32, © (2011), with permission from Elsevier.

critically function in both the peripheral and central nervous systems, interacting with neurons and glia to contribute to nociceptive hypersensitivity following nerve injury.

The Flip-Side: The Protective Role of the Immune System Following Nerve Injury

Both astrocytes and microglia can release anti-inflammatory factors that facilitate the clearance of apoptotic cells and tissue debris, and that increase the expression of self-associated proteins to dampen and halt continued pro-inflammatory actions (Figure 9.3B). The balance between the protective and harmful effects of activated CNS glia is suspected to involve several anti-inflammatory molecules as well as adaptive immune responses to "self," "altered self," and "non-self" cues that favor the clearance of tissue debris and allow repair to occur. These factors often have protective roles that are dependent on the timing of release and possibly on the severity of the CNS injury (Milligan and Watkins, 2009). For example, studies with transgenic TNF-α KO mice have demonstrated that, although a major pro-inflammatory/nociceptive signal, the timing of endogenous microglial TNF-α is important for the resolution of an inflammatory response and excitotoxic cell death (Milligan and Watkins, 2009). *In vitro* neuronal modeling of differing levels of hypoxic injury due to glutamate and ATP revealed that microglia activated with media from moderately damaged neurons, and co-cultured with hypoxic neurons, were found to be neuro-protective. Neither media from mildly hypoxia-damaged neurons nor media from severely hypoxia-damaged neurons resulted in microglial neuroprotection. In a separate study of CNS damage produced by lipopolysaccharide (LPS) in combination with a surfactant compound that leads to cell lysis, TLR4 was shown to mediate microglial neuroprotection and lead to increased production of anti-inflammatory cytokine mRNA levels. Notably, in these studies both IL-6 and IL-10 were strongly upregulated following immune stimulation. IL-10 is a well-described anti-inflammatory cytokine that has been shown to prevent and reverse pathological pain, whereas IL-6 is a cytokine that has been shown to have both nociceptive and anti-nociceptive effects. However, the evidence predominantly indicates that IL-6 stimulates nociceptive transmission (Milligan and Watkins, 2009).

Similarly, a range of studies indicates that peripheral immune cells also play a protective role in the context of neuropathic pain (Grace, Rolan, and Hutchinson, 2011). For example, adoptive transfer of T_H2 cells attenuated allodynia in nerve-injured rats. The anti-inflammatory cytokine profile secreted by these cells has been independently identified in the dorsal spinal cords of nerve-injured rats in a separate study. Whilst there is some evidence that endogenous IL-2 is pro-inflammatory, exogenous administration has been shown to increase the nociceptive threshold in naïve rats, and intrathecal IL-2 gene therapy was shown to dose-dependently attenuate hyperalgesia in the nerve-injured rat. Other studies have shown that opioid-containing T-cells infiltrate the site of nerve injury and may protect against nociceptive hypersensitivity.

The Immune System as an Alternative Pharmacological Target for Neuropathic Pain

Medications currently prescribed to manage pain, for the most part, target neurons. Such approaches are associated with a poor likelihood for effective pain relief: 3–4 patients need to be treated (NNT) for one patient to achieve a 50% pain score reduction, meaning that the 2–3 unsuccessfully treated patients have to try other treatments. Therefore, alternative therapeutic strategies to control neuropathic pain states, such as targeting glial function, have attracted a lot of attention and are beginning to yield promising results (Milligan and Watkins, 2009). Although the animal studies discussed above have described a broad array of compounds that inactivate or disrupt glial function, most of them are not appropriate for human application. For example, fluorocitrate, although highly effective at blocking the onset of neuropathic pain, blocks glial uptake of excitatory amino acids and has a narrow dose range, with higher doses becoming neurotoxic. However, given that many animal models of neuropathic pain lead to the activation of microglia and astrocytes in the spinal cord, and given that IL-1β and TNF-α are crucially important for the initiation and maintenance of neuropathic pain, several compounds that specifically target microglia or the production of glial IL-1β and TNF-α continue to be explored.

The therapies being examined fall into three major categories: compounds that attenuate microglia and/or astrocyte activation, compounds that inhibit pro-inflammatory cytokine production, and anti-inflammatory compounds. Minocycline, a second-generation tetracycline antibiotic, selectively targets microglia and can cross the blood–brain barrier. In addition, minocycline prevents the production of pro-inflammatory cytokines and NO, and was recently shown to reduce microglial trafficking to injured neurons, supporting clinical utility. It should be noted that the minocycline doses attainable in humans are lower than can be reached in rodent models, which may have neuronal consequences that are paradoxically deleterious for neuropathic pain. Propentofylline, a methylxanthine derivative, suppresses astrocyte activation and is known to control pain behavior in rodent models of enhanced pain states. Other compounds, such as pentoxifylline and ibudilast (AV411/MN-166) are generally nonspecific cytokine and phosphodiesterase inhibitors that stimulate IL-10 production. Consequently, such drugs would also be expected to have deleterious consequences for neuropathic pain, due to neuronal hyperexcitability. Both are therapeutically effective in animal models of neuropathic pain. TLR4 blockade represents another avenue to attenuate glial activation, as it not only prevents the initial development of neuropathic pain (Tanga, Nutile-McMenemy, and DeLeo, 2005), but also reverses established neuropathic pain (Hutchinson *et al.*, 2011). The (+)-opioid antagonist naloxone, whilst inactive at the μ-opioid receptor, was shown to antagonize TLR4 activation (Hutchinson *et al.*, 2011). In targeting T-cells, immunosuppressants, such as rapamycin, leflunomide and methotrexate, have been shown to significantly attenuate hyperalgesia and allodynia in nerve-injured rodents (Grace, Rolan, and Hutchinson, 2011).

Although small molecules offer promising approaches to treat neuropathic pain, recent studies using gene-transfer techniques offer a unique advantage: targeted drug delivery to discrete areas of the pain pathway. Targeted and chronic spinal cord transgene expression may be an important mechanism by which to achieve long-term neuropathic pain control. Gene therapy has been gaining momentum as a tool by which to target neurons or glia for pain control. Intrathecal delivery of IL-10 or IL-2 genes reversed peripheral nerve injury-induced thermal hyperalgesia and mechanical allodynia for up to 4 weeks while leaving normal pain thresholds intact. In these studies, viral vectors were administered systemically and directly over the spinal cord for gene transfer to the CNS. Intramuscular or intrathecal gene transfer using viral vectors encoding IL-4 or IL-10, respectively, reversed neuropathic pain for 4 months (Milligan and Watkins, 2009).

Strategies to enhance the protective role of the immune system, such as providing anti-inflammatory cytokines (e.g. IL-10), or autologous transfer of anti-inflammatory T-cells, could be a more beneficial approach than administering antagonists of the pro-inflammatory cytokines themselves, or blocking the normal function of immune cells by globally preventing activation.

Future Directions

Recognition of the role of the immune system in the nociceptive hypersensitivity associated with neuropathic pain has raised a number of exciting implications that are currently being explored and are moving the field in new directions.

We have described a number of processes by which activated immune cells amplify the pain process after nerve injury. However, the clinical evidence clearly shows that the majority of patients with nerve injury will not go on to develop chronic pain. The question now being posed is "How and why does a patient subset transition from acute to chronic pain?" Evidence is accumulating from outside the pain field that prior microglial activation (e.g., trauma, inflammation, infection) can dramatically alter their response to new challenges. Preliminary evidence has shown that systemic low-dose LPS administration, which is insufficient to induce allodynia, preceded by laparotomy, for which allodynia had already resolved, caused exaggerated allodynia and microglial activation, well in excess of either challenge alone (Hains *et al.*, 2010). Further research may identify whether such mechanisms of glial sensitization underlie the transition from acute to chronic pain. In addition to this, and as discussed above, the contribution of T-cells to the maintenance of neuropathic pain requires clarification.

Much of the neurobiology research to date has focused on mechanisms in the spinal dorsal horn, dorsal root ganglia and the site of injury. However, these are not the only sites important for pain processing. To gain a more complete picture of how the immune system influences neuropathic pain, glial activation and peripheral immune cell infiltration should be explored in the pain matrix, and in the descending modulatory sites. Indeed, studies have already indentified glial activation in the PAG and RVM, following peripheral nerve injury (Wei *et al.*, 2008; Mor *et al.*, 2010). Since neuropathic pain is not "simply" an alteration in nociceptive signaling, but encompasses many other psychosocial components (e.g., depression, anxiety, sleep disturbance, substance abuse), investigation of these additional pain-relevant sites may provide further insight into such chronic pain co-morbidities. For example, the Keay group identified increased astrocyte activation in the PAG of nerve-injured rats with disability (altered social interaction and sleep–wake cycle) versus those with no or transient disability (Mor *et al.*, 2010). Sophisticated study designs, such as these, may continue to yield promising results.

It is now clear that the quest to pharmacologically treat neuropathic pain in a disease-modifying fashion is incomplete without targeting the immune system. In moving towards such a goal, the many preclinical therapies, described above, require translation in clinical populations. The only major clinical trial to date, in which propentofylline, a drug that may not be a suitable glial modulator in humans, was trialed in 143 postherpetic neuralgia patients (ClinicalTrials.gov NCT00813826) has been disappointing, as it failed to improve self-reported pain scores compared to placebo (Landry *et al.*, 2012). Given the multiple inherent design issues, from trialling a pain syndrome for which no data exist to support glial involvement, to stopping the dosing before reversal of long-standing pain with glial modulators would be expected, to no knowledge of whether the drug reached spinal cord in therapeutic levels, this trial raised far more questions than it resolved (Watkins *et al.*, 2012).

It is perhaps a lesson that Aventis, who trialed propentofylline for Alzheimer's disease with mixed success, refused to consider trialing it for pain, given problems they encountered with the drug in its present chemical form. Therefore, further clinical trials of improved design will be of immense value. It is likely, however, that the most satisfactory treatment outcomes will be therapies that combine immune targeting and other neuronal activation mechanisms.

Given the many challenges surrounding the clinical management of neuropathic pain, such as the inability to make mechanism-based diagnoses, the high number needed to treat, and the dearth of mechanism based therapies, there is growing interest in the development of objective biomarkers for chronic pain. The major limiting factor to any chronic pain biomarker is that many of the underlying mechanisms are considered to be inaccessible within the CNS. An appreciation of the role of the immune system may be of advantage in moving towards this goal: as circulating immune cells are likely to be in communication with glia and neurons in the CNS (Grace, Rolan, and Hutchinson, 2011), quantification of their activity may serve as useful biomarkers of chronic pain (e.g., Hutchinson and colleagues, (Hutchinson, La Vincente, and Somogyi, 2004)). Such an approach is particularly amenable to translational study designs, where putative biomarkers can be derived in animal models to facilitate a targeted search in humans.

After two decades of glial research in neuropathic pain, enormous gains have been made in understanding how glia become activated and signal to each other, to other immune cells and to neurons. However, we have only scratched the surface of the glial response repertoire. For example, we need to develop more sophisticated tools and approaches in order to understand the differences between rodent and human glial cells. Furthermore, the glial activation phenotype can lead to vastly different outcomes in terms of neuronal consequences. Investigation of these activation subtleties, such as specific glial cell populations, their locations and temporal profiles, will enable us to target and manipulate these processes in a more sophisticated manner, with the ultimate goal of better treatment outcomes for chronic pain sufferers world-wide.

References

Abbadie, C., Bhangoo, S., De Koninck, Y., Malcangio, M., Melik-Parsadaniantz, S., and White, F. A. (2009). Chemokines and pain mechanisms. *Brain Research Reviews*, 60(1), 125–34.

Araque, A., Parpura, V., Sanzgiri, R. P., and Haydon, P. G. (1999). Tripartite synapses: glia, the unacknowledged partner. *Trends in Neuroscience*, 22(5), 208–215.

Austin, P. J. and Moalem-Taylor, G. (2010). The neuro-immune balance in neuropathic pain: involvement of inflammatory immune cells, immune-like glial cells and cytokines. *J Neuroimmunology*, 229(1–2), 26–50.

Cao, L. and Deleo, J. A. (2008). CNS-infiltrating $CD4^+$ T lymphocytes contribute to murine spinal nerve transection-induced neuropathic pain. *European Journal of Immunology*, 38(2), 448–458.

Costigan, M., Scholz, J., and Woolf, C. J. (2009). Neuropathic pain: a maladaptive response of the nervous system to damage. *Annual Review of Neuroscience*, 32, 1–32.

Coull, J. a. M., Beggs, S., Boudreau, D., Boivin, D., Tsuda, M., Inoue, K., Gravel, C. et al. (2005). BDNF from microglia causes the shift in neuronal anion gradient underlying neuropathic pain. *Nature*, 438(7070), 1017–1021.

Descartes, R. (1972). *Treatise of Man*, Cambridge, MA: Harvard University Press.

Garrison, C. J., Dougherty, P. M., and Carlton, S. M. (1994). GFAP expression in lumbar spinal cord of naive and neuropathic rats treated with MK-801. *Expperimental Neurology*, 129 237–243.

Garrison, C. J., Dougherty, P. M., Kajander, K. C., and Carlton, S. M. (1991). Staining of glial fibrillary acidic protein (GFAP) in lumbar spinal cord increases following a sciatic nerve constriction injury. *Brain Research*, 565(1), 1–7.

Grace, P. M., Hutchinson, M. R., Bishop, A., Somogyi, A. A., Mayrhofer, G., and Rolan, P. E. (2011). Adoptive transfer of peripheral immune cells potentiates allodynia in a graded chronic constriction injury model of neuropathic pain. *Brain, Behavior, Immunity*, 25(3), 503–513.

Grace, P. M., Rolan, P. E., and Hutchinson, M. R. (2011). Peripheral immune contributions to the maintenance of central glial activation underlying neuropathic pain. *Brain, Behavior, Immunity*, 25(7), 1322–1332.

Guo, W., Wang, H., Watanabe, M., Shimizu, K., Zou, S., LaGraize, S. C. et al. (2007). Glial–cytokine–neuronal interactions underlying the mechanisms of persistent pain. *Journal of Neuroscience*, 27(22), 6006–6018.

Hains, L. E., Loram, L. C., Weiseler, J. L., Frank, M. G., Bloss, E. B., Sholar, P. et al. (2010). Pain intensity and duration can be enhanced by prior challenge: initial evidence suggestive of a role of microglial priming. *Journal of Pain*, 11(10), 1004–1014.

Hutchinson, M. R., La Vincente, S. F., and Somogyi, A. A. (2004). In vitro opioid induced proliferation of peripheral blood immune cells correlates with in vivo cold pressor pain tolerance in humans: a biological marker of pain tolerance. *Pain*, 110(3), 751–755.

Hutchinson, M. R., Shavit, Y., Grace, P. M., Rice, K. C., Maier, S. F., and Watkins, L. R. (2011). Exploring the neuroimmunopharmacology of opioids: an integrative review of mechanisms of central immune signaling and their implications for opioid analgesia. *Pharmacological Reviews*, 63(3), 772–810.

Kim, D., Kim, M. A., Cho, I. H., Kim, M. S., Lee, S., Jo, E. K. et al. (2007). A critical role of toll-like receptor 2 in nerve injury-induced spinal cord glial cell activation and pain hypersensitivity. *Journal of Biological Chemistry*, 282(20), 14975–14983.

Landry, R. P., Jacobs, V. L., Romero-Sandoval, E. A., and DeLeo, J. A. (2012). Propentofylline, a CNS glial modulator does not decrease pain in post-herpetic neuralgia patients: in vitro evidence for differential responses in human and rodent microglia and macrophages. *Experimental Neurology*,234, 340–350.

Meller, S. T., Dykstra, C., Grzybycki, D., Murphy, S., and Gebhart, G. F. (1994). The possible role of glia in nociceptive processing and hyperalgesia in the spinal cord of the rat. *Neuropharmacology*, 33(11), 1471–1478.

Melzack, R. and Wall, P. D. (1965). Pain mechanisms: a new theory. *Science*, 150(699), 971–9.

Milligan, E. D., O'Connor, K. A., Nguyen, K. T., Armstrong, C. B., Twining, C., Gaykema, R. P. et al. (2001). Intrathecal HIV-1 envelope glycoprotein gp120 induces enhanced pain states mediated by spinal cord proinflammatory cytokines. *Journal of Neuroscience*, 21(8), 2808–2819.

Milligan, E. D. and Watkins, L. R. (2009). Pathological and protective roles of glia in chronic pain. *Nature Reviews Neuroscience*, 10(1), 23–36.

Mor, D., Bembrick, A. L., Austin, P. J., Wyllie, P. M., Creber, N. J., et al. (2010). Anatomically specific patterns of glial activation in the periaqueductal gray of the sub-population of rats showing pain and disability following chronic constriction injury of the sciatic nerve. *Neuroscience*, 166(4), 1167–1184.

Nicotra, L., Loram, L. C., Watkins, L. R., and Hutchinson, M. R. (2012). Toll-like receptors in chronic pain. *Experimental Neurology*, 234(2), 316–329.

Obata, K., Katsura, H., Miyoshi, K., Kondo, T., Yamanaka, H., Kobayashi, K. et al. (2008). Toll-like receptor 3 contributes to spinal glial activation and tactile allodynia after nerve injury. *Journal of Neurochemistry*, 105(6), 2249–2259.

Raghavendra, V., Tanga, F., and Deleo, J. A. (2003). Inhibition of microglial activation attenuates the development but not existing hypersensitivity in a rat model of neuropathy. *Journal of Pharmacology and Experimental Therapeutics*, 306(2), 624–630.

Sherrington, C. S. (1906). *The Integrative Action of the Nervous System*, New York, Scribner.

Tanga, F. Y., Nutile-Mcmenemy, N., and Deleo, J. A. (2005). The CNS role of Toll-like receptor 4 in innate neuroimmunity and painful neuropathy. *Proceedings of the National Academy of Sciences, USA*, 102(16), 5856–5861.

Tanga, F. Y., Raghavendra, V., and Deleo, J. A. (2004). Quantitative real-time RT-PCR assessment of spinal microglial and astrocytic activation markers in a rat model of neuropathic pain. *Neurochemistry International*, 45(2–3), 397–407.

Tsuda, M., Shigemoto-Mogami, Y., Koizumi, S., Mizokoshi, A., Kohsaka, S. et al. (2003). P2X4 receptors induced in spinal microglia gate tactile allodynia after nerve injury. *Nature*, 424(6950), 778–83.

Watkins, L. R., Hutchinson, M. R., Johnson, K. W. (2012). Commentary on Landry *et al.*: "Propentofylline, a CNS glial modulator, does not decrease pain in post-herpetic neuralgia patients: in vitro evidence for differential responses in human and rodent microglia and macrophages". *Experimental Neurology*, 234, 351–353.

Watkins, L. R., Wiertelak, E. P., Goehler, L. E., Mooney-Heiberger, K., Martinez, J. et al. (1994). Neurocircuitry of illness-induced hyperalgesia. *Brain Research*, 639, 283–299.
Wei, F., Guo, W., Zou, S., Ren, K., and Dubner, R. (2008). Supraspinal glial–neuronal interactions contribute to descending pain facilitation. *Journal of Neuroscience*, 28(42), 10482–10495.
Woolf, C. J. (1983). Evidence for a central component of post-injury pain hypersensitivity. *Nature*, 306(5944), 686–688.
Woolf, C. J. and Ma, Q. (2007). Nociceptors – noxious stimulus detectors. *Neuron*, 55(3), 353–364.

10

Stress and Neuroendocrine–Immune Interaction

A Therapeutic Role for β-endorphin

Olivia Wynne and Dipak K. Sarkar

Endocrinology Program and Department of Animal Sciences, Rutgers, The State University of New Jersey, New Brunswick, NJ, USA

Physiology of Stress: General Overview

Stress can be defined as a threat or a challenge to the survival of an animal (Weiner, 1991); it can be physical (infection or fatigue), psychological (separation and loss), or perceived (the threat of war or predators). Stress can be acute such as brief public speaking or chronic such as disease. What is considered stressful depends on the prior experience of the animal and the perceived outcome of the event (Weiner, 1991). Experience determines the way the stress is perceived, as do ontogenetic variables, such as prenatal programming, nutritional factors, and hormonal development (Levine, 1991). The degree to which the body reacts is determined by the effectiveness of the stress response. Furthermore, social factors also play a role with social interaction and support being beneficial in reducing the stress response (Berk, 2003).

Whilst what constitutes "stress" is not easily defined, the psychological response to stress is stable and well-characterized. Physiologically, this is reflected by activation of the hyothalamus and hypothalamic–pituitary–adrenal (HPA) axis, which plays a major role in allostasis. The hypothalamus controls the basic mechanisms of survival, i.e., reproduction, food and fluid intake, control of the body's temperature, instigation of attack and defense, metabolism and growth, as well as aspects of memory (FitzGerald, 1996). The hypothalamus forms a major part of the neuroendocrine communication with the central and peripheral immune systems. For example, the increase in body temperature indicative of sickness is controlled by the hypothalamus. Fever, due to infectious agents, is caused by macrophages in the hypothalamus releasing a protein that causes the thermostat of the hypothalamus to be reset to a higher than homeostatic value in an effort to eradicate the infection (FitzGerald, 1996).

Stressors can be categorized according to the relative duration of the exposure. Acute stress generally means a single exposure to a single stressor. The duration of the challenge can be experimentally manipulated, i.e., restraint, cold, and foot shock. In other cases the acute stress initiates the stress response, e.g., insulin-induced hypoglycemia (Kovacs, Miklos, and Bali, 2005). Chronic stress generally refers to continuous exposure to a stressor, for example, alcohol abuse; or continuous social conflict or disease states, such as arthritis. Experimentally

The Wiley-Blackwell Handbook of Psychoneuroimmunology, First Edition. Edited by Alexander W. Kusnecov and Hymie Anisman.

induced states such as adrenalectomy could also be regarded as a chronic stressor because of the physiological imbalance caused by the intervention (Kovacs, Miklos, and Bali, 2005). An animal's response to stress can also include activation of the immune system and sympathetic nervous system. This chapter is focused on the neuroendocrine response to stress and its potential to be programmed by early-life events.

Regardless of the source of the stress, the same physiological response occurs: the HPA axis initiates a reliable hormonal cascade that results in glucocorticoids (GC) being released into circulation. In humans the main GC is cortisol, while in rodents it is corticosterone. Cortisol inhibits allergic and inflammatory responses, exerting an immunosuppressive action, and stimulating the "fight or flight" response of the sympathetic nervous system; such actions help the animal survive a stressor. The HPA-axis-driven stress response starts when the paraventricular nucleus of the hypothalamus (PVN) produces corticotrophin-releasing hormone (CRH; also known as CRF, for corticotropin release factor) and vasopressin, which stimulate the anterior pituitary to synthesize proopiomelanocortin (POMC), and release adrenocorticotropic hormone (ACTH), which initiates the synthesis and release into blood of cortisol from the adrenal cortex.

As steroid hormones, glucocorticoids have direct access to the brain (Levine, 2005), and participate in the control of protein, carbohydrate, and lipid metabolism, as well as promoting the breakdown of protein and reducing the synthesis of proteins in skeletal muscle. In the liver, GCs stimulate glycogen synthesis, increase gene expression, and activate multiple enzymes. In humans, GCs at normal levels are necessary for fetal organ maturation (Rhoades and Pflanzer, 2003), but excessive exposure has been linked to a number of growth abnormalities (Sun, Yang, and Challis, 1997). During development, glucocorticoids have key functions in cell division, differentiation and maturation. However, in excess GCs can have negative effects on brain development by slowing down neurogenesis, prematurely stopping cell division, and inhibiting dendritic and axonal cell growth, thereby reducing brain size and leading to abnormalities of behavior (Robson, Leckie, Seckl, and Holmes, 1998).

The other main physiological aspect of the stress response is the autonomic nervous system (ANS). The ANS has the capacity to trigger two opposing responses- the "flight or flight" of the sympathetic nervous system (SNS), or the "tend and mend" of the parasympathetic nervous system. The activation of the sympathetic nervous system causes the release of catecholamines from the medulla of the adrenal glands. Catecholamines such as epinephrine (E) and norepinephrine (NE) trigger the familiar feeling of decreased saliva, increases in respiration, perspiration, and heart rate. The SNS is the first line of defense against a stressor, traditionally allowing escape from the immediate threat. Such a response cannot be physiologically maintained for long periods of time, as demonstrated by the early findings of Hans Selye.

As part of the HPA and SNS response to stress, the opioid peptide β-endorphin (BEP) is generated from the propeptide, POMC, and has been implicated in the behavioral as well as the biological response associated with stress stimuli. The best studied effect of BEP is its ability to modulate pain, but the peptide has also been implicated in the central regulation of ACTH (Fratta, Rossetti, Poggioli, and Gessa, 1981) and hypothalamic CRH (Appel and Van Loon, 1986; Khachaturian, Lewis, Alessi, and Watson, 1985; Plotsky, 1986). Indeed, BEP has been shown to play a critical role in bringing the stress response to a state of homoeostasis. In response to stress, the secretion of CRH and catecholamines stimulate the synthesis of BEP and other POMC-derived peptides from the hypothalamus, which in turn inhibit the activity of the HPA axis (Boyadjieva *et al.*, 2009). Central BEP binds to δ- and μ-opioid receptors, and modulates the ANS via neurons within the PVN of the hypothalamus. The β-endorphin produced from pituitary POMC is primarily regulated by CRH and AVP and has less impact on ANS function.

The activity of the HPA axis response to stress is tightly regulated because extended tissue exposure to cortisol can result in damage to organs and tissues in the body. This regulation is carried out by a feedback system via glucocorticoid receptors (GRs) in the PVN, and mineralocorticoid receptors (MRs) and GRs in the hippocampus. Glucocorticoid receptors inhibit HPA axis activity; because at basal levels of cortisol, the MRs are occupied while GRs are mostly unoccupied. However, when there are elevated levels of plasma cortisol, as during a period of stress, there is an increased occupation of GRs (Reul and de Kloet, 1985). It is the increased occupation of GRs that triggers the negative feedback. The glucocorticoids released by the adrenal cortex interact with the GRs in the pituitary, hypothalamus and hippocampus; so any overactivity results in feedback, causing a reduction in circulating CRH (Bertram and Hanson, 2002), thereby "switching off" the stress response. This effect by GCs can involve fast, intermediate, and slow modes of feedback. Fast feedback is mediated at the cell membrane and occurs in seconds to minutes. Intermediate feedback can last hours and occurs 30 minutes after a pulse or continuous exposure to GCs, and slow feedback occurs when there is supraphysiological exposure to exogenous GCs for days or weeks (Dallman, 2000).

Stress Effects on Development: Critical Periods

Prenatal period

There are a number of periods during development in which environmental insult can have long-lasting effects on functioning. The impact of prenatal maternal stress in programming the offspring phenotype has been reinforced by many human and animal studies looking at the effects of stressors as varied as physiological prenatal stress in the form of exposure to excess GCs, maternal substance abuse (Weinberg, Sliwowska, Lan, and Hellemans, 2008), undernutrition (Hales and Barker, 2001), overnutrition (Armitage, Taylor, and Poston, 2005) and infection (Ebert and Kotler, 2005). Psychological stressors have also been investigated, with studies on the effects of depression (Davis *et al.*, 2007b), civil war (Malaspina *et al.*, 2008), a specific isolated terrorist attack (Engel *et al.*, 2005; Lederman *et al.*, 2004; Yehuda *et al.*, 2005), and anxiety (Brouwers, van Baar, and Pop, 2001). All studies show a long-lasting effect of early-life stress on the quality of life of the offspring. Generally, prenatal stress results in offspring with predispositions to cardiovascular disease, type 2 diabetes, hypertension, and obesity. Prenatal stress has also been linked to psychological disorders such as anxiety and depression, as well as behavioral and cognitive deficits.

Alcohol abuse during pregnancy is well known to cause major problems, such as fetal alcohol syndrome (FAS). Nevertheless, alcohol exposure at lower levels can result in increased risk of seizures (Sun *et al.*, 2009); and, when controlling for IQ, adults exposed to prenatal alcohol exposure are more susceptible to mental illnesses such as depression, substance abuse, and psychotic disorders (Famy, Streissguth, and Unis, 1998). The majority of studies have looked at levels of alcohol exposure that result in disorders in the FAS spectrum owing to the empirical difficulties in studying mild-to-moderate exposure. However, at least one study has found a positive correlation with higher alcohol exposure related to higher cortisol activity, negative affect and elevated heart rate (Taylor, Branch, Van Zuylen, and Redei, 1988).

Prenatal maternal depression excluding the postnatal maternal state has been shown to negatively affect offspring temperament (Davis *et al.*, 2007a). Offspring of mothers with high anxiety during pregnancy have lower mental development scores (Brouwers, 2001). In rhesus monkeys, prenatal maternal psychological stress, in the form of acoustic startle, resulted in offspring with significantly reduced focused exploration, increased non-directed locomotor behavior (i.e., pacing), in addition to significantly increased cortisol and decreased hippocampal neurogenesis and volume (Coe *et al.*, 2003). Implicitly and explicitly in some cases, the variable that all these studies have in common is an increase in maternal circulating cortisol. Regardless of whether the stress is physiological or psychological, the maternal stress response is triggered resulting in excesses of cortisol. The broad finding is maternal stress negatively impacts the offspring's health and behavior both in the short and long term.

Postnatal period

Environmental factors are known to affect the development of psychopathology during postnatal life, infancy and childhood (Rutter, 2005). Human studies suffer from the complex interaction of genes and environment (Kramer, 2005), in addition to exposure to multiple stressors over long periods of time. Stressors such as family conflict, maternal psychopathology and low socioeconomic status do not happen in isolation or within short timeframes, so the identification of the detrimental type, timing and dose of the stressor are difficult to determine in human studies. Animal models provide more genetic and environmental control; and when assessing outcomes at the molecular level are suitable substitutes for humans.

The level of development in the neonatal period in rodents is thought to roughly translate to the third trimester of pregnancy in humans (Clancy, Darlington, and Finlay, 2001), as such rodent models investigating late prenatal paradigms carry out their manipulation on neonatal rodents. It is a period unique to altricial animals – dependent on the dam for food, warmth and protection, developmentally immature but physically separate from the dam. Many studies take advantage of the pups' dependence on the dam to induce a stressor known as maternal deprivation.

Studies investigating postnatal stressors in animals use either models of neonatal infection or maternal deprivation. One study exposing postnatal day (PND) 3 rats to maternal deprivation found sex specific alterations to GR and MR regulation and binding affinity in the brain (Sutanto, Rosenfeld, de Kloet, and Levine, 1996). Males exposed to deprivation, or deprivation with ACTH injection, showed a reduction in GRs and MRs; while females exposed to deprivation and saline or ACTH injections showed increased GR capacity with no changes to MRs. The binding affinity of the receptors was also affected (Sutanto, Rosenfeld, de Kloet, and Levine, 1996). Maternal separation has also been linked to increased basal corticosterone and an attenuated corticosterone response to stress at 3 months of age, with decreases in GR binding and abundance in the hippocampus in adulthood (Workel *et al.*, 2001). Other outcomes of maternal separation include impaired fear conditioning (Kosten, Lee, and Kim, 2006), increased basal corticosterone and decreased GRs in the hippocampus (Aisa *et al.*, 2007).

Period of adolescence

Any period of significant growth and development is vulnerable to the detrimental effects of stress. The focus of much research is the perinatal period, while less is known about the effects of stress during adolescence. Generally, stress during childhood has been linked with metabolic disorders such as obesity, and psychological disorders such as depression and anxiety. However, data for direct relations between symptoms of stress, circulating levels of stress mediators and later morbidity are scarce for adolescents. Evidence indicates that neonatal and adolescent stress exposure can result in significant impairments to subsequent neuroplasticity, cognitive ability, and emotional behavior that do not occur under similar conditions in adults (McCormick, Mathews, Thomas, and Waters, 2010; McCormick and Mathews, 2010; Buwalda, Geerdink, Vidal, and Koolhaas, 2011). For example, children with PTSD show a significant divergence in their NE and cortisol profile (Pervanidou *et al.*, 2007). Adolescence is also a time when psychological disorders manifest for the first time, indicating a period of vulnerability for the HPA/stress response system. Perhaps most important in terms of long-term effects of stress, studies show that adolescents do not habituate to stress like adults (Romeo, Lee, and McEwen, 2004b; Romeo *et al.*, 2004a; Doremus-Fitzwater, Varlinskaya, and Spear, 2009), meaning there is potentially a longer period of exposure to the detrimental effects of stress during a critical time of development.

Stress Effects on Immune Function

The HPA axis and sympathetic nervous system are major pathways by which the brain regulates immune processes (see Figure 10.1). The first indication of such communication was noted by Selye, who recorded that rats exposed to a large variety of stressors simultaneously developed large adrenal glands and shrunken thymuses and lymph nodes, which suggested the former secreting a hormone that suppressed the latter (Selye, 1998). Immune cells have receptors to bind with a number of hormones, neuropeptides, and neurotransmitters (Bellinger, Ackerman, Felten, and Felten, 1992; Haas and Schauenstein, 1997); therefore, changes in neuroendocrine and/or autonomic activities may lead to modulation of immune responses. For example, tumor necrosis factor α (TNF-α), IL-1, and IL-6 act upon the HPA axis and sympathetic nervous system locally and via the central nervous system (Pickering, Cumiskey, and O'Connor, 2005; Besedovsky and del Rey, 1996; Wilder, 1995). Furthermore, CRH has a variety of effects on immune cells (Elenkov, Webster, Torpy, and Chrousos, 1999) and modulates immune/inflammatory responses through receptor-mediated actions of GCs on target immune cells (Tsigos and Chrousos, 2002). GCs prevent the migration of leukocytes from circulation into extravascular regions, reduce accumulation of monocytes and granulocytes, and suppress the production and/or action of many cytokines and inflammatory mediators (Hermann, Beck, and Sheridan, 1995; Zhang *et al.*, 1998; Sheridan *et al.*, 1998). Therefore, GCs inhibit the immune system response protecting the animal from potentially toxic inflammatory processes.

Cytokines released in response to infection stimulate the stress response, releasing GCs which then downregulate the cytokines. This negative feedback prevents an overreaction of the stress response to infection by intricately regulating the cytokine response to immune stimuli. GCs are known to be anti-inflammatory and have been used clinically as such for decades. The exact mechanism(s) of action is still being elucidated. It is known that GCs inhibit a number of cytokines including Interleukin (IL)-1α, IL-1β, IL-6, IL-12, IFN-γ, TNF-α, granulocyte-macrophage colony-stimulating factor (GM CSF) and chemokine (C-C motif) ligand 5 (RANTES) (Wiegers, Stec, Sterzer, and Reul, 2005). Glucocorticoids inhibit cytokines at multiple levels: transcription, translation, mRNA stability, secretion, and combinations of levels mentioned (Sapolsky, Romero, and Munck, 2000). They are not always inhibitory, for example, GCs can increase the activity of transforming growth factor β (TGFβ) by activating a latent form of the cytokine (Oursler, Riggs, and Spelsberg, 1993) which may indirectly form part of the immune response, because TGFβ inhibits activation of T-cells and macrophages. GCs also increase production of IL-10, which inhibits antigen presentation and T-cell activation (de Waal Malefyt *et al.*, 1991). It is worth noting that IFN-γ, TNF-α, GM CSF, IL-1, IL-2, and IL-6 are toxic at high levels (Munck and Naray-Fejes-Toth, 1994). Glucocorticoids inhibit pro-inflammatory cytokine synthesis and/or induce cytokines that have immunosuppressive potential, further supporting the idea that GCs act to protect against hyperactivation of the stress response.

Role of β-endorphin in the Control of the Stress Response

The peptide, β-endorphin, is known to have the ability to inhibit stress hormone production, produce analgesia and promote a feeling of wellbeing (Akil *et al.*, 1984). It is an endogenous opioid polypeptide, primarily produced by the hypothalamus and pituitary gland, derived as a cleavage product of POMC, which is also the precursor hormone for ACTH and α-melanocyte-stimulating hormone (α-MSH). β-endorphin neuronal cell bodies are primarily localized in the arcuate nuclei of the hypothalamus, with terminals distributed throughout the central nervous system (CNS), including the PVN of the hypothalamus (Appel and Van Loon, 1986; Plotsky, 1986). Via the neuronal circuitry within the PVN, BEP has also been found to regulate the immune system. For example, BEP binds to δ- and μ-opioid receptors, and modulates the neurotransmission in sympathetic neurons to alter NK cell cytolytic functions in the spleen (Boyadjieva, Advis, and Sarkar, 2006; Boyadjieva *et al.*, 2009).

The peripheral actions of β-endorphin are well known. Release of BEP from the pituitary has an established analgesic action, inhibiting pain sensation thereby reducing the stress caused by physical injury. Less studied are the central actions of BEP. Within the CNS, BEP functions as a neurotransmitter regulating the HPA axis (see Figure 10.1). Specifically, in the PVN, BEP neurons innervate CRH neurons and inhibit CRH release (Kawano and Masuko, 2000). Conversely, a μ-opioid receptor antagonist increases CRH release (Boyadjieva, Advis, and Sarkar, 2006). Indeed, during stressor exposure, secretion of CRH and catecholamines stimulates secretion of hypothalamic BEP and other POMC-derived peptides, which in turn inhibit the activity of the stress system (Boyadjieva, Advis, and Sarkar, 2006). However, abnormalities in BEP neuronal function are correlated with a higher incidence of cancers and infections in patients with schizophrenia, depression, and obesity, as well as in individuals with fetal alcohol syndrome (Lissoni *et al.*, 1987; Bernstein *et al.*, 2002). Whereas low levels of central BEP have been linked with depression, schizophrenia, and post-traumatic stress disorder (Darko, Risch, Gillin, and Golshan, 1992; Bernstein *et al.*, 2002).

Role of β-endorphin in the Control of Immune Regulation

β-endorphin has been shown to inhibit T-cell proliferation (van den Bergh, Rozing, and Nagelkerken, 1993), and can also inhibit antibody production (Morgan, McClurg, and Janda,

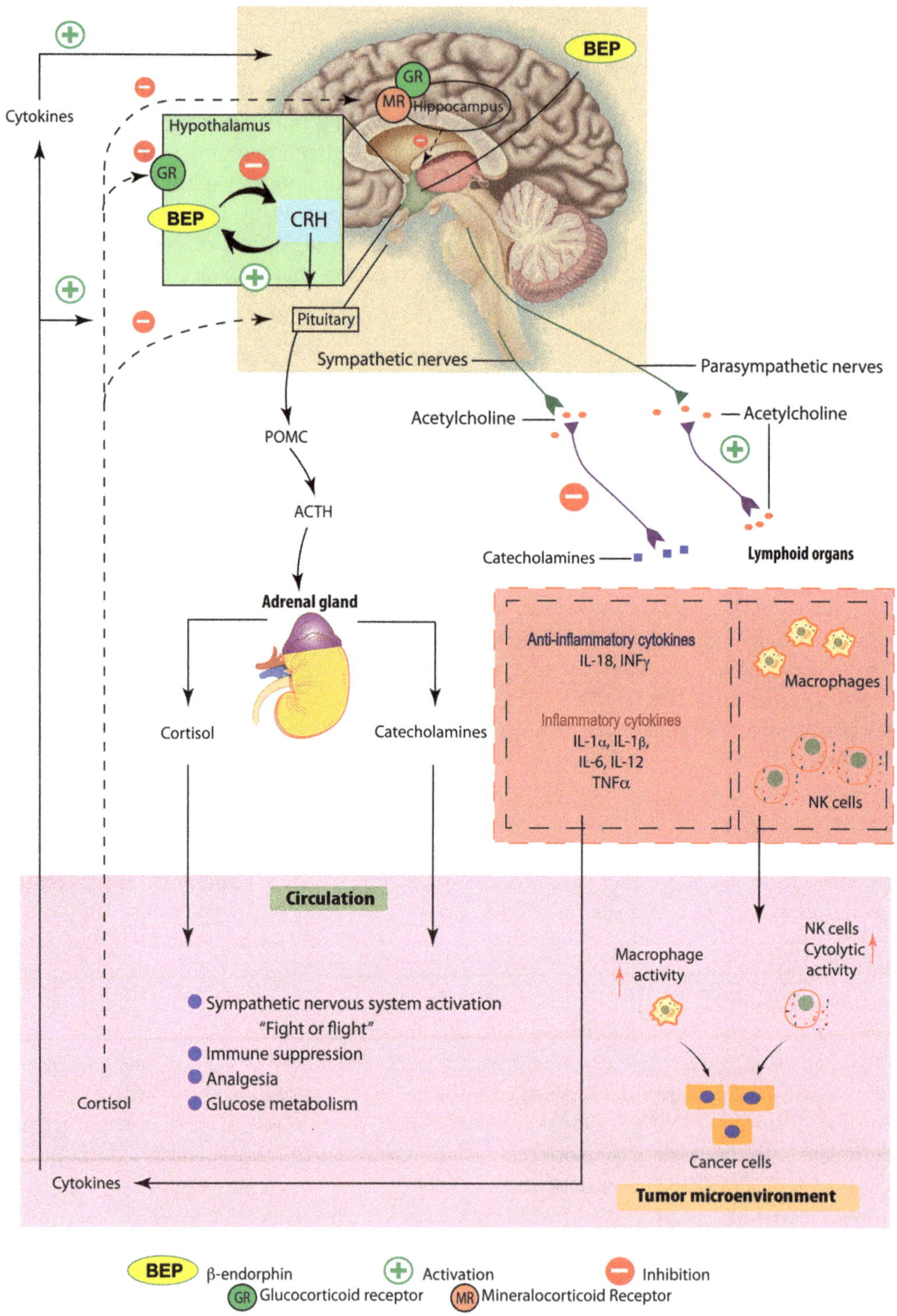

Figure 10.1 The bi-directional communication between the brain and the immune system, highlighting the influence of ß-endorphin (BEP). Stress signals reach the hypothalamus, causing a secretion of corticotrophin-releasing hormone (CRH) from the neurons of the hypothalamus. CRH induces the

1990). If incubated with human PMNC or NK-enriched cell populations, BEP enhances NK cell activity (Mathews, Froelich, Sibbitt, and Bankhurst, 1983). In animal models, chronic intracerebroventricular infusion of BEP enhances NK cell activity *in vivo*, and this effect is eliminated by the opioid antagonist, naloxone (Jonsdottir *et al.*, 1996). This result is due to the actions of central BEP, as shown by the finding that BEP in the same dose administered peripherally does not alter *in vivo* NK cell cytotoxicity.

β-endorphin is also known to play a role in cancer progression (see below). The BEP neuron in the hypothalamus influences neurotransmission of the ANS and activates immune cells. The effects of such modulation include the stimulation of the sympathetic nervous system, and the subsequent release of norepinephrine leading to the activation of innate immune cells including macrophages and NK cells of the lymphoid system, and anti-inflammatory cytokine levels in circulation. In a tumor microenvironment, these immune cell and cytokine changes suppress cancer growth and progression by increasing apoptotic death of tumor cells and reducing inflammation-mediated epithelial–mesenchymal transition that is a key step for carcinogenesis. Collectively, these outcomes create a hostile environment for tumor initiation, growth and progression.

β-endorphins as Treatment

Given the connections between the HPA/immune system and BEP, it stands to reason that BEP may have therapeutic applications. Indeed, previous studies from our group using the rat model have shown that after BEP neurons derived from neural stem cells have been transplanted into the PVN, animals show decreased lipopolysaccaride (LPS)-induced levels of hypothalamic CRH and plasma corticosterone, increased NK cell cytolytic function, and anti-inflammatory cytokine production in response to an immune challenge, and suppressed carcinogen-induced prostate cancer and breast cancer development (Boyadjieva *et al.*, 2009; Sarkar *et al.*, 2008). Importantly, the exogenous BEP cells remained at the site of transplantation. While it has been shown that BEP neuronal terminals innervate the PVN, BEP cell bodies do not naturally occur there. The endurance of the implanted cells has positive implications for potential therapeutic options. Another exciting result from our group has demonstrated that supplementation of BEP neurons, through the above-mentioned transplants, prevents mammary tumor growth, progression and metastasis. Of therapeutic importance is that when the BEP

Figure 10.1 (*continued*) synthesis of proopiomelanocortin (POMC) and the secretion of adrenocorticotropic hormone (ACTH) from the pituitary, and then ACTH elicits secretion of cortisol from the adrenal gland. Cortisol crosses the blood–brain barrier and activates specific receptors in the hippocampus and other regions, leading to regulation by negative inhibition. The brain modulates immune functions via the hypothalamic–pituitary–adrenal (HPA) axis and sympathetic neurons, and the immune-cell-derived cytokines affect neuroendocrine function via the CNS and peripheral organs. In the hypothalamus, the interaction of CRH and BEP involves negative inhibition; CRH increases the secretion of BEP, while BEP inhibits the secretion of CRH. Specific to cancer, BEP suppresses sympathetic nervous system control but activates the parasympathetic nervous system control of lymphoid organs, activating innate immune cells (macrophages and NK cells) and increasing anti-inflammatory cytokine levels in circulation. BEP neuronal cells in the hypothalamus control the neoplastic growth and progression of tumor cells likely by modulating one or more of the factors indicated. (Sarkar, Murugan, Zhang, and Boyadjieva, 2012).

transplants were given at the early stage of tumor development, many tumors were destroyed and the surviving tumors lost their ability to progress to high-grade cancer, due to the BEP cells' suppressive effects on inflammation-induced epithelial-mesenchymal transition regulators (Sarkar *et al.*, 2011).

Stress Effects on Health

Stress is catabolic, and GCs by their very nature break down tissue to produce energy. As discussed above, stress inhibits the immune system, but also depletes hormones and increases blood pressure. Therefore, stress exacerbates many diseases, from the common cold to HIV to cardiovascular disease (McEwen and Gianaros, 2010; Cohen, Janicki-Deverts, and Miller, 2007). However, stress and excess GCs are not believed to cause disease; rather they "leave the door open" for the disease to gain a foothold.

Briefly, the sum of the actions of excess GCs includes: increasing blood glucose concentrations via actions in the liver, and inhibiting glucose uptake and utilization in peripheral tissues such as muscles; deposition of adipose tissue is stimulated. Glucocorticoids cause catabolic changes in muscle, skin, and connective tissue, and also inhibit epidermal cell division and DNA synthesis, as well as reducing collagen synthesis and production (Stewart,2003). Excess GCs cause muscle atrophy, but not necrosis, and reduce muscle protein synthesis. Osteoblast function is impaired by excess GCs, leading to reduced bone density, in addition to GCs causing a negative calcium balance by inhibiting calcium absorption and increasing renal calcium excretion (Stewart, 2003). The anti-inflammatory actions of GCs are vital to maintain allostasis; however, an imbalance in GCs can lead to detrimental outcomes.

Studies have also shown that stress may have effects on carcinogenesis indirectly, through poor destruction or elimination of abnormal cells by reduced natural killer (NK) cell activity. Decreased NK cell activity is also associated with growth and progression of a variety of cancers in animals and humans, because NK cells appear to represent a first line of defense against the metastatic spread of tumor cells. Stress is associated with altered inflammatory and anti-inflammatory cytokine ratio in systemic circulation. It increases expression of IL-1β and TNF-α, and reduced expression of IL-2 and IFN-γ. Sustained elevation of TNF-α is known to inhibit the activity of protein tyrosine phosphatase (PTPase), causing reduced production of MHC class I antigen of the cell surface and leading to malignant cells escaping immune surveillance. Although there are many specific details yet to be delineated, it is becoming increasingly clear that stressful life events can impact health by modulating the nervous, endocrine and immune systems of body (Sarkar, Murugan, Zhang, and Boyadjieva, 2012).

References

Aisa, B., Tordera, R., Lasheras, B., del Rio, J., and Ramirez, M.J. (2007). Cognitive impairment associated to HPA axis hyperactivity after maternal separation in rats. *Psychoneuroendocrinology*, 32 (3), 256–266. doi: 10.1016/j.psyneuen.2006.12.013.

Akil, H., Watson, S.J., Young, E., Lewis, M.E., Khachaturian, H., and Walker, J.M. (1984). Endogenous opioids: biology and function. *Annual Review of Neuroscience*, 7, 223–255. doi: 10.1146/annurev.ne.07.030184.001255.

Appel, N.M. and Van Loon, G.R. (1986). beta-Endorphin-induced stimulation of central sympathetic outflow: inhibitory modulation by central noradrenergic neurons. *The Journal of Pharmacology and Experimental Therapeutics*, 237 (3), 695–701.

Armitage, J.A., Taylor, P.D. and Poston, L. (2005). Experimental models of developmental programming: consequences of exposure to an energy rich diet during development. *The Journal of Physiology*, 565 (Pt 1), 3–8. doi: 10.1113/jphysiol.2004.079756.

Bellinger, D.L., Ackerman, K.D., Felten, S.Y., and Felten, D.L. (1992). A longitudinal study of age-related loss of noradrenergic nerves and lymphoid cells in the rat spleen. *Experimental Neurology*, 116 (3), 295–311.

Berk, L.E. (2003). *Child Development.* 6th ed. Boston, MA: Allyn and Bacon.

Bernstein, H.G., Krell, D., Emrich, H.M., Baumann, B., Danos, P., Diekmann, S., and Bogerts, B. (2002). Fewer beta-endorphin expressing arcuate nucleus neurons and reduced beta-endorphinergic innervation of paraventricular neurons in schizophrenics and patients with depression. *Cellular and Molecular Biology*, 48 Online Pub:OL259-65.

Bertram, C.E., and Hanson, M.A. (2002). Prenatal programming of postnatal endocrine responses by glucocorticoids. *Reproduction*, 124 (4), 459–467.

Besedovsky, H.O., and del Rey, A. (1996). Immune–neuro–endocrine interactions: facts and hypotheses. *Endocrine Reviews*, 17 (1), 64–102.

Boyadjieva, N., Advis, J.P., and Sarkar, D.K. (2006). Role of beta-endorphin, corticotropin-releasing hormone, and autonomic nervous system in mediation of the effect of chronic ethanol on natural killer cell cytolytic activity. *Alcoholism, Clinical and Experimental Research*, 30 (10), 1761–1767. doi: 10.1111/j.1530-0277.2006.00209.x.

Boyadjieva, N.I., Ortiguela, M., Arjona, A., Cheng, X., and Sarkar, D.K. (2009). Beta-endorphin neuronal cell transplant reduces corticotropin releasing hormone hyperresponse to lipopolysaccharide and eliminates natural killer cell functional deficiencies in fetal alcohol exposed rats. *Alcoholism, Clinical and Experimental Research*, 33 (5), 931–937. doi: 10.1111/j.1530-0277.2009.00911.x.

Brouwers, E.P.M., van Baar, A.L., and Pop, V.J.M. (2001). Maternal anxiety during pregnancy and subsequent infant development. *Infant Behavior and Development*, 24, 95–106.

Buwalda, B., Geerdink, M., Vidal, J., and Koolhaas, J.M. (2011). Social behavior and social stress in adolescence: a focus on animal models. *Neuroscience and Biobehavioral Reviews*, 35 (8), 1713–1721. doi: 10.1016/j.neubiorev.2010.10.004.

Clancy, B., Darlington, R.B., and Finlay, B.L. (2001). Translating developmental time across mammalian species. *Neuroscience*, 105 (1), 7–17.

Coe, C.L., Kramer, M., Czeh, B., Gould, E., Reeves, A.J., Kirschbaum, C., and Fuchs, E. (2003). Prenatal stress diminishes neurogenesis in the dentate gyrus of juvenile rhesus monkeys. *Biological Psychiatry*, 54 (10), 1025–1034.

Cohen, S., Janicki-Deverts, D., and Miller, G.E. (2007). Psychological stress and disease. *Journal of the American Medical Association*, 298 (14), 1685–1687.

Dallman, M.F. (2000). Glucocorticoid negative feedback. In *Encyclopedia of Stress*, edited by G. Fink, 224–228. San Diego, CA: Academic Press.

Darko, D.F., Risch, S.C., Gillin, J.C., and Golshan, S. (1992). Association of beta-endorphin with specific clinical symptoms of depression. *The American Journal of Psychiatry*, 149 (9), 1162–1167.

Davis, E.P., Glynn, L.M., Schetter, C.D., Hobel, C., Chicz-Demet, A., and Sandman, C.A. (2007a). Prenatal exposure to maternal depression and cortisol influences infant temperament. *Journal of the American Academy of Child and Adolescent Psychiatry*, 46 (6), 737–746. doi: 10.1097/chi.0b013e318047b775.

Davis, E.P., Glynn, L.M., Schetter, C.D., Hobel, C., Chicz-Demet, A., and Sandman, C.A. (2007b). Prenatal exposure to maternal depression and cortisol influences infant temperament. *Journal of the American Academy of Child and Adolescent Psychiatry*, 46 (6), 737–746.

de Waal Malefyt, R., Haanen, J., Spits, H., Roncarolo, M.G., te Velde, A., Figdor, C. et al. (1991). Interleukin 10 (IL-10) and viral IL-10 strongly reduce antigen-specific human T cell proliferation by diminishing the antigen-presenting capacity of monocytes via downregulation of class II major histocompatibility complex expression. *Journal of Experimental Medicine*, 174 (4), 915–924.

Doremus-Fitzwater, T.L., Varlinskaya, E.I., and Spear, L.P. (2009). Social and non-social anxiety in adolescent and adult rats after repeated restraint. *Physiology and Behavior*, 97 (3–4), 484–494. doi: 10.1016/j.physbeh.2009.03.025.

Ebert, T., and Kotler, M. (2005). Prenatal exposure to influenza and the risk of subsequent development of schizophrenia. *Israel Medical Association Journal*, 7 (1), 35–38.

Elenkov, I.J., Webster, E.L., Torpy, D.J., and Chrousos, G.P. (1999). Stress, corticotropin-releasing hormone, glucocorticoids, and the immune/inflammatory response: acute and chronic effects. *Annals of the New York Academy of Sciences*, 876, 1–11; discussion 11–13.

Engel, S.M., Berkowitz, G.S., Wolff, M.S., and Yehuda, R. (2005). Psychological trauma associated with the World Trade Center attacks and its effect on pregnancy outcome. *Paediatric and Perinatal Epidemiology*, 19 (5), 334–341.

Famy, C., Streissguth, A.P., and Unis, A.S. (1998). Mental illness in adults with fetal alcohol syndrome or fetal alcohol effects. *American Journal of Psychiatry*, 155 (4), 552–554.

FitzGerald, M.J.T. (1996). *Neuroanatomy : Basic and Clinical.* 3rd ed. London: W.B. Saunders.

Fratta, W., Rossetti, Z.L., Poggioli, R., and Gessa, G.L. (1981). Reciprocal antagonism between ACTH1-24 and beta-endorphin in rats. *Neuroscience Letters*, 24 (1), 71–74.

Haas, H.S., and Schauenstein, K. (1997). Neuroimmunomodulation via limbic structures – the neuroanatomy of psychoimmunology. *Progress in Neurobiology*, 51 (2), 195–222.

Hales, C.N., and Barker, D.J. (2001). The thrifty phenotype hypothesis. *British Medical Bulletin*, 60, 5–20.

Hermann, G., Beck, F.M., and Sheridan, J.F. (1995). Stress-induced glucocorticoid response modulates mononuclear cell trafficking during an experimental influenza viral infection. *Journal of Neuroimmunology*, 56 (2), 179–186.

Jonsdottir, I. Johansson, H.C., Asea, A., Hellstrand, K., Thoren, P., and Hoffmann, P. (1996). Chronic intracerebroventricular administration of beta-endorphin augments natural killer cell cytotoxicity in rats. *Regulatory Peptides*, 62 (2–3), 113–118.

Kawano, H., and Masuko, S. (2000). Beta-endorphin-, adrenocorticotrophic hormone- and neuropeptide y-containing projection fibers from the arcuate hypothalamic nucleus make synaptic contacts on to nucleus preopticus medianus neurons projecting to the paraventricular hypothalamic nucleus in the rat. *Neuroscience*, 98 (3), 555–565.

Khachaturian, H., Lewis, M.E., Alessi, N.E., and Watson, S.J. (1985). Time of origin of opioid peptide-containing neurons in the rat hypothalamus. *Journal of Comparative Neurology*, 236 (4), 538–546. doi: 10.1002/cne.902360409.

Kosten, T.A., Lee, H.J., and Kim, J.J. (2006). Early life stress impairs fear conditioning in adult male and female rats. *Brain Research*, 1087 (1), 142–150. doi: 10.1016/j.brainres.2006.03.009.

Kovacs, K.J., Miklos, I.H.,and Bali, B. (2005). Psychological and physiological stressors. In T. Steckler, N.H. Kalin and J.M.H.M. Reul (Eds.), *Handbook of Stress and the Brain* (pp. 775–792). Amsterdam: Elsevier.

Kramer, D.A. (2005). Commentary: Gene–environment interplay in the context of genetics, epigenetics, and gene expression. *Journal of the American Academy of Child and Adolescent Psychiatry*, 44 (1), 19–27.

Lederman, S.A., Rauh, V., Weiss, L., Stein, J.L., Hoepner, L.A., Becker, M., and Perera, F.P. (2004). The effects of the World Trade Center event on birth outcomes among term deliveries at three lower Manhattan hospitals. *Environmental Health Perspectives*, 112 (17), 1772–1778.

Levine, S. (2005). Stress: An historical perspective. In T. Steckler, N.H. Kalin, and J.M.H.M. Reul (Eds.), *Handbook of Stress and the Brain* (pp. 3–23). Amsterdam: Elsevier.

Levine, S., and Ursin, H. (1991). What is stress? In G.F. Koob M.R. Brown, and C. Rivier (eds.), *Stress: Neurobiology and Neuroendocrinology* (pp. 3–21). New York: Marcel Decker, Inc.

Lissoni, P., Barni, S., Paolorossi, F., Crispino, S., Rovelli, F., Ferri, L. et al. (1987). Evidence for altered opioid activity in patients with cancer. *British Journal of Cancer*, 56 (6), 834–837.

Malaspina, D., Corcoran, C., Kleinhaus, K.R., Perrin, M.C., Fennig, S., Nahonet, D. et al. (2008). Acute maternal stress in pregnancy and schizophrenia in offspring: a cohort prospective study. *BMC Psychiatry*, 8, 71.

Mathews, P.M., Froelich, C.J., Sibbitt, W.L. Jr, and Bankhurst, A.D. (1983). Enhancement of natural cytotoxicity by beta-endorphin. *Journal of Immunology*, 130 (4), 1658–1662.

McCormick, C.M., and Mathews, I.Z. (2010). Adolescent development, hypothalamic–pituitary–adrenal function, and programming of adult learning and memory. *Progress in Neuropsychopharmacology and Biological Psychiatry*, 34 (5), 756–765. doi: 10.1016/j.pnpbp.2009.09.019.

McCormick, C.M., Mathews, I.Z., Thomas, C., and Waters, P. (2010). Investigations of HPA function and the enduring consequences of stressors in adolescence in animal models. *Brain and Cognition*, 72 (1), 73–85. doi: 10.1016/j.bandc.2009.06.003.

McEwen, B.S., and Gianaros, P.J. (2010). Central role of the brain in stress and adaptation: links to socioeconomic status, health, and disease. *Annals of the New York Academy of Sciences*, 1186, 190–222.

Morgan, E.L., McClurg, M.R., and Janda, J.A. (1990). Suppression of human B lymphocyte activation by beta-endorphin. *Journal of Neuroimmunology*, 28 (3), 209–217.

Munck, A., and Naray-Fejes-Toth, A. (1994). Glucocorticoids and stress: permissive and suppressive actions. *Annals of the New York Academy of Sciences*, 746, 115–30; discussion 131–133.

Oursler, M.J., Riggs, B.L., and Spelsberg, T.C. (1993). Glucocorticoid-induced activation of latent transforming growth factor-beta by normal human osteoblast-like cells. *Endocrinology*, 133 (5), 2187–2196.

Pervanidou, P., Kolaitis, G., Charitaki, S., Margeli, A., Ferentinos, S., Bakoula, C. et al. (2007). Elevated morning serum interleukin (IL)-6 or evening salivary cortisol concentrations predict posttraumatic stress disorder in children and adolescents six months after a motor vehicle accident. *Psychoneuroendocrinology*, 32 (8–10), 991–999. doi: 10.1016/j.psyneuen.2007.07.001.

Pickering, M., Cumiskey, D., and O'Connor, J.J. (2005). Actions of TNF-alpha on glutamatergic synaptic transmission in the central nervous system. *Experimental Physiology*, 90 (5), 663–670.

Plotsky, P.M. (1986). Opioid inhibition of immunoreactive corticotropin-releasing factor secretion into the hypophysial–portal circulation of rats. *Regulatory Peptides*, 16 (3–4), 235–242.

Reul, J.M., and de Kloet, E.R. (1985). Two receptor systems for corticosterone in rat brain: microdistribution and differential occupation. *Endocrinology*, 117 (6), 2505–2511.

Rhoades, R., and Pflanzer, R.G. (2003). *Human Physiology*. 4th ed. Pacific Grove, CA: Thomson Learning; Brooks/Cole.

Robson, A.C., Leckie, C.M., Seckl, J.R., and Holmes, M.C. (1998). 11 Beta-hydroxysteroid dehydrogenase type 2 in the postnatal and adult rat brain. *Brain Research, Molecular Brain Research*, 61 (1–2), 1–10.

Romeo, R.D., Lee, S.J., Chhua, N., McPherson, C.R., and McEwen, B.S. (2004a). Testosterone cannot activate an adult-like stress response in prepubertal male rats. *Neuroendocrinology*, 79 (3), 125–132. doi: 10.1159/000077270.

Romeo, R.D., Lee, S.J.,and McEwen, B.S. (2004b). Differential stress reactivity in intact and ovariectomized prepubertal and adult female rats. *Neuroendocrinology*, 80 (6), 387–393. doi: 10.1159/000084203.

Rutter, M. (2005). Environmentally mediated risks for psychopathology: research strategies and findings. *Journal of the American Academy of Child and Adolescent Psychiatry*, 44 (1), 3–18.

Sapolsky, R.M., Romero, L.M., and Munck, A.U. (2000). How do glucocorticoids influence stress responses? Integrating permissive, suppressive, stimulatory, and preparative actions. *Endocrine Reviews*, 21 (1), 55–89.

Sarkar, D.K., Boyadjieva, N.I., Chen, C.P., Ortiguela, M., Reuhl, K., Clement, E.M. et al. (2008). Cyclic adenosine monophosphate differentiated beta-endorphin neurons promote immune function and prevent prostate cancer growth. *Proceedings of the National Academy of Sciences of the USA*, 105 (26), 9105–9110. doi: 10.1073/pnas.0800289105.

Sarkar, D.K., Murugan, S., Zhang, C., and Boyadjieva, N. (2012). Regulation of Cancer Progression by beta-Endorphin Neuron. *Cancer Research*, 72 (4), 836–840. doi: 10.1158/0008-5472.CAN-11-3292.

Sarkar, D.K., Zhang, C., Murugan, S., Dokur, M., Boyadjieva, N.I., Ortiguela, M. et al. (2011). Transplantation of beta-endorphin neurons into the hypothalamus promotes immune function and restricts the growth and metastasis of mammary carcinoma. *Cancer Research*, 71 (19), 6282–6291. doi: 10.1158/0008-5472.CAN-11-1610.

Selye, H. (1998). A syndrome produced by diverse nocuous agents. (1936). *Journal of Neuropsychiatry and Clinical Neuroscience*, 10 (2), 230–231.

Sheridan, J.F., Dobbs, C., Jung, J., Chu, X., Konstantinos, A., Padgett, D., and Glaser, R. (1998). Stress-induced neuroendocrine modulation of viral pathogenesis and immunity. *Annals of the New York Academy of Sciences*, 840, 803–808.

Stewart, P.M. (2003). The Adrenal Cortex. In P.R. Larsen, H.M. Kronenberg, S. Melmed and K. S. Polonsky (Eds.), *Williams Textbook of Endocrinology* (pp. 491–546). London: W. B. Saunders.

Sun, K., Yang, K., and Challis, J.R. (1997). Differential expression of 11 beta-hydroxysteroid dehydrogenase types 1 and 2 in human placenta and fetal membranes. *Journal of Clinical Endocrinology and Metabolism*, 82 (1), 300–305.

Sun, Y., Strandberg-Larsen, K., Vestergaard, M., Christensen, J., Nybo Andersen, A.M. et al. (2009). Binge drinking during pregnancy and risk of seizures in childhood: a study based on the Danish National Birth Cohort. *American Journal of Epidemiology*, 169 (3), 313–322.

Sutanto, W., Rosenfeld, P., de Kloet, E.R., and Levine, S. (1996). Long-term effects of neonatal maternal deprivation and ACTH on hippocampal mineralocorticoid and glucocorticoid receptors. *Brain Research. Developmental Brain Research*, 92 (2), 156–163.

Taylor, A.N., Branch, B.J., Van Zuylen, J.E., and Redei, E. (1988). Maternal alcohol consumption and stress responsiveness in offspring. *Advances in Experimental Medicine and Biology*, 245, 311–317.

Tsigos, C., and Chrousos, G.P. (2002). Hypothalamic–pituitary–adrenal axis, neuroendocrine factors and stress. *Journal of Psychosomatic Research*, 53 (4), 865–871.

van den Bergh, P., Rozing, J., and Nagelkerken, L. (1993). Identification of two moieties of beta-endorphin with opposing effects on rat T-cell proliferation. *Immunology*, 79 (1), 18–23.

Weinberg, J., Sliwowska, J.H., Lan, N., and Hellemans, K.G. (2008). Prenatal alcohol exposure: foetal programming, the hypothalamic–pituitary–adrenal axis and sex differences in outcome. *Journal of Neuroendocrinology*, 20 (4), 470–488.

Weiner, H. (1991). Behavioral biology of stress and psychosomatic medicine. In M.R. Brown, G.F. Koob, and C. Rivier (Eds.), *Stress: Neurobiology and Neuroendocrinology* (pp. 23–51). New York: Marcel Decker, Inc.

Wiegers, G.J., Stec, I.E.M., Sterzer, P., and Reul, J.M.H.M. (2005). Glucorticoids and the immune response. In T Steckler, N.H. Kalin, and J.M.H.M. Reul (Eds.), *Handbook of Stress and the Brain. Part 2: Intergrative and Clinical Aspects* (pp. 175–191). Amsterdam: Elsevier.

Wilder, R.L. (1995). Neuroendocrine–immune system interactions and autoimmunity. *Annual Review of Immunology*, 13, 307–338.

Workel, J.O., Oitzl, M.S., Fluttert, M., Lesscher, H., Karssen, A., and de Kloet, E.R. (2001). Differential and age-dependent effects of maternal deprivation on the hypothalamic–pituitary–adrenal axis of brown norway rats from youth to senescence. *Journal of Neuroendocrinology*, 13 (7), 569–580.

Yehuda, R., Engel, S.M., Brand, S.R., Seckl, J., Marcus, S.M., and Berkowitz, G.S. (2005). Transgenerational effects of posttraumatic stress disorder in babies of mothers exposed to the World Trade Center attacks during pregnancy. *Journal of Clinical Endocrinology and Metabolism*, 90 (7), 4115–4118.

Zhang, D., Kishihara, K., Wang, B., Mizobe, K., Kubo, C., and Nomoto, K. (1998). Restraint stress-induced immunosuppression by inhibiting leukocyte migration and Th1 cytokine expression during the intraperitoneal infection of Listeria monocytogenes. *Journal of Neuroimmunology*, 92 (1–2), 139–151.

11

Assessing Neuroendocrine-Mediated Modulation of Immunity to Infection in Animals

Caveats and Methodological Issues

Jodi L. Yorty[1] and Robert H. Bonneau[2]

[1]*Department of Biology, Elizabethtown College, Elizabethtown, PA, USA*
[2]*Department of Microbiology and Immunology, The Pennsylvania State University College of Medicine, Milton S. Hershey Medical Center, Hershey, PA, USA*

Introduction to Stress–Neuroendocrine–Immune Interactions

The impact of psychological stress on human health has been recognized for quite some time. Support for the existence of this stress–health relationship was initially based primarily on anecdotal evidence; however, recent technological advances, and an increased knowledge of the structure and function of the various organ systems of the body at both the cellular and molecular level, have provided us with compelling scientific evidence that a relationship between stress and health does exist. This relationship is manifested in part by the function, or in some cases *dysfunction*, of the nervous, endocrine, and/or immune systems. The field of psychoneuroimmunology (PNI) seeks to understand the complex, bidirectional communication that exists between the nervous, endocrine, and immune systems. This chapter will describe the development and use of experimental animal models of stress and infection – animal models have been and continue to be invaluable in contributing to the field of PNI by delving deeper into the mechanisms that are involved in this intriguing, yet very complex, relationship.

Human Studies – A Broad Perspective

A variety of real-life stressors

Studies in both humans and animals have contributed significantly to our knowledge of the vast and complex levels of communication that exist among the nervous, endocrine, and immune systems. These human-based studies have shown that stressors of varying types, magnitude, and duration across the lifespan have the potential to modulate immune function (Glaser,

The Wiley-Blackwell Handbook of Psychoneuroimmunology, First Edition. Edited by Alexander W. Kusnecov and Hymie Anisman.

2005). This modulation affects one's susceptibility to pathogens and other diseases that are immunologically resisted. A variety of stressful situations have been studied in humans: the taking of academic examinations, feeling grief, being afflicted with a chronic illness, and serving as a caregiver for a relative with Alzheimer's disease, to name a few. These and other stressors have provided the framework for additional studies designed to decipher the impact of stress on immune function.

Stress-mediated modulation of immune function

The immune system plays an important role in determining the ability to ward off a variety of pathogens to which an individual has been exposed. In the absence of medical intervention (e.g., antibiotics), a highly functioning immune system is essential for the effective and timely resolution of an infection. However, the ability of some stressors to suppress one or more of the many components of a pathogen-specific immune response may increase one's susceptibility to acquiring an infection, and the subsequent morbidity and mortality that is associated with some infections. Although extremely limited in number and conducted under very carefully controlled conditions, there have been studies in which individuals exhibiting positive/negative emotional style, or experiencing psychological stress, were assessed for their resistance to illness after experimental exposure to rhinovirus (one of the causative agents of the common cold) and influenza A virus (Cohen *et al.*, 2006; Cohen, Tyrrell, and Smith, 1991). More typical are those studies in which the immune response is determined following vaccination.

The design and utilization of vaccines to confer protection from diseases caused by pathogens is one of the most important medical advances of the twentieth century. While vaccines against the human immunodeficiency virus (HIV), herpes simplex virus (HSV), and parasites belonging to the genus *Plasmodium* (the causative agent of malaria) have remained elusive, illnesses caused by a variety of other bacterial, viral, and fungal pathogens are now prevented through vaccination. One generally *assumes* that vaccination results in a robust immune response and confers protection from the disease that the pathogen elicits. However, individuals experiencing psychological stress or anxiety at or near the time of vaccination are suppressed in their ability to generate vaccine-induced immunity (e.g. antibody production) to pathogens such as hepatitis B virus and influenza virus (Glaser *et al.*, 1992; Yang and Glaser, 2002). Interestingly, the ability to cope with the stressor, and the availability of social support during the time of the stressful experience, can counter this immunosuppressive effect.

Limitations of human studies

Studying the human immune system in the context of real-life stressors and clinically relevant pathogens provides us with data that are germane to our understanding of the relationship among stress, neuroendocrine function, immunity, and human health. Despite the applicability of such studies to the human condition, there are some potentially significant limitations to these studies. For example, it is difficult to control many of the variables that alone have the potential to influence the function of the nervous, endocrine, and immune systems. Some of these variables are behavioral in nature (diet, alcohol and drug use and abuse, smoking, and sleep) while others are medical conditions (heart disease, diabetes, obesity, pregnancy, and chronic infection). Even in those studies in which behavioral and medical variables are well controlled, there is still the likelihood for significant genetic (including epigenetic) variability among individuals within a given study. Additionally, analysis of immune function in humans is typically limited to those cells and molecules that are located in the peripheral blood, and are thus readily accessible for collection and analysis. However, many of the major steps in the development of an immune response to a pathogen occur primarily within the spleen and the lymph nodes. Lastly, although there is a particular interest in determining the impact of stress and its associated neuroendocrine activity on the kinetics and magnitude of the immune response to clinically relevant pathogens, ethical reasons preclude their study in humans. Combined, these limitations may compromise one's ability to correctly interpret the results that are obtained, fail to take into account components of immune function that are critical for the resolution of a specific infection, and/or not allow for the study of those pathogens which are responsible for a significant level of morbidity and mortality in humans.

Animal Studies – A Broad Perspective

Strengths of animal studies

Despite some of their inherent limitations, human-based studies using a variety of real-life stressors have provided both the foundation and impetus for determining the cellular and molecular mechanisms underlying stress–neuroendocrine–immune interactions. However, in order to delineate these mechanisms as well as to understand the broader aspects of the complex relationships that exist among the nervous, endocrine, and immune systems, a number of animal models of stress and immunity have been developed and used extensively. Table 11.1 compares some of the characteristics inherent in human and animal studies. As is described

Table 11.1 Benefits and Caveats to Consider in Evaluating Stress/Neuroendocrine-Mediated Modulation of Immunity to Infection in Humans and Animals

Human studies	*Animal studies*
• Individual differences in behaviors, medical conditions, and genetic composition increase intersubject experimental variability.	• Experimenter control over behavioral, environmental, and genetic variables decreases intersubject experimental variability.
• The study of relevant, "real-life" stressors allows for a direct association between the experimental results obtained and the human condition.	• The lack of a perfect "animal model" of human anatomy and physiology results in a less-than-perfect extrapolation of experimental results to the human condition.
• Restricted access to immune cells and tissues limit the extent of immune function analysis.	• Widespread access to immune cells and tissues allows for a comprehensive analysis of immune function throughout the organism.
• Ethical concerns limit the use of many clinically relevant experimental pathogens.	• The ability to use a wide variety of experimental pathogens allows for a broad assessment of immune–pathogen relationships; however, the dose and route of pathogen administration may not mimic precisely the human condition.

below, one key advantage of using animal models is decreased experimental variability. The use of animal models also allows for a more comprehensive analysis of the immune response to those pathogens which cause significant morbidity and mortality in humans. With both advances in technology and our increasing knowledge of organ systems, animal models have become increasingly more complex. This complexity has been beneficial by providing an excellent opportunity to conduct a more in-depth analysis of the intricate degree of inter-organ system communication and the impact of this communication on human health.

Decreased experimental variability

The availability of animal models takes advantage of test subjects who, as compared to their human counterparts, exhibit less variability between one another from environmental, behavioral, and genetic perspectives. For example, from an environmental perspective, researchers are able to control the temperature, humidity, and lighting in the animal housing area. They can also regulate the type, nutritional content, and amount of food that each animal is provided. Although these factors may appear to be relatively innocuous, each has the *potential* to affect neuroendocrine activity and, in turn, immune function. Many animal studies, particularly those in which mice and rats are used, take advantage of the widespread availability of genetically inbred strains. These inbred strains are useful in that they eliminate the variability that can be caused by the large number of genetic polymorphisms that exist among animals of the same species. In addition, there are other highly specialized strains (e.g., knockout mice) in which certain genes that are associated with a particular neuroendocrine and/or immune phenotype have been manipulated at the molecular level so that they have been deleted (knocked out) or engineered such that they are able to be turned on or off at will. In many instances, these specialized strains provide a direct approach for deciphering the cellular and molecular components that are critical in mediating the interactions between stress, neuroendocrine activity, and immune function.

Increased opportunity to assess immune function

In research using animals, unlike human studies, the effect of stress on immune function can be assessed at sites within the body that extend beyond the peripheral blood, thus providing a much more comprehensive analysis of the neuroendocrine–immune relationship. It is in the secondary lymphoid tissues (i.e., spleen and lymph nodes) where the relatively few T- and B-lymphocytes – cells that have been programmed in the thymus and bone marrow, respectively, to recognize and respond to a particular antigen – undergo activation. Determining the extent of this activation often requires that the spleen and lymph nodes be removed in order to quantify the pathogen-specific lymphocytes. An additional benefit of animal studies is that the magnitude of the pathogen-specific immune response can be assessed in the tissue(s) where the pathogen resides, replicates, and causes pathology. For example, the immune response to a respiratory infection, such as influenza virus, can be studied by analyzing the number and function of influenza-virus specific lymphocytes and antibody levels in the lungs (Sheridan, Stark, Avitsur, and Padgett, 2000). With the exception of performing tissue biopsies, studies of the immune response within a particular tissue are extremely limited in humans.

Choice of experimental pathogen

Humans have the potential to be afflicted with a number of bacterial, viral, fungal, and parasitic pathogens. However, as noted above, the ability to deliberately infect individuals for experimental purposes has significant limitations. Thus, the use of animal models of infection and immune responsiveness have served the research community well by allowing us to decipher the impact of stress on those pathogens that cannot be administered experimentally to humans. Although the design of such models can be difficult, they do allow us to gain a better understanding of stress–immune relationships and to extrapolate the findings using these models to the human condition. Some of the difficulties and other important issues to consider in developing and using such animal models are outlined below.

Developing Animal Models of Stress

Introduction

The use of animal models has served the scientific community well in demonstrating the impact of stress on the immune response to pathogens and in deciphering the role that the nervous and endocrine systems play in this stress–immune interaction. Such animal models often contain a number of individual components, each of which must be modeled appropriately. If even one of these components is significantly flawed, the usefulness of the model as a basis for conclusions drawn from the collected data may be compromised. However, it should be emphasized that there are no *perfect* models – that is why they are referred to as models. This section describes factors that should be considered when developing animal-based studies that are designed to determine the impact of experimental stressors on immune function (Figure 11.1).

Choosing the species

The vast majority of animal-based studies in the field of PNI have used mice and rats. Rodents such as these have historically been the animal of choice given their small size, ease of handling, and anatomical and physiological similarities to humans – particularly that of the neuroendocrine and immune systems. The use of mice and rats is also a function of the wide array of methods, including commercially-available kits, for measuring the various stress-associated hormones. Mice are particularly valuable given the plethora of species-specific reagents (e.g. monoclonal antibodies) that are available for not only quantifying the various types of immune cells but also determining their function both *in vivo* and *in vitro*.

Other species of animals such as non-human primates (e.g. mandrills, macaques, rhesus monkeys, squirrel monkeys), rabbits, guinea pigs, cows, poultry, and pigs have also been used as model organisms in stress-related studies, but in far smaller numbers than rodents. As with humans, there are significant limitations in being able to assess, qualitatively and quantitatively, a broad-range of immune functions, particularly those functions that are responses to an experimentally administered pathogen. These limitations are directly related to the need not to remove lymphoid and/or any other tissues in which an immune response may be occurring so as not to cause harm to the animal. Even if these tissues were to be used, the lack of immunological reagents for measuring immune cell number and function in some of these species is of concern. Lastly, compared to humans, some species have vastly different levels of

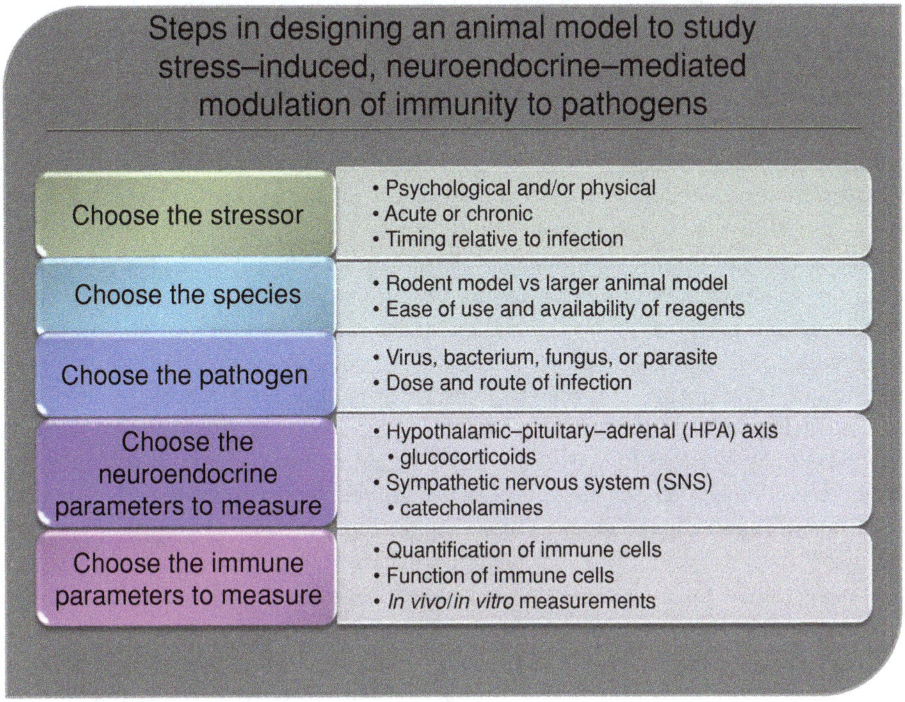

Figure 11.1 Steps in designing an animal model to study stress-induced, neuroendocrine-mediated modulation of immunity to pathogens.

susceptibility and immune responses to pathogens and thus would not serve as valid models for studying the impact of stress on the immune response.

Types of experimental stressors

Stress is a natural and pervasive component of the day-to-day life experiences of nearly all animals. As defined by Walter Cannon in the early twentieth century, stress is any stimulus which alters the homeostasis of an organism (Cannon, 1935). Whereas Cannon's definition of stress is centered on the *alteration* that occurs upon experiencing a stressor, Hans Selye's classic definition of stress is focused on the non-specific *response* of the body to the stressor (Selye, 1936). This ability to respond to a stressor, regardless of its type, is critical for the wellbeing, and in some cases survival, of the animal.

There are a variety of experimental methods that can be used to elicit a stress response in animals. Although the focus of this chapter is on the use of psychological stress, it should be noted that some stressors have both a psychological and a physical component. Some commonly used psychological/physical combination stressors include confinement, restraint, electric footshock, forced treadmill running, sleep deprivation, and cold-water swim. In those studies in which the physical component is relatively minor (e.g. confinement) the alterations are likely to be primarily a function of hypothalamic–pituitary–adrenal (HPA) axis and sympathetic nervous system (SNS) activation alone, thereby simplifying the interpretation of the data collected. The main end-products of these two pathways, both of which modulate the immune response, are the glucocorticoids (cortisol in humans, corticosterone in rodents) and catecholamines (epinephrine and norepinephrine), respectively. However, when the stressor includes a physical component (e.g., forced treadmill running), hormones such as growth hormone and endorphins may also be produced and, in turn, modulate aspects of the immune response. The potential importance of the physical component of these stressors is a function of their intensity and duration, and may need to be taken into account when determining exactly which factors are responsible for mediating stress-induced alterations in immune function.

Experimental stressors are typically viewed as events which elicit a stress response by some type of deliberate experimental manipulation. However, it is important to recognize that even the routine handling of an animal that occurs as a function of day-to-day animal husbandry activities may also be perceived by the animal as a stressor (Misslin, Herzog, Koch, and Ropartz, 1982). Examples of such stressors include the daily examination of animals for illnesses and/or any other unusual conditions, and the changing of animals' cages. In the later case, an event as simple as placing rodents into a freshly washed cage containing clean bedding material may be perceived initially by these animals as a stressful situation. Other unintended but potentially significant stressors may include disruption of an animal's environment by the repeated and frequent entry of individuals into the room as well as the performing of procedures on *other animals* within the same room. Experimentally necessary procedures such as weighing an animal or observing it for illness-induced behavioral changes may be viewed as a stressor by the animal. However, the levels of stress that are associated with these latter two examples may be relatively minor as compared to some of the other experimental stressors mentioned above. However, depending on the duration and frequency of these procedures, the cumulative effects may be significant enough to have an effect on neuroendocrine activity and, subsequently, on immune function.

Duration/frequency of stress – acute versus chronic

Regardless of the method that is used to elicit a stress response, stressors are generally defined as being either acute or chronic. The criteria that are used to define each of these stressors are somewhat imprecise: they take into account not only the duration of the stressor (e.g. minutes to hours per day) and the frequency with which the stressor is administered (e.g., once, a few times, many times), but also the combination of this duration and frequency. As can probably be imagined, there are many such combinations. For example, an acute stressor may be viewed as one that is applied for a short duration only once, for a short duration on a number of successive days, or for a long duration either once or on just a few successive days. Although the first scenario clearly represents an acute stressor, the latter two scenarios could be viewed by some as chronic stressors, depending on how a chronic stressor is defined. A chronic stressor might be defined as one that is applied for a long duration on a number of successive days. However, whether or not a stressor of a long duration administered either once or on just a few successive days or for a short duration on a number of successive days is to be considered chronic is subject to debate.

Unique features of a chronic stressor

The desire to use a chronic stress model, regardless of the type, duration, and frequency of the stressor being applied, must be carefully evaluated before being used in an experimental study. This evaluation is necessary since it is possible for an animal to acclimate to some events (e.g. confinement) which it perceives as being stressful when applied in the short term, but which, when applied over the long term (for a long duration and/or repeatedly), the animal may become acclimated to (Melia *et al.*, 1994). Thus, activation of the HPA axis and/or the SNS may not occur. If the use of a chronic stressor is desired, it may be necessary to design the experimental studies so that the type of stressor is periodically varied so as to prevent the animal acclimating to the stressor. The use of a chronic stress model may also result in the HPA axis lacking sensitivity to feedback mechanisms that regulate its functioning. In humans, this acclimatization to potentially chronically stressful conditions and regulation of HPA axis activity may function as a defense mechanism, allowing individuals who are experiencing a chronic stressor (e.g. long-term care of a chronically ill relative) to retain a level of immune function that is sufficient to ward off those pathogens that might inflict disease under immunosuppressive conditions.

Using Animal Models to Study Stress-Induced Neuroendocrine-Activation

Introduction

Studies in the field of PNI are difficult, as they involve not only a number of complex organ systems (e.g. nervous, endocrine, immune) and the integration of these organ systems, but also a variety of experimenter-chosen variables. Such variables must be carefully selected, particularly if one wants to extrapolate the results from animal-based studies to the human condition. However, it is equally important to select assay methods that will allow for an accurate assessment of the function of each of these systems. As described in this section, the selection of appropriate methods is key to achieving a better understanding of the role of the nervous and endocrine systems in stress-mediated modulation of resistance to pathogens.

Assessing neuroendocrine involvement in stress–immune interactions

A variety of experimental approaches have been used to identify which neuroendocrine components elicited in response to a particular stressor modulate a component of an immune response and alter susceptibility to a specific pathogen. Most of these approaches center around the glucocorticoids and catecholamines produced by the HPA axis and SNS, respectively. Immune cells express an intracellular glucocorticoid receptor and, to varying degrees, the adrenergic receptors that bind the catecholamines. Thus, stress-induced activation of both the HPA axis and SNS has the potential to alter the immune response in animals.

One of the most common methods used to determine the role of corticosterone (CORT) is to subject animals to bilateral adrenalectomy. This surgical procedure eliminates an animal's ability to produce CORT under both stress and non-stress conditions. Although adrenalectomy is an effective method of eliminating the production of adrenal cortex-derived CORT, it is important to note that it also results in the loss of the adrenal medulla-derived catecholamines (epinephrine and norepinephrine). These catecholamines are released into the bloodstream where they bind to adrenergic receptors on cells, including cells of the immune system. The effect of these blood-derived catecholamines on immune cells is essentially the same as those catecholamines that come in contact with immune cells via direct sympathetic nerve fiber innervation in the secondary lymphoid tissues. Therefore, although adrenalectomized mice are typically used to determine the impact of stress-induced elevations in CORT on immune function, a limitation of using these mice is the inability to attribute effects on immune function to *only* CORT. An alternative, yet less often used method for reducing CORT levels is though the use of the CORT synthesis inhibitor metyrapone. Unlike adrenalectomy, metyrapone does not directly affect catecholamine production.

It should be noted that the ability to interpret the data obtained from adrenalectomized and metyrapone-treated animals may be somewhat complicated in that in response to the lowered serum levels of CORT there may be a compensatory increase in release of corticotropin-releasing hormone (CRH) from the hypothalamus and adrenocorticotropic hormone (ACTH) from the pituitary. Not only are both of these hormones involved in CORT production but, they are also alone able to modulate various aspects of immune function. Therefore, alternations in immune function that may seem logical to associate with decreases in CORT may be due, in part, to increases in CRH and/or ACTH. One way to prevent these compensatory CRH and ACTH increases in adrenalectomized and metyrapone-treated animals is to maintain baseline, non-stress levels of CORT through the use of implantable, time-release, low-dose CORT-containing pellets. Alternatively, baseline levels of CORT can be maintained by providing CORT in the drinking water. However, although these two methods are able to prevent gross dysregulation of the HPA axis, neither reproduces the changes in CRH, ACTH, and CORT associated with circadian rhythm.

As an alternative to using adrenalectomy or CORT synthesis inhibitors to determine the contribution of CORT to stress-induced modulation of immune function, one can also use glucocorticoid receptor antagonists. Two commonly used glucocorticoid receptor antagonists are RU486 (mifepristone), a type II glucocorticoid receptor-specific antagonist, and spironolactone, a type I glucocorticoid receptor-specific antagonist. Because these substances are administered systemically and do not discriminate between type I and type II receptors on immune cells and other cells within the body, their effects can be widespread.

As is noted above, sympathetic nerve fibers innervate the thymus, lymph nodes, and spleen. It is in these lymphoid tissues that nerve fiber termini come in close contact with immune cells, thus releasing catecholamines in the proximity of these cells. However, these nerve fibers can be effectively ablated via systemic administration of 6-hydroxydopamine (6-OHDA; 2,4,5-trihydroxyphenethylamine). Therefore, by subjecting 6-OHDA-treated animals to stress, it is possible to determine the role that direct sympathetic innervation plays in stress-induced immunomodulation. It has been shown in mice that the levels of CORT rise significantly when 6-OHDA is first administered (Leo, Callahan, and Bonneau, 1998). However, these elevated levels of CORT return to baseline in a few days.

Using Animal Models to Study Stress-Induced, Neuroendocrine-Mediated Modulation of the Immune Response to Infections

Introduction

The numerous cells and proteins that comprise the immune system generally protect humans and other animals from infection by a wide variety of viruses, bacteria, fungi, and parasites. For many of these pathogens, there already exist one or more animal models. The nature of the immune response that is elicited in response to infection depends on a variety of factors including the category to which the pathogen belongs, the specific pathogen within that category, the site of infection, and the age of the infected individual.

Both the innate and adaptive components of the immune response play an important role in overall defense against pathogens. Although relatively non-specific, cells of the innate immune system (e.g. macrophages, neutrophils, dendritic cells) recognize conserved pathogen-associated molecular patterns (PAMPs) via pattern recognition receptors (PRRs). Following this recognition, a series of complex intracellular biochemical events leads to activation of the innate immune cell. These activated cells begin producing cytokines, and often phagocytose the pathogen. Peptides (antigens) that are derived from the proteins which are made by the pathogen and, in some cases, are part of its structure, are then presented together with major histocompatibility complex (MHC) molecules on the surface of a subset of innate immune cells (macrophages and DCs) known as antigen-presenting cells (APC). The main function of these APCs is to present these peptide-MHC complexes to T-lymphocytes (T-cells), an important component of the adaptive immune system. The adaptive immune system is responsible for development of pathogen-specific immunity both at the time of initial infection (primary immune response) and upon subsequent encounter with the same or closely-related pathogen at a later date (secondary or memory immune response). In contrast to T-cells, B-lymphocytes (B-cells) are able to directly recognize pathogens through the B-cell receptor. However, B-cell activation and production of pathogen-specific antibody often requires help, in the form of cytokines, from activated T-cells, particularly $CD4^+$ T-helper cells.

It is important to emphasize that there are very few lymphocytes that are specific for any given pathogen prior to an individual being infected with the pathogen for the first time. Thus, in order to mount an effective defense against the pathogen, the number of pathogen-specific lymphocytes must increase substantially. This increase occurs when one or more lymphocytes are activated by their encounter with APC and undergo multiple rounds of cell division. In an ideal immune response, this series of events results in a sufficient number of cells to effectively eliminate the pathogen and/or to inhibit further development of infection. The impact of stress and its associated neuroendocrine-derived products on the immune response can be quantified simply by counting the number of lymphocytes that are generated within the secondary lymphoid tissues. However, thanks to technological advances such as those described below, and our detailed knowledge of the series of events that lead up to and are involved in lymphocyte activation and proliferation, we are also able to quantify the number of lymphocyte receptors and intracellular signaling molecules, and the synthesis and release of cytokines by lymphocytes and other cells of the immune system. These and other measures allow us to delve deeper into the cellular and molecular mechanisms that affected by stress.

Assessing immune function

The study of immune function generally relies upon measurement of the number of immune cells, the molecules that they produce, and/or the microbicidal activities that they perform (e.g. killing of virus-infected cells, phagocytosis of bacteria). Because relatively few pathogen-specific immune cells are present in secondary lymphoid organs and infected tissues, even after their expansion *in vivo*, most early studies relied on removing these immune cells and further expanding their numbers *in vitro* (often for several days) prior to assessing their function. It is fortunate that some of the effects of stress-induced, neuroendocrine-derived peptides

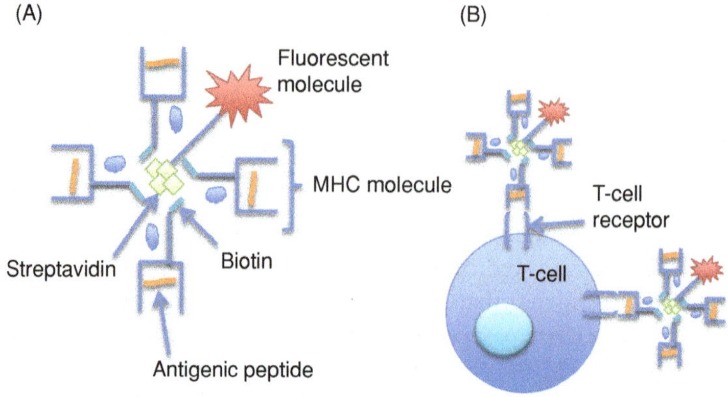

Figure 11.2 Tetramer technology quantifies antigen-specific T-cells. A) Basic diagram of a tetramer. B) Tetramer binding to an antigen-specific T-cell. T cells that bind to the tetramer are then quantified using flow cytometry.

and hormones on immune cell function are long-lived. Otherwise, one might incorrectly conclude that stress has no effect on immune function. However, it is still quite likely that the culture of those cells *in vitro*, outside of the secondary lymphoid organs, infected tissues, and neuroendocrine system, mask or alter the effects of stress and thus result in less-than-accurate conclusions regarding the relationship between stress and immune function. During the past decade, newer and more exquisitely sensitive technologies have been developed which allow for the assessment of immune cell numbers and function directly ex vivo with little to no incubation time required prior to analysis. Examples of these newer methods, each of which rely on the use of fluorescent flow cytometry (commonly referred to as flow cytometry), include tetramer analysis, intracellular cytokine staining, and a degranulation assay.

A tetramer is a cluster of four biotinylated MHC molecules linked together by stretpavidin and attached to a molecule which fluoresces when exposed to a specific wavelength of light. Each of these molecules is also bound to a specific, pathogen-derived peptide that elicits a T-cell immune response (Figure 11.2A). These tetramers are briefly incubated *in vitro* with lymphocytes, some of which are expected to be T-cells that have specificity for, and thus bind to, the MHC-peptide complex (Figure 11.2B). These T-cell–tetramer complexes are quantified by virtue of the fluorescent molecule that is coupled to the tetramer. Thus, tetramer analysis is a powerful technique that has revolutionized our ability to quantify both $CD4^+$ and $CD8^+$ pathogen-specific T-cell responses (Appay and Rowland-Jones, 2002).

Not only is it important to quantify the number of pathogen-specific cells, but it is also important to assess their function. One critical function of immune cells is their production of cytokines. The quantification of cytokine-producing cells can be achieved through intracellular cytokine staining (ICS). As with tetramer analysis, ICS uses a fluorescing molecule. However, unlike tetramer analysis, this fluorescing molecule is attached to a monoclonal antibody that binds with high affinity to a specific cytokine. By permeabilizing the immune cell membrane, these monoclonal antibodies are able to gain access to the cytoplasm and bind to cytokines within the cell. Thus, if an immune cell is producing the cytokine of interest, the cell fluoresces when examined by flow cytometry (Appay and Rowland-Jones, 2002).

In addition to producing cytokines, $CD8^+$ T-cells mediate their antipathogen defense mechanisms in a more direct fashion by destroying cells of the host that have been infected with a virus. The failure to destroy these cells can result in the production of significant quantities of progeny virus. The lytic activity of $CD8^+$ T-cells has typically been quantified by ^{51}Cr-release assay, whereby $CD8^+$ T-cells are incubated *in vitro* with target cells that have been infected with a virus and labeled with a radioisotope of chromium (^{51}Cr). The ability of these $CD8^+$ T-cells to recognize and lyse the target cells is directly proportional to the amount of ^{51}Cr that is released from the target cells (Brunner, Mauel, Cerottini, and Chapuis, 1968). The lysis of target cells by $CD8^+$ T-cells is mediated, in part, by the synthesis and release of cytotoxic molecules that are located within granules in the cells. The release of these granules has allowed for the development of yet another flow-cytometry-based assay known as a degranulation assay (Betts *et al.*, 2003). Unlike the ^{51}Cr-release assay, the degranulation assay does not require the use of radioactive reagents yet it still retains the ability to determine the number and functional capacity of virus-specific $CD8^+$ T-cells.

Although the above ex vivo methods represent a clear advantage over those methods that require an extended period of *in vitro* lymphocyte incubation, they still do not determine the number and function of these cells in a living animal. However, this deficit has been overcome by the recent development of sophisticated *in vivo* methods that allow for a more direct assessment of the effects of stress-induced activation of the HPA axis and SNS on the immune response to pathogens. These new methods include *in vivo* killing assays, *in vivo* ICS, and intravital microscopy. Together, the above methods have already and will continue to expand our knowledge of the relationship among stress, neuroendocrine activation, and immune-mediated protection against infectious diseases.

Assessing Immune Involvement in Stress–Immune–Pathogen Interactions

Infection as a modulator of immune function

If stress, as defined by Cannon, is truly any stimulus that alters the homeostasis of an organism, then the presence of an infection *alone* must be considered a stressor. Indeed, infections have been shown to activate the HPA axis resulting in increased levels of glucocorticoids (Perez, Bottasso, and Savino, 2009). This activation is thought to occur via the release of interleukin-1β (IL-1β) from activated immune cells and its binding to IL-1 receptor-expressing cells located throughout the brain. This HPA axis activation and subsequent release of glucocorticoids plays a truly homeostatic role by controlling the extent and duration of the inflammatory response to infection. Support for this role is provided by studies which show that a lack of glucocorticoids increases the damage resulting from a strong inflammatory reaction to infection (Tait, Butts, and Sternberg, 2008). Thus, when assessing the impact of stress on the immune response to a pathogen, one should also consider the role that the infection itself may have on neuroendocrine-mediated modulation of immunity.

Stress as a modulator of immune function

It has been clearly established that psychological stress induces activation of the HPA axis and SNS and thus increases the circulating levels of the glucocorticoids and catecholamines. Because cells of the immune system express glucocorticoid and adrenergic receptors, these cells are susceptible to modulation by glucocorticoids and catecholamines. These neuroendocrine-derived products typically function to suppress the immune response, thus increasing one's susceptibility to infection. A few examples of this stress–immune–infection relationship are provided below, along with a primer for the type of immune response that is effective in controlling the various types of infections that occur in animals.

Viral infections The elimination of viral infections requires cooperation between the innate and adaptive components of the immune system. Virus-infected cells release interferon-α and -β and may be recognized by natural killer (NK) cells — the cytotoxic cell of the innate immune system. Cooperation and communication between the innate and adaptive response is nicely coordinated by the release of inflammatory cytokines (e.g. IFN-γ, IL-12) from activated innate cells and the subsequent cytokine-aided activation and proliferation of virus-specific T- and B-cells. After several days of proliferation, the activated $CD8^+$ T-cells migrate to the site of infection where they destroy virus-infected cells and, as is noted above, eliminate the source of progeny virus. As another antiviral defense mechanism, activated $CD4^+$ T-cells provide the necessary cytokine-mediated help to B-cells to secrete virus-specific antibody which can neutralize the virus and lead to viral clearance.

As is briefly alluded to above, there are a variety of innate and adaptive immune components that play a role in the immune response to a virus infection. Stress-induced activation of the HPA axis and SNS and release of glucocorticoids and catecholamines have the potential to alter many of these components through their ability to modulate the transcription and translation of cytokines, the activation and subsequent proliferation of T- and B-cells, and the trafficking of immune cells to the site of infection. Indeed, it is well established that stress increases the susceptibility of humans and animals to viral infections through its ability to alter several aspects of the viral-specific immune response.

Many of the mechanisms by which stress alters the immune response to viral infection have been elucidated though the use of mouse models. For example, restraint stress has been shown to diminish the proliferation of immune cells in the lymph node(s) near the site of HSV infection (Bonneau, Sheridan, Feng, and R. Glaser, 1991). Stress also decreases the magnitude of the cytotoxic immune response by decreasing the number of NK cells and $CD8^+$ T-cells responding to both HSV and influenza virus infection (Bonneau, Sheridan, Feng, and R. Glaser, 1991; Dobbs Feng, Beck, and Sheridan, 1996). Often, such a decrease is the result of reduced production of inflammatory cytokines during the innate phase of the immune response. Restraint stress decreases the number of antibody-secreting B-cells responding to influenza virus infection and therefore diminishes the concentration of antibody in the lungs of infected mice. Restraint-stressed mice also exhibit delayed antibody isotype class switching (Feng *et al.*, 1991). Another interesting virus infection model uses Thelier's murine encephalomyelitis virus (TMEV), a natural pathogen of mice that causes demyelination (Welsh *et al.*, 2009). Because demyelination results in the destruction of the protective myelin that surrounds neurons, infection with TMEV serves as a model for the autoimmune disease multiple sclerosis. Similarly to both HSV and influenza virus infections, restraint stress of TMEV-infected mice suppresses aspects of both the innate and adaptive immune response. For example, decreased NK cell cytotoxicity, decreased production of the inflammatory cytokine IFN-γ, and reduced $CD4^+$ and $CD8^+$ T-cell responses to known TMEV-specific antigens have been observed in mice subjected to restraint stress (Welsh *et al.*, 2010). As would be expected, suppression of this antiviral immune response leads to increased viral replication in the brain and an increased extent of demyelination. Some of these negative effects of stress have been shown to involve both the HPA axis and SNS, as the use of both glucocorticoid-receptor and adrenergic-receptor antagonists have been shown to abrogate the stress-induced immune suppression. Overall, stress-induced effects on immune function result in a higher level of virus and, in turn, an increase in viral-associated pathogenesis in the host.

Bacterial infections As described earlier, phagocytic innate immune cells are critical for the initial immune recognition of bacteria through PAMPs such as lipopolysaccharide and lipoteichoic acids in the bacterial cell wall. Following this recognition and subsequent bacterial phagocytosis, phagocytic cells such as macrophages and neutrophils generate reactive oxygen species and nitric oxide, both of which are bactericidal and aid in clearing the infection. However, restraint-stressed mice infected with *Listeria monocytogenes* exhibit a decrease in the migration of these phagocytic cells to the site of infection and altered production of inflammatory cytokines and reactive oxygen species (Zhang *et al.*, 1998). Additionally, decreased bacterial antigen presentation by macrophages and B-cells also affects the ability of the adaptive immune response to clear infection in restraint-stressed mice. A similar effect of stress-induced neuroendocrine activation on production of TNF-α and nitric oxide has been shown in a mouse model of mycobacteria infection (Zwilling, Brown, and Pearl, 1992).

It should be noted that although most animal models of stress are typically immunosuppressive, there are some models that actually enhance the immune response to infection (Dhabhar, 2009). For example, a social disruption stressor has been shown to enhance cytokine production and the bactericidal activity of macrophages responding to *E. coli* infection (Bailey *et al.*, 2007). This enhancement occurs via a stress-induced increase in cell surface Toll-like receptor (TLR) expression on macrophages. These TLRs are a subset of receptors critical for recognizing PAMPS within the bacterial cell wall. Immune enhancement can also occur when the stressor causes a redistribution of immune cells such that the density of cells in compartments such as the skin is increased. Hence, an immune response that develops following wounding and/or a skin infection may be enhanced.

Fungal and parasitic infections Although perhaps not as common as viral and bacterial infections, infections with fungi and parasites are generally more difficult to treat once they are established and therefore rely on adequate immune function for clearance. Thus, the use of animal models to determine the impact of stress on the immune response to such infections has been invaluable. For example, the ability of macrophages to respond to and eliminate the fungus *Candida albicans* was studied in rats exposed to a varied stressor (Rodriguez-Galan *et al.*, 2003). In this model, rats were infected intraperitoneally with *C. albicans* and subjected to 5 minutes of cold-water swim on day 1, 2 hours of restraint on day 2, and 24 hours of food deprivation on day 3. Macrophages from these stressed rats exhibited decreased phagocytic and fungicidal activity and produced decreased amounts of nitric oxide and less TNF-α and IL-1β upon *in vitro* culture. As a result, stressed rats exhibited a higher fungal burden in multiple organs (Rodriguez-Galan *et al.*, 2010). The immune response to parasitic infection of animals is also affected by stress. For example, heat stress was shown to suppress the immune response to *Toxoplasma gondii* in mice as exhibited by lower levels of *T. gondii*-specific antibody and altered cytokine profiles as compared to non-stressed, infected mice (Nishiya *et al.*, 2005). As would be expected, these heat-stressed mice had higher levels of *T. gondii* in tissue samples and exhibited increased *T. gondii*-associated mortality.

The studies described above represent only a sampling of how the field of PNI has markedly advanced our understanding of how stress-induced activation of the HPA axis and SNS affects the immune response to infection in animals. The various animal models of stress used and types of infections and immune responses studied have clearly demonstrated that stress-induced suppression of the immune system can increase the susceptibility of animals to infectious disease.

The role of experimental variables in defining the nature of neuroendocrine–immune interactions

Animal models of stress and infection have served us well in defining the effects of stress-induced activation of the HPA axis and SNS and their associated neuroendocrine-derived products on the immune response to pathogens. As noted earlier, animal models have some clear advantages over human subject studies, particularly with respect to being able to better control some of the variables that have the potential to affect neuroendocrine-immune activity (Table 11.1). However, there are some variables that may initially appear to be so innocuous that they are not even recognized as being variables. For example, the type of cage (e.g., metal, plastic), number of animals per cage, and presence of environmental enrichment devices (e.g., plastic/paper tunnels and igloos for rats and mice; balls, bells, and chew toys for larger animals) can potentially affect neuroendocrine activity. Even the ability/inability of animals to socialize with other animals as well as with the humans who care for them are important factors that can influence their behavior and, in turn, the production of neuroendocrine-derived peptides and hormones. These and other relatively subtle experimental variables have the potential to affect the results of a study, and thus may have a major impact on the conclusions that are drawn. As a result, such conclusions may not be congruent with the results of other similar studies, thus leading to multiple conclusions, and possibly confusion, regarding the nature of neuroendocrine–immune interactions.

The ability of investigators to readily alter various components of an experimental stressor in animal models represents an important variable which can have a significant impact on determining the cellular and molecular mechanisms underlying neuroendocrine–immune interactions. Subtle differences in the type of stressor, the degree and extent to which it is applied, and when it is applied relative to infection can have a significant effect on the results obtained and the interpretation of these results. For example, restraint stress of mice infected with influenza virus has been shown to be immunosuppressive and increase the susceptibility of the mice to infection. In contrast, a social disruption stressor has been shown to increase the ability of DCs to present influenza virus antigen to T-cells, thus resulting in an enhanced virus-specific T-cell response (Powell *et al.*, 2011). An example of the importance of the timing of stress relative to infection is illustrated by an experiment in which social disruption was applied to mice either prior to or concurrently with lymphocytic choriomeningitis virus (LCMV) infection (Sommershof *et al.*, 2011). When applied prior to infection, a reduced LCMV-specific T-cell response was observed. However, when applied at the same time of infection, virus-specific T-cell responses were not altered. These examples illustrate that the type and time of stress application, relative to the time of infection, can differentially affect the immune response. This differential effect on immunity is a function of the relationship between the timing of stress-induced HPA axis and SNS activation and the number, type, and sequence of events that must occur to generate an immune response to infection.

The use of animals to study the impact of stress on the immune response to, and pathogenesis of, microorganisms has been a powerful resource in furthering our understanding of the relationship among stress, immune function, and resistance to infection in humans.

Unfortunately, the ability to directly extrapolate the findings from these animal studies to the human condition may be somewhat compromised by one or more unintentional flaws in the design of the experimental model. For example, in an effort to elicit a readily measurable immune response, the dose of infecting pathogen used in animals often far exceeds that with which a human would be infected under natural conditions. Even the route of infection used (e.g. intraperitoneal, intravenous, subcutaneous) may not be one that occurs naturally in humans but instead is chosen by an investigator to elicit an immune response in a readily accessible lymphoid tissue and/or cause an infection at a site where the degree of pathology can be easily quantified. The ability of stress to enhance or suppress an immune response may be a function of not only the dose of pathogen used but also the particular strain (virus) or subtype (bacteria) of pathogen used, as the kinetics and magnitude of infection among microorganisms of even the same species can vary tremendously. Although this latitude in experimental design is somewhat commonplace, it is important to realize that there are limitations which must be considered when interpreting the results from past studies and in designing future studies.

There are many variables that must be considered in the design and utilization of any experimental model. In the case of animal models associated with the field of PNI, this consideration increases in importance as a consequence of the complexity of the interactions between the nervous, endocrine, and immune systems. As is alluded to above, some of these variables must be considered when attempting to draw broad-based conclusions from the data obtained using these models and in applying these conclusions to the various species, including humans, that are subject to stress-induced modulation of immunity to pathogens.

Recent Developments and Future Directions

Introduction

The field of PNI has made tremendous progress in understanding the complex relationships that exist between the nervous, endocrine, and immune systems. With the rapid technological advances that are occurring in cellular and molecular biology, this field is well poised to embark upon exciting and innovative research studies using animal models. Although certainly not exhaustive, this section highlights some of the active areas of research that have built upon our current foundation of knowledge. Whereas some of these studies have delved deeper into the mechanisms by which stress-induced glucocorticoids and catecholamines affect immune function, other studies have sought ways in which to alleviate the negative effects of stress on the immune response to infection.

Cellular and molecular immune cell changes

As is described above, early experiments in PNI utilized surgical (e.g., adrenalectomy) and pharmacological approaches (e.g., receptor antagonists) to study the effects of the neuroendocrine system on immune function. Many of the broad questions addressing *which* immune cells are affected and, in general, *how* immune cells are affected by stress-induced HPA axis and SNS activation have been answered. Recent research has focused on the cellular and molecular mechanisms that are associated with these changes. Many of these mechanisms involve increases or decreases in the rate of gene transcription and subsequent mRNA translation and protein production. Thus, stress-induced neuroendocrine activation has the potential to significantly alter the level of cytokines, cell-surface receptors, and other proteins that play critical roles in an immune response. As noted above, a recent study showed that social disruption stress enhances macrophage killing of *E. coli*. At the cellular level, this enhancement was shown to be the result of significantly increased levels of TLR2 and TLR4 on macrophages, which resulted in enhanced recognition and elimination of the bacteria (Bailey *et al.*, 2007). Like macrophages, the function of DCs is also altered at the molecular level. For example, *in vitro* studies have demonstrated that exposure of DCs to CORT diminishes activation-induced expression of MHC molecules and other receptors required for activation of T-cells (Elftman, Norbury, Bonneau, and Truckenmiller, 2007). Thus, DCs isolated from mice infected with HSV and exposed to stress have a decreased ability to process and present HSV antigens and are less able to stimulate the proliferation of HSV-specific T-cells (Elftman *et al.*, 2010).

Stress-induced cellular and molecular changes, particularly at the level of gene transcription, are being elucidated through *in vitro* studies and subsequently the biological effects of these changes are being studied in animal models. The examples described above are representative of an active and ongoing area of research, and it is likely that comparable changes in gene expression will be identified in other immune cells. Having a detailed understanding of the cellular and molecular mechanisms by which stress alters immune cell function may allow for the development of strategies to prevent these stress-induced changes at the cellular and molecular level.

Cell-to-cell interactions

The development of a protective immune response requires extensive communication between various immune cells. For example, the type of cytokines produced by cells of the innate immune system dictate whether $CD8^+$ or $CD4^+$ T-cells are the predominant cell type involved in the adaptive immune response. Additionally, cytokines instruct B-cells to produce specific isotypes of antibody. Thus, even if stress-induced products of the HPA axis and SNS do not directly interact with the receptor within a given immune cell type, that cell type may *still* be affected indirectly if these products modulate the communication between immune cells.

One way to study these 'indirect effects' of stress is to simply prevent stress-induced glucocorticoids and catecholamines from interacting with a specific immune cell type. In a recent study, T-cells were adoptively transferred into mice that had been administered CORT prior to transfer. Even though this CORT administration had been terminated prior to adoptive transfer, significantly fewer of the transferred cells underwent antigen-specific proliferation as determined by carboxyfluorescein succinimydyl ester (CFSE) labeling (Yorty, unpublished observation). These findings suggest that the effects of the CORT were not on the T-cell themselves but rather some other immune cell that played a supplemental role in this proliferation.

Maternal–fetal programming

A new and exciting area of study is the role that maternal behavior plays in the programming of the developing fetus and newborn. For example, maternally influenced prenatal and early postnatal life events have been shown to affect disease susceptibility of the offspring. Some possible aspects of maternal behavior during both pregnancy and the postpartum period which may affect fetal development include nutrition, levels of stress, and drug use/abuse. These maternal factors have the potential to alter the offspring's susceptibility to disease by not only directly affecting the development and function of its immune system, but also the reprogramming of its HPA axis.

One well-studied example of maternal–fetal programming is fetal alcohol syndrome (Zhang, Sliwowska, and Weinberg, 2005). Although it is known that children born to mothers who use alcohol during pregnancy have an increased susceptibility to recurrent viral and bacterial infection, animal models allow for a more detailed analysis of the effects of alcohol consumption on the immune response. For example, the use of animal models has shown that fetal alcohol syndrome affects the adaptive immune response more so than it does the innate immune response. In one specific study, neonatal rats who were exposed to ethanol prenatally exhibited diminished T-cell and B-cell responses to *Trichinella spiralis* infection and had elevated numbers of these worms in their intestinal tract (Seelig, Steven, and Stewart, 1996). Whereas deficits in immune cell function and increased susceptibility to infection may not be apparent in the offspring under non-stress conditions, these traits may be observed when the offspring is exposed to a stressor (Zhang, Sliwowska, and Weinberg, 2005). These immune deficits may be related to alterations in the responsiveness of the HPA axis via epigenetic mechanisms.

Through the use of mouse models, maternal stress has been shown to alter fetal and neonatal serum antibody levels which, in turn, increases the susceptibility of the offspring to infection. For example, in the absence of maternal stress, HSV-specific antibody present in the breast milk of mothers who have previously been infected with HSV protects approximately 55% of neonates from HSV-associated mortality. In contrast, neonates who nursed on mothers provided with CORT in their drinking water exhibit a marked increase in the rate and extent of mortality as compared to those neonates who nursed mothers without elevated CORT (Yorty, Schultz, and Bonneau, 2004). This increase in mortality correlated with a reduction in both total and HSV-specific antibody (IgG isotype) in the neonate. These findings suggest that postnatal maternal CORT decreases the transmammary transfer of antibody. Indeed, neonates who receive HSV-specific antibody from CORT-treated mothers exhibit an increase in survival if the neonate receives HSV-specific antibody. This study is just one example of how maternal stress-induced activation of the HPA axis and SNS can alter susceptibility to infection in the offspring.

Technological advances

The discovery of unique cell surface and intracellular proteins has provided a means for identifying and discriminating between a variety of immune cell subsets. By developing protein-specific monoclonal antibodies and using them in flow-cytometry-based applications, these subsets can be detected, quantified, and purified. For example, we now recognize that in addition to the classic $CD4^+$ T helper 1 (T_H1) and T helper 2 (T_H2) subsets there are also $CD4^+$ T_H17 cells, follicular T helper cells (T_{FH}), and $CD4^+$ regulatory T-cells. Even memory T-cells are now classified as either effector memory (T_{EM}) or central memory (T_{CM}) cells based upon their distribution throughout the body and their differential expression of a series of cell-surface proteins. Newly identified DC subsets are also emerging, as are the specific role that each subset plays in overall immune defense. For example, plasmacytoid DCs are recognized as being critical for recognition of viral infection and the development of T-cell-based immune responses. Whereas some immune cell subsets can be identified by the presence of only a few unique proteins, other subsets require significantly more proteins for accurate identification. Technological advances in flow cytometry that allow for the detection of up to 35 different molecules on a single cell, although not a common practice, have made such identification possible. Given this increased knowledge of immune cell subsets and their function, future studies in PNI could begin to elucidate whether there are differences in how stress-induced glucocorticoids and catecholamines affect the number and function of these various immune cell subsets and their role in the immune response to pathogens.

Even when the appropriate subsets of immune cells for providing defense against pathogens are present, the functional ability of these cells often relies on their physical interaction with other immune cells. Moreover, their ability to migrate to the site of infection is critical to their function. The use of intravital microscopy, a relatively new technique, allows one to visualize biological processes as they occur *in vivo* within a living animal. This type of microscopy combines strong resolving power with time-lapse video imaging to track the movement and interactions of immune cells. This technology has already been used to monitor the interactions between APCs and T-cells within a lymph node and provides an amazing real-time view within secondary lymphoid organs during the immune response (Mempel, Henrickson, and Von Andrian, 2004). Such technology could be used to gain insight into the mechanisms by which stress and stress-associated peptides and hormones modulate the immune response to pathogens.

The ability to manipulate the murine genome through transgenic and knockout technology has provided researchers with numerous lines of mice in which a specific gene has been either deleted or overexpressed, often in a cell- or tissue-specific fashion. One such example is a mouse line which lacks expression of the glucocorticoid receptor, but *only* in T-cells (Brewer *et al.*, 2003). Thus, the use of this mouse model eliminates any potential direct affects of glucocorticoid–glucocorticoid receptor interactions on the T-cells themselves. Studies using these mice have demonstrated that exposure of DCs to glucocorticoids *in vivo* hinders the development of the DC from its splenic-derived precursor. This reduced number of DCs and the impairment in their ability to process and present antigen results in a decreased *in vivo* T-cell response. Using a model in which these mice are also infected with HSV leads to increased infectious HSV and more severe lesions in stressed mice. Thus, although the T-cells are not directly affected by glucocorticoids, cellular and molecular changes within the DCs decreases the antiviral response of the T-cells.

There is another mouse line which has been engineered to lack expression of the μ-opioid receptor – a receptor which plays a role in HPA axis activation (Mague *et al.*, 2009). The development of additional mouse lines that lack receptors for other stress-associated peptides and hormones would also be valuable. For example, the ability to target deletions to specific immune cells such as macrophages, DCs, or B-cells will allow us to determine the cells that are not only most affected by glucocorticoids and catecholamines but that also play a critical role in stress-induced modulation of the immune response. Overall, technologies such as these will serve to better define the roles of the nervous, endocrine, and immune systems in stress-mediated modulation of defense against pathogens.

Counteracting the effects of stress on immune function

Research during the past two decades has clearly demonstrated that stress affects many components of the immune response to infection. More recent studies have allowed us to begin to understand the cellular and molecular mechanisms that are, in part, responsible for these effects. Given this understanding, we are now well poised to determine the best ways to counteract the effects of stress on immune function.

The most obvious way to prevent stress-induced effects on immune function is to eliminate the stressor itself. Although this is not always possible, the use of interventional strategies such as social support and counseling may serve to diminish the extent of HPA axis and SNS activation and thus the impact of the stressor on immune function. The use of glucocorticoid- and catecholamine-receptor antagonists can also reduce the effects of stress on immune function. However, it is important to note that these systemically administered antagonists have the potential to block receptors not only on immune cells but also on all cells that express the glucocorticoid and catecholamine receptors and to which the antagonists have access. Other pharmacological approaches are also being studied. For example, animal models have been used to evaluate whether treatment with the common antidepressant, fluoxetine (Prozac®), can reduce the negative effects of stress on the immune response. Indeed, daily fluoxetine treatment of auditory-stressed mice partially restored both NK cell and CD8$^+$ T-cell cytotoxicity (Nunez *et al.*, 2006). These studies were recently extended to show that fluoxetine partially reduces the effects of auditory stress on the immune response to *C. albicans* infection in rats (Nunez *et al.*, 2010).

Conclusions

The development and use of animal models of stress and infection have contributed significantly to our understanding of the cellular and molecular mechanisms that are involved in the relationship between stress, the nervous and the endocrine systems, and the immune response to pathogens. This understanding is a function, in part, of the numerous advantages of animal models over that of human subject studies. Although there are many variables that are inherent to the use of animal models, such models have served and will continue to serve the PNI research community. To date, animal-based studies have been instrumental in demonstrating that stress-induced activation of the HPA axis and SNS and subsequent release of glucocorticoids and catecholamines, respectively, often impairs the development of an immune response to a variety of pathogens, leading to increased morbidity and mortality. Technological advances in each of the individual disciplines that are associated with the study of stress–neuroendocrine–immune interactions have already and will continue to allow us to better understand the nature of these interactions. Such an understanding may eventually allow us to design strategies to block the negative effects of stress on immune function and thus prevent the all-too-common adverse effects that stress has on susceptibility to infection.

References

Appay, V., and Rowland-Jones, S.L. (2002). The assessment of antigen-specific CD8$^+$ T cells through the combination of MHC class I tetramer and intracellular staining. *Journal of Immunological Methods*, 268(1), 9–19.

Bailey, M.T., Engler, H., Powell, N.D., Padgett, D.A., and Sheridan, J.F. (2007). Repeated social defeat increases the bactericidal activity of splenic macrophages through a Toll-like receptor-dependent pathway. *American Journal of Physiology, Regulatory, Integrative, and Comparative*, 293(3), R1180–1190.

Betts, M.R., Brenchley, J.M., Price, D.A., De Rosa, S.C., Douek, D.C., Roederer, M., and Koup, R.A. (2003). Sensitive and viable identification of antigen-specific CD8$^+$ T cells by a flow cytometric assay for degranulation. *Journal of Immunological Methods*, 281(1–2), 65–78.

Bonneau, R.H., Sheridan, J.F., Feng, N.G., and Glaser, R. (1991). Stress-induced suppression of herpes simplex virus (HSV)-specific cytotoxic T lymphocyte and natural killer cell activity and enhancement of acute pathogenesis following local HSV infection. *Brain, Behavior, Immunity*, 5(2), 170–192.

Brewer, J.A., Khor, B., Vogt, S.K., Muglia, L.M., Fujiwara, H., Haegele, K.E., Sleckman, B.P., and Muglia, L.J. (2003). T-cell glucocorticoid receptor is required to suppress COX-2-mediated lethal immune activation. *Nature Medicine*, 9(10), 1318–1322.

Brunner, K.T., Mauel, J., Cerottini, J.C., and Chapuis, B. (1968). Quantitative assay of the lytic action of immune lymphoid cells on 51-Cr-labelled allogeneic target cells in vitro; inhibition by isoantibody and by drugs. *Immunology*, 14(2), 181–196.

Cannon, W. (1935). Stresses and strains of homeostasis. *American Journal of Medical Science*, 89, 1–14.

Cohen, S., Alper, C.M., Doyle, W.J., Treanor, J.J., and Turner, R.B. (2006). Positive emotional style predicts resistance to illness after experimental exposure to rhinovirus or influenza a virus. *Psychosomatic Medicine*, 68(6), 809–815.

Cohen, S., Tyrrell, D.A., and Smith, A.P. (1991). Psychological stress and susceptibility to the common cold. *New England Journal of Medicine*, 325(9), 606–612.

Dhabhar, F.S. (2009). Enhancing versus suppressive effects of stress on immune function: implications for immunoprotection and immunopathology. *Neuroimmunomodulation*, 16(5), 300–317.

Dobbs, C.M., Feng, N., Beck, F.M., and Sheridan, J.F. (1996). Neuroendocrine regulation of cytokine production during experimental influenza viral infection: effects of restraint stress-induced elevation in endogenous corticosterone. *Journal of Immunology*, 157(5), 1870–1877.

Elftman, M.D., Hunzeker, J.T., Mellinger, J.C., Bonneau, R.H., Norbury, C.C., and Truckenmiller, M.J. (2010). Stress-induced glucocorticoids at the earliest stages of herpes simplex virus-1 infection suppress subsequent antiviral immunity, implicating impaired dendritic cell function. *Journal of Immunology*, 184(4), 1867–1875.

Elftman, M.D., Norbury, C.C., Bonneau, R.H., and Truckenmiller, M.E. (2007). Corticosterone impairs dendritic cell maturation and function. *Immunology*, 122(2), 279–290.

Feng, N., Pagniano, R., Tovar, C.A., Bonneau, R.H., Glaser, R., and Sheridan, J.F. (1991). The effect of restraint stress on the kinetics, magnitude, and isotype of the humoral immune response to influenza virus infection. *Brain, Behavior, Immunity*, 5(4), 370–382.

Glaser, R. (2005). Stress-associated immune dysregulation and its importance for human health: a personal history of psychoneuroimmunology. *Brain, Behavior, Immunity*, 19(1), 3–11.

Glaser, R., Kiecolt-Glaser, J.K., Bonneau, R.H., Malarkey, W., Kennedy, S., and Hughes, J. (1992). Stress-induced modulation of the immune response to recombinant hepatitis B vaccine. *Psychosomatic Medicine*, 54(1), 22–29.

Leo, N.A., Callahan, T.A., and Bonneau, R.H. (1998). Peripheral sympathetic denervation alters both the primary and memory cellular immune responses to herpes simplex virus infection. *Neuroimmunomodulation*, 5(1–2), 22–35.

Mague, S.D., Isiegas, C., Huang, P., Liu-Chen, L.Y., Lerman, C., and Blendy, J.A. (2009). Mouse model of OPRM1 (A118G) polymorphism has sex-specific effects on drug-mediated behavior. *Proceedings of the National Academy of Sciences of the USA*, 106(26), 10847–10852.

Melia, K.R., Ryabinin, A.E., Schroeder, R., Bloom, F.E., and Wilson, M.C. (1994). Induction and habituation of immediate early gene expression in rat brain by acute and repeated restraint stress. *Journal of Neuroscience*, 14(10), 5929–5938.

Mempel, T.R., Henrickson, S.E., and Von Andrian, U.H. (2004). T-cell priming by dendritic cells in lymph nodes occurs in three distinct phases. *Nature*, 427(6970), 154–159.

Misslin, R., Herzog, F., Koch, B., and Ropartz, P. (1982). Effects of isolation, handling and novelty on the pituitary–adrenal response in the mouse. *Psychoneuroendocrinology*, 7(2–3), 217–221.

Nishiya, K., Norose, K., Aosai, F., Chen, M., Mun, H.S., Kang, H.K., Miyazaki, M., and Yano, A. (2005). Heat stress-induced modulation of host defense against *Toxoplasma gondii* infection in mice. *Journal of Parasitology*, 91(3), 702–706.

Nunez, M.J., Balboa, J., Rodrigo, E., Brenila, J., Gonzalez-Peteiro, M., and Freire-Garabal, M. (2006). Effects of fluoxetine on cellular immune response in stressed mice. *Neuroscience Letters*, 396(3), 247–251.

Nunez, M.J., Novio, S., Suarez, J.A., Balboa, J., and Freire-Garabal, M. (2010). Effects of psychological stress and fluoxetine on development of oral candidiasis in rats. *Clinical and Vaccine Immunology*, 17(4), 668–673.

Perez, A.R., Bottasso, O., and Savino, W. (2009). The impact of infectious diseases upon neuroendocrine circuits. *Neuroimmunomodulation*, 16(2), 96–105.

Powell, N.D., Mays, J.W., Bailey, M.T., Hanke, M.L., and Sheridan, J.F. (2011). Immunogenic dendritic cells primed by social defeat enhance adaptive immunity to influenza A virus. *Brain, Behavior, Immunity*, 25(1), 46–52.

Rodriguez-Galan, M.C., Sotomayor, C., Costamagna, M.E., Cabanillas, A.M., Renteria, B.S., Masini-Repiso, A.M., and Correa, S.G. (2003). Immunocompetence of macrophages in rats exposed to *Candida albicans* infection and stress. *American Journal of Physiology. Cell Physiology*, 284(1), C111–118.

Rodriguez-Galan, M.C., Sotomayor, C.E., Cano, R., Porporatto, C., Renna, M.S., Paraje, M.G., Cejas, H., and Correa, S.G. (2010). Immune neuroendocrine interactions during a fungal infection in immunocompetent or immunosuppressed hosts. *Neuroimmunomodulation*, 17(3), 188–191.

Seelig, L.L., Jr., Steven, W.M., and Stewart, G.L. (1996). Effects of maternal ethanol consumption on the subsequent development of immunity to *Trichinella spiralis* in rat neonates. *Alcoholism: Clinical and Experimental Research*, 20(3), 514–522.

Selye, H. (1936). A syndrome produced by diverse nocuous agents. *Nature*, 138, 32–33.

Sheridan, J.F., Stark, J.L., Avitsur, R., and Padgett, D.A. (2000). Social disruption, immunity, and susceptibility to viral infection. Role of glucocorticoid insensitivity and NGF. *Annals of the New York Academy of Sciences*, 917, 894–905.

Sommershof, A., Basler, M., Riether, C., Engler, H., and Groettrup, M. (2011). Attenuation of the cytotoxic T lymphocyte response to lymphocytic choriomeningitis virus in mice subjected to chronic social stress. *Brain, Behavior, Immunity*, 25(2), 340–348.

Tait, A. S., Butts, C.L., and Sternberg, E.M. (2008). The role of glucocorticoids and progestins in inflammatory, autoimmune, and infectious disease. *Journal of Leukocyte Biology*, 84(4), 924–931.

Welsh, C.J., Steelman, A.J., Mi, W., Young, C.R., Dean, D.D., Storts, R., Welsh, T.H., Jr, and Meagher, M.W. (2010). Effects of stress on the immune response to Theiler's virus-implications for virus-induced autoimmunity. *Neuroimmunomodulation*, 17(3), 169–172.

Welsh, C.J., Steelman, A.J., Mi, W., Young, C.R., Storts, R., Welsh, T.H., Jr, and Meagher, M.W. (2009). Neuroimmune interactions in a model of multiple sclerosis. *Annals of the New York Academy of Sciences*,1153, 209–219.

Yang, E.V., and Glaser, R. (2002). Stress-associated immunomodulation and its implications for responses to vaccination. *Expert Review of Vaccines*, (4), 453–459.

Yorty, J. L., Schultz, S.A., and Bonneau, R.H. (2004). Postpartum maternal corticosterone decreases maternal and neonatal antibody levels and increases the susceptibility of newborn mice to herpes simplex virus-associated mortality. *Journal of Neuroimmunology*, 150(1–2), 48–58.

Zhang, D., Kishihara, K., Wang, B., Mizobe, K., Kubo, C., and Nomoto, K. (1998). Restraint stress-induced immunosuppression by inhibiting leukocyte migration and Th1 cytokine expression during the intraperitoneal infection of *Listeria monocytogenes*. *Journal of Neuroimmunology*, 92(1–2), 139–151.

Zhang, X., Sliwowska, J.H., and Weinberg, J. (2005). Prenatal alcohol exposure and fetal programming: effects on neuroendocrine and immune function. *Experimental Biology and Medicine*, 230(6), 376–388.

Zwilling, B. S., Brown, D., and Pearl, D. (1992). Induction of major histocompatibility complex class II glycoproteins by interferon-gamma: attenuation of the effects of restraint stress. *Journal of Neuroimmunology*, 37(1–2), 115–122.

12

Approaches to Assessing Stressor-Induced Cytokine and Endocrine Changes in Humans

Kim Matheson and Hymie Anisman

Departments of Neuroscience and Psychology, Carleton University, Ottawa, Ontario, Canada

Stressful events elicit a wide variety of pathological conditions, likely stemming from the neuroendocrine, neurotransmitter, metabolic, and immunological processes that are provoked. Based on studies in animals it is known that various factors related to the stressor itself (severity, controllability, predictability, chronicity), as well as factors related to the organism (gender, age, strain, or species) and previous experiences (both pre- and postnatally) influence vulnerability or resilience to the negative impact of stressors. Studies in humans have also revealed the profound effects of stressors at various stages of life, and like the animal studies, indicated that stressors in early life may affect the trajectory of biological changes (Lupien *et al.*, 2011), and hence vulnerability to later pathology.

For obvious reasons, studies in humans cannot be conducted to measure the impact of stressors on specific brain neurochemical systems. Likewise, the controlled analyses of how particular events influence behavioral and biochemical processes are not amenable to studies in humans. Yet, the richness of data that can be obtained from human studies far exceeds that which can be gleaned from animal research, including an understanding of the contribution of complex cognitive processes, as well as the role of personality variables and certain emotional responses (e.g., self esteem, self- vs other-directed anger, shame, guilt). In addition, there are certain stressors that do not occur in animals, such as the response to discrimination and stigmatization, job-related distress, and numerous others, that play a fundamental role in shaping human behaviors.

The present chapter will provide a broad overview of approaches that can be taken to assess the impact of stressors on behavioral and biological processes that have implications for wellbeing. The analysis of stressor effects on immune and cytokine functioning in humans has been fairly impressive, but neither the breadth nor depth of these studies has been as extensive as those that have involved the analysis of neuroendocrine changes exerted by stressors. Thus, in this chapter we will not focus exclusively on immunologically related studies, but will also borrow from other related research literatures to point to possibilities that might be considered in the assessment of cytokine changes associated with environmental triggers. Indeed, stressful experiences have multiple adverse consequences (as well as some positive outcomes), and it has been argued that some of these, including psychological illnesses, such as depression,

The Wiley-Blackwell Handbook of Psychoneuroimmunology, First Edition. Edited by Alexander W. Kusnecov and Hymie Anisman.

burnout, anxiety, and post-traumatic stress disorder, as well as physical disorders, including Type 2 diabetes, heart disease, immunologically related illnesses (e.g., susceptibility to virally related illnesses, autoimmune disorders), and neurodegenerative disorders (e.g., Alzheimer's, Parkinson's disease, poststroke recovery and poststroke depression) may involve overlapping biological processes. In this regard, it was suggested that the frequent comorbidity that has been observed between many of these disturbances (e.g., depression and heart disease as well as neurodegenerative disorders that likely involve inflammatory processes) might involve brain cytokine release from microglia (Anisman, Merali, and Hayley, 2008). This makes it all the more important to consider multiple factors, in parallel or sequentially, in assessing the impact of stressors.

Stressor Appraisals and Coping in Humans

Before embarking on a description of different approaches to assessing the consequences of stressors, it is necessary to describe, in a general way, the stress process. In humans, stressful events, more often than not, are fairly chronic, especially when one considers that apparently acute stressors have enduring psychological repercussions (e.g., rumination and a variety of other emotional responses). Depending on the nature of stressors, they may engage different processes, and call upon a wide array of resources. For instance, interpersonal problems (family disputes, divorce, fight with your best friend), illness, financial or work-related issues, traumatic experiences or reminders of trauma, as well as those related to ego insults (e.g., public humiliation or shame, loss of face or self-esteem) likely engage different behavioral and cognitive processes, and it can be expected that they might have different health-related repercussions. Indeed, studies in animals have indicated that different neural circuits may be engaged in response to physical and psychological stressors, and to innate versus learned stressors (Anisman, Merali, and Hayley, 2008), and thus it should come as no surprise that the circuitry associated with different stressors in humans would vary as well.

According to the transaction model of stress (Lazarus and Folkman, 1984), in response to potential stressors (threats), individuals appraise the situation (primary appraisals that essentially determine whether the event is a threat or a challenge) followed by a secondary appraisal that entails an analysis of whether resources to contend (cope) with the stressor are available. Once appraisals of the stressor have been made, particular coping responses will be used to deal with it. In part, these coping methods may be dispositional propensities (i.e., styles of coping, wherein individuals are more likely to engage in a particular method of coping), although it seems that the actual coping strategy endorsed will vary across situations and may change over time as the stressor evolves. Broadly speaking, these coping methods fall into three categories, namely problem-coping, emotion-coping, and avoidant-coping, each of which subsumes several specific strategies. Although it is often said that problem-focused coping is "adaptive" and emotion- and avoidant-focused coping are maladaptive, this is likely an oversimplification, as there are instances in which problem-focused coping may not be productive, whereas emotional-focused or avoidant-coping is adaptive (e.g., in response to a diagnosis of an incurable form of cancer) (Stanton and Franz, 1999). We have suggested that the most effective method of coping may involves being flexible in the adoption of particular strategies, being prepared to change from one strategy to another as the situation demands, and to use coping strategies in effective combinations (e.g., rumination is often thought of being a poor method of coping, but it might be effective if combined with problem solving or cognitive restructuring, such as finding meaning in a tragedy) (Matheson and Anisman, 2011). This, too, is a bit of an oversimplification, as factors related to attributional style, as well as the inferences (expectancies) made on the basis of the attributions, together with factors such as self-esteem, mastery, hardiness, optimism, and other personality dimensions likely contribute to the appraisal-coping process.

Along with these cognitive processes, several neuroendocrine and neurotransmitter changes occur that facilitate the ability to deal with the stressor. Among other things, they might initiate behavioral responses to limit the impact of the stressor, blunt the emotional consequences of the challenge, and limit activation of still other biological systems that threaten to become excessive (e.g., exaggerated immune activation may have adverse repercussions). These biological reactions are influenced by psychosocial factors and appraisal-coping processes, and conversely, the neurobiological changes may also affect the way individuals appraise and behaviorally respond to stressors.

It is important to consider the differential impacts of acute and chronic stressors. When a stressor is acute, of moderate severity, and is controllable, a series of neuroendocrine and hormonal changes occur that facilitate the organism's ability to contend with the challenge. If the stressor is more intense, and especially if it is uncontrollable and occurs on a chronic or sustained basis, then a further series of biological changes occurs, including compensatory changes of certain neurotransmitters, as well as variations of receptor sensitivity. Often, the varied emotional, behavioral and biological resources available might diminish the impact of severe challenges, thus maintaining wellbeing (Anisman and Matheson, 2005). However, the effectiveness of these processes can go only so far. If the stressor persists long enough and is sufficiently intense, then allostatic overload occurs, in which biological coping systems become overly taxed, rendering individuals especially vulnerable to pathology (McEwen, 2000). For example, the immune activation that has been reported following an acute stressor (although suppression has also been reported) might not be evident with a chronic stressor, and indeed, in the latter instance immune functioning may be impaired. Alternatively, the beneficial biological effects of an acute stressor (e.g., release of glucocorticoids) might, in response to chronic stressors, come to have adverse consequences (e.g., sustained cortisol release may provoke cell loss within the hippocampus, and might thus contribute to cognitive and behavioral disturbances; McEwen, 2000).

One final point warrants consideration before turning to the methods used to assess how stressors affect immune activity. Typically, when the impact of stressors is considered, we think in terms of the immediate effects engendered, and we might assume that they are self-limiting. However, it is fairly certain that stressful events, particularly those encountered early in life (including adolescence), as well as prenatal challenges in a pregnant mom, may have enduring effects so that behavioral and emotional responses, as well as health risks, might be exceptionally persistent. Such changes could come about through epigenetic processes wherein stressful events might suppress gene functioning (permanently, although not necessarily irreversibly) so that adult responses to stressors might be altered, as might responses in ensuing generations that inherit the turned-off genes. In this regard, studies in humans have implicated epigenetic processes in affecting both glucocorticoid and GABAA receptor functioning (Szyf, 2011), both of which are highly related to stress responses, and have been implicated in depression and anxiety.

In addition to epigenetic processes, or perhaps tied to them, it seems that potent stressors provoke the "sensitization" of several neurochemical systems, so that when these stressors (or reminders of these stressors) are subsequently encountered, exaggerated neurochemical responses are elicited (Anisman, Hayley, and Merali, 2003). These sensitized responses likely reflect neuronal plasticity related to synaptic strength or receptor variations (as opposed to sensitization in the immunological sense that involves memory immune cells), and may be fundamental in the provocation of depression and illness recurrence (Post, 1992). Thus, analyses of the impact of stressors on wellbeing might not only consider the short-term changes evoked, but also those that might be elicited long after the initial stressor was encountered.

Laboratory-based Stressor Paradigms

Field studies assessing the impact of stressors on immune and endocrine functioning are certainly more relevant to the analysis of wellbeing than studies conducted in contrived laboratory settings. However, the rigor of the experiment is often not possible, with stressor variables within a study differing with respect to their duration, chronicity, predictability, and intermittence. Moreover, the ethics involved in exposing humans to particular stressors precludes certain studies in naturalistic settings. Thus, laboratory studies using stressors of limited severity have often been used as a practical alternative.

The neuroendocrine responses, such as cortisol release, as well as immune responses elicited by stressors, likely reflect adaptive changes. In this regard, cortisol release in response to a challenge ought to be dictated, to a considerable extent, by appraisals and coping responses. Yet, because the release of corticotropin releasing hormone (CRH), which triggers ACTH and hence cortisol release, occurs as rapidly as it does (see Sapolsky, Romero, and Munck, 2000), there might not be sufficient time for the lengthy processes that might be associated with secondary appraisals ("do I have control over this situation?"). Instead, it might be most adaptive for the system to respond quickly to anything that seems like a challenge, and then if it looks like the threat is not all that great, and is appraised as being one that can be dealt with behaviorally, the extent of the cortisol response should be dampened. In contrast, if the threat turns out to be substantial, it might be expected that the cortisol rise would be elevated and would be longer lasting relative to that elicited by a moderate threat. However, this, too, is a somewhat simplified characterization of the cortisol response, as there are occasions (e.g., response to chronic stressors, or traumatic events leading to post-traumatic stress disorder) wherein the cortisol response is blunted (Yehuda, 2009).

Trier Social Stress Test (TSST)

One frequently used method to evaluate stressor effects in a laboratory setting is the Trier Social Stress Test (TSST). In this paradigm, individuals are asked to prepare a 5-minute speech (say, for example, concerning a would-be job interview), and then to present it (without notes) to a panel of judges. This is followed by an arithmetic task with or without distractions present. This paradigm elicits a marked rise of cortisol (Kirschbaum and Hellhammer, 1994): in some studies the rise was of the magnitude of 100%, and even 300%, but it is more common to see a rise of 40–80%. Importantly, the cortisol rise was shown to vary with numerous factors that would be expected to influence stress responses, such as previous stressful experiences, as well as other biological processes such as those related to whether women were using oral contraceptives, and as a function of menstrual cycle (Foley and Kirschbaum, 2010).

The magnitude of the cortisol rise associated with the TSST stands in marked contrast to the 600–800% corticoid rise ordinarily seen in rodents, and is also very different from the 30% change associated with anticipation of real-life stressors, such as open heart surgery, or the anxiety among students about to walk into their MS or PhD thesis oral exam (reviewed in Michaud, Matheson, Kelly, and Anisman, 2008). At first blush, these results seem paradoxical – do they mean that open heart surgery is appraised as less stressful than the TSST? Obviously, this is not the case, but the finding makes it clear that there is more to the cortisol response than just the stressor appraisal. Presumably, participants in the TSST are not aware of the procedure before they get to the experimental setting, whereas surgery patients likely had been forewarned about the procedures and some degree of "adaptation" may have occurred. Furthermore, cortisol levels in the former instance was determined in blood (or saliva) taken after the stressor test, whereas in the case of the heart surgery or the academic oral examination, blood samples were taken before (i.e., in anticipation) the primary stressor event.

In their evaluation of the processes responsible for the cortisol rise elicited by the TSST, Dickerson and Kemeny (2004) suggested that it was essential to consider the emotional and cognitive sequelae of the different stressors. They suggested that public speaking (which is a component of the TSST) involves social evaluation (being judged by others) and elicits feelings of shame, and it is this emotion that is primarily responsible for the cortisol changes. In effect, it is not the stressor itself, or the anticipation of the stressor, but the emotional responses that accompany the stressor that promote the cortisol variations. Our own findings have largely been in line with those reported by Dickerson and Kemeny. In our studies the TSST was associated with several emotional responses (anxiety, anger, shame), but it was shame that increased to the greatest extent. However, it seemed that anger (likely self-directed anger – "I could have done better"; "I'm such a dope") was the factor that accounted for the greatest amount of unique variance in relation to the cortisol levels (Raspopow, Abizaid, Matheson, and Anisman, 2010), although we would not by any means dismiss an important function for shame in eliciting neuroendocrine responses. Indeed, the self-directed anger may have been a reflection of the shame experienced. The important issue here is that some brain changes are closely tied to particular emotions that give rise to corticoid variations.

There have been a few studies that assessed the impact of the TSST on immune functioning. For instance, this stressor was found to reduce the delayed-type hypersensitivity response (Buske-Kirschbaum, Kern, Ebrecht, and Hellhammer, 2007), increased circulating leukocyte subpopulations as well as mitogen-stimulated interferon (IFN)-γ and interleukin (IL)-2, and reduced production of the anti-inflammatory cytokine IL-10 (Buske-Kirschbaum, Kern, Ebrecht, and Hellhammer, 2007). There have also been reports of elevated IL-6 in response to single or multiple sessions of the TSST (von Känel *et al.*, 2006), and to a considerable extent, the cytokine variations were related to the mood state elicited by the stressor. In addition, in some instances, the immune changes associated with stressors were unique to certain individuals. By example, plasma IL-6 levels were not influenced in the TSST among healthy participants, but were elevated in depressed individuals (Pace *et al.*, 2006). Likewise, the TSST has been reported to produce a modest rise of IL-6 in a control set of healthy participants, but to elicit a much greater rise among individuals who had experienced childhood maltreatment (Carpenter *et al.*, 2010). It was similarly reported that a mental stress task (i.e., a modified version of the Stroop color naming test as well as mirror drawing) promoted increased IL-6, whereas TNF-α and C-reactive protein were unaffected by this stressor (Steptoe *et al.*, 2001). In contrast to the changes of IL-6, mitogen-stimulated TNF-α production following a speech challenge was reduced shortly after stress in chronic fatigue syndrome patients, whereas it was modestly elevated in healthy controls (Gaab *et al.*, 2005).

In a relatively sophisticated analysis in which participants were required to make a speech about an alleged transgression (shoplifting or traffic violation) it was observed that IL-6 levels were elevated following the task, but that this varied with individuals' mood. Specifically, task-related increases of anger and anxiety were associated with increasing levels of IL-6, and it appeared that these affective responses were independent predictors of change in IL-6 (Carroll *et al.*, 2011). It was similarly observed that hostility elicited in relation to the TSST predicted elevated levels of circulating IL-6 (Brydon *et al.*, 2010). Moreover, it appeared that in response to a speech task, greater self-esteem was associated with smaller rise of TNF-α and that of the IL-1 receptor antagonist (IL-1Ra). It also appeared that the cytokine changes associated with the TSST depended on the individuals coping style. Specifically, it was reported (Master *et al.*, 2009) that engagement in the TSST resulted in elevated levels of the soluble receptor for tumor necrosis factor-α (sTNF-αRII) in saliva, but the extent of the rise was less pronounced among individuals with higher emotional-approach coping (this comprised intentional efforts to identify, process, and express emotions associated with stressors).

Summarizing, it seems clear that stressful events within a laboratory context might influence aspects of immune functioning, just as these stressors influence cortisol responses. Moreover, these outcomes vary with the nature of the coping responses that are elicited. Furthermore, it seems that the effects of the stressors on these immune changes are linked to the emotional responses elicited. This included not only shame as purportedly a main element in accounting for the cortisol changes associated with the TSST, but also anger and anxiety that are provoked. To be sure, these emotions are highly intercorrelated and it might be that although they might each contribute to certain outcomes (and unique variance might only be attributable to one of these factors), it is equally possible their effects on different biological systems might not be identical.

Together, these findings suggest that the TSST is a potent stressor that not only influences cortisol release, but also increases the circulating levels of several cytokines. These elevations, like some of the cortisol changes reported, may be dependent on the nature of the emotional and cognitive responses elicited by the stressor. This conclusion is largely based on studies that assessed correlations between mood states and emotional responses, and few (but see Slavich, Way, Eisenberger, and Taylor, 2010) attempted to directly manipulate the effects of mood changes on the provocation of immune or cytokine alterations.

To a significant extent, the TSST has become a favorite tool because it is fairly easy to administer (provided that a panel of judges is available, as simple video monitoring or even virtually reality settings do not provide all that strong a response) and analyses of cortisol can be conducted in saliva samples that had been collected with limited intrusiveness. Yet, the TSST, especially if it relies only on saliva as a biological sample, has its shortcomings. Saliva can be used to obtain some biological indices (e.g., cortisol, alpha amylase, and an index of some immunoglobulins, and there have been demonstrations showing adequate measurement of IL-6 and sTNF-αRII), but more informative immune indices cannot be obtained, necessitating the collection of blood. Further, the TSST is essentially an acute stressor, and thus may have little bearing on the influence of chronic stressor effects on the development of neuroendocrine or immune changes, or for that matter on the development of pathological conditions.

The TSST may be a very good method of evaluating stress reactivity, particularly in relation to individual differences in mood state, previous stressful experiences, and the presence of pathology, or in relation to particular moods instigated by a treatment that involves an evaluative stressor. In a sense, the TSST is able to provide information about stress sensitivity/vulnerability, just as a stress test (treadmill running) can help to determine whether a cardiac problem exists. However, it needs to be remembered that the TSST may not be representative of other stressors. If Dickerson and Kemeny (2004) are correct that this stressor's effects lie in its capacity to act as a self-evaluative threat, then one needs to consider that: a) not all individuals appraise public speaking as equally stressful; and b) it has little bearing with respect to the vast number of other stressors that can influence neuroendocrine and immune responses, although the paradigm can incorporate other stressors, for example, by having participants give a speech regarding their own stressful experiences.

Social rejection

Some of the most potent stressors that social beings, like us, can encounter are those that involve social challenges. Of the many social stressors that can be encountered, social rejection can be especially damaging. For instance, groups of individuals can be rejected, as seen in cases of discrimination related to gender, sexual orientation, race, or religion. The rejection can also be at a personal level, as in the case of stigmatization and discrimination against those with particular illness, such as AIDS or mental disorders. Social rejection can also occur in the absence of these factors, occurring either because the individual is somewhat different from the rest of their ingroup or is viewed as being an embarrassment to the group. This is often referred to as the black sheep effect, where members of the ingroup do not want their group's identity tarnished by a particular individual. As some parents will know, a child (whether when young or as an adolescent) might also encounter situations where best friends turn on, or simply ignore, him/her, leaving them out of social events and generally diminishing them. In general, unsupportive relationships, especially those that involve targeted rejection, can be especially damaging, and have been linked to exacerbation of depressive feelings in a variety of contexts (e.g., Slavich *et al.*, 2009). Indeed, it has been suggested that social pain and physical pain may share common underlying neural processes (Eisenberger, 2012).

The fear of social rejection is tied to depression, and is known to influence cortisol levels. In this regard, this fear is accompanied by reduced levels of cortisol, much like that seen in relation to chronic distress and PTSD. Thus, it was proposed that fear of social rejection reflects a trait that is accompanied by chronic distress, leading to an adaptation in the form of inhibited cortisol output (Tops *et al.*, 2008). However, in acute laboratory conditions (e.g., online interaction regarding dating) social rejection was accompanied by elevated cortisol levels in those with low self-esteem, but not among individuals with high self-esteem (Blackhart, Eckel, and Tice, 2007; Ford and Collins, 2010).

Given the powerful effects of social rejection, efforts at assessing this in a laboratory context have been undertaken. One recent and increasingly popular approach to studying this is a computer (or web) game, referred to as cyberball. In this paradigm a virtual ball is tossed between three characters; one of these virtual characters is controlled by the participant, and the others by presumably are controlled by other individuals involved in the study. Initially, the ball is tossed evenly between the players, but shortly afterward, it passed between the other two virtual participants and the actual participant is excluded. In this instance, negative ruminative thoughts, altered mood, hostility (in males) and elevated cortisol levels, particularly among women in their luteal phase of the menstrual cycle have been reported (Zwolinski, 2012).

Social rejection in the cyberball paradigm has marked effects on brain processes associated with appraisals and decision making, as well as inducing depressed mood. Specifically, it has been reported that rejection is accompanied self-reported distress and by increased activity (as measured by fMRI) in the dorsal anterior cingulate cortex (dACC) (Eisenberger, Lieberman, and Williams, 2003). Moreover, rich social support in the days prior to testing attenuated the dACC variations otherwise associated with social rejection (Eisenberger *et al.*, 2007). Predictably, the effects of social rejection in the cyberball test were marked in adolescents, and this was especially apparent in those with higher rejection sensitivity and high in social competence who may be particularly vigilant regarding peer acceptance (Masten *et al.*, 2009).

Of particular relevance to the present review was the finding that cyberball rejection also affected cytokine levels. Specifically, it was demonstrated that both saliva IL-6 and sTNF-αRII were elevated in response to the social rejection. Interestingly, the extent of the brain changes correlated with the stressor elicited variations of sTNF-αRII (Slavich, Way, Eisenberger, and Taylor, 2010). Thus, these investigators suggested that a neurocognitive pathway might contribute to inflammatory changes elicited by evaluative stressors as well as those that involve social rejection. Furthermore it was demonstrated that social exclusion that occurred following intravenous endotoxin treatment elicited self-reported signs of depression. Moreover, in females (but not males) the increased levels of plasma IL-6 elicited by the endotoxin were associated with increased social pain and feelings of depression that were mediated by neuronal activity within the dACC and anterior insula (Eisenberger *et al.*, 2009). On the basis of a series of studies, it was suggested that social rejection promoted self-conscious emotions (e.g., humiliation, shame) and negative self-referential cognitions that were mediated by the dACC and the insula, which might have influenced HPA functioning, inflammatory processes and promotion of depressive disorder (Slavich, Way, Eisenberger, and Taylor, 2010).

Reminders of a stressful event

An alternative method of evaluating stressor effects is to place individuals in a situation in which stressful events are portrayed visually. Gruesome scenes (car accidents), objects that promote disgust, some degree of repulsion (e.g., a tangle of snakes), or anger typically do not have much of an effect on cortisol levels. This is not particularly surprising as one sees so many more disturbing scenarios (e.g., in movies and television), most people have likely become inured to such visual stimuli so that they no longer elicit the response that one would need to elicit a meaningful and detectable biological change.

A slightly modified version of this stressor test can be conducted to elicit greater effects. In this instance, stimuli are presented that remind participants of a previous stressful event relevant to their own experiences, and are asked to comment on the scenario. For instance, just as expected, when responding to a questionnaire regarding their own past trauma experiences, it was observed that among women who had been in abusive dating relationships, cortisol levels varied in an inverted U-shape fashion in relation to their PTSD scores. Specifically, cortisol increased in relation to PTSD scores up to a point (moderate levels of PTSD), after which cortisol levels were lower with more extreme scores. It is of particular interest, however, that when women with PTSD symptoms who had been in an abusive relationship were shown a video clip that portrayed abuse, their plasma cortisol levels were exceptionally high (Matheson and Anisman, 2011). Essentially, these data are in keeping with the finding that hypothalamic–pituitary–adrenal (HPA) functioning is downregulated among individuals with PTSD, possibly to deal with the adverse effects of persistent cortisol elevations (Yehuda, 2009). However, in the presence of relevant (meaningful) stimuli, activation of certain brain regions that might be pertinent to memories of aversive events (e.g., prefrontal cortex, amygdala) might have the effect of promoting HPA activation even in the face of downregulated functioning. To our knowledge, similar studies have not been conducted to evaluate the impact of visual reminders of trauma on immune or cytokine functioning in blood samples.

Another approach that can be used to assess the influence of relevant and meaningful cues on hormone and cytokine/immune activity has involved having participants: a) complete a questionnaire concerning trauma they experienced, and then either in written format or verbally, describe the specific trauma that they considered the most stressful; or b) read a script that portrays a stressful event that is relevant versus irrelevant to their own experiences (or a control script) and then comment on this scenario (orally or in written form). Considering the neuroendocrine changes that have been associated with the specific mood elicited by stressors, it has been of particular interest in our studies to determine the relations between trauma reminders, mood elicited by these cues, and hormone and/or cytokine variations (Danielson, Matheson, and Anisman, 2011). Figure 12.1 shows the plasma IL-6 levels evident after reading a script about a woman talking to her friend about plans she made with her boyfriend. The script was either innocuous (control) or indicated abuse from the boyfriend. Figure 12.1 (top left panel) shows the plasma IL-6 levels among women that had not been in an abusive relationship and who were asked to read a control script. Although this script was expected not to be stressful, for some women it was clearly associated with negative mood. Further, in this condition, the level of IL-6 was positively associated with self-reported anger or sadness, but not with shame or anxiety. A similar, but subdued profile of relations was apparent among nonabused women asked to read the script that portrayed an abusive interaction (see top-right panel). In contrast, as seen in the two lower panels of Figure 12.1, these relations were largely absent among women who were in abusive dating relationships and who read the control scenario; among the abused women shown the abuse scenario, a modest relationship between IL-6 and mood intensity was evident, but this was apparent regardless of the nature of the mood they expressed. The important points for the present purpose are that: a) this paradigm revealed cytokine variations that were tied to both stressor experiences and to the mood associated with these experiences; and b) the IL-6 response associated with mood changes disappeared with more intense stressful experiences. It is as if the cytokine levels are ordinarily tied to certain types of emotions (anger and sadness) but, like the cortisol elevations described earlier, these relations disappear with greater stressor severity.

Acute Versus Chronic Stressor Experiences and the Morning Cortisol Rise

In rodents, acute and chronic stressor treatments have different effects on immune and cytokine functioning. Acute stressors of moderate severity increase, whereas severe stressors may reduce cytokine levels, as might a chronic stressor regimen. In humans, it is much more difficult to identify the impact of acute and chronic stressors in natural settings, as the acuteness of the stressor and its severity are often entwined. In particular, a strong stressor may have repercussions on mood (and rumination), finances, lifestyle and so on, so that it essentially comprises a compound stressor. Acute events might also entail rumination and other downstream mood effects (e.g., shame), and thus these events might also have a chronic component. Essentially, while participants can be asked to describe the severity or duration of stressful experiences,

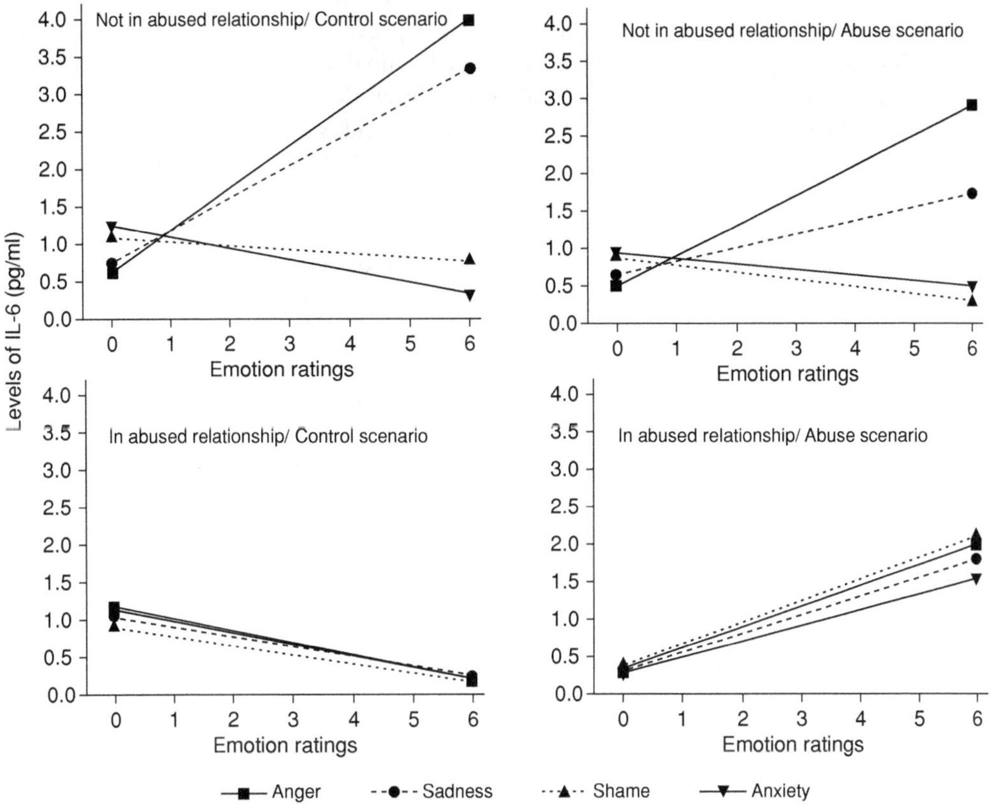

Figure 12.1 Unstandardized regression lines depicting the relations between the extent to which women reported each emotion (anger, sadness, shame, and anxiety) and levels of IL-6 as a function of abuse in their own dating relationships and the stressor condition (abuse vs control scenario). Women who had or had not been in an abusive relationship read a script depicting an abusive relationship, or a situation that was not deemed to be as stressful. Among women who were not in an abusive relationship, feelings of anger or sadness were directly related to plasma IL-6 levels. This was not apparent in relation to either shame or anxiety. Among women in an abusive relationship, the IL-6 response elicited by the scenario that they read, particularly one about abuse, was markedly blunted. (From Danielson *et al.*, 2011.)

these might not necessarily coincide with the experimenter's preconceived notions or those that appear on standard questionnaires. In fact, participants themselves might not be consciously aware of the chronic or complex nature of a given stressor experience.

These limitations notwithstanding, various attempts have been made to assess the impact of life stressors on biological responses. As already indicated, it is virtually impossible to assess such outcomes immediately after a traumatic event (given that most researchers will not be in a position to chase ambulances, nor should they be), and at lengthier intervals most biological responses will not be apparent, but there are some exceptions in this regard. However, it has been reported that the diurnal cortisol fluctuations that ordinarily occur can be influenced by stressor experiences. Specifically, cortisol levels are fairly high at awakening and rise over the subsequent 30 minutes, after which levels decline, eventually reaching their nadir in the late evening or early morning. Among individuals who are stressed to a moderately high degree, the initial morning cortisol rise increases appreciably. However, among individuals who experienced a chronic strong stressor, or in those individuals who displayed PTSD symptomatology, the morning cortisol rise is blunted and the afternoon levels slightly elevated (the diurnal curve is thus flattened to a degree) (Michaud, Matheson, Kelly, and Anisman, 2008). These findings are particularly interesting in that they suggest that aspects of HPA functioning can be tied to stressful experiences and that the nature of the HPA changes vary with different stressor-provoked pathologies. In effect, the relation between stress and diurnal cortisol changes is not a simple one, but instead varies as a function of the mood or pathological condition evoked.

A serious problem with studies that rely on participants providing saliva samples at predetermined times in order to establish diurnal profiles, is that it counts on accuracy (and truthfulness) on the part of the participant. Specifically, the participant is required to provide a saliva sample immediately upon awakening and at 30 min post-awakening. But, how reliable are participants in doing this? For example, there is often confusion, indeed ambiguity, between time of awakening and time of arising. As a result, if the first sample is taken 15 minutes after awakening, then the rise of cortisol will already be half-way to its peak, and if the next sample is provided 30 minutes later (45 minutes after awakening) this sample might reflect descending cortisol levels, thereby minimizing the difference that might exist. A variety of techniques have been used to have participants provide accurate reports as to when samples were taken (e.g., containers that record the time at which the salivette used for sample collection is opened), but these methods do not assure that the initial sample was actually provided immediately after awakening. Compliance can be improved by enhancing participant commitment to the study, and by giving them a detailed explanation regarding the importance of precision in sample collection, and to indicate accurately their time of awakening and the time at which samples were taken, even if they have not fully complied with the experimental protocol. Because of the variability in participant responses, most investigators will obtain samples over several (two or three) weekdays (cortisol levels during weekdays and weekends, workdays vs off days may differ), which is certainly useful. Ultimately, however, the participant's behavior is governed only by that participant, and variability can be expected in this regard.

Like other biological factors, inflammatory markers may vary over the course of the day, and may be associated with illnesses, such as those related to coronary dysfunction (Dominguez-Rodriguez, Abreu-Gonzalez, and Kaski, 2009). It has, however, been reported that neither TNF-α nor IL-6 varied over the course of the day following endotoxin administration. This said, it might be important to consider the time of day at which the challenge is administered. Specifically, the response to the endotoxin (in terms of body temperature, ACTH and cortisol) was greatest when it was administered in the evening relative to that evident following morning administration (Pollmächer *et al.*, 1996). It is possible that the effects of stressful experiences might interact with the time at which the challenge is administered. To the best of our knowledge the influence of stressors on diurnal cytokine variations have not been assessed, although subjective wellbeing was reported to be related to a more pronounced decline of nocturnal IL-6 and epinephrine levels (Rief *et al.*, 2010). It is important to underscore that in studies that attempted to assess diurnal cytokine variations (e.g., in relation to sleep) it was reported that simply maintaining an intravenous catheter necessary for repetitive sampling caused an increase of IL-6 levels, likely reflecting local inflammation associated with the continued presence of a needle. In fact a single stick procedure to obtain blood from the other arm provided serum with lower cytokine levels than that seen in the arm that had the catheter in place (Haack *et al.*, 2002). In some studies, researchers did not indicate the time of day at which blood samples for cytokine analyses were collected, thus potentially limiting the relevance of the study and the conclusions that can actually be made. At this point it is not known whether the variations of cytokines or immune factors are preferentially influenced in relation to particular times of day, or whether stressful events alter normal circadian rhythms. Accordingly, researchers need to either collect samples within a narrow time-window, or collect samples across numerous times with an N sufficiently large to include time of day as an independent variable.

Pre–Post Paradigms in Natural Settings

As indicated earlier, it is difficult to determine responses to naturally occurring stressors (earthquake, floods) as obtaining blood samples at such times are clearly not possible. Likewise, waiting at hospital emergency centers is often not functionally effective given that samples would be taken at various times after events, the presence of wounds may affect immune factors, and patients may not be keen to discuss research at these times. Despite these difficulties, there have been reports of cytokine changes that occur in relation to trauma, such as motor vehicle accidents. In one such study it was found that within the first 24 hours after the accident, IL-6 levels were higher in children that sustained physical or emotional injury than in control participants (Pervanidou *et al.*, 2008), whereas cortisol was elevated only in children that sustained physical injury. Interestingly, those children with the highest IL-6 levels were most likely to subsequently develop PTSD (Pervanidou *et al.*, 2007). It still remains to be established whether circulating IL-6 levels are a reliable biomarker of later PTSD development, but it does seem that plasma levels of this cytokine are exquisitely sensitive to stressors, and could potentially serve in this capacity (although the argument could be made that IL-6 is actually too sensitive to stressors and might thus not distinguish between subtle factors that would be important in predicting later pathology).

Another approach to assess cytokine levels in relation to stressors involves measuring these cytokines immediately prior to an anticipated aversive event (or after the event) relative to that evident at the same time of day, but during a more quiescent period. In effect, one takes advantage of the knowledge of an impending stressor in a natural setting, but one that allows for enhanced experimental control of the situation (as much as it can be). Using this approach, for instance, it was reported that among patients with rheumatoid arthritis who were to undergo total knee or hip arthroplasties (blood was drawn when patients were already on the operating table, but prior to the anesthetic being administered), the levels of IL-6 and cortisol were elevated relative to that evident 24 hours earlier, and declined 30 minutes following the anaesthetic being administered (Hirano, Nagashima, Ogawa, and Yoshino, 2001). Along the same lines, it was reported that perceived stress, anxiety, and mood disturbance among women who were to have breast biopsies were elevated relative to those behavioral and mood changes seen previously. These mood alterations were accompanied by reduced natural killer (NK) cell activity and IFN-γ production as well as increased levels of the anti-inflammatory cytokines IL-4 and IL-10, and that of the pro-inflammatory IL-6. These cytokine variations were evident irrespective of the cancer diagnosis, and, remarkably, persisted for at least a month (Witek-Janusek, Gabram, and Mathews, 2007).

In line with these findings, it was reported that men who received two sessions of stress management training prior to prostatectomy exhibited higher levels of NK cell cytotoxicity and IL-1β levels than they had one month earlier, as well as higher IL-1β levels than those of men in a standard care group (Cohen *et al.*, 2011). Predictably, these patients also exhibited superior mood scores than did those that had not received the stress management training. Once more, these data point to a link between psychological wellbeing and immune and cytokine variations, and importantly, they indicate that cytokine levels are modifiable on the basis of an individual's ability to deal with the stressor.

Individual Difference Factors that Influence Stress Responses

The point was made earlier that the effects of stressors on various behavioral and biological outcomes are moderated by factors related to how individuals appraise and cope with stressful events, as well as a constellation of personality variables and previous stressor experiences. In this regard, it has been shown that in a laboratory context, stressor controllability was related to plasma IL-6 changes (Peters *et al.*, 1999). In a naturalistic setting, the response to stressors among elderly caregivers varied as a function of the interaction between perceived self-efficacy and stress experiences. When self-efficacy was low, stressful experiences were related to elevated IL-6 levels, but this cytokine was not elevated in association with stressor experiences among individuals who reported high self-efficacy (Mausbach *et al.*, 2011). Similarly, among men, job stress (quantitative workload, mental demand) and positive coping styles were related to higher IFN-γ and IL-4, whereas in the presence of low job demands the levels of these cytokines were also low (Sakami *et al.*, 2004). It was also observed that with increasing levels of stress among breast cancer patients, levels of NKCA and IFN-γ were diminished. However, these low levels of NK cell activity were not apparent among those women who were found to exhibit high levels of dispositional optimism (Von Ah, Kang, and Carpenter, 2007).

Not only do stressors influence circulating cytokine levels, it seems that factors that reduce distress, including those related to altering appraisals of stressors, were found to diminish stress responses. In this regard, a prospective analysis revealed that breast cancer patients who engaged in increased social activities or who expressed satisfaction with these activities, displayed higher levels of mitogen-stimulated lymphocyte activity than those who did not have social resources available to them (Marucha, Crespin, Shelby, and Andersen, 2005). Likewise, cognitive behavioral therapy and mindfulness training for pain associated with rheumatoid arthritis improved coping abilities, and promoted reductions of IL-6 that were not evident in patients who simply received education related to their illness (Zautra *et al.*, 2008). It was similarly observed that among women newly diagnosed with breast cancer, low levels of blood NK cell activity and IFN-γ production were present, whereas IL-4, IL-6, and IL-10 production and plasma cortisol levels were high. While immune disturbances persisted in women who did not receive any stress reduction training, among those who engaged in mindfulness-based stress reduction, NK cell activity and cytokines reverted to normal levels (Witek-Janusek *et al.*, 2008). Paralleling such findings, it was reported that among women recruited 4–8 weeks after breast cancer surgery, cognitive behavioral stress management intervention resulted in psychosocial adaptation, reflected by both lower reported cancer-specific anxiety by patients and by interviewer-rated general anxiety symptoms. Significantly, these anxiety changes were also accompanied by several changes of neuroendocrine and immune functioning. Specifically, relative to a control condition, among these women, cortisol levels were lower and interleukin-2 and interferon-γ production was elevated (Antoni *et al.*, 2009). Once again, these data speak to the link between stress-related mood changes and cytokine levels, and point to the fact that these immune changes are affected by cognitive behavioral stress management procedures.

Summary

One of the best known characteristics of the stress response in humans is that it varies appreciably across individuals. They might appraise stressors differently, and exhibit varied ways of coping with adverse events; variations in emotional responses are common. Moreover, at least some of these emotional responses are linked to neuroendocrine changes associated with certain stressful situations: this occurs within both a laboratory context and within natural settings. Thus, in assessing the impact of stressors on biological substrates it might be advantageous to assess these in the context of stressors that are relevant to the individual, considering several variables that are cogent in determining the emotional responses elicited. There has, in recent years, been an effort to promote individualized treatment in relation to psychopathology wherein treatments are administered on the basis of behavioral symptoms presented together with the presence of particular biomarkers. It is reasonable to expect that research regarding the impact of stressors would endorse a similar individualized strategy that aims to define the conditions under which stressors elicit different types or degrees of responsivity. In this regard, however, it might not only be important to consider just individual difference characteristics, but also earlier stressor experiences (both acute and chronic), as well as the specific characteristics of the stressor, their appraisals, and the emotions that they elicit.

Acknowledgements

The author's research is supported by grants from the Canadian Institutes of Health Research. HA holds a Canada Research Chair in Neuroscience.

References

Anisman, H., and Matheson, K. (2005). Anhedonia and depression: Caveats concerning animal models. *Neuroscience and Biobehavioral Reviews*, 29, 525–546.

Anisman, H., Merali, Z., and Hayley, S. (2008). Neurotransmitter, peptide and cytokine processes in relation to depressive disorder: Comorbidity of depression with neurodegenerative disorders. *Progress in Neurobiology*, 85, 1–74.

Anisman, H., Hayley, S., and Merali, Z. (2003). Sensitization associated with stressors and cytokine treatments. *Brain, Behavior, Immunity*, 17, 86–93.

Antoni, M., Lechner, S., Diaz, A., Vargas, S., Holley. H., and Phillips, K. (2009). Cognitive behavioral stress management effects on psychosocial and physiological adaptation in women undergoing treatment for breast cancer. *Brain, Behavior, Immunity*, 23, 580–591.

Blackhart, G.C., Eckel, L.A., and Tice, D.M. (2007). Salivary cortisol in response to acute social rejection and acceptance by peers. *Biological Psychology*, 75, 267–276.

Brydon, L., Strike, P., Bhattacharyya, M., Whitehead, D., McEwan, J., Zachary, I., and Steptoe, A. (2010). Hostility and physiological responses to laboratory stress in acute coronary syndrome patients. *Psychosomatic Research*, 68, 109–116.

Buske-Kirschbaum, A., Kern, S., Ebrecht, M., and Hellhammer, D. (2007). Altered distribution of leukocyte subsets and cytokine production in response to acute psychosocial stress in patients with psoriasis vulgaris. *Brain, Behavior, Immunity*, 21, 92–99.

Carpenter, L., Gawuga, C., Tyrka, A., Lee, J., Anderson, G., and Price, L. (2010). Association between plasma IL-6 response to acute stress and early-life adversity in healthy adults. *Neuropsychopharmacology*, 35, 2617–2623.

Carroll, J., Low, C., Prather, A., Cohen, S., Fury, J., Ross, D., and Marsland, A. (2011). Negative affective responses to a speech task predict changes in interleukin (IL)-6. *Brain, Behavior, Immunity*, 25, 232–238.

Cohen, L., Parker, P., Vence, L., Savary, C., Kentor, D., Pettaway, C., Babaian, R., Pisters, L., Miles, B., Wei, Q., Wiltz, L., Patel, T., and Radvanyi, L. (2011). Presurgical stress management improves postoperative immune function in men with prostate cancer undergoing radical prostatectomy. *Psychosomatic Medicine*, 73, 218–225.

Danielson, A., Matheson, K., and Anisman, H. (2011). Cytokine levels at a single time point following a reminder stimulus among women in abusive dating relationships: Relationship to emotional states. *Psychoneuroendocrinology*, 36, 40–50.

Dickerson, S., and Kemeny, M. (2004). Acute stressors and cortisol responses: a theoretical integration and synthesis of laboratory research. *Psychological Bulletin*, 130, 355–391.

Dominguez-Rodriguez, A., Abreu-Gonzalez, P., and Kaski, J. (2009). Inflammatory systemic biomarkers in setting acute coronary syndromes – effects of the diurnal variation. *Current Drug Targets*, 10, 1001–1008.

Eisenberger, N.I. (2012).The neural bases of social pain: evidence for shared representations with physical pain. *Psychosomatic Medicine*, 74, 126–135.

Eisenberger, N.I., Inagaki, T.K., Rameson, L.T., Mashal, N.M., and Irwin, M.R. (2009). An FMRI study of cytokine-induced depressed mood and social pain: the role of sex differences. *Neuroimage*, 47, 881–890.

Eisenberger, N.I., Lieberman, M.D., and Williams, K.D. (2003). Does rejection hurt? An FMRI study of social exclusion. *Science*, 302, 290–292.

Eisenberger, N.I., Taylor, S.E., Gable, S.L., Hilmert, C.J., and Lieberman, M.D. (2007). Neural pathways link social support to neuroendocrine stress responses. *Neuroimage*, 35, 1601–1612.

Foley, P., and Kirschbaum, C. (2010). Human hypothalamus–pituitary–adrenal axis responses to acute psychosocial stress in laboratory settings. *Neuroscience and Biobehavioral Reviews*, 35, 91–96.

Ford, M.B., and Collins, N.L. (2010). Self-esteem moderates neuroendocrine and psychological responses to interpersonal rejection. *Journal of Personality and Social Psychology*, 98, 405–419.

Gaab, J., Rohleder, N., Heitz, V., Engert, V., Schad, T., Schürmeyer, T., and Ehlert, U. (2005). Stress-induced changes in LPS-induced pro-inflammatory cytokine production in chronic fatigue syndrome. *Psychoneuroendocrinology*, 30, 188–98.

Haack, M., Kraus, T., Schuld, A., Dalal, M., Koethe, D., and Pollmächer, T. (2002). Diurnal variations of Interleukin-6 plasma levels are confounded by blood drawing procedures. *Psychoneuroendocrinology*, 27, 921–931.

Hirano, D., Nagashima, M., Ogawa, R., and Yoshino, S. (2001). Serum levels of Interleukin 6 and stress related substances indicate mental stress condition in patients with rheumatoid arthritis. *Rheumatology*, 28, 490–495.

Kirschbaum, C., and Hellhammer, D. (1994). Salivary cortisol in psychoneuroendocrine research: recent developments and applications. *Psychoneuroendocrinology*, 19, 313–333.

Lazarus, R., and Folkman, S. (1984). *Stress, Appraisal, and Coping*. New York: Springer.

Lupien, S., Parent, S., Evans, A., Tremblay, R., Zelazo, P., Corbo, V., Pruessner, J.C., and Séguin, J. (2011). Larger amygdala but no change in hippocampal volume in 10-year-old children exposed to maternal depressive symptomatology since birth. *Proceedings of the National Academy of Sciences of the USA*, 108, 14324–14329.

Marucha, P., Crespin, T., Shelby, R., and Andersen, B. (2005). TNF-alpha levels in cancer patients relate to social variables. *Brain, Behavior, Immunity*, 19, 521–525.

Masten, C.L., Eisenberger, N.I., Borofsky, L.A., Pfeifer, J.H., McNealy, K., Mazziotta, J.C., and Dapretto, M. (2009). Neural correlates of social exclusion during adolescence: understanding the distress of peer rejection. *Social Cognitive and Affective Neuroscience*, 4, 143–157.

Master, S., Amodio, D., Stanton, A., Yee, C., Hilmert, C., and Taylor, S. (2009). Neurobiological correlates of coping through emotional approach. *Brain, Behavior, Immunity*, 23, 27–35.

Matheson, K., and Anisman, H. (2011). Biological and psychosocial responses to discrimination. In J. Jetten, A. Haslam, and C. Haslam (Eds.). *The Social Cure* (pp. 133–154). New York: Psychology Press.

Mausbach, B., Von Känel, R., Roepke, S., Moore, R., Patterson, T., Mills, P., Dimsdale, J., Ziegler, M., Ancoli-Israel, S., Allison, M., and Grant, I. (2011). Self-efficacy buffers the relationship between dementia caregiving stress and circulating concentrations of the proinflammatory cytokine Interleukin-6. *American Journal of Geriatric Psychiatry*, 19, 64–71.

McEwen, B. (2000). Allostasis and allostatic load: implications for neuropsychopharmacology. *Neuropsychopharmacology*, 22, 108–124.

Michaud, K., Matheson, K., Kelly, O., and Anisman, H. (2008). Impact of stressors in a natural context on release of cortisol in healthy adult humans: a meta-analysis. *Stress Amsterdam*, 11, 177–197.

Pace, T., Mletzko, T., Alagbe, O., Musselman, D., Nemeroff, C., Miller, A., and Heim, C. (2006). Increased stress-induced inflammatory responses in male patients with major depression and increased early life stress. *American Journal of Psychiatry*, 163, 1630–1633.

Pervanidou, P., Kolaitis, G., Charitaki, S., Margeli, A., Ferentinos, S., Bakoula, C., Lazaropoulou, C., Papassotiriou, I., Tsiantis, J., and Chrousos, G. (2007). Elevated morning serum Interleukin (IL)-6 or evening salivary cortisol concentrations predict posttraumatic stress disorder in children and adolescents six months after a motor vehicle accident. *Psychoneuroendocrinology*, 32, 991–999.

Pervanidou, P., Margeli, A., Lazaropoulou, C., Papassotiriou, I., and Chrousos, G. (2008). The immediate and long-term impact of physical and/or emotional stress from motor vehicle accidents on circulating stress hormones and adipo-cytokines in children and adolescents. *Stress*, 11, 438–447.

Peters, M., Godaert, G., Ballieux, R., Brosschot, J., Sweep, F., Swinkels, L., Van Vliet, M., and Heijnen, C. (1999). Immune responses to experimental stress: Effects of mental effort and uncontrollability. *Psychosomatic Medicine*, 61, 513–524.

Pollmächer, T., Mullington, J., Korth, C., Schreiber, W., Hermann, D., Orth, A., Galanos, C., and Holsboer, F. (1996). Diurnal variations in the human host response to endotoxin. *Journal of Infectious Diseases*, 174, 1040–1045.

Post, R. (1992). Transduction of psychosocial stress into the neurobiology of recurrent affective disorder. *American Journal of Psychiatry*, 149, 999–1010.

Raspopow, K., Abizaid, A., Matheson, K., and Anisman, H. (2010). Psychosocial stressor effects on cortisol and ghrelin in emotional and non-emotional eaters: Influence of anger and shame. *Hormones and Behavior*, 58, 677–684.

Rief, W., Mills, P., Ancoli-Israel, S., Ziegler, M., Pung, M., and Dimsdale, J. (2010). Overnight changes of immune parameters and catecholamines are associated with mood and stress. *Psychosomatic Medicine*, 72, 755–762.

Sakami, S., Maeda, M., Maruoka, T., Nakata, A., Komaki, G., and Kawamura, N. (2004). Positive coping up- and down-regulates in vitro cytokine productions from T cells dependent on stress levels. *Psychotherapy and Psychosomatics*, 73, 243–251.

Sapolsky, R., Romero, L., and Munck, A. (2000). How do glucocorticoids influence stress responses? Integrating permissive, suppressive, stimulatory, and preparative actions. *Endocrinology Reviews*, 21, 55–89.

Slavich, G.M., Thornton, T., Torres, L.D. Monroe, S.M., and Gotlib, I.H. (2009). Targeted rejection predicts hastened onset of major depression. *Journal of Social and Clinical Psychology*, 28, 223–243.

Slavich, G., Way, B., Eisenberger, N., and Taylor, S. (2010). Neural sensitivity to social rejection is associated with inflammatory responses to social stress. *Proceedings of the National Academy of Sciences of the USA*, 107, 14817–14822.

Stanton, A., and Franz, R. (1999). Focusing on emotion: an adaptive coping strategy? In C.R. Snyder (Ed.), *Coping. The Psychology of What Works* (pp. 90–118). New York: Oxford University Press.

Steptoe, A., Willemsen, G., Owen, N., Flower, L., and Mohamed-Ali, V. (2001). Acute mental stress elicits delayed increases in circulating inflammatory cytokine levels. *Clinical Science*, 101, 185–192.

Szyf, M. (2011). The early life social environment and DNA methylation; DNA methylation mediating the long-term impact of social environments early in life. *Epigenetics*, 6, 971–978.

Tops, M., Riese, H., Oldehinkel, A.J., Rijsdijk, F.V., and Ormel, J. (2008). Rejection sensitivity relates to hypocortisolism and depressed mood state in young women. *Psychoneuroendocrinology*, 33, 551–559

Von, Ah, Kang, D., and Carpenter, J. (2007). Stress, optimism, and social support: impact on immune responses in breast cancer. *Research in Nursing and Health*, 30, 72–83.

Von Känel, R., Kudielka, B., Preckel, D., Hanebuth, D., and Fischer, J. (2006). Delayed response and lack of habituation in plasma Interleukin-6 to acute mental stress in men. *Brain, Behavior, Immunity*, 20, 40–48.

Witek-Janusek, L., Albuquerque, K., Chroniak, K., Chroniak, C., Durazo-Arvizu, R., and Mathews, H. (2008). Effect of mindfulness based stress reduction on immune function, quality of life and coping in women newly diagnosed with early stage breast cancer. *Brain, Behavior, Immunity*, 22, 969–981.

Witek-Janusek, L., Gabram, S., and Mathews, H. (2007). Psychological stress, reduced NK cell activity, and cytokine dysregulation in women experiencing diagnostic breast biopsy. *Psychoneuroendocrinology*, 32, 22–35.

Yehuda, R. (2009). Status of glucocorticoid alterations in post-traumatic stress disorder. *Annals of the New York Academy of Sciences*, 1179, 56–69.

Zautra, A., Davis, M., Reich, J., Nicassario, P., Tennen, H., Finan, P., Kratz, A., Parrish, B., and Irwin, M. (2008). Comparison of cognitive behavioral and mindfulness meditation interventions on adaptation to rheumatoid arthritis for patients with and without history of recurrent depression. *Journal of Consulting and Clinical Psychology*, 76, 408–421.

Zwolinski, J. (2012). Psychological and neuroendocrine reactivity to ostracism. *Aggressive Behavior*, 38(2), 108–125.

13

Stress and Immune Function in Humans

A Life-Course Perspective

Jan A. Moynihan, Kathi L. Heffner, Mary T. Caserta, and Thomas G. O'Connor

Department of Psychiatry, University of Rochester, Medical Center, Rochester, NY, USA

Psychoneuroimmunology studies in humans have shown many of the same relationships that have long been observed in animal models, despite the significant variability inherent in the inability to control the genetics and environment of a pool of human subjects. Studies of *psychological stress* (as well as intervention studies aimed at ameliorating the stress) and immunity have provided the majority of the data illuminating the bidirectional communication between the central nervous system (CNS) and the immune system in humans. As has been shown in animal models, stress-induced changes in human immune responses are not only a function of trait individual differences, but are also a function of the previous history of the individual, the nature, intensity and chronicity of the stressor, and the individual's perception of the stressor as stressful. The aims of this chapter are to: a) review the emerging work on PNI in pediatric samples; b) to discuss PNI and how it relates to aging and immunosenescence; and c) to examine candidate mechanisms accounting for the links between stress and compromised immune function that have been widely reported in older adults, but less studied in children and adolescents.

Early Childhood Stress and Inflammation

The sum of a lifetime of stressors may predispose an individual to immunologic dysregulation, such as is observed in individuals with high allostatic load, a term coined by McEwen and colleagues (McEwen, 1998). Allostatic load refers to the persistent activation of bodily systems that results from repeated or prolonged exposure to stressors, and leads to a state of chronic inflammation, with elevated levels of pro-inflammatory cytokines, particularly interleukin (IL)-6, and the acute phase reactant C-reactive protein (CRP). While allostatic load may be most evident in older adults, the wear and tear provoked by stressors may begin accumulating in childhood and has been reported in young adults. Numerous studies show that childhood stresses are associated with many of the common inflammatory diseases of aging in adulthood, including cardiovascular disease, diabetes, and metabolic syndrome, as well as specific markers

The Wiley-Blackwell Handbook of Psychoneuroimmunology, First Edition. Edited by Alexander W. Kusnecov and Hymie Anisman.

of inflammation. For example, in a longitudinal-prospective study, Danese *et al.* (2009) found that childhood maltreatment predicted low-grade inflammation (increased CRP) by age 32, even after controlling for co-occurring childhood risks, health-damaging behaviors, and indicators of adult stress. Among adults *without* physical and mental health symptoms, Carpenter *et al.* (2010) observed that histories of childhood maltreatment predicted greater IL-6 acute release and concentrations over time in response to a social stress test, and Kiecolt-Glaser *et al.* (2011) recently observed that childhood abuse was associated with increased levels of circulating IL-6 and tumor necrosis factor (TNF)-α levels in older adults.

There are three main unresolved developmental questions from this work. The first is that research has not yet established that stress exposures in childhood have immediate-term effects. That is, childhood adversities are widely reported to be associated with adult illness, but we do not yet know if the characteristic signs and symptoms of stress on the immune system have a childhood onset. It may be that the effects of the wear and tear on the body's immune system and physiology are evident only after prolonged exposure. A second, related question has to do with the timing of exposure of stresses. It is as yet not clear that there is anything particular about *early* exposure to stress, if it is the persistence of exposure throughout childhood, or whether it is the more immediate stress context that is most predictive of changes in immune outcomes. Studies in rats (Meaney, 2010) show that early variations in maternal care are associated with stable epigenetic changes in glucocorticoid receptor gene expression in the hippocampus of rat pups, affecting their behavior and stress responsivity as adults, and data indicate that early child maltreatment is associated with similar epigenetic changes in post-mortem brains of suicide completers (McGowan *et al.*, 2009). These findings would suggest that early childhood is, then, a period of particular sensitivity to the effects of environment on the maturation of brain regions and neural circuitries – with downstream consequences for the immune system. It is tempting to conclude that there may be a parallel sensitive period in human development – such a notion is found in the burgeoning research on developmental programming, for example – but inferences about developmental timing of exposure across species are especially dubious. This underscores the need for developmental research on PNI that integrates pediatric samples.

A third development question for research on PNI is whether or not the same mechanisms operating in the adult (model) extend to pediatric samples. For instance, we reported, in an ambulatory sample of 5–10-year-olds assessed on seven occasions, that parental psychiatric symptoms predicted *enhanced* natural killer (NK) cell function independent of recent illnesses. That latter finding hints that there may be, in early development, activation of the immune system in response to early stress that only later takes the form of downregulation. The implication is that research on PNI in adult and old-age samples would be informed by research on the mechanisms underlying PNI that occur much earlier in development.

In addition to changes in glucocorticoid receptor expression in the brain, cells of the immune system may also become cortisol resistant in response to chronic stress-induced production of cortisol by the adrenal cortex, thereby providing a mechanism for the link between stress and immune responses. That is, glucocorticoids can downregulate glucocorticoid receptor expression, and pro-inflammatory cytokines can activate transcription pathways that inhibit glucocorticoid receptor signaling. Indeed, Miller and colleagues (Miller and Chen 2010) have shown that over a period of 1.5 years, adolescent girls living in an environment marked by chronic family stress showed increasing production of IL-6 and associated glucocorticoid resistance that mirrored the inflammatory profile. Further, they have observed (Miller *et al.*, 2009) that dysregulated gene expression – favoring glucocorticoid receptor downregulation and elevated inflammatory cytokine levels – occurs in specific immune cell subtypes, specifically, plasmacytoid dendritic cells, monocytes (antigen presenting cells (APC)) and B-lymphocytes.

Additional lifetime stressors accrued after childhood may serve to further magnify these inflammatory processes, as noted by Kiecolt-Glaser and colleagues (Kiecolt-Glaser *et al.*, 2011). One meta-analysis found that childhood abuse conferred a risk for poor health outcomes in adults equal to the risk for poor psychological outcomes (Wegman and Stetler, 2009); among individual health outcomes, neurological, musculoskeletal, respiratory, cardiovascular, and gastrointestinal disorders (the majority with inflammatory/immunological bases) were most strongly associated with childhood abuse (effect sizes ranging from 0.37 to 0.94).

Despite the deleterious effects of early adversity discussed to this point, it is important to reiterate that there is significant variability in individual responses to stress, even stress as severe as early institutional rearing (e.g., O'Connor *et al.*, 2003). Accordingly, models and analyses examining stress–immune function links in children must attend to the multivariate nature of the mechanisms involved, including the possibility of protective factors. Specific protective factors such as maternal warmth, cognitive agency/efficacy, and support can moderate the effects of stress on stress physiology and immunity in children. For example, Caserta *et al.*, (2011) found children's higher self-efficacy to be associated with lower IL-6 concentrations, and in a study by Fuligni *et al.* (2009), role fulfillment moderated a link between family burden and IL-6 and CRP in children.

Inflammatory cytokines and depression

Inflammatory cytokines are not only associated with physical illness, but may play a role in mental illness as well. Over the last decade, studies provide the foundation for the prevailing theory that psychological distress has innate immunological underpinnings. At least some types of depression may be causally mediated by chronic increases in proinflammatory cytokines (Raison and Miller, 2011), which not only act as messengers to cells of the immune system, but also instruct the hypothalamus to initiate a robust constellation of depressive-like symptoms, including fever, fatigue, anhedonia, and decreased activity, originally known as "sickness behavior." Why some individuals and not others are particularly vulnerable to development of depressive symptoms in response to inflammatory cytokines such as IL-6 and interferon (IFN)-α is currently unknown.

Psychoneuroimmunology and Adaptive Immunity

In addition to central nervous system links with inflammation, there is a large literature exploring the bidirectional communication between the brain and the adaptive arm of the immune system in humans. In a seminal paper, Cohen, Tyrrell, and Smith (1991) showed that psychological stress was associated in a dose-dependent manner with increased risk of infection by respiratory viruses following deliberate nasal challenge with viruses.

Studies such as the Cohen "hotel studies," which require that subjects remain sequestered in a hotel for 7 days or more, are extremely costly and difficult to conduct. While the data they have provided have been central to our understanding of human PNI, an alternative approach is to study immune responses to vaccination in the "real world." One of the first human PNI vaccine studies was Glaser *et al.* (1992), which examined the responses of stressed medical students to the hepatitis B vaccine series (usually three immunizations). Approximately 21% of the students developed a protective antibody response after the initial immunization; notably these students reported significantly lower anxiety levels as captured by the Profile of Mood State (POMS) compared to the students who seroconverted (as defined by a greater than four-fold increase in titer) only after a second immunization.

A recent review of the adult literature (Powell *et al.*, 2011) concluded that chronic stressors are consistently associated with decreased antibody responses to vaccines. Although little is currently known about the immunological mechanisms underlying these reduced antibody titers in humans, in mouse model systems, the initial defect in the immune response appears to be the downregulation of antigen-presenting dendritic cells by stress-induced corticosteroids. *In vitro*, glucocorticoids interfere with dendritic cell processing, and presentation of viral antigens to cytotoxic $CD8^+$ T-cells, and likely would have the same effect on helper $CD4^+$ T-cell function and B-cell antibody production (Powell *et al.*, 2011).

The Neuroendocrine Stress Response and Immunity

In response to both physical and psychological stressors, there is an orchestrated neuroendocrine stress response. In this chapter, we will consider three hormones which have, over the course of decades, been shown not only to play important roles in stress physiology but to also have wide-ranging immunoregulatory properties: cortisol, catecholamines, and dehydroepiandrosterone (DHEA).

Following stress exposure, the adrenal cortex produces glucocorticoids, of which cortisol is the primary stress hormone secreted in humans. Other androgens can be released as well, including DHEA, an endogenous hormone that regulates activities of cortisol. In parallel, sympathetic activation results in release from the adrenal medulla of the catecholamines epinephrine (EP), and norepinephrine (NE) into the circulation. Together, cortisol and epinephrine upregulate glucose metabolism and cardiovascular activity to support fight or flight. Cortisol and catecholamines also modulate immune activity, whereas DHEA may serve to moderate these immunosuppressive affects, as DHEA antagonizes the effects of glucocorticoids.

Cortisol Glucocorticoids are well-known for their anti-inflammatory and immunosuppressive properties; we have already discussed the consequences of too much cortisol exposure and the development of glucocorticoid resistance in certain immune cell types. Cortisol can have powerful effects on the adaptive immune response, by inhibiting production of IL-12 (Elenkov, Chrousos, and Wilder, 2000), a major inducer of T helper (T_H)1 responses (which are critical for cell-mediated adaptive immunity) and also suppressing T_H1 cytokines directly, including production of IFN-γ and IL-2, and leaving intact or increasing production of T_H2 cytokines, including IL-4 and IL-10. As a result, glucocorticoids alter the T_H1/T_H2 balance, suppressing anti-viral immune effector functions and enhancing T_H2-induced production of immunoglobulin E (IgE).

DHEA Like cortisol, DHEA is secreted by the adrenal cortex in response to corticotrophin releasing hormone (CRH) and adrenocorticotropic hormone (ACTH) stimulation, and there is evidence that both pharmacological challenges and psychological stressors provoke increases in circulating and salivary levels of DHEA(S) in humans (Hazeldine, Arlt, and Lord, 2010). DHEA has direct effects on cytokine-producing monocytes and lymphocytes, and evidence suggests its potential role in reducing inflammation. *In vitro* studies with human peripheral blood mononuclear cells have shown that DHEA can upregulate production of IL-2, decrease production of IL-6, and augment cell-mediated cytotoxic responses to pathogens (reviewed by (Hazeldine, Arlt, and Lord, 2010)), although as is often the case, findings with IL-6 are somewhat mixed. In addition to direct effects of DHEA, the hormone may also affect inflammatory cytokine production indirectly through its suppressive effects on cortisol production (Hazeldine, Arlt, and Lord, 2010). In recent years, DHEA supplementation has been explored as an anti-aging therapy; despite mixed findings here as well, DHEA supplementation continues to be regarded as a promising approach to reduce age associated risks for inflammatory diseases.

Catecholamines Naïve human $CD4^+$ T-cells, T_H1 cells, and B-cells all express the β_2 adrenergic receptor (β_2 AR) but it is not clear if human T_H2 cells express the receptor. Kin and Sanders (2006) have elegantly reviewed findings from both non-human and human studies which show that the magnitude of a normal immune response in lymphoid tissues (which are innervated by sympathetic nervous system (SNS) fibers) appears to be dictated by the concentration of norepinephrine (the principal transmitter of the SNS) released after antigen exposure, which is a function of the degree of SNS innervation of lymphoid organs, and the level of receptor expression on immune cells. Activation of the SNS is generally associated with an anti-inflammatory response, although the effects on adaptive responses are mixed and may depend upon the antigen challenge.

Under basal conditions, epinephrine enhances lipopolysaccharide-induced production of the anti-inflammatory cytokine IL-10 by human monocytes, while inhibiting pro-inflammatory TNF-α and IL-12 (Elenkov, 2008), similar to norepinephrine. In contrast, *in vitro* studies indicate that both physiologic stress levels of glucocorticoids and epinephrine inhibit production of IL-12, the potent stimulator of T_H1 responses (Elenkov, 2008). Further, epinephrine and corticosteroids *in vitro* decrease T_H1 cytokine production and increase T_H2 cytokine production to a significantly greater degree than either adrenal hormone alone (Salicru, Sams, and Marshall, 2007).

Taken together, catecholamines, specifically epinephrine, play a role in both innate pro-inflammatory cytokine regulation, as well as adaptive T_H responses, and may act in concert with cortisol during stress to modulate cytokine activity. Indeed, hyporesponsiveness of the HPA axis *and* hyperresponsiveness of the sympathetic–adrenal–medullary (SAM) axis to psychological stress have been observed in patients with atopic dermatitis, a chronic inflammatory disease primarily mediated by T_H2 inflammatory responses (Buske-Kirschbaum *et al.*, 2002), further underscoring co-regulatory contributions of these stress hormones.

Acute stress and immune responses

In contrast to the concept of chronic stress and suppressed adaptive immunity, an acute stressor may have the opposite effect. Acute stressors will elicit a fight–flight response, resulting in a transient outpouring of epinephrine and norepinephrine by the sympathetic nervous system and cortisol by the adrenals. Although as with chronic stress, increases in proinflammatory IL-6 are observed following an acute laboratory stressor (Carpenter *et al.*, 2010), adaptive immune responses have been shown to be elevated by acute stress. Using a brief exercise (ergometer) task or a 45-minute mental arithmetic task, Edwards and colleagues (Edwards *et al.*, 2006) observed that women but not men in either acute stress group had significantly higher antibody responses to influenza vaccination at 4 and 20 weeks post-immunization compared to control subjects.

One of the more interesting and entertaining illustrations of the dynamic changes in immune response to acute stressors is a 1993 paper from Schedlowski and colleagues (Schedlowski, Jacobs, *et al.*, 1993). They monitored first time tandem parachutists from 2 hours prior to jumping to 1 hour after jumping out of the airplane. Not surprisingly, they observed a significant increase in epinephrine and norepinephrine during the jump, and cortisol was elevated shortly after jumping. Natural killer (NK) cell cytotoxicity in peripheral blood was significantly elevated immediately after the jump, but was then significantly decreased below their starting levels 1 hour after jumping; the changes were correlated with norepinephrine levels. Indeed, injection of catecholamines mimicked this stressor exposure, with circulating NK cell numbers elevated 5 minutes after injection, peaking 15 to 30 minutes postinjection, and declining to baseline values at 1 hour (Schedlowski, Falk, *et al.*, 1993).

Aging and Immunosenescence

Studies of the aged and aging provide important information about the ultimate consequences of a lifetime of stressors on the immune system, which controls longevity in the elderly (Pawelec, Larbi, and Derhovanessian, 2010). Immunosenescence has become the most common immunodeficiency state in humans, occurring in more than 30% of the community-dwelling elderly, and greater than 90% of elderly who are ill, taking medication, or residing in long-term care facilities (Shen, Kim, and Weksler, 1999). Immunosenescence is characterized by two major imbalances in healthy, normal immune function: a) a chronic inflammatory state; and b) a decline in adaptive immunity (Pawelec, Larbi, and Derhovanessian, 2010).

Neuroendocrine changes and aging

Immunosenescence may reflect tandem changes in neuroendocrine responses. We summarize aging-related changes in cortisol, DHEA and catecholamines which Straub and colleagues (Straub, Miller, Scholmerich, and Zietz, 2000) hypothesize set up a "vicious cycle of endocrinosenescence and immunosenescence," which is depicted in Figure 13.1.

Cortisol Evidence suggests that glucocorticoid levels remain constant throughout adulthood and may even increase, although observed diurnal increases may be more evident among distressed older adults (Bauer *et al.*, 2000). Other studies indicate higher nocturnal levels of cortisol among older compared to younger adults (Ferrari *et al.*, 2001), resulting in greater overall cortisol circulation across the diurnal cycle. Further, cortisol remains elevated relative to age-related declines in other adrenal hormones (Straub, Miller, Scholmerich, and Zietz, 2000).

Aging also appears to affect glucocorticoid output in response to HPA activation, although evidence is mixed and may depend on the source of activation as well as subject characteristics. Some psychological challenge studies support age-related increases in cortisol response (Kudielka, Buske-Kirschbaum, Hellhammer, and Kirschbaum, 2004), while others show no age differences (Rohleder *et al.*, 2002) or reduced responsiveness in older adults (Nicolson,

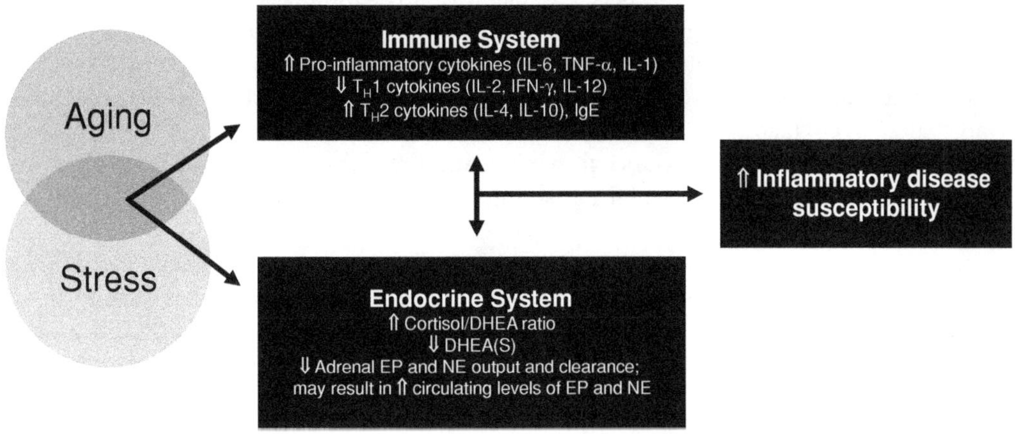

Figure 13.1 Aging and stress both impact endocrine and immune function, affecting regulation of inflammatory mediators and adrenal stress hormones. Stress-related dysregulation of these systems may combine with age-related dysregulation to render older adults particularly vulnerable to inflammatory disease. *Abbreviations*: IL, interleukin; TNF, tumor necrosis factor; T_H, T helper; Ig, immunoglobulin; DHEA(S), dehydroepiandrosterone (sulfate); EP, epinephrine; NE, norepinephrine.

Storms, Ponds, and Sulon, 1997). There are apparent gender differences, as well as other moderators of aging effects on cortisol response, such as fitness level. In a recent meta-analysis (Otte *et al.*, 2005), age had stronger effects on cortisol responses to pharmacological and psychosocial challenges in women compared to men. However, older men overall show larger cortisol responses to psychological stress compared to older women (Kudielka, Buske-Kirschbaum, Hellhammer, and Kirschbaum, 2004), a gender effect consistently observed across the age range. Mixed findings from stress reactivity studies comparing men versus women, and older and younger adults, may be due to a host of factors. For example, there is evidence that sex steroids, which, of course, vary by age and gender, modulate HPA reactivity (Kudielka, Buske-Kirschbaum, Hellhammer, and Kirschbaum, 2004). Further, different kinds of stressors (e.g., interpersonal versus cognitive) and other psychosocial factors (e.g., social environment) modulate cortisol reactivity differently in men versus women (Stroud, Salovey, and Epel, 2002), and older versus younger adults. Thus, the nature of the stressor used in research must be considered when interpreting age and gender differences.

DHEA Dehydroepiandrosterone (DHEA) and its inactive precursor, DHEA sulfate (DHEAS) are the most abundant adrenal steroid hormones in circulation in humans, and their steady decline with advancing age is a well-recognized pattern (Straub, Miller, Scholmerich, and Zietz, 2000). DHEA/DHEAS peak during the third decade of life, and by the end of the eighth decade are at 10–30% of peak levels (Ferrari *et al.*, 2001). In two studies, women showed less decline relative to men (Kahonen *et al.*, 2000; Tannenbaum, Barrett-Connor, Laughlin, and Platt, 2004), though Mazat *et al.* (2001) found greater decline in women. Older individuals show reduced DHEA secretion in response to ACTH stimulation compared to younger individuals (Parker, Mixon, Brissie, and Grizzle, 1997); however, little is known about stress-responsivity and DHEA(S) in aging.

Catecholamines The sympathetic nervous system (SNS) shows changes with as a function of age, higher basal circulating levels of NE are observed in older compared to younger men (Kudielka *et al.*, 2000). In contrast, EP output by the adrenal medulla under resting conditions was shown to decline with age (Esler *et al.*, 2002), whereas others had reported a slight decline or no change in circulating levels of EP with aging (Franco-Morselli *et al.*, 1977). However, age-related reductions in EP clearance from circulation can obscure interpretations about EP output by the adrenal medulla when measuring circulating catecholamine levels (Seals and Esler, 2000).

The same interpretation constraints may also contribute to mixed findings regarding age effects on sympathetic adrenal medullary (SAM) responses to stress. Adrenal catecholamine output in response to stress also appears to decline with age (Esler *et al.*, 2002; Seals and Esler, 2000). Again, however, age-related declines in catecholamine clearance may have led to the larger increases in circulating levels of NE observed in older relative to younger adults following physical and psychological stressors (Aslan, Nelson, Carruthers, and Lader, 1981). In addition, NE spillover from neuroeffector junctions into circulation increases with age (Seals and Esler, 2000); thus it is unclear whether circulating levels of NE are more a function of spillover or age-related changes in NE output by the adrenal medulla.

In sum, relatively little is known about the effects of age on SAM activity during stress, but evidence suggests there may be age-related differences in adrenal output and clearance of catecholamines. The health implications of these age-related changes remain to be determined.

Inflammation and aging

The low-level, chronic increase in the innate, inflammatory response observed in older adults ultimately results in tissue damage and disease; the key inflammatory mediators in this process are CRP, nuclear factor (NF)-κB, IL-1β, IL-6, TNF-α, cyclooxygenase-2 (COX-2), and inducible nitric oxide (NO) synthase (Chung *et al.*, 2002). As discussed previously, stress, including the stress of caring for a spouse with dementia (Bauer *et al.*, 2000), is associated with the development of resistance to the anti-inflammatory effects of glucocorticoids (Miller *et al.*, 2009; Miller and Chen, 2010). Further, glucocorticoid inhibition of IL-6 production was observed to be lower in older compared to younger men following psychological stress-induced HPA activation (Rohleder, Wolf, and Kirschbaum, 2003); treatment with testosterone diminished the age-related reduction in stress-induced glucocorticoid resistance.

Earlier in this chapter, we reviewed evidence that early adversity and chronic stress set the stage for the chronic inflammatory response observed in adults. Franceschi hypothesizes that the immune system itself contributes to this inflammation (Franceschi *et al.*, 2007). He suggests that chronic exposure to antigens, and in particular to viruses such as cytomegalovirus, for periods of time longer than that predicted by evolution, results in chronic, low grade inflammation, a term he has called "inflammaging." Thus, according to Franceschi, inflammation results from "...the fact that the most important network of defense of the body is overstimulated as a whole during aging." In addition to the notion of chronic inflammation, there is also evidence that a large expansion of late effector CMV-specific cells that are $CD8^+CD28^-CD57^+$ T-cells occurs at the expense of naïve cell pools – a process termed "memory inflation"; these memory cells are associated with poor response to other viral infections and immunization in the elderly (Waller, Day, Sissons, and Wills, 2008). Notably, Caserta *et al.* (2008) reported a significant association between parental psychiatric symptoms and the frequency of these

$CD8^+CD28^-CD57^+$ T-cells in a sample of CMV seropositive children, perhaps reflecting the beginning of the process of immunosenescence.

Inflammation and shortened telomeres As a result of inflammation, lymphocytes are induced to replicate faster, resulting in accelerated loss of telomere length, which is associated with cellular senescence or biological aging (reviewed in De Meyer, 2011). Shortened telomeres (the protective ends of chromosomes) have been observed in peripheral blood mononuclear cells from highly stressed populations; in one study, shorter telomeres and lower telomerase activity (the enzyme which adds DNA to the ends of chromosomes) were shown to be associated with increased concentrations of the stress hormones cortisol, epinephrine and norepinephrine in response to a laboratory stressor (Epel *et al.*, 2006).

It is noteworthy that signs of telomere attrition are not only observed in adult populations, but can also be observed in children. That is, in a study of 5- and 6-year-old kindergarten students (Kroenke *et al.*, 2011), those students who had evidence of high sympathetic activation, parasympathetic withdrawal, and high cortisol reactivity had shorter buccal cell telomere length (which is correlated with PBMC telomere length). Further, internalizing behaviors (associated with depressive symptoms and anxiety) in the children were also inversely related to telomere length.

Thus, accelerated aging of the cells of the immune system is a complex process involving psychological, physiological/endocrine, and inflammatory pathways. The shortening of telomeres, placing cells at risk for replicative senescence, may be the ultimate biological insult.

Adaptive immunity and aging

In contrast to the increased innate inflammatory response, acquired or antigen-specific immune function declines with age from adulthood to old age, and the hardest-hit immune effector function is cell-mediated immunity (Pawelec, Larbi, and Derhovanessian, 2010). T_H1 and T_H2 cytokines are mutually inhibitory, and, ideally, maintain a homeostatic equilibrium between cell-mediated and humoral responses (Amsen, Spilianakis, and Flavell, 2009). Aging, however, is associated with a decline in this equilibrium. T_H1 cytokine secretion declines with advancing age, especially impaired expression of IL-2, and there is a shift toward a greater T_H2 response (reviewed by Straub, Miller, Scholmerich, and Zietz, 2000). Along with the chronic elevation in proinflammatory cytokines, these T_H1–T_H2 cytokine shifts are linked to increased risk for or exacerbation of diseases of aging, including atherosclerosis, diabetes, osteoporosis, asthma, and autoimmunity (Franceschi *et al.*, 2007).

To illustrate the decline in specific immunity in the aged, we discuss studies that have compared immune responses to influenza vaccination in the elderly and young adults. Influenza-specific antibody titer, T-cell proliferation and cytokine production are significantly lower in the elderly (Murasko *et al.*, 2002). Further, compared to young adults there is a significant reduction in the percentage of elderly seroconverting after vaccination. It is estimated that a positive response to vaccination occurs in as low as 33% of elderly, compared to 70–90% of young–middle-aged adults (Murasko *et al.*, 2002; Ginaldi *et al.*, 2001). Not surprisingly, the risk of contracting influenza following immunization is greatest among seniors with poor antibody and cell-mediated immune responses (Murasko *et al.*, 2002). Most importantly, it is estimated that 90% of the deaths caused by influenza annually in the United States occur in seniors 65 and older (Ginaldi *et al.*, 2001).

Many factors influence the rate of decline of immune function; chief among these are genetics and environment, including health behaviors such as diet and exercise (van Loveren *et al.*, 2001). Prior research (Schulz *et al.*, 1996) suggests smaller associations between psychological variables, such as optimism or hope, and good health outcomes with increasing age. An alternative perspective suggests that perceived stress would have a more significant impact in older adults (Kiecolt-Glaser, McGuire, Robles, and Glaser, 2002), as their immune systems are already in decline, compared to healthy, middle-aged adults. With less "immunological reserve," it may take less stress, for example, to cause a deviation from immunological homeostasis in the elderly, amplifying the effects of stress on immune function. Just as the adverse effects of stress might become more pronounced with age, the beneficial effects of stress-reducing treatments might also increase across the lifespan.

Psychosocial Interventions and Immunological Outcomes

There is a growing literature on interventions to prevent the deleterious effects of stress on immune function, with interventions ranging from stress-reduction to exercise. In one study (Kiecolt-Glaser *et al.*, 1985), geriatric residents of independent-living facilities were randomly assigned to relaxation therapy, social support, or control groups. Relaxation therapy, but not the other two conditions, led to decreased distress and an increase in T-cell proliferation to the mitogen phytohemagglutinin. A brief intervention involving expressive writing about stressful life events also led to positive changes in immune function, including a decrease in overall rheumatoid arthritis disease activity in patients (Smyth, Stone, Hurewitz, and Kaell, 1999) and higher antibody responses to hepatitis B vaccine in medical students (Petrie *et al.*, 1995). Antoni and colleagues determined that cognitive behavioral therapy or relaxation/stress management for HIV-positive subjects was associated with reconstitution of relevant immune functions, including increases in naïve $CD4^+$ T-cells (Antoni *et al.*, 2002). These studies suggest that interventions aimed at patients with disease, a significant stress burden, or elderly individuals may confer significant benefit.

Irwin and colleagues have offered compelling support for the role of behavioral interventions in slowing the process of immunosenescence. They examined the effects of a 15-week Tai Chi Chih (TCC) program on cell-mediated immunity to varicella zoster virus (VZV) in volunteers (mean age of 70.9 years) (Irwin, Pike, Cole, and Oxman, 2003). In comparison to wait list controls, TCC participants showed greater increases in cell-mediated immunity to VZV and in health functioning (as measured by the Medical Outcomes Short Form (SF-36)). Consistent with the idea that interventions tend to benefit those in greatest need, effects were greatest in those subjects who reported the most impairment in physical functioning at recruitment. Further, Irwin and Olmstead (2011) recently observed that TCC reduced circulating levels of IL-6 most dramatically in the older adults who initially had the most elevated levels of the cytokine.

Finally, exercise has immune-enhancing effects, especially in older adults. In a study of influenza vaccine response, previously sedentary older adults who were randomized to cardiovascular exercise versus flexibility and balance training (both arms engaged in the activities 3 days/week) had longer-lasting seroprotection at 24 weeks post-vaccination (Woods *et al.*, 2009). Although reports of influenza infection did not differ between the two groups, the subjects who engaged in cardiovascular exercise had significantly reduced illness severity. In addition, the cardio group also reported less sleep disturbance, less fatigue and fewer headaches.

Exercise not only improves the antibody response to influenza vaccination, but can also decrease inflammation in older adults. Kohut *et al.* (2006) observed that cardiovascular exercise versus flexibility training (3 days/week, 45 minutes/day for 10 months) for previously sedentary older adults resulted in significant reductions in proinflammatory serum CRP, IL-6, and IL-18 even after adjustment for body mass index (BMI), which is positively associated with inflammatory cytokines and CRP. Psychosocial measures of depression, optimism and sense of coherence improved in both the cardiovascular exercise and flexibility groups, suggesting that the improvement in inflammation was not mediated by the psychological factors that were measured.

Given the controlling role of the immune system in health status and longevity, interventions that improve immune functioning are clearly desirable. Further, given that cardiovascular exercise decreases cardiovascular risk factors, including inflammation, obesity, hypertension, dyslipidemia and glucose intolerance, it would seem that older adults – even older adults with no history of exercise – should be encouraged to adopt a physically active lifestyle.

Conclusion

Human studies in psychoneuroimmunology underscore the multiple ways in which the bidirectional influence of the central nervous system and immune system impacts well-being. Further, human studies indicate that stress-induced changes in immune function – including shortened telomere length and increased inflammation – begin to accumulate in early childhood. There are individual differences which protect some people from the stressors and strains, and it will be important to better determine what those factors are, as well as to identify the biological mechanisms of protection and those at risk who might benefit from early behavioral interventions.

References

Amsen, D., Spilianakis, C.G., and Flavell, R.A. (2009). How are T(H)1 and T(H)2 effector cells made? *Current Opinion in Immunology*, 21, 153–160.

Antoni, M.H., Cruess, D.G., Klimas, N., Maher, K., Cruess, S., Kumar, M. et al. (2002). Stress management and immune system reconstitution in symptomatic HIV-infected gay men over time: effects on transitional naive T cells (CD4(+)CD45RA(+)CD29(+). *American Journal of Psychiatry*, 159 (1), 143–145.

Aslan, S., Nelson, L., Carruthers, M., and Lader, M. (1981). Stress and age effects on catecholamines in normal subjects. *Journal of Psychosomatic Research*, 25 (1), 33–41.

Bauer, M.E., Vedhara, K., Perks, P., Wilcock, G.K., Lightman, S.L., and Shanks, N. (2000). Chronic stress in caregivers of dementia patients is associated with reduced lymphocyte sensitivity to glucocorticoids. *Journal of Neuroimmunology*, 103 (1), 84–92.

Buske-Kirschbaum, A., Geiben, A., Hollig, H., Morschhauser, E., and Hellhammer, D. (2002). Altered responsiveness of the hypothalamus–pituitary–adrenal axis and the sympathetic adrenomedullary system to stress in patients with atopic dermatitis. *Journal of Clinical Endocrinology and Metabolism*, 87 (9), 4245–4251.

Carpenter, L.L., Gawuga, C.E., Tyrka, A.R., Lee, J.K., Anderson, G.M., and Price, L.H. (2010). Association between plasma IL–6 response to acute stress and early-life adversity in healthy adults. *Neuropsychopharmacology*, 35, 2617–2623.

Caserta, M.T., O'Connor, T.G., Wyman, P.A., Wang, H., Moynihan, J., Cross, W. et al. (2008). The associations between psychosocial stress and the frequency of illness, and innate and adaptive immune function in children. *Brain, Behavior, and Immunity*, 22 (6), 933–940. doi: 10.1016.

Caserta, M.T., Wyman, P.A., Wang, H., Moynihan, J., and O'Connor, T.G. (2011). Associations among depression, perceived self-efficacy and immune function and health in preadolescent children. *Development and Psychopathology*, 23 (4), 1139–1147

Chung, H.Y., Kim, H.J., Kim, K.W., Choi, J.S., and Yu, B.P. (2002). Molecular inflammation hypothesis of aging based on the anti-aging mechanism of calorie restriction. *Microscopy Research and Technique*, 59 (4), 264–272.

Cohen, S., Tyrrell, D.A.J., and Smith, A.P. (1991). Psychological stress and susceptibility to the common cold. *New England Journal of Medicine*, 325, 606–612.

Danese, A., Moffitt, T.E., Harrington, H., Milne, B.J., Polanczyk, G., Pariante, C.M. et al. (2009). Adverse childhood experiences and adult risk factors for age-related disease: depression, inflammation, and clustering of metabolic risk markers. *Archives of Pediatric and Adolescent Medicine*, 163, 1135–1143.

De Meyer, T. (2011). Telomere length integrates psychological factors in the successful aging story, but what about the biology? *Psychosomatic Medicine*, 73 (7), 524–527. doi: 10.1097.

Edwards, K.M., Burns, V.E., Reynolds, T., Carroll, D., Drayson, M., and Ring, C. (2006). Acute stress exposure prior to influenza vaccination enhances antibody response in women. *Brain, Behavior, and Immunity*, 20 (2), 159–168. doi: 10.1016.

Elenkov, I.J. (2008). Neurohormonal–cytokine interactions: implications for inflammation, common human diseases and well-being. *Neurochemistry International*, 52, 40–51.

Elenkov, I.J., Chrousos, G.P., and Wilder, R.L. (2000). Neuroendocrine regulation of IL-12 and TNF-alpha/IL-10 balance. Clinical implications. [Review]. *Annals of the New York Academy of Sciences*, 917, 94–105.

Epel, E.S., Lin, J., Wilhelm, F.H., Wolkowitz, O.M., Cawthon, R., Adler, N.E. et al. (2006). Cell aging in relation to stress arousal and cardiovascular disease risk factors. *Psychoneuroendocrinology*, 31 (3), 277–287.

Esler, M., Lambert, G., Kaye, D., Rumantir, M., Hastings, J., and Seals, D.R. (2002). Influence of ageing on the sympathetic nervous system and adrenal medulla at rest and during stress. *Biogerontology*, 3 (1–2), 45–49.

Ferrari, E., Cravello, L., Muzzoni, B., Casarotti, D., Paltro, M., Solerte, S.B. et al. (2001). Age-related changes of the hypothalamic–pituitary–adrenal axis: pathophysiological correlates. *European Journal of Endocrinology*, 144 (4), 319–329.

Franceschi, C., Capri, M., Monti, D., Giunta, S., Olivieri, F., Sevini, F. et al. (2007). Inflammaging and anti-inflammaging: a systemic perspective on aging and longevity emerged from studies in humans. *Mechanisms of Ageing and Development*, 128, 92–105.

Franco-Morselli, R., Elghozi, J.L., Joly, E., Di Giuilio, S., and Meyer, P. (1977). Increased plasma adrenaline concentrations in benign essential hypertension. *British Medical Journal*, 2 (6097), 1251–1254.

Fuligni, A.J., Telzer, E.H., Bower, J., Irwin, M.R., Kiang, L., and Cole, S.W. (2009). Daily family assistance and inflammation among adolescents from Latin American and European backgrounds. *Brain, Behavior, and Immunity*, 23 (6), 803–809. doi: 10.1016.

Ginaldi, L., Loreto, M.F., Corsi, M.P., Modesti, M., and De Martinis, M. (2001). Immunosenescence and infectious diseases. *Microbes and Infection*, 3, 851–857.

Glaser, R., Kiecolt-Glaser, J.K., Bonneau, R.H., Malarkey, W.B., Kennedy, S., and Hughes, J. (1992). Stress-induced modulation of the immune response to recombinant hepatitis B vaccine. *Psychosomatic Medicine*, 54, 22–29.

Hazeldine, J., Arlt, W., and Lord, J.M. (2010). Dehydroepiandrosterone as a regulator of immune cell function. *Journal of Steroid Biochemistry and Molecular Biology*, 120 (2–3), 127–136. doi: 10.1016.

Irwin, M.R., and Olmstead, R. (2011). Mitigating Cellular Inflammation in Older Adults: A Randomized Controlled Trial of Tai Chi Chih. *American Journal of Geriatric Psychiatry*, doi: 10.1097.

Irwin, M.R., Pike, J.L., Cole, J.C., and Oxman, M.N. (2003). Effects of a behavioral intervention, Tai Chi Chih, on varicella-zoster virus specific immunity and health functioning in older adults. *Psychosomatic Medicine*, 65 (5), 824–830.

Kahonen, M.H., Tilvis, R.S., Jolkkonen, J., Pitkala, K., and Harkonen, M. (2000). Predictors and clinical significance of declining plasma dehydroepiandrosterone sulfate in old age. *Aging (Milano)*, 12 (4), 308–314.

Kiecolt-Glaser, J.K., Glaser, R., Williger, D., Stout, J., Messick, G., Sheppard, S. et al. (1985). Psychosocial enhancement of immunocompetence in a geriatric population. *Health Psychology*, 4 (1), 25–41.

Kiecolt-Glaser, J.K., Gouin, J.P., Weng, N.P., Malarkey, W.B., Beversdorf, D.Q., and Glaser, R. (2011). Childhood adversity heightens the impact of later-life caregiving stress on telomere length and inflammation. *Psychosomatic Medicine*, 73, 16–22.

Kiecolt-Glaser, J.K., McGuire, L., Robles, T.F., and Glaser, R. (2002). Emotions, morbidity, and mortality: new perspectives from psychoneuroimmunology. *Annual Review of Psychiology*, 53, 83–107.

Kin, N.W., and Sanders, V.M. (2006). It takes nerve to tell T and B cells what to do. *J Leukocyte Biology*, 79 (6), 1093–1104.

Kohut, M.L., McCann, D.A., Russell, D.W., Konopka, D.N., Cunnick, J.E., Franke, W.D. et al. (2006). Aerobic exercise, but not flexibility/resistance exercise, reduces serum IL-18, CRP, and IL-6 independent of beta-blockers, BMI, and psychosocial factors in older adults. *Brain, Behavior, and Immunity*, 20 (3), 201–209.

Kroenke, C.H., Epel, E., Adler, N., Bush, N.R., Obradovic, J., Lin, J.et al. (2011). Autonomic and adrenocortical reactivity and buccal cell telomere length in kindergarten children. *Psychosomatic Medicine*, 73 (7), 533–540. doi: 10.1097.

Kudielka, B.M., Buske-Kirschbaum, A., Hellhammer, D.H., and Kirschbaum, C. (2004). HPA axis responses to laboratory psychosocial stress in healthy elderly adults, younger adults, and children: impact of age and gender. *Psychoneuroendocrinology*, 29 (1), 83–98.

Kudielka, B.M., Schmidt-Reinwald, A.K., Hellhammer, D.H., Schurmeyer, T., and Kirschbaum, C. (2000). Psychosocial stress and HPA functioning: no evidence for a reduced resilience in healthy elderly men. *Stress*, 3 (3), 229–240.

Mazat, L., Lafont, S., Berr, C., Debuire, B., Tessier, J.F., Dartigues, J.F., and Baulieu, E.E. (2001). Prospective measurements of dehydroepiandrosterone sulfate in a cohort of elderly subjects: relationship to gender, subjective health, smoking habits, and 10-year mortality. *Proceedings of the National Academy of Sciences of the USA*, 98 (14), 8145–8150. doi: 10.1073.

McEwen, B.S. (1998). Stress, adaptation, and disease. Allostasis and allostatic load. [Review]. *Annals of the New York Academy of Sciences*, 840, 33–44.

McGowan, P.O., Sasaki, A., D'Alessio, A.C., Dymov, S., Labonte, B., Szyf, M. et al. (2009). Epigenetic regulation of the glucocorticoid receptor in human brain associates with childhood abuse. *Nature Neuroscience*, 12, 342–348.

Meaney, M.J. (2010). Epigenetics and the biological definition of gene x environment interactions. *Child Development*, 81, 41–79.

Miller, G.E., and Chen, E. (2010). Harsh family climate in early life presages the emergence of a proinflammatory phenotype in adolescence. *Psychological Science*, 21, 848–856.

Miller, G.E., Chen, E., Fok, A.K., Walker, H., Lim, A., Nicholls, A.F. et al. (2009). Low early-life social class leaves a biological residue manifested by decreased glucocorticoid and increased proinflammatory signaling. *Proceedings of the National Academy of Sciences of the USA*, 106, 14716–14721.

Murasko, D.M., Bernstein, E.D., Gardner, E.M., Gross, P., Munk, G., Dran, S., and Abrutyn, E. (2002). Role of humoral and cell-mediated immunity in protection from influenza disease after immunization of healthy elderly. *Experimental Gerontology*, 37 (2–3), 427–439.

Nicolson, N., Storms, C., Ponds, R., and Sulon, J. (1997). Salivary cortisol levels and stress reactivity in human aging. *Journal of Gerontology Series A: Biological Sciences and Medical Sciences*, 52 (2), M68–75.

O'Connor, T.G., Marvin, R.S., Rutter, M., Olrick, J.T., and Britner, P.A. (2003). Child–parent attachment following early institutional deprivation. *Developmental Psychopathology*, 15 (1), 19–38.

Otte, C., Hart, S., Neylan, T.C., Marmar, C.R., Yaffe, K., and Mohr, D.C. (2005). A meta-analysis of cortisol response to challenge in human aging: importance of gender. *Psychoneuroendocrinology*, 30 (1), 80–91. doi: 10.1016/j.

Parker, C.R., Jr, Mixon, R.L., Brissie, R.M., and Grizzle, W.E. (1997). Aging alters zonation in the adrenal cortex of men. *Journal of Clinical Endocrinology and Metabolism*, 82 (11), 3898–3901.

Pawelec, G., Larbi, A., and Derhovanessian, E. (2010). Senescence of the human immune system. *Journal of Comparative Pathology*, 142 Suppl 1, S39–S44.

Petrie, K.J., Booth, R.J., Pennebaker, J.W., Davison, K.P., and Thomas, M.G. (1995). Disclosure of trauma and immune response to a hepatitis B vaccination program. *J Consulting and Clinical Psychology*, 63 (5), 787–792.

Powell, N.D., Allen, R.G., Hufnagle, A.R., Sheridan, J.F., and Bailey, M.T. (2011). Stressor-induced alterations of adaptive immunity to vaccination and viral pathogens. *Immunology and Allergy Clinics of North America*, 31 (1), 69–79. doi: 10.1016.

Raison, C.L., and Miller, A.H. (2011). Is Depression an Inflammatory Disorder? *Current Psychiatry Reports*, 13 (6), 467–475. doi: 10.1007/s11920-011-0232-0.

Rohleder, N., Kudielka, B.M., Hellhammer, D.H., Wolf, J.M., and Kirschbaum, C. (2002). Age and sex steroid-related changes in glucocorticoid sensitivity of pro-inflammatory cytokine production after psychosocial stress. *Journal of Neuroimmunology*, 126 (1–2), 69–77.

Rohleder, N., Wolf, J.M., and Kirschbaum, C. (2003). Glucocorticoid sensitivity in humans – interindividual differences and acute stress effects. *Stress*, 6 (3), 207–222. doi: 10.1080.

Salicru, A.N., Sams, C.F., and Marshall, G.D. (2007). Cooperative effects of corticosteroids and catecholamines upon immune deviation of the type-1/type-2 cytokine balance in favor of type-2 expression in human peripheral blood mononuclear cells. *Brain, Behavior, and Immunity*, 21, 913–920.

Schedlowski, M., Falk, A., Rohne, A., Wagner, T.O., Jacobs, R. et al. (1993). Catecholamines induce alterations of distribution and activity of human natural killer (NK) cells. *Journal of Clinical Immunology*, 13, 344–351.

Schedlowski, M., Jacobs, R., Alker, J., Prohl, F., Stratmann, G., Richter, S. et al. (1993). Psychophysiological, neuroendocrine and cellular immune reactions under psychological stress. *Neuropsychobiology*, 28, 87–90.

Schulz, R., Bookwala, J., Knapp, J.E., Scheier, M.F., and Williamson, G.M. (1996). Pessimism, age, and cancer mortality. *Psychology and Aging*, 11, 304–309.

Seals, D.R., and Esler, M.D. (2000). Human ageing and the sympathoadrenal system. *Journal of Physiology*, 528 (Pt 3), 407–417.

Shen, S.S., Kim, J.S. and Weksler, M.E. (1999). Effect of age on thymic development, T cell immunity, and helper T cell function. [Review]. *Reviews of Physiology, Biochemistry & Pharmacology*, no 139, 123–139.

Smyth, J.M., Stone, A.A., Hurewitz, A., and Kaell, A. (1999). Effects of writing about stressful experiences on symptom reduction in patients with asthma or rheumatoid arthritis: a randomized trial.[comment]. *Journal of the American Medical Association*, 281 (14), 1304–1309.

Straub, R.H., Miller, L.E., Scholmerich, J., and Zietz, B. (2000). Cytokines and hormones as possible links between endocrinosenescence and immunosenescence. *Journal of Neuroimmunology*, 109 (1), 10–15.

Stroud, L.R., Salovey, P., and Epel, E.S. (2002). Sex differences in stress responses: social rejection versus achievement stress. *Bioogical Psychiatry*, 52 (4), 318–327.

Tannenbaum, C., Barrett-Connor, E., Laughlin, G.A., and Platt, R.W. (2004). A longitudinal study of dehydroepiandrosterone sulphate (DHEAS) change in older men and women: the Rancho Bernardo Study. *European Journal of Endocrinology*, 151 (6), 717–725.

van Loveren, H., Van Amsterdam, J.G., Vandebriel, R.J., Kimman, T.G., Rumke, H.C., et al. (2001). Vaccine-induced antibody responses as parameters of the influence of endogenous and environmental factors. *Environmental Health Perspectives*, 109 (8), 757–764.

Waller, E.C., Day, E., Sissons, J.G., and Wills, M.R. (2008). Dynamics of T cell memory in human cytomegalovirus infection. *Medical Microbiology and Immunology*, 197 (2), 83–96. doi: 10.1007.

Wegman, H.L., and Stetler, C. (2009). A meta-analytic review of the effects of childhood abuse on medical outcomes in adulthood. *Psychosomatic Medicine*, 71, 805–812.

Woods, J.A., Keylock, K.T., Lowder, T., Vieira, V.J., Zelkovich, W., Dumich, S. et al. (2009). Cardiovascular exercise training extends influenza vaccine seroprotection in sedentary older adults: the immune function intervention trial. *Journal of the American Geriatric Society*, 57 (12), 2183–2191. doi: 10.1111.

14

Predicting Health

The Role of the Early-Life Environment

Luba Sominsky,[1] Adam K. Walker,[2] and Deborah M. Hodgson[1]

[1] *Laboratory of Neuroimmunology, School of Psychology, Faculty of Science and IT, The University of Newcastle, New South Wales, Australia*
[2] *Integrative Immunology and Behavior Program, Department of Animal Sciences and Department of Medical Pathology, University of Illinois at Urbana–Champaign, Urbana, IL, USA*

Perinatal Programming

Who we become as a person in adulthood is typically considered to be a function of our environment – factors such as our parental, filial, and social relationships. In contrast, our physical appearance and health status are often thought to be biologically determined. What is becoming increasingly important to our understanding is the nature of the interaction between the environment and our biology, and how that impacts on all aspects of our lives. It is now clear that the distinction, between "nature" and "nurture," limits the degree to which we can understand the human condition. Indeed, we now know that we can view our biological composition as the pages on which the environment writes the script of our development. This interaction between the environment and our biology is the focus of ever-expanding research, which has indicated that the degree of influence the environment holds over biological and psychological development is dependent upon the timing of exposure and the nature of environmental events that we are exposed to. One period known to be particularly sensitive to environmental factors is the perinatal period, during which an organism is highly vulnerable, with many systems undergoing critical phases of development. An area of research which focuses on the impact of environmental stimuli at or around the time of birth is known as perinatal programming.

The sensitivity of organisms to environmental input during early development ensures that certain stimuli presented to the infant during this time can "set the tone" of functioning for many systems. This process has typically been referred to as "programming" in the literature. This is particularly important as the predisposition to certain diseases may originate from this early perinatal programming. While there is evolutionary value for fetal and neonatal biological systems to respond to environmental cues in preparation for the birth environment, and hence enhance survival probabilities, in some cases the outcomes are not adaptive. It

The Wiley-Blackwell Handbook of Psychoneuroimmunology, First Edition. Edited by Alexander W. Kusnecov and Hymie Anisman.

has been suggested that this maladaptive programming may lead to increased risk of disease in later life. The first person to formally present the potential for perinatal environmental factors to explain the causation of later life health- and disease-states was epidemiologist Professor David Barker. Barker proposed that adult disease states may have their origins in the early developmental period, and initially published findings showing that death by stroke was more closely correlated to maternal mortality than any other cause of death, suggestive that maternal health was closely linked to the risk of disease in their offspring (Barker and Osmond, 1987). His subsequent studies demonstrated relationships between low birth weight and high placental weight with increased adult systolic blood pressure (Barker *et al.*, 1989; Barker, Bull, Osmond, and Symmonds, 1990). Taken together, these data were the first to clearly connect the perinatal experience with later disease susceptibility, and eventually led to the ***developmental origins of health and disease*** (DOHaD) hypothesis. The DOHaD hypothesis provides a framework in which to understand human life-long development, stating that the long-term health or (susceptibility to) illness of an individual is strongly determined by the perinatal experiences of that individual (see Figure 14.1).

The mechanism underpinning the DOHaD hypothesis can be seen as perinatal programming, whereby environmental factors predispose to later health outcomes via a shift in the functional "tone" of physiological systems. Thus, the developing organism "senses" the early life environment and uses this information to systematically establish homeostatic set points (Davies and Norman, 2002; Welberg and Seckl, 2001). This involves the organization of specific tissues and gene expression to optimize environmental adaptedness (Meaney, Szyf, and Seckl, 2007). Environmental factors are both intracellular and extracellular, given that both exert demands on cell output (Maes *et al.*, 2009), and influence the development of whole organisms, systems, tissues, cells and molecules. Thus, programming persistently organizes and imprints the development of bodily systems, consequently influencing physiology and behavior.

The increased sensitivity of the perinatal organism to environmental inputs is due to its high degree of developmental plasticity. Plasticity refers to the way the brain and other tissues can

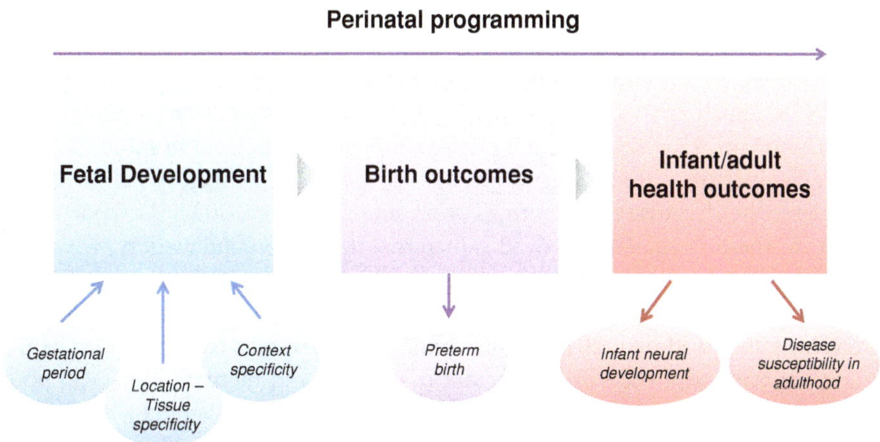

Figure 14.1 Developmental model of adult health and disease. The impact of early life environment on fetal development, birth outcomes and later life health status, via the process of perinatal programming.

modify their phenotype in response to environmental pressure. While environmental regulation of phenotype is a life-long process, development of neural and peripheral tissue occurs at an alarmingly high rate during early life, with each system demonstrating a critical period of enhanced sensitivity, after which the level of plasticity becomes more limited (Nelson, 2000). Hence, environmental factors can exert the greatest influence in perinatal life during these critical periods of development. Once these critical periods have passed, reversal of the established phenotype becomes more difficult, explaining how the early life environment can induce persistent changes in morphology and function.

Professor Barker demonstrated that early environmental factors can influence metabolic disease outcomes, and as such, there has been a great degree of research implicating the perinatal period in the predisposition to obesity, cancer, asthma, and reproductive diseases among others. More recently, the field has begun to address the impact the early environment has on the development of emotionality and behavior. In fact, stress or trauma during infancy is considered one of the largest risk factors for the development of psychiatric disorders, in particular affective disorders such as anxiety and depression. It is the role that the perinatal environment plays on later psychological outcomes that will be the focus of this chapter.

Predisposition to Psychopathology can Develop Early in Life

Stressful or traumatic events experienced during early life have been demonstrated to facilitate the onset of later-life psychopathologies, supportive of the notion that environmental factors during critical periods of development can set the tone of emotional and behavioral function. Epidemiological studies have reported that sexual, physical, and emotional abuse in childhood correlates with earlier onset and elevated severity of depression (Heim, Plotsky, and Nemeroff, 2004), with women being at higher risk than men (Weiss, Longhurst, and Mazure, 1999). For instance, women who have been exposed to some form of abuse in childhood are more likely to experience depressive and anxiety symptoms, as well as difficulties in interpersonal and sexual relations (Mullen *et al.*, 1996).

Abuse is typically more prominent in families from disadvantaged socioeconomic backgrounds. Social disadvantage is a significant burden in these families, and represents a source of consistent stress, which compromises emotional wellbeing of both parents and children (McLoyd, 1998). Such environmental adversity often hinders healthy parent–child interactions and attachments. Unstable parental relationships and household dysfunction are known to detrimentally affect psychological and physiological development in the child and increase the risk for later life depression (Rapetti, Taylor, and Seeman, 2002). A major contributor to instability for the maternal–infant dyad is maternal depression and anxiety, which dramatically reduces the quality of caregiving. Poor maternal care is associated, in the offspring, with increased stress and decreased immune competence, resulting in negative short- and long-term outcomes (Davis and Sandman, 2010; Essex *et al.*, 2002). Its long-term effect on neurodevelopment and behavior, and the subsequent risk of physical and mental illness, can potentially render similar patterns of parenting style in the second generation. Parents who were exposed to early traumatic or abusive experiences may exhibit anxious and unstable parenting behavior themselves (Main and Hesse, 1990). Examination of the long-term effects of extreme trauma among Holocaust survivors has also been shown to increase levels of psychological stress and impaired parental attachments in families of second- and third-generation offspring (Scharf, 2007).

These human findings have been supported by preclinical studies using animal models, which have shown that maternal care produces profound changes in infant biology that are proposed to be responsible for the enhanced predisposition to psychiatric illness in later life. Maternal separation in rodents, for instance, leads to altered neuroendocrine stress reactivity and increased anxiety-like behaviors in these offspring when they reach adulthood, corresponding with increased levels of corticotropin-releasing hormone (CRH) in the paraventricular nucleus (PVN), amygdala and locus coeruleus (Kalinichev, Easterling, Plotsky, and Holtzman, 2002; Plotsky *et al.*, 2005). Pivotal work from Michael Meaney's laboratory has demonstrated that poor maternal care in rats causes increased defensive responses and anxiety-like behavior, which results from non-genomic modulation of the hypothalamic–pituitary–adrenal (HPA) axis (Weaver *et al.*, 2004). The underlying mechanisms are proposed to include altered serotonin (5-HT) activity at 5-HT7 receptors as well as downregulation of glucocorticoid receptor (GR) density via hypomethylation of the CPG site on the exon 17 GR promoter. Importantly, these effects can be reversed by early postnatal cross-fostering (Weaver *et al.*, 2004).

Although psychological stress experienced in early life is clearly a substantial contributor to the development of later-life psychopathologies, another important factor, and the focus of this chapter, is exposure to immunological stressors. The multidimensional relationship between the peripheral immune system and the brain creates a potential pathway through which later-life physiological and behavioral alterations may occur.

The Early Microbial Environment as a Critical Factor in the Development of Mood and Behavior

The notion that the immune system plays a critical role in psychopathology is quite a new concept. The first convincing evidence emerged in the 1980s when it was observed that newly cloned recombinant cytokines that were administered to patients for therapeutic purposes could induce depressive-like symptoms and activate stress responses (Besedovsky, del Rey, Sorkin, and Dinarello, 1986; Sapolsky *et al.*, 1987). Many papers have since been published linking inflammation to the onset of depression, the focus of which is to be dealt with in other chapters of this book. What is of interest here is the relationship between the innate immune system during perinatal life with the onset of psychopathology in later life. To understand the progression of research within the framework of psychoneuroimmunology we must first acknowledge work that occurred prior to the 1980s outside this field.

It was in 1929 that the first epidemiological evidence emerged which some believe implicated the early microbial environment with the incidence of schizophrenia. Tramer (1929) reported that individuals born in the winter months were several-fold more likely to develop schizophrenia. This "seasonality of birth" observation has been replicated many times, and has been accounted for with many proposed explanations including vitamin D deficiency (Mackay-Sim *et al.*, 2004) and meteorological factors (Tochigi, Okazaki, Kato, and Sasaki, 2004). One proposed explanation for this phenomenon has been the viral hypothesis of schizophrenia, which proposes that the predisposition to schizophrenia may have viral roots, given that influenza and other viruses are common during winter months (Brown and Derkits, 2010). A large body of work has been devoted to studying this proposition; however, it was not until the co-emergence of clinical findings linking immunotherapies to depression in the 1980s that a paradigm was created in which the emerging areas of psychoneuroimmunology and DOHaD could exist together as a platform from which to study immune involvement in the development of psychopathology.

Clinical Studies

Since the emergence of PNI and DOHaD, numerous human studies have attempted to establish a link between prenatal or postnatal immune status with psychopathology. The findings of these studies have been strongly supportive, indicating the neurodevelopmental origin of psychopathologies. For instance, maternal infectious illnesses, including viral (e.g., influenza), bacterial (e.g., pneumonia) or parasitic-related (e.g., toxoplasmosis) diseases, are associated with an increased risk of schizophrenia and other psychosis-related disorders in the offspring. (Brown and Derkits, 2010). Higher incidences of psychiatric disorders were also demonstrated among children born to HIV-infected mothers (Gaughan *et al.*, 2004). Maternal reports of fever during the second-trimester were found to be associated with altered psychological and behavioral outcomes in children, such as negative emotionality, lack of task persistence and poor school achievements (Dombrowski, Martin, and Huttunen, 2003). Respiratory diseases in childhood predicted higher incidence of panic disorders in adulthood (Craske, Poulton, Tsao, and Plotkin, 2001). In addition, epidemiological evidence suggests a link between viral exposure during early life and the development of autism, although this still requires further verification (Libbey, Sweeten, McMahon, and Fujinami, 2005).

While revealing this association between the perinatal microbial environment and psychopathological development is valuable, human studies are often limited in their ability to target mechanisms owing to the ethical restraints of invasive procedures on humans. It is for this reason that preclinical experimentation on animals is required. Rodent studies allow researchers to examine biological mechanisms involved in the programming phenomenon. In the following section we will discuss the common preclinical models employed in examining the role of perinatal immune activation on psychopathology.

Preclinical Models of Perinatal Immune Activation and Psychopathology

Preclinical research on the neurobiology of psychopathology is typically employed both in the search for potential therapeutic agents and as a tool to investigate underlying mechanisms and pathways. The common view is that psychiatric disorders are characterized by a dysfunction of neuronal systems in both animals and humans. Animal models of psychopathology are not intended to present a complete animal equivalent of the human disorder, but rather focus on specific behaviors, and are usually designed to examine a certain causative or mechanistic hypothesis. Rodent models of anxiety are typically optimized to take advantage of avoidance of open spaces, risk assessment or hypervigilance, escape latencies, fear of novelty, reduced exploration, or habituation to fear-provoking stimuli. Behaviors assessed in rodents that are proposed to model to depressive symptoms are associated with anhedonia, learned helplessness and immobility, as well as loss of motivation, and reduced sexual interest and social decline.

Models of schizophrenia assess both anxiety and depressive-related behaviors but also utilize measures assessing cognitive performance including prepulse inhibition (PPI) and latent inhibition (LI).

Animal models examining the effects of early-life immunological stress on the development of psychopathology involve perinatal exposure to immune stimulators and later-life assessments of physiology and behavior. These models utilize administration of cytokines, bacterial and viral agents including mimetics, (e.g., lipopolysaccharide (LPS), polyinosinic:polycytidylic acid (poly I:C)), live reagents (e.g., *Escherichia coli (E. coli))*, and other agents, such as toxins (i.e., endotoxins and exotoxins). Both central and peripheral administration is employed, in order to target specific immune-related pathways involved in activation of neural systems responsible for generating behavioral outcomes. Prenatal and postnatal models of immune activation target different critical time points of development relevant to specific physiological and neural systems. The importance of these time-points will be discussed later.

Prenatal models of immune activation

Maternal immune activation in pregnant rodents typically induces behavioral abnormalities associated with symptoms of schizophrenia and autism. Administration of poly I:C, a viral mimetic, to pregnant dams on distinct gestational days has been repeatedly shown to modulate active avoidance learning, PPI and LI in adult offspring, reflecting a common endophenotype of schizophrenia. Prenatal immune stimulation increases amphetamine-induced locomotor activity in adulthood and produces histopathological abnormalities in the hippocampus and the entorhinal cortex, similar to the well-known mesolimbic dopaminergic and temporolimbic pathology in schizophrenia (Meyer, Feldon, and Yee, 2009; Smith, Hsiao, and Patterson, 2010; Zuckerman, Rehavi, Nachman, and Weiner, 2003). Rodent models utilizing perinatal immune challenge suggest that behavioral and neurodevelopmental abnormalities in the offspring are induced by the activation of the maternal immune system, such as increased levels of proinflammatory cytokines, rather than the infection per se. For instance, a single administration of interleukin 6 (IL-6) in pregnant mice has been reported to result in decreased PPI and LI in adult offspring, while administration of anti-IL-6 antibody in poly I:C-treated dams prevented the PPI and LI deficits. Maternal poly I:C administration in IL-6 knockout mice did not generate the above-mentioned behavioral changes, implicating IL-6 in the regulation of the behavioral symptoms of schizophrenia.

Activation of the immune system promotes HPA axis activation, and thus maternal immune stimulants can also result in changes in offspring behavior and physiology via exposure to elevated maternal glucocorticoids. Although the fetus is relatively protected from high maternal glucocorticoid levels by the placental enzyme 11β-hydroxysteroid hydroxylase, which converts active hydroxylated corticosteroids to inactive 11 ketone compounds, a reduction in expression or activity of the enzyme may lead to increased transplacental crossing of active glucocorticoids. Maternal exposure to glucocorticoids in rats results in increased anxiety-like behaviors in adult offspring, as well as elevated plasma corticosterone levels and altered GR and MR mRNA expression in the hippocampus (Harris and Seckl, 2011). Prenatal glucocorticoid exposure also affects the development of the dopaminergic system, implicating its developmental relevance to schizo-affective disorders. Offspring born to corticosterone-treated mothers displayed enhanced spontaneous and apomorphine-induced locomotor activity (Diaz, Brown, and Seckl, 1998). Prenatal corticosterone administration during the last week of gestation may also lead to an impairment in selective association learning indicative of impaired cognitive development (Shalev and Weiner, 2001).

Postnatal models of immune activation

In rodents, the early postnatal period is associated with increased rates of neurogenesis, neuronal migration, and cell apoptosis, while circulating corticosterone levels are low. Acute exposure to glucocorticoids during this critical period causes reductions in brain weight and myelination, producing detrimental effects on brain development (Huang, 2011). In addition to administration of glucocorticoid agonists (e.g., dexamethasone or corticosterone), administration of immune activators is known to lead to an increased HPA axis activity. As such, neonatal LPS exposure has been widely employed in a range of studies exploring the effects of neonatal immune challenge on later life development. As demonstrated in Figure 14.2, administration of LPS in rodents, in particular during the first week of life, corresponding with the critical period of the HPA axis development, is known to result in increased levels of circulating corticosterone following the drug exposure (Walker, F., Brogan, Smith, and Hodgson, 2004a; Walker, A. *et al.*, 2009). Moreover, neonatal LPS exposure has been shown to be associated with increases in anxiety-related behavior in adulthood. Several studies from this and other laboratories have reported that LPS-exposed neonatal rats exhibit, in adulthood, reduced exploration and increased avoidance of aversive areas and stimuli (Breivik *et al.*, 2002, Walker, F., March, and Hodgson, 2004b; Walker, Knott, and Hodgson, 2008; Walker, A. *et al.*, 2009). These findings, however, are less consistent in juvenile and adolescent animals, when neonatal LPS exposure was reported to result in either no anxiety-related behaviors (Walker, F., March, and Hodgson, 2004b), or fewer (Fan, Mitchell, Rhodes, and Cai, 2008; Rico, Ferraz, Ramalho-Pinto, and Morato, 2010). A number of articles have suggested that this effect may be mediated by altered maternal care of LPS-treated neonates. Maternal care has been reported to be reduced in dams of LPS-treated pups (Walker, F., March, and Hodgson, 2004b), which may amplify the stress-related behavioral effects observed in the offspring

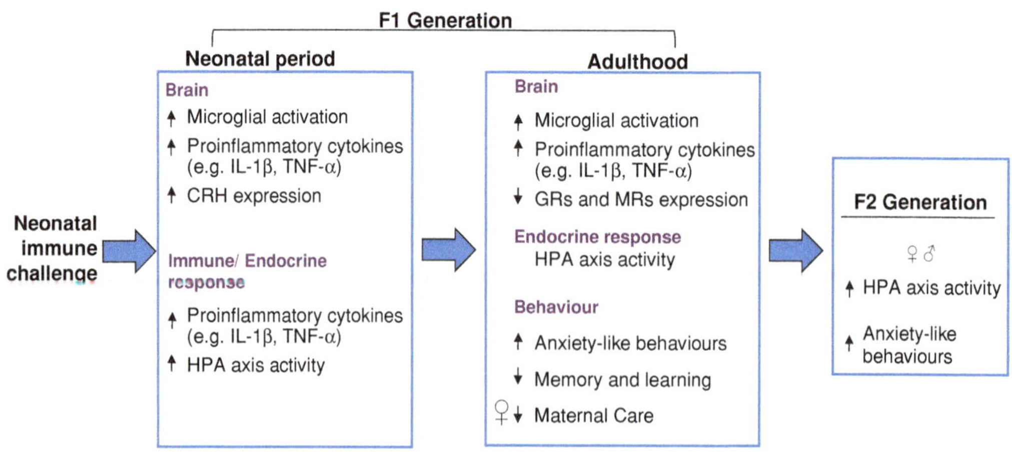

Figure 14.2 Summary of major outcomes from animal models of neonatal immune challenge – the impact of early microbial environment on immune, neuroendocrine and behavioral responses in the first (F1) and second (F2) generations.

(Hood, Dreschel, and Granger, 2003; Lucchina, Carola, Pitossi, and Depino, 2010). Although these studies seem to indicate that maternal care may interact with the immunostimulating effects of LPS, inconsistencies regarding this explanation remain (Spencer, Martin, Mouihate, and Pittman, 2006). Currently, the extent to which physiological processes are affected by potential changes in maternal care of LPS-treated offspring is unknown.

Finally, neonatal immune challenge has been shown to impact largely on cognition. The majority of this research has employed rat models using live bacterial infection. Such studies have been instrumental in indicating neuroimmune pathways through which cognition can be disrupted following early-life immune activation. These studies are consistent with the LPS-based models investigating behavioral perturbations. Neonatal *Escherichia coli* (*E. coli*) exposure has been demonstrated to impair learning and memory in adult rats (Bilbo *et al.*, 2005, 2007, 2008). Such research has indicated the involvement of hippocampal glial cell reactivity, pro-inflammatory cytokines, and brain-derived neurotrophic factor (BDNF) in producing these cognitive impairments (Bland *et al.*, 2010a, b). Interestingly, the strongest data have occurred in the presence of a secondary immune challenge in adulthood (Bilbo *et al.*, 2005; Bilbo, Rudy, Watkins, and Maier, 2006), indicative of the requirement of a second hit to produce observable perturbations (i.e., double-hit paradigm; Maynard, Sikich, Lieberman, and Lamantia, 2001). Importantly, this suggests that the secondary stressor may also amplify the behavioral alterations observed in the LPS-based studies. One study has investigated this double-hit hypothesis in regard to a secondary restraint stressor and found that the anxiety-related behaviors observed in neonatally LPS-treated rats are exacerbated (Walker, A., *et al.*, 2009).

In sum, these studies clearly indicate that animal models of prenatal and neonatal immune activation are effective tools in which to examine later-life behavioral outcomes. Furthermore, they allow for greater examination of the underlying mechanisms involved in the programming of psychopathology. The importance of using both prenatal and postnatal models becomes clear when we understand the importance of the timing of inflammation for various neural networks as related to their specific periods of vulnerability.

The Critical Issue of Timing

Environmental stressors experienced in early life vary in their ability to produce different functional outcomes according to the developmental stage of the organism at the time of exposure. The cause for this variability is the stage-specific order of critical periods of development for different physiological systems (see Figure 14.3). Accordingly, it is possible that while some neural networks are more susceptible to the impact of immune activation during the early prenatal period, others may be more vulnerable during the postnatal period. Prenatal and postnatal models of immune activation are therefore broad categories, whereas the specific timing of an insult within each model can render variations in functional outcomes as discussed below.

The early gestational period is by far the most vulnerable period of fetal development. In humans, the first trimester of pregnancy, between the 2nd and 8th weeks of embryonic development, is extremely vulnerable to teratogenic damage, which often results in termination of the pregnancy or major birth defects (Rice and Barone, 2000). Research using rodents has indicated that elevations in pro-inflammatory cytokine production following activation of the innate immune system leads to pregnancy termination through inhibition of the hypothalamic–pituitary–gonadal (HPG) axis. For instance, forced ligation of CD40 (tumor necrosis factor (TNF) superfamily member) with agonistic anti-CD40 antibodies, inducing

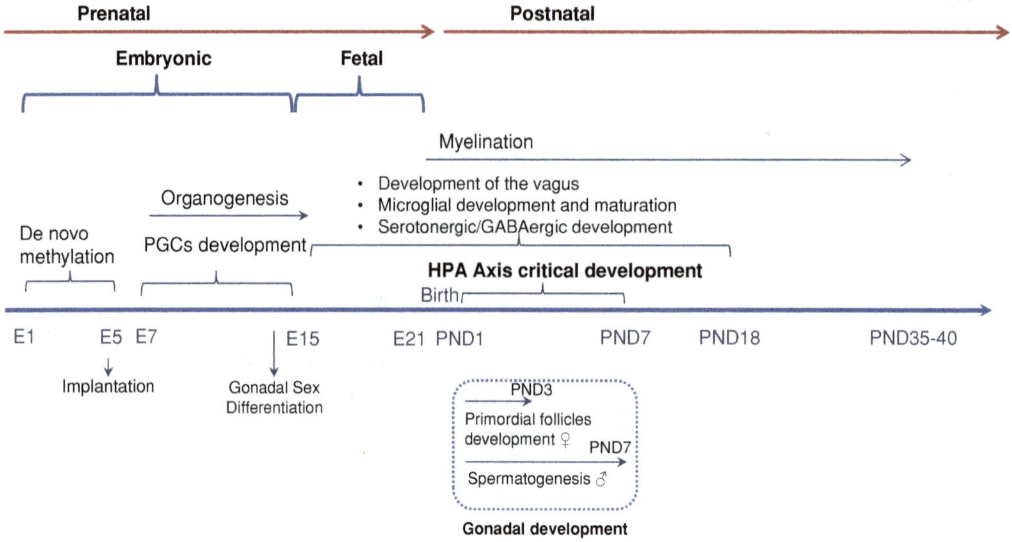

Figure 14.3 The prenatal and postnatal development of the rat. During the early embryonic period, germ cells undergo a pre-implantation wave of de novo methylation followed by primordial germ cells (PGCs) development, organogenesis and gonadal sex differentiation. During the fetal period, development of higher structures and systems begins, including the vagus, microglial network, serotonergic and GABAergic systems. These systems continue their development after birth. The early postnatal period is a critical period of the HPA axis development. In the rat ovary, primordial follicles are formed by PND3. In the testes, gonocytes resume mitosis and differentiate into spermatogonia during the first week of life.

exaggerated immune response, has been shown to result in systemic inflammation during pregnancy, ovarian resistance to the gonadotropic effects of prolactin and impaired progesterone production, leading to pregnancy failure (Erlebacher, Zhang, Parlow, and Glimcher, 2004). Administration of LPS in pregnant mice was reported to induce fetal reabsorption, and to be associated with increased levels of TNF-α in the amniotic fluid. However, reabsorption rates were dependent on the timing of exposure, with highest rates occurring when LPS was administered on gestational day 8 (Gendron, Nestel, Lapp, and Baines, 1990). Elevated levels of TNF-α in the amniotic fluid, as a result of abnormal immune system activation, was suggested to mediate pregnancy loss and fetal growth retardation (Gorivodsky, *et al.*, 1998; Heyborne, Witkin, and McGregor, 1992). Furthermore, increased expression of proinflammatory molecules (e.g., TNF-α,) was associated with diabetes-induced teratogenicity in pregnant mice (Fein *et al.*, 2002).

However, despite the vulnerability of the fetus during the first trimester, there are a number of protective mechanisms in place to limit the degree to which environmental cues reach the developing fetus. Placental and maternal factors protect the fetus to a large extent from deleterious environmental exposures. It is later in prenatal development, such as during the second and, particularly, third trimesters, that the developing fetus is better equipped to respond to a multitude of signals from the environment which assist in "fine-tuning" developmental trajectories. As such, the maternal immune response, rather than the effects of direct infection, appear responsible for the increased incidence of the psychopathology in the offspring of mothers exposed to infection in pregnancy (Patterson, 2002).The critical factors mediating the maternal immune response are circulating cytokines. Animal studies have shown altered cytokine levels in the maternal serum, amniotic fluid, and fetal brain as a result of maternal immune activation, with a particular influence being exerted by IL-6 (Smith, Garbett, Mirnics, and Patterson, 2007). There is currently conflicting evidence regarding the ability of cytokines to cross the placenta. However, some animal and ex vivo human studies indicate the bidirectional transfer of proinflammatory cytokines across the placenta (Dahlgren, Samuelsson, Jansson, and Holmäng, 2006; Zaretsky, Alexander, Byrd, and Bawdon, 2004). Essentially, the placenta functions to limit fetal exposure to adverse environmental conditions experienced by the mother; however, its protective capacity is not absolute and often can only act as a first line of defense. Therefore, the potential for subtle environmental cues to be transferred to the fetus and induce changes to developing systems remains. In contrast, during the very early stages of pregnancy the common outcome of exposure to an environmental stressor will be death or malformation – phenomena which largely exist outside the realm of perinatal programming, which focuses not on the outcome of exposure to teratogenic factors, but subtle changes in physiology induced by environmental factors that have prolonged effects.

While the placenta plays a strong role in regulating fetal programming during prenatal life, postnatal models represent a more direct route to the infant. Nevertheless, programming targets more advanced developmental stages, affecting different aspects of neural and behavioral development. In this regard, it is important to understand the relative timing of development, given that developmental trajectories are species-dependent and can vary significantly. The timing of the brain growth spurt relative to birth can be considered an important marker of developmental age among species and is crucial for understanding vulnerability of the developing brain to early life adversity. While some species are precocial, such as guinea pig, sheep, or monkey, others, like the rat, mouse, or rabbit, are altricial, born underdeveloped with their eyes shut (Clancy, Finlay, Darlington, and Anand, 2007). Hence, postnatal infections in some species can produce long-term outcomes analogous to prenatal infections in humans. Despite the timing of critical periods of development relative to parturition being species-dependent, the sequence of these periods is highly conserved and comparable across species. Therefore, both models of perinatal programming act rather complementarily than distinctively, and allow for investigation of similar as well as disparate questions.

Subtle alterations to the functional set points of developing systems, which is the focus of perinatal programming, can result in greater propensities towards pathology later in life rather than in immediate defects in the organism. As such, models of perinatal programming investigate how subtle developmental insults may initiate a cascade of effects which may not be detected immediately, but may manifest at a later time-point subsequent to the critical developmental window when the exposure occurred.

Brain–Immune Communication in the Adult

Most infections begin in the periphery, and therefore, several sophisticated signaling pathways have evolved to allow communication between the peripheral immune system and the brain. As it is not the focus of this chapter, we will only briefly outline the major pathways through which peripheral immune activation signals the brain.

Peripheral immune challenge generates an immediate acute-phase reaction of the immune system, indicated by an increased release of pro-inflammatory cytokines, such as IL-6, interleukin-1β (IL-1β) and TNF-α. These pro-inflammatory agents activate the entire network of the immune system, inducing additional release of pro-inflammatory cytokines, such as interleukin 12 (IL-12) and interferon-gamma (IFN-γ) by antigen presenting cells (APCs) and natural killer (NK) cells. Further release of these cytokines stimulates the differentiation of T-helper 1(T_H) cells, inducing the functional activity of macrophages, T-cytotoxic, and NK cells, which are the major components of the cell-mediated immunity (CMI). Moreover, activation of the peripheral immune response is known to trigger cytokine-specific regulation of the HPA axis, cause neurotransmitter functional alterations and induce sickness behavior, indicated by fever, fatigue, reduced appetite, and decreased libido.

In response to an infection, IL-1β stimulates receptors expressed within the sensory neurons of the vagus, which projects the signal to the brain where the vagus primarily innervates with the nucleus of the tractus solitarius (NTS) and medulla. Norepinephrinergic activation then occurs, projecting towards the PVN and hippocampus where glial cells synthesize and release IL-*1*β and other cytokines. The dual action of norepinephrine and cytokine release activates the HPA axis (Konsman, Parnet, and Dantzer, 2002; Goehler *et al.*, 1999; Watkins, Maier, and Goehler, 1995). Peripheral cytokines can directly cross the blood–brain barrier (BBB) via specific cytokine transport mechanisms (Banks, 2005), and can directly enter the brain in areas where the BBB is absent, known as circumventricular organs. These cytokines can stimulate the release of secondary messengers in blood vessel-associated cells, such as nitric oxide and cyclooxygenase 2 (COX-2) (Vitkovic, Bockaert, and Jacque, 2000), which can then propagate to nearby target sites involved in HPA axis and body temperature regulation, including the PVN, and the catecholaminergic brainstem nuclei (Dantzer *et al.*, 2008; Konsman, Parnet, and Dantzer, 2002; Watkins, Maier, and Goehler, 1995). COX-2 is the prostaglandin synthesizing enzyme, and prostaglandin E2 (PGE2) synthesis is associated with cytokine-induced febrile response and HPA axis activation (Boissé, Mouihate, Ellis, and Pittman, 2004). Cytokines that reach the brain via these pathways disperse into the parenchyma via a process known as volume transmission, and thus activate all brain regions with receptors available to cytokines. Finally, the brain can induce cytokine synthesis itself for responding, regulating and initiating immune signaling.

Brain-immune communication in early life

The pathways discussed above are largely developed at birth. However, some important differences exist during this early period of life which are pertinent to our discussion of behavioral programming by immune pathways. There is a conflicting body of evidence regarding the permeability of the blood–brain barrier (BBB) during the neonatal period. While some suggest that increased potential for immune molecules to be present in the brain at this period is driven by underdeveloped BBB and therefore its greater permeability (Foust *et al.*, 2009; Ek, Dziegielewska, Stolp, and Saunders, 2006), others suggest that the elevated potential for neuroinflammation in early life is due to the less mature network of glia and astrocytes at this time (Lowenstein, 2009; Saunders, Ek, and Dziegielewska, 2009). Pertinent to animal models, astrocyte development in rodents occurs postnatally and is complete only at 3 weeks of age (Calley and Maxwell, 1970), and there is a higher ratio of neurons to glia in the developing brain. Thus, the endothelium of adult brains is tighter, owing to the presence of more fully developed astrocytic endfeet that regulate biological transport and inhibit further transduction beyond the glial barrier (Lowenstein, 2009; Saunders, Ek, and Dziegielewska, 2009). Notably, while severe insults in neonates, such as meningitis and asphyxia, can increase BBB permeability (Anagnostakis, Messaritakis, Damianos, and Mandyla, 1992; van der Flier *et al.*, 2001), it is more likely that elevated trafficking of cytokines to the brain following a more subtle immune challenge is mediated by glial and astrocytic genesis.

The development of the vagus proceeds through all embryonic stages and postnatally, followed by further establishment of vagal sensorimotor circuitry. However, the human vagus is only partially myelinated at birth and its myelination continues during the first postnatal months. Preterm infants are born with an underdeveloped vagus and largely rely on the SNS and on the umyelinated vagus to regulate visceral states. It is possible that due to its early maturational state, the vagus is more susceptible to an immune challenge during early development, particularly for preterm infants. Intratracheal LPS administration in rat pups resulted in increased mRNA expression of proinflammatory cytokines in medulla oblongata, which was attenuated following vagotomy (Balan *et al.*, 2011). Therefore, while much of these immune-brain pathways of communication are already apparent early in development, there is some degree of immaturity that remains. This is suggestive of the potential for elevated rates of cytokine and chemokine trafficking to the brain during perinatal life – the implications of which point towards an increased ability for immune agents to regulate brain ontogeny and thus changes in behavior later in life.

Mechanisms of Perinatal Programming Induced by Immunological Challenge for the Predisposition to Psychopathology

The HPA axis

The HPA axis is particularly vulnerable to environmental influences during the neonatal period (Karrow, 2006). Glucocorticoids are important for normal brain maturation, but elevated glucocorticoid levels perturb normal brain development and functioning (Lupien, McEwen, Gunnar, and Heim, 2009). Hence, stress exposure during the neonatal period has been demonstrated to produce life-long perturbations to the functioning of the HPA axis, especially in relation to negative feedback. Excess perinatal glucocorticoid exposure has been shown to downregulate mineralocorticoid receptors (MRs) and GRs (Shanks, Larocque, and Meaney, 1995; Weaver *et al.*, 2004), resulting in hypersecretion of glucocorticoids in response to later aversive stimuli (Shanks, Larocque, and Meaney, 1995; Welberg and Seckl, 2001; Witek-Janusek, 1988). However, this profile of peripheral glucocorticoid secretion has been found to be largely dependent on the timing, strength, type, and duration of exposure to not only the initial stressor but also a secondary stressor. Chronic-type stress exposures have typically been shown to produce blunted glucocorticoid output (Rich and Romero, 2005), which can be maladaptive at times of stress. Animals exposed to brief periods of handling as neonates, exhibit a decrease in corticosterone secretion and increased GR expression in the hippocampus in adulthood compared to non-handled animals (Liu *et al.*, 1997). The increased hippocampal GR expression is results in increased feedback inhibition of CRH synthesis and reduced levels of ACTH and corticosterone when compared to non-handled animals during stress exposure. Thus, the sensitivity of the HPA axis is directly programmed by the degree of stress exposure during development.

Many studies have implicated the endocrine system in the programming of later-life function following perinatal immune activation, focusing on enzymes, hormones, and receptors (Boissé, Mouihate, Ellis, and Pittman, 2004; Hodgson, Knott, and Walker, 2001; Iwasa *et al.*, 2009; Jaworek *et al.*, 2007; Li *et al.*, 2007; Reul *et al.*, 1994; Shanks, Larocque, and Meaney, 1995; Spencer, Martin, Mouihate, and Pittman, 2006; Spencer, Field, and Pittman, 2010; Walker, F., Brogan, Smith, and Hodgson, 2004a). Long-term HPA axis perturbations following neonatal LPS administration (i.e., on postnatal days (PNDs) 3 and 5) have been widely demonstrated, with alterations to ACTH and corticosterone secretion during stress commonly reported (Hodgson, Knott, and Walker, 2001; Li *et al.*, 2007; Shanks, Larocque, and Meaney, 1995; Walker, F., Brogan, Smith, and Hodgson, 2004a). For instance, Walker, A. *et al.* (2009) administered LPS to Wistar neonates on PNDs 3 and 5, which resulted in immediate activation of the HPA axis. In adulthood, these animals demonstrated increased anxiety-related behaviors including hypervigilance, avoidance of open spaces, and failure to habituate to startle. Importantly, these findings were exacerbated in response to a 3-day restraint and isolation stress protocol in adulthood, and were associated with blunted corticosterone responses, suggestive of their failure to mount an appropriate neuroendocrine response to stress. Conversely, the same neonatal protocol was associated with potentiated and prolonged corticosterone responses when rats were exposed to an acute restraint protocol (Walker, A., Nakamura, and Hodgson, 2010). These findings suggest that neonatal immune activation programs the developing HPA axis to an exaggerated response to acute stress in later life. However, this potentiation is severe enough to switch the response to a blunted response after only 3 days of restraint exposure, mimicking findings typically observed following severe chronic stress exposures. Hence, the sensitivity to later-life stressors is greatly enhanced and can be considered as a fundamental component of the ***double-hit hypothesis***, which will be discussed in greater detail later in this chapter.

Negative-feedback sensitivity has also been observed to be altered in animals exposed to LPS during the neonatal period (Shanks, Larocque, and Meaney, 1995). The seminal 1995 study by Shanks and colleagues found that neonatally LPS-treated rats show only minimal inhibition of ACTH responses to acute restraint stress when pre-treated with dexamethasone. These rats also exhibit reduced GR density in the hippocampus, hypothalamus, and frontal cortex.

Other HPA-axis-related findings have demonstrated basal expression of urocortin 2 (UCN-2) and CRH-r2 mRNA to be significantly higher in animals postnatally exposed to LPS (Iwasa *et al.*, 2009). Similarly, resting median eminence levels of CRH and AVP are significantly elevated in rats exposed to LPS during the neonatal period (Shanks, Larocque, and Meaney, 1995). This indicates that a large reservoir of these hormones is available in these rats for quick and elevated release in response to a stressor in later life. Additionally, these neuropeptides are important in stress-induced suppression of the HPG axis. This hyper-responsive HPA axis is believed to cause increased neuronal cell loss in the hippocampus (Sapolsky, 1996) in postnatally LPS-treated animals.

Therefore, the HPA axis appears to be an integral player in the pathogenesis of affective disorders following perinatal infection. Typically a hyper-responsive HPA axis is produced with prolonged and potentiated downstream glucocorticoids being secreted. However, under certain conditions blunted and inappropriate excitation of the HPA axis response can result. These discrepancies are largely dependent on subsequent adversity but, at any rate, indicate that central and peripheral HPA axis alterations contribute to increased anxiety-related behaviors following perinatal immune activation.

Neuroimmune mechanisms

The ability of cytokines to induce changes in mood and cognition is well known. For instance, 30–45% of individuals receiving cytokine therapy for cancer or viral diseases have been shown to develop symptoms of depression (Valentine *et al.*, 1998; Capuron, Ravaud, and Dantzer, 2000). Furthermore, chronic inflammatory diseases typically associated with altered cytokine profiles, such as arthritis, cardiovascular or inflammatory bowel diseases, exhibit high rates of comorbidity with anxiety and depression (Kurina, Goldacre, Yeates, and Gill, 2001). There is also a growing body of evidence implicating the role of cytokines in neurodegenerative diseases, such as Alzheimer's disease and dementia (Wilson, Finch, and Cohen, 2002). Animal studies have supported these findings, with peripheral and central administration of IL-1β and TNF-α, or LPS in rodents, inducing behavioral symptoms of sickness and depression (Kent, Kelley, and Dantzer, 1992; O'Connor *et al.*, 2009; Yirmiya, 1996). Importantly, central administration of pro-inflammatory cytokines induce profound behavioral changes at doses significantly lower than those required when peripheral immune challenge is applied (Banks, Farr, La Scola, and Murphy, 2001). Animals administered either IL-1β or TNF-α (centrally or peripherally) show significant reductions in locomotor activity, memory function, and interest in their environment, along with reduced food and water consumption (Bluthé, Michaud, Poll, and Dantzer, 2000). Intracerebroventricular administration of IL-1β receptor antagonists have been shown to reverse the behavioral and physiological effects induced by systemic injection of IL-1, indicating an important role for IL-1 in mediating local and systemic responses to inflammation(Kent, Kelley, and Dantzer, 1992).

The contribution of cytokines to long-term behavioral changes in early development is currently a focus of research. Indeed, peripheral immune challenge in early life leads to altered cytokine production, both peripherally and centrally (Walker, F. *et al.*, 2004; Walker, A., Nakamura, and Hodgson, 2010). Epidemiological studies have demonstrated that bacterial exposure in childhood can enhance allergy-protective type-1 immune responses (Braun-Fahrlander *et al.*, 2002; Gereda *et al.*, 2000; Litonjua *et al.*, 2002), but predispose to exaggerated peripheral inflammatory responses in later life in both human (Finch and Crimmins, 2004) and animal models (Shanks *et al.*, 2000). The inflammatory hypothesis, introduced by Caleb Finch, proposes that inflammatory markers (i.e. C-reactive protein, IL-6, TNF-α) become elevated after early life infection, and this can drive later life morbidity and mortality (Finch and Crimmins, 2004). It is important to note that although improved public health and hygiene, including immunization and the use of antibiotics, significantly decrease the impact of early-life inflammatory exposure, other sources of inflammation, such as exposure to high fat diet, or malnutrition, are of increasing concern worldwide and especially pertinent to the Western countries.

Several laboratories investigating the developmental impact of early-life immune activation have demonstrated that neonatal LPS exposure results in changes in cytokine activity. Ellis and colleagues found reduced circulating levels of IL-1β, TNF-α and IL-6 in adult rats, neonatally exposed to LPS, following a secondary immune challenge in adulthood, which reached significance for TNF-α and IL-6. In line with these findings a reduction in the activity of peripheral NF-κB, responsible for much of the LPS-induced cytokine production, has been observed (Ellis, Mouihate, and Pittman, 2005). Additionally, natural killer (NK) cells, a major component of cell-mediated immunity which are known to be responsive to cytokine signaling, were found to exhibit reduced cytotoxicity leading to increased susceptibility to tumor metastasis following neonatal endotoxin challenge (Hodgson, Knott, and Walker, 2001; Hodgson and Knott, 2002). These alterations in cytokine function also represent implications for mood, cognition, and behavior. Our laboratory has demonstrated that rats exposed to LPS on days 3 and 5 postpartum present with elevated anxiety-related behaviors in adulthood including avoidance, startle, immobility, risk assessment and reduced exploration (Walker, F. *et al.*, 2004; Walker A. *et al.*, 2009; Walker, Nakamura, and Hodgson, 2010; Walker, A, Hawkins, Sominsky, and Hodgson, 2012; Sominsky *et al.*, 2012). These rats also exhibit elevated hippocampal TNF-α and IL-1β protein concentrations in response to acute restraint stress in adulthood (Walker, Nakamura, and Hodgson, 2010). These elevated brain cytokine levels were associated with a potentiated and prolonged corticosterone response to stress, suggestive of the potential co-regulatory nature of these neuroimmune and neuroendocrine systems for behavior. Findings from the Bilbo laboratory have also demonstrated that neonatal exposure to *E. coli* increases hippocampal gene expression of IL-1β at 24 hours post administration (Bilbo *et al.*, 2005). In adulthood, these animals exhibited increased IL-1β production within the hippocampus and parietal cortex in response to a subsequent LPS challenge in adulthood, which was associated with memory impairments. Importantly, these memory impairments were abrogated in the presence of a caspase-1 inhibitor, which prevents the synthesis of IL-1β (Bilbo *et al.*, 2005). These data directly support the notion that early immune activation shifts the long-term functional tone of cytokine action, which has direct implications for behavior.

Models of prenatal inflammation have also produced reliable changes in cytokine expression in both maternal and fetal compartments (Ashdown *et al.*, 2006; Cai *et al.*, 2000). Maternal LPS exposure on gestational day 18 in mice resulted in dose-dependent increases in IL-1β and TNF-α mRNA levels in the fetal brain (Cai *et al.*, 2000). Similar findings have been observed following exposure of pregnant dams to the viral mimetic, poly I:C (Gilmore, Jarskog, and Vadlamudi, 2005). Notably, the impact of the immune challenge appears to differ depending on whether it occurs during middle or late gestation, again highlighting the critical importance of timing. Furthermore, the variation in timing of maternal inflammation yielded divergent behavioral outcomes, such that administration of Poly I:C in mice in mid pregnancy resulted in reduced open-field exploration by the adult offspring, while immune challenge in late pregnancy induced a perseverative phenotype, as was demonstrated on a water T-maze (Meyer *et al.*, 2006).

Thus, it appears that perinatal immune challenge induces replicable central proinflammatory cytokine responses, which affect multiple aspects of neuronal development and can drive behavioral perturbations. Increasing evidence implicates resident immune cells in the brain, particularly microglia, as the putative candidate responsible for such alterations in cytokine production. Glia have become increasingly recognized as important players in the operation of central nervous system (CNS) function, and are now acknowledged to exhibit a high degree of plasticity. Glia are involved in maintaining the integrity of synapses through the release of neurotransmitters and immune proteins, acting as a tissue alarm system, and potentially controlling synaptogenesis in addition to their well-established supportive and housekeeping functions (Graeber, 2010; Miller, 2005). Of the various subtypes of glial cells, microglia are the major immunocompetent brain cells, and have been implicated in a range of CNS pathologies (Miller, 2005), including psychiatric disorders, due largely to their release of cytokines (Bilbo and Schwarz, 2009).

Early-life immune activation has been shown to induce a strong microglial response, which persists into adulthood, following live infection with *E. coli* (Bland *et al.*, 2010b) as well as neonatal LPS challenge (Sominsky *et al.*, 2012). Interestingly, a comparison between these two common models of early-life immune activation revealed distinct and divergent activation of inflammatory pathways. While *E.coli* infection provokes neuroinflammation via an

IL-1-predominant pathway, LPS appears to produce a less focused and more profound central immune response, affecting a broader spectrum of inflammatory gene expression. These results suggest that LPS uncovers the myriad of ways in which life-long microglial activity can be shifted following neonatal inflammation, while *E.coli* represents an infection-specific, IL-1-mediated mechanism. (Schwarz and Bilbo, 2011; Bilbo, Smith, and Schwarz, 2012).

Microglia play an important role in neural circuitry formation by mediating synaptic pruning and maturation during embryonic and postnatal development. Factors regulating microglial development, such as chemokines, growth factors, and hormones, can disrupt microglial function and lead to synaptic abnormalities evident in neurodevelopmental disorders (Lewis, 2011; Paolicelli *et al.*, 2011). Such abnormalities in the pruning process are associated with neurodevelopmental and psychiatric disorders (e.g. autism and schizophrenia) as well as impaired cognitive function and early stages of neurodegenerative disease. (e.g., Alzheimer's disease) (Bilbo *et al.*, 2011). Therefore, environmental stressors during early development, such as infection, bear the capacity to alter synaptic formation via changes in glial function. This, in turn, further programs the individual for possible later-life adversity. The impact of early-life experiences on microglial development and their role in cognitive and mental health function is thoroughly discussed in Chapter 15 by Schwarz and Bilbo. However, given the known impact of cytokine activity on programming behavioral outcomes it is necessary to understand the plastic nature of microglia, given they are largely responsible for cytokine secretion and activity.

Neuronal and neurotransmitter mechanisms

The reported increased risk of developing psychiatric disorders, such as schizophrenia or autism, following perinatal infection indicates the profound impact that the early immune system has on higher-order neural structures. During periods of neurodevelopmental plasticity, adverse experiences influence developing neurons. In the human brain, synaptic formation starts in the second trimester of pregnancy and continues well after birth (Glover, 2011). This extensive neurodevelopmental window creates the potential risk for environmental miscues to affect later-life neuronal functioning. Early-life insults initiate a continuous interaction between innate and adaptive immune responses, affecting brain development over a prolonged time period (Malaeb and Dammann, 2009). Direct inflammation of the brain has profound effects on the development of severe neurological abnormalities, whereas mild changes in the pre- or postnatal microbial environment may affect some neural functional properties via activation of an immune response, i.e. cytokine release. Kinase pathways involved in cytokine signaling, such as NF-κB, MAPK, and JAK/STAT, also control neuronal differentiation, migration, axon pathfinding, and synaptic formation during periods of brain development. In addition, neuronal expression of cytokine receptors can cause further morphological and functional alterations as a result of an exposure to inflammatory stimulus (Bauer, Kerr, and Patterson, 2007).

Animal models of programming following immune activation during perinatal life directly implicate the role of cytokine response in subsequent neurodevelopmental changes. For example, prenatal exposure to LPS has been shown to alter brain-derived neurotrophic factor (BDNF) and nerve-growth factor (NGF) in the developing fetal and neonatal brain (Gilmore, Jarskog, and Vadlamudi, 2003). Cytokines have similarly been implicated in the development of hippocampal and cortical neurons (Bauer, Kerr, and Patterson, 2007). Hippocampal neuronal alterations have been shown to occur as a result of maternal LPS exposure, demonstrating increase in pyramidal and granular cell numbers and shrinkage of pyramidal neurons in the hippocampus of adult offspring These morphological changes were associated with impairments in learning and memory but not locomotion, indicating particular sensitivity of the hippocampus to inflammatory stimuli during early development (Golan *et al.*, 2005). Maternal poly I:C exposure causes deficits in Purkinje cells, hippocampal synaptic dysfunction, changes in dopaminergic activity, and increased GABA-A receptor expression in the adult offspring. These animals demonstrate deficits in PPI, LI and other behavior alterations typically associated with schizophrenia (Smith, Hsiao, and Patterson, 2010). Neonatal intracerebral LPS administration results in dopaminergic neuronal injury in the adolescent and adult rat brain, reduced tyrosine hydroxylase immunoreactive neurons in the substantia nigra, (which results in reduced catecholaminergic and dopaminergic activity), and elevated microglial activation and central release of IL-1β and TNF-α, indicating a robust effect of neonatal immune challenge on the developing brain (Fan *et al.*, 2005; Fan, Mitchell, Rhodes, and Cai, 2008). Interestingly, deficits in locomotor activity in LPS-treated animals induced by neuroinflammation recovered by adulthood, suggesting that inflammation may have a detrimental effect on neuronal functioning, but it may also initiate endogenous repair mechanisms, such as the release of neurotrophic factors (Malaeb and Dammann, 2009). It appears that in the adult brain, the immune compartment supports the maintenance of hippocampal neurogenesis. Therefore, careful control of immune activity is critical, as both deficient and exaggerated immune responses may lead to impaired neurogenesis and impaired cognitive performance (Ziv and Schwartz, 2008).

Early-life immune activation also has an impact on the development of the serotonergic system, which has been strongly implicated in anxiety, depression, and other psychiatric disorders. Exposure to stress during postnatal period has been shown to result in decreased neural activity of 5-HT and altered 5-HT1A autoreceptor sensitivity (Bambico, Nguyen, and Gobbi, 2009). Moreover, the serotonergic system is known to be sensitive to proinflammatory cytokines, and such exposure can cause degeneration of serotonergic axons (Ishikawa, Ishikawa, and Nakamura, 2007). Prenatal high-fat diet consumption, a known source of inflammation in the developing fetus, causes perturbations to the fetal serotonergic system (Hassanain and Levin, 2002). Increased expression of TPH2, the rate-limiting enzyme in serotonin synthesis, and increased levels of the inhibitory 5-HT_{1A}autoreceptor were found in the rostral raphe of non-human primate offspring born to mothers that received high-fat diet in pregnancy (Sullivan *et al.*, 2010). Similarly, a recent paper (Lin, Lin and Wang, 2012) has shown that rats prenatally exposed to LPS develop anxiety-like behavior. Importantly, these rats also exhibit reductions in DA in the nucleus accumbens and 5-HT in the mPFC, corresponding to reduced DA and 5-HT_{1A} receptors. A few human studies have also implicated serotoninergic involvement following perinatal infection. For instance, epidemiological studies, suggesting an infectious basis for the development of autism, demonstrate serotonin disturbances, associated with elevated serotonin levels (reviewed in Hornig and Lipkin, 2001).

Epigenetic mechanisms in perinatal programming

An exciting area of research in the field of perinatal programming is epigenetics. Psychopathology, including depression, schizophrenia and anxiety disorders, has been well-documented to transmit down filial lines (Baron, Gruen, Asnis, and Lord, 1985; Cadoret, O'Gorman, Heywood, and Troughton, 1985; Merikangas and Swendson, 1997). However, the mechanisms underlying this apparent heritability have proven to be elusive. For instance, studies showing increased prevalence of sharing a psychological disorder for identical versus fraternal twins (Plomin, Owen, and McGuffin, 1994) have arguably demonstrated genetic influences for this phenomenon. However, genome mapping has failed to definitively isolate any gene which is responsible for the behavioral sequelae characterized by any psychological condition. Furthermore, the suggestion that environmental factors alone are responsible for transgenerational transmittance of psychopathology becomes less convincing in light of studies showing identical twins separately adopted at birth share a mental health condition (e.g. McGuffin and Owen, 1995). However, the discovery of non-genomic, or *epigenetic*, influences on gene expression has proven to be a potential explanation for demonstrating how environmental and genetic influences can interact to produce a heritable vulnerability to mental health.

Epigenetics refers to the environmental modification of gene activation without altering the underlying DNA sequence (Meaney and Ferguson-Smith, 2010; Skinner and Guerrero-Bosagna, 2009). A number of these changes are mitotically or meiotically heritable (Meaney and Ferguson-Smith, 2010). Thus, epigenetics provides a mechanism for experience-dependent phenotypic plasticity that can transmit intergenerationally. Two of the most widely investigated epigenetic mechanisms are DNA methylation and histone acetylation, which both alter gene transcription.

Genomic DNA in eukaryotes is packaged with histones to form chromatin (Bulger, 2005). Gene activation is largely dependent on the relative condensation of chromatin around the DNA, whereby decondensed chromatin allows for access by RNA polymerase and transcription factors to the gene. Thus, condensation of the chromatin limits availability to the gene to be transcribed, usually resulting in silenced expression. Methylation and acetylation refer to the modification of chromatin structure by the addition (or removal) of a methyl or acetyl group to the amino-terminal tail domains of the core histones by specific enzymes (Bulger, 2005). Methylation therefore, works to condense the chromatin, thus silencing gene expression. Conversely, demethylation refers to the removal of a methyl group and opening up of the chromatin. Histone acetylation, on the other hand, activates gene expression by the addition of histone acetyltransferases, which remodel the chromatin to a decondensed form (Cheung, Allis, and Sassone-Corsi, 2000; Zhang and Meaney, 2010). Histone deacetylases remove acetyl groups, condense the chromatin, and produce transcriptional silencing.

Numerous studies have demonstrated that environmental factors can influence chromatin remodeling, which appears to be particularly susceptible to stress (Hinwood, Tynan, Day, and Walker, 2010; Hunter *et al.*, 2009; Reul, Hesketh, Collins, and Mecinas, 2009). Epigenetics therefore, potentially explains how stressful early-life events can program sustained changes in phenotype. Research into the perinatal environmental regulation of the epigenome is scarce; however, pivotal work from the Meaney laboratory has established a rat model of maternal care which demonstrates epigenetic regulation of the HPA axis. Rat offspring of low-maternal-care-providing mothers exhibit comparatively reduced GR expression (and thus reduced negative-feedback sensitivity) and elevated HPA axis responses to stress (Francis *et al.*, 1999; Liu *et al.*, 1997). These epigenetic modifications to GR abundance are also associated with increased anxiety-related behavior (Weaver *et al.*, 2006). These findings have been shown to be the result of hypermethylation of the exon 1_7 GR promoter and associated hypoacetylation of histone H3-lysine (K)-9 and reduced binding to nerve growth factor-inducible protein-A (NGFI-A) (Weaver *et al.*, 2004). Furthermore, reversibility of this hyper-responsive HPA axis and anxiety-related behavioral phenotype is possible with histone deacetylase (HDAC) inhibitor administration (Weaver *et al.*, 2006).

Recent data from our laboratory have uncovered the potential for neonatal immune activation to produce transgenerational changes in behavior, suggestive of epigenetic modifications. That is, rats exposed to LPS during the neonatal period not only show increased anxiety-like behavior in adulthood but their offspring also exhibit anxiety-related phenotypes despite not being exposed to the LPS directly (Walker, Hawkins, Sominsky, and Hodgson, 2012). However, in order to understand these findings more fully, a distinction must be made between post-translational epigenetics and germ line epigenetics. Skinner and Guerrero-Bosagna (2009) highlight that the majority of environmentally-induced epigenetic modifications involve somatic cells and do not result in transgenerational phenotypes. Hence, the transgenerational findings in regards to maternal care quality rely on the offspring learning either "high" or "poor" maternal care from their mothers and transferring this to their offspring and so on. Therefore, without the continued generational maternal behavior, the epigenetic modification will be lost. In contrast, epigenetic changes to the germ line can produce an intrinsic transgenerational epigenetic phenomenon. This has been highlighted by Michael Meaney's laboratory whereby offspring of "poor" maternal care providing mothers were fostered to "high" maternal care providing mothers and vice versa (Francis, Diorio, Liu, and Meaney, 1999; Weaver *et al.*, 2004). After cross-fostering the intergenerational effects were attenuated.

In contrast to post-translational epigenetic modifications, germ line epigenetics can occur only in the germ cells for experience-dependent modifications to passed from one generation to the next. Embryonic development sees primordial germ cells migrate to the developing gonad where global demethylation of the genome occurs, thus erasing the previous generation's epigenome (Morgan *et al.*, 2005). Following sexual differentiation, meiosis begins in females. Mitosis continues until meiotic division at puberty in males. During sexual differentiation and meiosis, the genome becomes remethylated (Surani, 2001). It is during the early period surrounding its demethylation and remethylation that the genome appears to be most sensitive to environmental effects (Skinner and Guerrero-Bosagna, 2009).

In the study reported by Walker, Hawkins, Sominsky, and Hodgson (2012), neonatal rats were exposed to 0.05 mg/kg LPS or an equivolume of saline. In adulthood, LPS-treated rats exhibited increased anxiety-like behaviors and altered neuroendocrine responsivity to stress compared to saline-treated controls. Interestingly, when these rats were bred with untreated partners, their offspring also exhibited increased anxiety-like behavior. The mechanism along the maternal line appears to coincide with the altered maternal care findings reported by Meaney (discussed above). LPS-treated dams provided lower-quality care to their offspring, who, in turn, exhibited exaggerated HPA axis responses to stress and anxiety-like behavior. This effect was reversed, however, in the presence of cross-fostering. Importantly, while the increased anxiety-like phenotype was also observed in offspring of LPS-treated males, there were no differences in maternal care provided by the untreated females they were mated with. This suggests the potential for genomic epigenetic inheritance. At this stage these putative mechanisms still require confirmation. However, clearly the potential exists for the neonatal immune system to produce long-lasting and intergenerational changes in mood and behavior via these non-genomic pathways.

So, Why Aren't We All Sick?

The impact of the perinatal microbial environment on later-life health outcomes described in this chapter raises important questions. Most pertinent is how this phenomenon, designed to enhance adaptedness, and which has been laid down early in evolution, holds ecological relevance in contemporary populations. For instance, if infections are a common occurrence during such a vulnerable period of life, what makes some of us more susceptible than others to experience behavioral and physiological alterations in response to adversity later in life? Is this phenotypic variability necessarily maladaptive? And why is it still important to consider this risk given the advances in public health, such as immunization programs, and antibiotics? Finally, does exposure to environmental stressors, such as infection, produce deleterious outcomes or rather aim to produce adaptive changes relevant to the present context?

The mismatch and double-hit hypotheses

In all living species survival is an ultimate goal. One of the fundamental principles of enhancing survival is the ability to adapt to a changing environment. The genetic foundation that allows for adaptive phenotypic plasticity is the basic concept of Darwinism, ensuring survival of the fittest. In humans, the challenges to survival gradually extended from natural predators, to wars, poverty, famine, poor natural resources and more. However, still the fundamentally greatest challenge to human mortality is infection and disease. Advances in science have substantially increased the human lifespan, and medicine is now equipped with effective tools to combat pathogenic assaults. However, a new range of diseases and health complications have arisen in the modern age, which challenge human health during this extended lifespan. It is possible that much of this can be attributed to early-life experiences, and the phenomenon of perinatal programming which is designed to enhance immediate survival and increase the chances of reaching reproductive age. Evolution has instilled these survival mechanisms to enable us to have progeny, with health and wellbeing after reaching reproductive age being of lesser concern. As such, if the environmental cues provided in early life do not match with those in later life, maladaptation may occur – even if the later-life environment provides more opportunities to improve wellbeing. For instance, being born in a nutrient-restricted environment requires us to be able to control our growth in order to survive. During pregnancy, if the mother has limited access to food, we will restrict our growth in utero and alter metabolic conditions to enhance our chances of survival in an environment with limited nutrient supplies. However, if these cues do not match our later nutritional experience, we may become susceptible to metabolic dysfunction, and more susceptible to a range of diseases, including, but not limited to, mental health and behavioral problems (Schlotz and Phillips, 2009). Therefore the "mismatch hypothesis" of development demonstrates that the specific developmental outcome is not completely dependent on the early-life experiences, but on the degree of match or mismatch between these and later-life environmental demands.

While the mismatch hypothesis accounts for how these programming consequences can become maladaptive, it does not answer the question directly as to why some of us are more susceptible than others to diseases. Discrepancies between in-utero and ex-utero environments are not limited to nutritional factors, but extend to other potential impacts, such as mental states. When born and raised in a stressful and unpredictable environment, more cautious behavior may prove beneficial. The HPA axis and the SNS are programmed during development to allow for quicker and more efficient responses to environmental change. Therefore, such a vigilant phenotype can improve adjustment to a variable environment. However, when no immediate danger is likely to occur, greater alertness and vigilance may evolve into anxious and psychotic symptoms. Often the transition into a psychopathological state occurs long after the perinatal experience. This sudden emergence of a maladaptive phenotype can be explained by the double-hit hypothesis of psychopathology. This posits that an insult, whether genetic or environmental, experienced in early life alters the developing infant and sets up a pre-existing vulnerability. However, the individual may show no maladaptive phenotypic outcomes unless confronted with a secondary insult. Studies from a number of laboratories utilizing neonatal immune challenge during critical periods of limbic and neuroendocrine development have demonstrated that while neonatal immune challenge can induce an increase in anxiety-related behavior and neuroendocrine disturbance, the effects are exacerbated and more robust in the presence of a secondary stressor in adulthood (Walker, A., *et al.*, 2009). As such, it appears that it is the cumulative effects of stress throughout the lifespan which contribute to the pathogenesis of anxiety or depression. However, the vulnerability to experience these disorders can be set up by immune activation in early life.

Context specificity

It is also important to note that these programming consequences need to be viewed in a context-specific manner. Early-life developmental plasticity allows an organism to shape its unique phenotypic characteristics in response to given environmental conditions. Hence it is important to view perinatal programming initially as a regulatory mechanism, the goal of which being to increase adaptation and enhance survival. As mentioned previously, correspondence between early-life and later-life environments, whether favorable or adverse, promotes physiological and behavioral adaptation. However, when a mismatch occurs, and the programmed function is no longer beneficial in a given environment – that is when the risk for adverse consequences increases. Champagne and colleagues (2008) demonstrated in rodents that cognitive functioning of animals exposed to poor maternal care is optimal in the context of high stress in adulthood, while it is diminished otherwise. These results were opposite for animals that received a high level of maternal care.

Contextual differences also need to be considered on a broader perspective of time. Behavioral and physiological functions that were necessary for survival in the past may not be beneficial in modern society. Given that the traditional threats to survival in the Western world have altered compared to early subsistence conditions, behavioral outcomes of perinatal stress and anxiety, such as increased vigilance or easily distracted attention, may not serve the same purpose for an individual these days as in our ancestral environment.

However, we need also to acknowledge this phenomenon at a population-based level. Early-life adversity may elicit expression of divergent genotypes and thus have different consequences for individuals in later life, while increasing phenotypic variability in a general population. This way, developmental plasticity of an organism allows for variability in responses to the same environmental condition. From an evolutionary perspective, individual variability has always had a beneficial impact on the survival of the group. Thus increased susceptibility of some individuals to diseases and psychopathologies, or, in particular, increased susceptibility to the effects of programming, may be a disadvantage from an individual perspective, but may have a favorable effect for the group. For example, increased hyperactivity and impulsiveness of some individuals can lead to engagement in dangerous activities, with severe outcomes, which will serve as a warning to others. On the other hand, increased hypervigilance and decreased novelty-seeking may prevent individuals falling into potentially harmful situations. Therefore, transgenerational transmission of these diverse phenotypes has an evolutionary importance in preserving living organisms in a constantly changing environment, while also providing phenotypic variability in case of habitat change. We will explore this more thoroughly by speculating about some findings from our laboratory. We have recently shown that the increased anxiety-related behaviors commonly observed following neonatal LPS exposure can be transmitted to the subsequent generation (Walker, Hawkins, Sominsky, and Hodgson 2012). While transmission of the anxiety-like phenotype through the maternal line was directly influenced by changes in maternal behavior, transmission via the paternal line suggests the potential for epigenetic germ line modifications. More importantly, the diverse strategies and pathways that are involved in transmission of this supposedly maladaptive phenotype suggest an importance in its preservation across generations. This notion is supported by recently documented findings showing that rats treated neonatally with LPS exhibit a subfertile phenotype, such that within a population of LPS-treated and non-treated rats, they would yield fewer total offspring overall (Walker *et al.*, 2011). This allows for the potentially deleterious phenotype to be limited within the population ***but also maintained*** in case the environmental conditions change such that elevated caution and vigilance becomes adaptive. If this were to happen, then Darwinian principles would dictate that more of the non-treated rats would not survive to reproductive age, while the LPS-treated line would increase. Therefore, the general proportion of the population would change, but the species would survive. This means that perinatal programming enables adaptedness at the population level many times faster than can occur with traditional Darwinian evolution. Hence the decision of whether programming outcomes are adaptive or maladaptive requires consideration in the precise context in which the phenomenon is occurring.

References

Anagnostakis, D., Messaritakis, J., Damianos, D., and Mandyla, H. (1992). Blood–brain barrier permeability in "healthy" infected and stressed neonates. *Journal of Pediatrics*, 121(2), 291–294.

Ashdown, H., Dumont, Y., Ng, M., Poole, S., Boksa, P., and Luheshi, G.N. (2006). The role of cytokines in mediating effects of prenatal infection on the fetus: implications for schizophrenia. *Molecular Psychiatry*, 11(1), 47–55.

Balan, K.V., Kc, P., Hoxha, Z., Mayer, C.A., Wilson, C.G., and Martin, R.J. (2011). Vagal afferents modulate cytokine-mediated respiratory control at the neonatal medulla oblongata. *Respiratory Physiology and Neurobiology*, 178(3), 458–464.

Bambico, F.R., Nguyen, N.T., Gobbi, G. (2009). Decline in serotonergic firing activity and desensitization of 5-HT1A autoreceptors after chronic unpredictable stress. *European Neuropsychopharmacology*, 19(3), 215–228.

Banks, W.A., Farr, S.A., La Scola, M.E. and Morley, J.E. (2001). Intravenous human interleukin-1a impairs memory processing in mice: Dependence on blood–brain barrier transport into posterior division of the septum. *Journal of Pharmacology and Experimental Therapeutics*, 299(2), 536–541.

Barker, D.J., and Osmond, C. (1987). Death rates from stroke in England and Wales predicted from past maternal mortality. *British Medical Journal (Clinical Research Ed.)*, 295(6590), 83–86.

Barker, D.J., Osmond, C., Golding, J., Kuh, D., and Wadsworth, M.E. (1989). Growth in utero, blood pressure in childhood and adult life, and mortality from cardiovascular disease. *British Medical Journal*, 298(6673), 564–567.

Barker, D.J., Bull, A.R., Osmond, C., and Symmonds, S.J. (1990). Fetal and placental size and risk of hypertension in adult life. *British Medical Journal*, 301(6746), 259–262.

Baron, M., Gruen, R., Asnis, U., and Lord, S. (1985). Familial transmission of schizotypal and borderline personality disorders. *American Journal of Psychiatry*, 142(8), 927–934.

Bauer, S., Kerr, B.J., and Patterson, P.H. (2007). The neuropoietic cytokine family in development, plasticity, disease and injury. *Nature Reviews*, 8(3), 221–32.

Besedovsky, H., del Rey, A., Sorkin, E., and Dinarello, C.A. (1986). Immunoregulatory feedback between interleukin-1 and glucocorticoid hormones. *Science*, 233(4764), 652–654.

Bilbo, S.D., Biedenkapp, J.C., Der-Avakian, A., Watkins, L.R., Rudy, J.W., and Maier, S.F. (2005). Neonatal infection-induced memory impairment after lipopolysaccharide in adulthood is prevented via caspase-1 inhibition. *Journal of Neuroscience*, 25(35), 8000–8009.

Bilbo, S.D., Rudy, J.W., Watkins, L.R., and Maier, S.F. (2006). A behavioural characterization of neonatal infection-facilitated memory impairment in adult rats. *Behavioral Brain Research*, 169(1), 39–47.

Bilbo, S.D., Newsum, N.J., Sprunger, D.B., Watkins, L.R., Rudy, J.W., and Maier, S.F. (2007). Differential effects of neonatal handling on early life infection-induced alterations in cognition in adulthood. *Brain, Behavior, and Immunity*, 21(3), 332–342.

Bilbo, S.D., Yirmiya, R., Amat, J., Paul, E.D., Watkins, L.R., and Maier, S.F. (2008). Bacterial infection early in life protects against stressor-induced depressive-like symptoms in adult rats. *Psychoneuroendocrinology*, 33(3), 261–269.

Bilbo, S.D., and Schwarz, J.M. (2009). Early-life programming of later-life brain and behavior: a critical role for the immune system. *Frontiers in Behavioral Neuroscience*, 3(14), 1–14.

Bilbo, S.D., Smith, S.H., and Schwarz, J.M. (2012). A lifespan approach to neuroinflammatory and cognitive disorders: A critical role for glia. *Journal of Neuroimmune Pharmacology*, 7(1), 24–41 DOI: 10.1007/s11481-011-9299-y.

Bland, S.T., Beckley, J.T., Young, S., Tsang, V., Watkins, L.R., Maier, S.F., and Bilbo, S.D. (2010a). Enduring consequences of early-life infection on glial and neural. *Brain, Behavior, and Immunity*, 24(3), 329–338.

Bland, S.T., Beckley, J.T., Watkins, L.R., Maier, S.F., and Bilbo, S.D. (2010b). Neonatal *Escherichia coli* infection alters glial, cytokine, and neuronal gene expression in response to acute amphetamine in adolescent rats. *Neuroscience Letters*, 474(1), 52–57.

Bluthé, R.M., Michaud, B., Poli, V., and Dantzer, R. (2000). Role of IL-6 in cytokine-induced sickness behavior: A study with IL-6 deficient mice. *Physiology and Behavior*, 70(3–4), 367–373.

Boissé, L., Mouihate, A., Ellis, S., and Pittman, Q.J. (2004). Long-term alterations in neuroimmune responses after neonatal exposure to lipopolysaccharide. *Journal of Neuroscience*, 24(21), 4928–4934.

Braun-Fahrländer, C., Riedler, J., Herz, U., Eder, W., Waser, M., Grize et al. (2002). Environmental exposure to endotoxin and its relation to asthma in school-age children. *New England Journal of Medicine*, 347(12), 869–877.

Breivik, T., Stephan, M., Brabant, G.E., Straub, R.H., Pabst, R., and von Horsten, S. (2002). Postnatal lipopolysaccharide-induced illness predisposes to periodontal disease in adulthood. *Brain, Behavior, and Immunity*, 16(4), 421–438.

Brown, A.S., and Derkits, E.J. (2010). Prenatal infection and schizophrenia: a review of epidemiological and translational studies. *American Journal of Psychiatry*. 167(3), 261–280.

Bulger, M. (2005). Hyperacetylated chromatin domains: Lessons from heterochromatin. *Journal of Biological Chemistry*, 280(23), 21689–21692.

Cadoret, R.J., O'Gorman, T.W., Heywood, E., and Troughton, E. (1985). Genetic and environmental factors in major depression. *Journal of Affective Disorders*, 9(2), 155–164.

Cai, Z., Pan, Z.L., Pang, Y., Evans, O.B., and Rhodes, P.G. (2000). Cytokine induction in fetal rat brains and brain injury in neonatal rats after maternal lipopolysaccharide administration. *Pediatric Research*, 47(1), 64–72.

Calley, D.W., and Maxwell, D.S. (1970). Development of the blood vessels and extracellular spaces during postnatal maturation of rat cerebral cortex. *Journal of Comparative Neurology*, 138(1), 31–48.

Capuron, L., Ravaud, A., and Dantzer, R. (2000). Early depressive symptoms in cancer patients rece1iving interleukin 2 and/or interferon alfa-2b therapy. *Journal of Clinical Oncology*, 18(10), 2143–2151.

Champagne, D.L., Bagot, R.C., van Hasselt, F., Ramakers, G., Meaney, M.J., de Kloet, E.R., Joels, M., and Krugers, H. (2008). Maternal care and hippocampal plasticity: evidence for experience-dependent structural plasticity, altered synaptic functioning, and differential responsiveness to glucocorticoids and stress. *Journal of Neuroscience*, 28(23), 6037–6045.

Cheung, P., Allis, C.D., and Sassone-Corsi, P. (2000). Signaling to chromatin through histone modifications. *Cell*, 103(2), 263–271.

Clancy, B., Finlay, B.L., Darlington, R.B., and Anand, K.J. (2007). Extrapolating brain development from experimental species to humans. *Neurotoxicology*, 8(5), 931–937.

Craske, M.G., Poulton, R., Tsao, J.C., and Plotkin, D. (2001). Paths to panic disorder/agoraphobia: An exploratory analysis from age 3 to 21 in an unselected birth cohort. *Journal of the American Academy of Child & Adolescent Psychiatry*, 40(5), 556–563.

Dahlgren, J., Samuelsson, A.M., Jansson, T., and Holmäng, A. (2006). Interleukin-6 in the maternal circulation reaches the rat fetus in mid-gestation. *Pediatric Research*, 60(2), 147–151.

Dantzer, R., O'Connor, J.C., Freund, G.C., Johnson, R.W., and Kelley. K.W. (2008). From inflammation to sickness and depression: When the immune system subjugates the brain. *Nature Reviews Neuroscience*, 9(1), 46–57.

Davies, M.J., and Norman, R.J. (2002). Programming and reproductive functioning. *Trends in Endocrinology and Metabolism*, 13(9), 386–392.

Davis, E.P., and Sandman, C.A. (2010). The timing of prenatal exposure to maternal cortisol and psychosocial stress is associated with human infant cognitive development. *Child Development*, 81(1), 131–148.

Diaz, R., Brown, R.W., and Seckl, J.R. (1998). Distinct ontogeny of glucocorticoid and mineralocorticoid receptor and 11beta-hydroxysteroid dehydrogenase types I and II mRNAs in the fetal rat brain suggest a complex control of glucocorticoid actions. *The Journal of Neuroscience*, 18(7), 2570–2580.

Dombrowski, S.C., Martin, R.P., and Huttunen, M.O. (2003). Association between maternal fever and psychological/behavioral outcomes: An hypothesis. *Birth Defects Research. Part A, Clinical and Molecular Teratology*, 67(11), 905–910.

Ek, C.J. Dziegielewska, K.M., Stolp, H., and Saunders, N.R. (2006). Functional effectiveness of the blood–brain barrier to small water-soluble molecules in developing and adult opossum (*Monodelphis domestica*). *Journal of Comparative Neurology*, 496(1), 13–26.

Ellis, S., Mouihate, A., and Pittman, Q.J. (2005). Early life immune challenge alters innate immune responses to lipopolysaccharide: implications for host defense as adults. *The FASEB Journal*, 19(11), 1519–1521.

Erlebacher, A., Zhang, D., Parlow, A.F., and Glimcher, L.H. (2004). Ovarian insufficiency and early pregnancy loss induced by activation of the innate immune system. *Journal of Clinical Investigation*, 114(1), 39–48.

Essex, M.J., Klein, M.H., Cho, E., Kalin, N.H. (2002). Maternal Stress beginning in infancy may sensitize children to later stress exposure: Effects on cortisol and behaviour. *Biological Psychiatry*, 52(8), 776–784.

Fan, L.W., Pang, Y., Lin, S., Rhodes, P.G., and Cai, Z. (2005). Minocycline attenuates lipopolysaccharide-induced white matter injury in the neonatal rat brain. *Neuroscience*, 133(1), 159–168.

Fan, L.W., Mitchell, H.J., Rhodes, P.G., and Cai, Z. (2008). Alpha-Phenyl-n-tert-butyl-nitrone attenuates lipopolysaccharide-induced neuronal injury in the neonatal rat brain. *Neuroscience*, 151(3), 737–744.

Fein, A., Magid, N., Savion, S., Orenstein, H., Shepshelovich, J., Ornoy, A., Torchinsky, A., and Toder, V. (2002). Diabetes teratogenicity in mice is accompanied with distorted expression of TGF-beta2 in the uterus. *Teratogenesis, Carcinogenesis and Mutagenesis*, 22(1), 59–71.

Finch, C.E., and Crimmins, E.M. (2004). Inflammatory exposure and historical changes in human life-spans. *Science*, 305(5691),1736–1739.

Foust, K.D., Nurre, E., Montgomery, C.L., Hernandez, A., Chan, C.M., and Kaspar, B.K. (2009). Intravascular AAV9 preferentially targets neonatal neurons and adult astrocytes. *Nature Biotechnology*, 27(1), 59–65.

Francis, D., Diorio, J., Liu, D., and Meaney, M.J. (1999). Nongenomic transmission across generations of maternal behavior and stress responses in the rat. *Science*, 286(5442), 1155–1158.

Gaughan, D.M., Hughes, M.D., Oleske, J.M., Malee, K., Gore, C.A., and Nachman, S. (2004). Psychiatric hospitalizations among children and youths with human immunodeficiency virus infection. 113(6), e544–551.

Gendron, R.L., Nestel, F.P., Lapp,W.S., and Baines, M.G. (1990). Lipopolysaccharide induced fetal resorption in mice is associated with the intrauterine production of tumor necrosis factor alpha. *Journal of Reproduction and Fertility*, 90(2), 395–402.

Gereda, J.E., Leung, D.Y., Thatayatikom, A., Streib, J.E., Price, M.R., Klinnert, M.D., and Liu, A.H. (2000). Relation between house-dust endotoxin exposure, type 1 T-cell development, and allergen sensitisation in infants at high risk of asthma. *Lancet*, 355(9216),1680–1683.

Gilmore, J.H., Jarskog, L.F., and Vadlamudi, S. (2003). Maternal infection regulates BDNF and NGF expression in fetal and neonatal brain and maternal–fetal unit of the rat. *Journal of Neuroimmunology*. 138(1–2), 49–55.

Gilmore, J.H., Jarskog, L.F., and Vadlamudi, S. (2005). Maternal poly I:C exposure during pregnancy regulates TNF alpha, BDNF, and NGF expression in neonatal brain and the maternal fetal unit of the rat. *Journal of Neuroimmunology*.159(1–2), 106–112.

Glover, V. (2011). Annual Research Review: Prenatal stress and the origins of psychopathology: an evolutionary perspective. *Journal of Child Psychology and Psychiatry*, 52(4), 356–367.

Goehler, L.E., Gaykema, R.P., Nguyen, K.T., Lee, J.E., Tilders, F.J., Maier, S.F., and Watkins, L.R. (1999). Interleukin-1beta in immune cells of the abdominal vagus nerve: a link between the immune and nervous systems? *Journal of Neuroscience*, 19(7), 2799–2806.

Golan, H.M., Lev, V., Hallak, M., Sorokin, Y., and Huleihel, M. (2005). Specific neurodevelopmental damage in mice offspring following maternal inflammation during pregnancy. *Neuropharmacology*, 48(6), 903–917.

Gorivodsky, M., Zemlyak, I., Orenstein, H., Savion, S., Fein, A., Torchinsky, A., and Toder, V. (1998). TNF-alpha messenger RNA and protein expression in the uteroplacental unit of mice with pregnancy loss. *Journal of Immunology*, 160(9), 4280–4288.

Graeber, M.B. (2010). Changing face of microglia. *Science*, 330(6005), 783–788.

Hassanain, M., and Levin, B.E. (2002). Dysregulation of hypothalamic serotonin turnover in diet-induced obese rats. *Brain Research*, 929(2), 175–180.

Harris, A., and Seckl, J. (2011). Glucocorticoids, prenatal stress and the programming of disease. *Hormones and Behavior*, 59(3), 279–289.

Heim, C., Plotsky, P.M., and Nemeroff, C.B. (2004). Importance of studying the contributions of early adverse experience to neurobiological findings in depression. *Neuropsychopharmacology*, 29(4), 641–648.

Heyborne, K.D., Witkin, S.S., and McGregor, J.A. (1992). Tumor necrosis factor-alpha in midtrimester amniotic fluid is associated with impaired intrauterine fetal growth. *American Journal of Obstetrics and Gynecology*, 167(4 Pt. 1), 920–925.

Hinwood, M., Tynan, R.J., Day, T.A., and Walker, F.R. (2011). Repeated social defeat selectively increases Delta FosB expression and histone H3 acetylation in the infralimbic medial prefrontal cortex. *Cerebral Cortex*, 21(2), 262–271.

Hodgson, D.M., Knott, B., and Walker, F.R. (2001). Neonatal endotoxin exposure influences HPA responsivity and impairs tumor immunity in Fischer 344 rats in adulthood. *Pediatric Research*, 50(6), 750–755.

Hodgson, D.M., and Knott, B. (2002). Potentiation of tumor metastasis in adulthood by neonatal endotoxin exposure: sex differences. *Psychoneuroendocrinology*, 27(7), 791–804.

Hood, K.E., Dreschel, N.A., Granger, D.A. (2003). Maternal behaviour changes after immune challenge of neonates with developmental effects on adult social behavior. *Developmental Psychobiology*, 42(1), 17–34.

Hornig, M., and Lipkin, I. (2001). Infectious and immune factors in the pathogenesis of neurodevelopmental disorders: epidemiology, hypotheses, and animal models. *Mental Retardation and Developmental Disabilities Research Review*, 7(3), 200–210.

Huang., L.T. (2011). The link between perinatal glucocorticoids exposure and psychiatric disorders. *Pediatric Research*, 69(5 Pt. 2), 19R–25R.

Hunter, R.G., McCarthy, K.J., Milne, T.A., Pfaff, D.W., and McEwen, B.S. (2009). Regulation of hippocampal H3 histone methylation by acute and chronic stress. *Proceedings of the National Academy of Sciences of the USA*, 106(49), 20912–20917.

Ishikawa, J., Ishikawa, A., and Nakamura, S. (2007). Interferon-alpha reduces the density of monoaminergic axons in the rat brain. *Neuroreport*, 18(2), 137–140.

Iwasa, T., Matsuzaki, T., Murakami, M., Kinouchi, R., Shimizu, F., Kuwahara, A., Yasui, T., and Irahara, M. (2009). Neonatal immune challenge affects the regulation of estrus cyclicity and feeding behavior in female rats. *International Journal of Developmental Neuroscience*, 27(1), 111–114.

Jaworek, J., Nawrot-Porabka, K., Leja-Szpak, A., Szklarczyk, J., Macko, M., Bonior, J. et al. (2007). Exposition of newborn rats to bacterial endotoxin impairs pancreatic enzyme secretion at adult age. *Journal of Physiology and Pharmacology*, 58(2), 287–302.

Kalinichev, M., Easterling, K.W., Plotsky, P.M., and Holtzman, S.G. (2002). Long-lasting changes in stress-induced corticosterone response and anxiety-like behaviors as a consequence of neonatal maternal separation in Long–Evans rats. *Pharmacology Biochemistry and Behavior*, 73(1), 131–140.

Karrow, N.A. (2006). Activation of the hypothalamic–pituitary–adrenal axis and autonomic nervous system during inflammation and altered programming of the neuroendocrine–immune axis during fetal and neonatal development: Lessons learned from the model inflammagen, lipopolysaccharide. *Brain, Behavior, and Immunity*. 20(2), 144–158.

Kent, S., Kelley, K.W., and Dantzer, R. (1992). Effects of lipopolysaccharide on food-motivated behavior in the rat are not blocked by an interleukin-1receptor antagonist. *Neuroscience Letters*, 145(1), 83–86.

Konsman, J., Parnet, P., and Dantzer, R. (2002). Cytokine-induced sickness behavior: Mechanisms and implications. *Trends in Neuroscience*, 25(3), 154–159.

Kurina, L.M., Goldacre, M.J., Yeates, D., and Gill, L.E. (2001). Depression and anxiety in people with inflammatory bowel disease. *Journal of Epidemiology and Community Health*, 55(10), 716–720.

Lewis, S. (2011). Development: Microglia go pruning. *Nature Reviews Neuroscience*, 12(9), 492–493.

Libbey, J.E., Sweeten, T.L., McMahon, W.M., and Fujinami, R.S. (2005). Autistic disorder and viral infections. *Journal of Neurovirology*, 11(1), 1–10.

Li, X.F., Kinsey-Jones, J.S., Knox, A.M., Wu, X.Q., Tahsinsoy, D., Brain, S.D., et al. (2007). Neonatal lipopolysaccharide exposure exacerbates stress-induced suppression of lutenizing hormone pulse frequency in adulthood. *Endocrinology*, 148(12), 5984–5890.

Lin, Y-L., Lin, S-Y., and Wang, S. (2012). Prenatal lipopolysaccharide exposure increases anxiety-like behaviors and enhances stress-induced corticosterone responses in adult rats. *Brain, Behavior, and Immunity*, 26(3), 459–468. DOI: 10.1016/j.bbi.2011.12.003.

Litonjua, A.A., Milton, D.K., Celedon, J.C., Ryan, L., Weiss, S.T., and Gold, D.R. (2002). A longitudinal analysis of wheezing in young children: The independent effects of early life exposure to house dust endotoxin, allergens, and pets. *Journal of Allergy and Clinical Immunology*, 110(5), 736–742.

Liu, D., Diorio, J., Tannenbaum, B., Caldji, C., Francis, D., Freedman, A., et al. (1997). Maternal care, hippocampal glucocorticoid receptors, and hypothalamic–pituitary–adrenal responses to stress. *Science*, 277(5332), 1659–1662.

Lowenstein, P.R. (2009). Crossing the Rubicon. *Nature Biotechnology*, 27(1), 42–44.

Lucchina, L., Carola, V., Pitossi, F., and Depino, A.M. (2010). Evaluating the interaction between early postnatal inflammation and maternal care in the programming of adult anxiety and depression-related behaviors. *Behavioral Brain Research*, 213(1), 56–65.

Lupien, S.J., McEwen, B.S., Gunnar, M.R., and Heim, C. (2009). Effects of stress throughout the lifespan on the brain, behaviour and cognition. *Nature Reviews Neuroscience*, 10(6), 434–445.

Mackay-Sim, A., Feron, F., Eyles, D., Burne, T., and McGrath, J. (2004). Schizophrenia, vitamin D, and brain development. *International Review of Neurobiology*, 59, 351–380.

Maes, M., Yirmiya, R., Noraberg, J., Brene, S., Hibbeln, J., Perini, G. (2009). The inflammatory and neurodegenerative (I&ND) hypothesis of depression: Leads for future research and new drug developments in depression. *Metabolic Brain Disease*, 24(1): 27–53.

Main, M., and Hesse, E. (1990). Parents' unresolved traumatic experiences are related to infant disorganized attachment status: Is frightened and/or frightening parental behavior the linking mechanism? In M. Greenberg, D. Cicchetti, and E.M. Cummings (Eds.), *Attachment in the Preschool Years: Theory, Research and Intervention* (pp. 161–184). University of Chicago Press.

Malaeb, S., and Dammann, O. (2009). Fetal inflammatory response and brain injury in the preterm newborn. *Journal of Child Neurology*, 24(9), 1119–1126.

Maynard, T.M., Sikich, L., Lieberman, J.A., and Lamantia, A.S. (2001). Neural development, cell–cell signaling, and the "Two-Hit" hypothesis of schizophrenia. *Schizophrenia Bulletin*, 27(3), 457–476.

McGuffin, P., Owen, M.J., and Farmer, A.E. (1995). Genetic basis of schizophrenia. *Lancet*, 346(8976), 678–682.

McLoyd, V.C. (1998). Socioeconomic disadvantage and child development. *American Psychologist*, 53(2), 185–204.

Meaney, M.J., Szyf, M., and Seckl, J.R. (2007). Epigenetic mechanisms of perinatal programming of hypothalamic–pituitary–adrenal function and health. *Trends in Molecular Medicine*, 13(7), 269–277.

Meaney, M.J., and Ferguson-Smith, A.C. (2010). Epigenetic regulation of the neural transcriptome: the meaning of the marks. *Nature Neuroscience*, 13(11), 1313–1318.

Merikangas, K.R., and Swendsen, J.D. (1997). Genetic epidemiology of psychiatric disorders. *Epidemiologic Reviews*, 19(1), 144–155.

Meyer, U., Nyffeler, M., Engler, A., Urwyler, A., Schedlowski, M., Knuesel, I., Yee, B.K., and Feldon, J. (2006). The time of prenatal immune challenge determines the specificity of inflammation-mediated brain and behavioral pathology. *Journal of Neuroscience*, 26(18), 4752–4762.

Meyer, U., Feldon. J., and Yee, B.K. (2009). A review of the fetal brain cytokine imbalance hypothesis of schizophrenia. *Schizophrenia Bulletin*, 35(5), 959–972.

Miller, G. (2005). The dark side of glia. *Science*, 308(5723), 778–781.

Morgan, H.D., Santos, F., Green, K., Dean, W., and Reik, W. (2005). Epigenetic reprogramming in mammals. *Human Molecular Genetics*, 14(1), R47–R58.

Mullen, P.E., Martin, J.L., Anderson, J.C., Romans, S.E., and Herbison, G.P. (1996). The long-term impact of the physical, emotional, and sexual abuse of children: A community study. *Child Abuse and Neglect*, 20(1), 7–21.

Nelson, C.A. (2000). Neural plasticity and human development: The role of early experience in sculpting memory systems. *Developmental Science*, 3(2), 115–136.

O'Connor, J.C., Lawson, M.A., André, C., Moreau, M., Lestage, J., Castanon, N. (2009). Lipopolysaccharide-induced depressive-like behavior is mediated by indoleamine 2,3-dioxygenase activation in mice. *Molecular Psychiatry*, 14(5), 511–522.

Paolicelli, R.C., Bolasco, G., Pagani, F., Maggi, L., Scianni, M., Panzanelli, P., et al. (2011). Synaptic pruning by microglia is necessary for normal brain development. *Science*, 333(6048): 1456–1458.

Patterson, P.H. (2002). Maternal infection: window on neuroimmune interactions in fetal brain development and mental illness. *Current Opinion in Neurobiology*, 12(1), 115–118.

Plomin, R., Owen, M.J., and McGuffin, P. (1994). The genetic basis of complex human behaviours. *Science.*, 264(5166), 1733–1739.

Plotsky, P.M., Thrivikraman, K.V., Nemeroff, C.B., Caldji, C., Sharma, S., and Meaney, M.J. (2005). Long-term consequences of neonatal rearing on central corticotrophin-releasing factor systems in adult male offspring. *Neuropsychopharmacology*, 30(12), 2192–2204.

Rapetti, R.L., Taylor, S.E., and Seeman, T.E. (2002). Risky families: Family, social environments and the mental and physical health of offspring. *Psychological Bulletin*. 128(2), 330–366.

Reul, J.M., Stec, I., Wiegers, G.J., Labeur, M.S., Linthorst, A.C.E., Arzt, E., and Holsboer, F. (1994). Prenatal immune challenge alters the hypothalamic–pituitary–adrenocortical axis in adult rats. *Journal of Clinical Investigation*, 93(6): 2600–2607.

Reul, J.M.,Hesketh, S.A., Collins, A., and Mecinas, M.G. (2009). Epigenetic mechanisms in the dentate gyrus act as a molecular switch in hippocampus-associated memory formation. *Epigenetics*, 4(7), 434–439.

Rice, D., and Barone, S. (2000). Critical periods of vulnerability for the developing nervous system: evidence from humans and animal models. *Environmental Health Perspectives*, 108(3), 511–533.

Rich, E.L., and Romero, L.M. (2005). Exposure to chronic stress downregulates corticosterone responses to acute stressors. *American Journal of Physiology. Regulatory, Integrative, Comparative Physiology*, 288(6), R1628–1636.

Rico, J.L., Ferraz, D.B., Ramalho-Pinto, F.J., and Morato, S. (2010). Neonatal exposure to LPS leads to heightened exploratory activity in adolescent rats. *Behavioural Brain Research*, 215(1), 102–109.

Sapolsky, R., Rivier, C., Yamamoto, G., Plotsky, P., and Vale, W. (1987). Interleukin-1 stimulates the secretion of hypothalamic corticotropin-releasing factor. *Science*, 238(4826), 522.

Sapolsky, R.M. (1996). Stress, Glucocorticoids, and Damage to the Nervous System: The Current State of Confusion. *Stress*, 1(1), 1–19.

Saunders, N.R., Ek, C.J., and Dziegielewska, K.M. (2009). The neonatal blood–brain barrier is functionally effective, and immaturity does not explain differential targeting of AAV9. *Nature Biotechnology*, 27(9), 804–805.

Scharf, M. (2007). Long-term effects of trauma: Psychosocial functioning of the second and third generation of Holocaust survivors. *Development and Psychopathology*, 19(2), 603–622.

Schlotz, W., and Phillips, D.I.W. (2009). Fetal origins of mental health: Evidence and mechanisms. *Brain, Behavior, and Immunity*, 23(7), 905–916.

Schwarz, J.M., and Bilbo, S.D. (2011). LPS elicits a much larger and broader inflammatory response than Escherichia coli infection within the hippocampus of neonatal rats. *Neuroscience Letters*, 497(2), 110–115.

Shalev, U., and Weiner, I. (2001). Gender-dependent differences in latent inhibition following prenatal stress and corticosterone administration. *Behavioral Brain Research*, 126(1–2), 57–63.

Shanks, N., Larocque, S., and Meaney, M.J. (1995). Neonatal endotoxin exposure alters the development of the hypothalamic–pituitary–adrenal axis: Early illness and later responsivity to stress. *Journal of Neuroscience*, 15(1 Pt. 1), 376–384.

Shanks, N., Windle, R.J., Perks, P.A., Harbuz, M.S. Jessop, D.S., Ingram, C.D., and Lightman, S.L. (2000). Early-life exposure to endotoxin alters hypothalamic–pituitary–adrenal function and predisposition to inflammation. *Proceedings of the National Academy of Sciences of the USA*, 97(10), 5645-5650.

Skinner, M.K., and Guerrero-Bosagna, C. (2009). Environmental signals and transgenerational epigenetics. *Epigenomics*, 1(1), 111–117.

Smith, S.E., Li, J., Garbett, K., Mirnics, K., and Patterson, P.H. (2007). Maternal immune activation alters fetal brain development through interleukin-6. *Journal of Neuroscience*, 27(40), 10695–10702.

Smith, S.E.P., Hsiao, E., and Patterson, P.H. (2010). Activation of the maternal immune system as a risk factor for neuropsychiatric disorders. In A.W. Zimmerman and S.I. Connors (Eds.). *Maternal Influences on Fetal Neurodevelopment. Clinical and Research Aspects* (pp. 97–115). New York: Springer Science Publishers.

Sominsky, L., Walker, A.K., Ong, L.K., Tynan, R.J., Walker, F.R., and Hodgson, D.M. (2012). Increased microglial activation in the rat brain following neonatal exposure to a bacterial mimetic. *Behavioral Brain Research*, 226(1), 351–356.

Spencer, S.J., Martin, S., Mouihate, A., and Pittman, Q.J. (2006). Early life immune challenge: defining a critical window for effects on adult responses to immune challenge. *Neuropsychopharmacology*, 31(9), 1910–1918.

Spencer, S.J., Field, E., and Pittman, Q.J. (2010). Neonatal programming by neuroimmune challenge: Effects on responses and tolerance to septic doses of lipopolysaccharide in adult male and female rats. *Journal of Neuroendocrinology*, 22(4), 272–281.

Sullivan, E.L., Grayson, B., Takahashi, D., Robertson, N., Maier, A., Bethea, C.L., Smith, M.S., Coleman, K., and Grove, K.L. (2010). Chronic consumption of a high-fat diet during pregnancy causes perturbations in the serotonergic system and increased anxiety-like behavior in nonhuman primate offspring. *Journal of Neuroscience*, 30(10), 3826–3830.

Surani, A.M. (2001). Reprogramming of genome function through epigenetic inheritance. *Nature*, 414(6859), 122–128.

Tochigi, M., Okazaki, Y., Kato, N., and Sasaki, T. (2004). What causes seasonality of birth in schizophrenia? *Neuroscience Research*, 48(1), 1–11.

Tramer, M. (1929). Ueber die biologische bedeutung des geburtsmonates insbesondere fuer die psychoseerkrankung, *Schweizer Archiv fuer Neurologie und Psychiatrie*, 24, 17–24.

Valentine, A.D., Meyers, C.A., Kling, M.A., Richelson, E., and Hauser, P. (1998). Mood and cognitive side effects of interferon-alpha therapy. *Seminars in Oncology*, 25(1 Suppl 1), 39–47.

van der Flier, M., Stockhammer, G., Vonk, G.J., Nikkels, P.G., van Diemen-Steenvoorde, R.A., van der Vlist, et al. (2001). Vascular endothelial growth factor in bacterial meningitis: detection in cerebrospinal fluid and localization in postmortem brain. *Journal of Infectious Diseases*, 183(1), 149–153.

Vitkovic, L., Bockaert, J., and Jacque, C. (2000). "Inflammatory" cytokines: neuromodulators in normal brain? *Journal of Neurochemistry*, 74(2), 457–471.

Walker, F.R., Brogan, A., Smith, R., and Hodgson, D.M. (2004a). A profile of the immediate endocrine, metabolic and behavioral responses following a dual exposure to endotoxin in early life. *Physiology and Behavior*, 83(3), 495–504.

Walker, F.R., March, J., and Hodgson, D.M. (2004b). Endotoxin exposure in early life alters the development of anxiety-like behaviour in the Fischer 344 rat. *Behavioral Brain Research*, 154(1), 63–69.

Walker, F.R., Knott, B., and Hodgson, D.M. (2008). Neonatal endotoxin exposure modifies the acoustic startle response and circulating levels of corticosterone in the adult rat but only following acute stress. *Journal of Psychiatric Research*, 42(13), 1094–1103.

Walker, A.K., Nakamura, T., Byrne, R.J., Naicker, S., Tynan, R.J., Hunter, M., and Hodgson, D.M. (2009). Neonatal lipopolysaccharide and adult stress exposure predisposes rodents to anxiety-like behavior and blunted corticosterone responses: implications for the double-hit hypothesis. *Psychoneuroendocrinology*, 34(10), 1515–1525.

Walker, A.K., Nakamura, T., and Hodgson, D.M. (2010). Neonatal lipopolysaccharide exposure alters central cytokine responses to stress in adulthood in Wistar rats. *Stress*, 13(6), 506–15.

Walker, A.K., Hiles, S.A., Sominsky, L., Mclaughlin, E.A., and Hodgson, D.M. (2011). Neonatal lipopolysaccharide exposure impairs sexual development and reproductive success in the Wistar rat. *Brain, Behavior, and Immunity*, 25(4), 674–684.

Walker, A.K., Hawkins, G., Sominsky, L., and Hodgson, D.M. (2012). Transgenerational transmission of anxiety induced by neonatal exposure to lipopolysaccharide: implications for male and female germ lines. *Psychoneuroendocrinology*, 37(8), 1320–1335.

Watkins, L.R., Maier, S.F., and Goehler, L.E. (1995). Cytokine-to-brain communication: A review and analysis of alternative mechanisms. *Life Sciences*, 57(11), 1011–1026.

Weaver, I.C., Cervoni, N., Champagne, F.A., D'Alessio, A.C., Sharma, S., Seckl, J.R., et al. (2004). Epigenetic programming by maternal behavior. *Nature Neuroscience*, 7(8), 847–854.

Weaver, I.C., Meaney, M.J., and Szyf, M. (2006). Maternal care effects on the hippocampal transcriptome and anxiety-mediated behaviors in the offspring that are reversible in adulthood. *Proceedings of the National Academy of Sciences of the USA*, 103(9), 3480–3485.

Weiss, E.L., Longhurst, J.G., and Mazure, C.M. (1999).Childhood sexual abuse as a risk factor for depression in women: Psychosocial and neurobiological correlates. *American Journal of Psychiatry*, 156(6), 816–828.

Welberg, L.A., and Seckl, J.R. (2001). Prenatal stress, glucocorticoids and the programming of the brain. *Journal of Neuroendocrinology*, 13(2), 113–128.

Wilson, C.J., Finch, C.E., and Cohen, H.J. (2002). Cytokines and cognition – the case for a head-to-toe inflammation paradigm. *Journal of the American Geriatric Society*, 50(12), 2041–2056.

Witek-Janusek, L. (1988). Pituitary–adrenal response to bacterial endotoxin in developing rats. *American Journal of Physiology*, 255(4 Pt. 2), E525–30.

Yirmiya, R. (1996). Endotoxin produces a depressive-like episode in rats. *Brain Research*, 711(1–2), 163–174.

Zaretsky, M.V., Alexander, J.M., Byrd, W., and Bawdon, R.E. (2004). Transfer of inflammatory cytokines across the placenta. *Obstetrics and Gynecology*, 103(3), 546–550.

Zhang, T.Y., and Meaney, M.J. (2010). Epigenetics and the environmental regulation of the genome and its function. *Annual Review of Psychology*, 61, 439–466.

Ziv, Y., and Schwartz, M. (2008). Immune-based regulation of adult neurogenesis: implications for learning and memory. *Brain, Behavior, and Immunity*, 22(2), 167–176.

Zuckerman, L., Rehavi, M., Nachman, R., and Weiner, I. (2003). Immune activation during pregnancy in rats leads to a postpubertal emergence of disrupted latent inhibition, dopaminergic hyperfunction, and altered limbic morphology in the offspring: a novel neurodevelopmental model of schizophrenia. *Neuropsychopharmacology*, 28(10), 1778–1789.

15

Microglia and Neurodevelopment

Programming of Cognition throughout the Lifespan

Jaclyn M. Schwarz[1] and Staci D. Bilbo[2]

[1]*Department of Psychology, University of Delaware, Newark, DE, USA*
[2]*Department of Psychology and Neuroscience, Duke University, Durham, NC, USA*

Introduction

Well-known for its critical role in host defense, the immune system also plays a critical role in brain development. The resident immune cells of the brain, microglia, and their releasable factors, cytokines and chemokines, have a central role in many processes of neural development, including cell proliferation, neurogenesis, synaptogenesis, and programmed cell death. In addition, the immune system represents a particularly critical interface between the environment, physiology, and brain of an individual, such that external stimuli can affect not only the immediate development but also the later-life function of the brain and behavior via activation of the immune system. Thus, neuroimmune activation during prenatal or early postnatal development can have profound and long-lasting effects on the brain. The purpose of this chapter will be to provide an up-to-date review of the *long-term effects* of early-life immune activation on adult cognition, a current perspective on the *long-term mechanisms* by which these effects are propagated from development to adulthood, and a brief primer on the techniques and methodology by which the long-term consequences of early-life immune activation on later-life cognition can be investigated in a rodent model.

Microglia and Neurodevelopment

Colonization of microglia in the developing rodent brain

Microglia originate early in the life of the rodent fetus and can be very long-lived, meaning that microglia are believed to reside in the brain for the entire life of the rodent. Microglial *progenitor cells* begin colonizing the rodent brain around embryonic day (E) 9–10 via the infiltration of primitive macrophage precursors from the yolk sac (Chan, Kohsaka, and Rezaie, 2007; Ginhoux *et al.*, 2010). Primitive microglia have been localized to subcortical regions of the developing brain including the hippocampus and the corpus callosum (Wang *et al.*, 2002; Xu, Kaur, and Ling, 1993), entering the brain parenchyma via the blood stream and ventricles

The Wiley-Blackwell Handbook of Psychoneuroimmunology, First Edition. Edited by Alexander W. Kusnecov and Hymie Anisman.

(Cuadros and Navascués, 1998). After their initial colonization of the brain, microglia migrate to their final destination within the brain, where they continue to proliferate throughout pre- and postnatal brain development.

To date, it is not well-known what factors drive the infiltration and migration of immature microglia into the brain parenchyma. Some researchers have noted that the invasion of microglia within the developing brain coincides with the naturally occurring programmed cell death during early brain development (Ashwell, 1991; Perry, Hume, and Gordon, 1985); however, very little is known about the exact relationship between developmental cell death in the brain and microglial colonization of neural tissues. While it is possible that the factors released from dying cells within the developing brain may in turn control the migration and infiltration of microglia into the parenchyma, it is also possible that other factors may attract the infiltration and migration of immature microglia throughout the developing nervous system. In fact, many chemokines (*chemo*tactic cyto*kines*) have a demonstrated role in microglial migration and neural development within the healthy brain (Cowell *et al.*, 2006; Cowell and Silverstein, 2003; Rezaie *et al.*, 2002), and a significant number of chemokines are highly upregulated within the rat hippocampus/cortex at birth, when compared to the adult brain. These include chemokine (C-C motif) ligand (CCL) 2, CCL3, CCL6, CCL7, and CCL12.

A few of these cytokines (CCL3, CCL5, and CCL7) are expressed by astrocytes and neural progenitor cells, and have a demonstrated role in regulating the development of microglial cells within the human brain (Hahn *et al.*, 2010; McKimmie and Graham, 2010; Rezaie *et al.*, 2002). Monocyte-chemoattractant protein (MCP)-1 (also known as CCL2), and intercellular cell adhesion molecule (ICAM)-2 may also play a role (Rezaie, Patel, and Male, 1999), and a recent report shows that mice lacking the receptor for colony-stimulating factor (CSF)-1 do not develop microglia (Ginhoux *et al.*, 2010). Thus, neural progenitor cells and immature astrocytes may release these chemokines, even in the absence of cell death, as a mechanism for attracting primitive macrophages and immature microglia into the developing brain.

Microglia have a distinct morphology throughout neural development

Developing microglia have a distinct morphology and function within the neonatal brain. Microglia shift morphology and function throughout brain development from an immature/amoeboid morphology to a mature/ramified morphology (Figure 15.1). This shift in microglial morphology occurs in an age- and brain region-dependent manner, such that microglial number, morphology, and cytokine/chemokine production coincide with the neural development of each brain region. For example, IL-1β is produced at detectable levels within the cortex from approximately E14 to postnatal day (P) 7 (Giulian *et al.*, 1988). In contrast, the cerebellum which develops significantly later, just prior to birth in rodents, has a peak in IL-1β levels that occurs from P2 to P14 (Giulian *et al.*, 1988). The developmental shift in microglial morphology and function is best-characterized within the hippocampus, cortex, and amygdala, brain regions that are important for cognitive processes such as learning, memory, attention, and a number of social behaviors in adulthood.

Within the embryonic hippocampus, cortex, and amygdala of the rat, microglia have a predominantly round amoeboid morphology, even days prior to birth. At this time, very few microglia have short, stout processes which extend from the enlarged soma. At birth, however, the microglial population begins to exhibit a significantly different morphology,

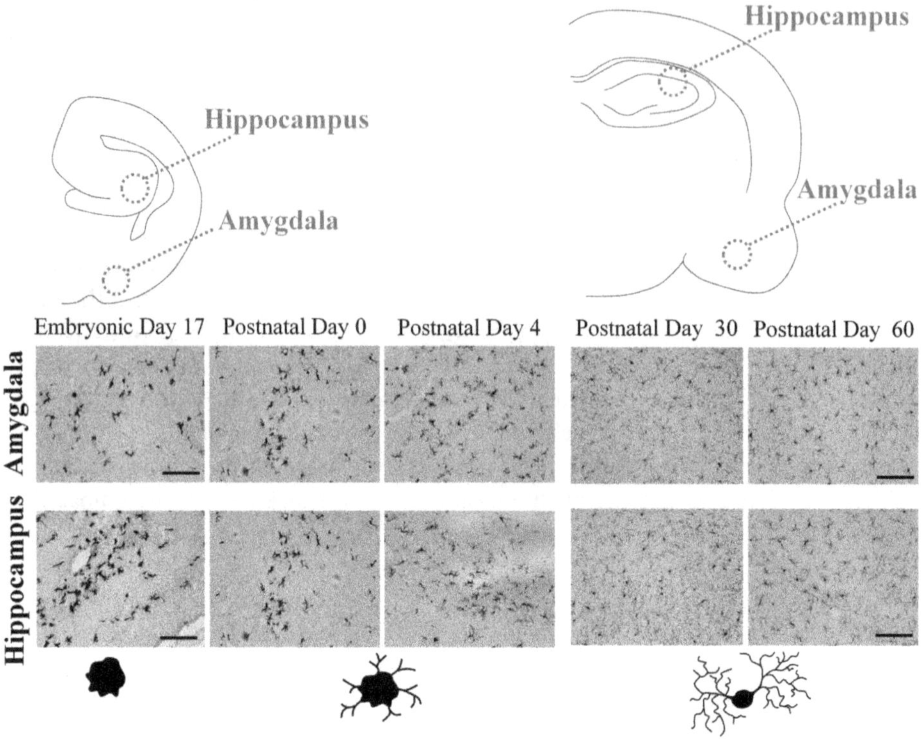

Figure 15.1 Microglia have a distinct morphology throughout early brain development. By embryonic day 17, microglia have heavily colonized the developing amygdala and hippocampus, two brain regions critical for cognition in adulthood, within the rat brain (scale bar = 50 μm). At birth (postnatal day 0) microglia begin to develop thick, short branches which elongate considerably by postnatal day 4. Later in development, by postnatal day 30, microglia have a more ramified morphology characterized by small cell bodies and thin, long processes, a morphology which is maintained into and throughout young adulthood, represented here at postnatal day 60 (scale bar = 50 μm). All photos taken at 20×.

as more microglia display short or long, thick processes at this time. Just four days later, on postnatal day (P) 4, there is a significant increase in the *number* of microglia within these brain regions and a dramatic shift in *morphology* such that microglia begin displaying smaller cell bodies and thinner processes. These findings indicate that, even at this early time point in neurodevelopment, microglia are rapidly maturing and shifting into a more ramified morphology.

Coincident with the striking difference in morphology, developing microglia also exhibit a significantly different biochemistry than microglia in the adult brain. For example, between birth and P4 the expression of Interleukin (IL)-1β, the enzyme which cleaves IL-1β into its active form (Caspase 1), and the IL-1 "decoy" receptor (IL1r2) are significantly increased approximately 6-, 6-, and 10-fold, respectively, when compared to the adult hippocampus and cortex, suggesting that immune molecules and signaling pathways such as these may have a more ubiquitous role within the brain than originally thought.

Further research must be done to expand the current knowledge of microglial ontogeny and function throughout the developing brain. Understanding the mechanisms of microglial colonization will lend greater insight into the mechanisms by which the brain develops under normal circumstances, and the mechanisms by which the developing brain might respond and subsequently be affected by an early-life immune challenge that occurs at the peak of microglial colonization, when cytokine and chemokine production are quite distinct from that in the adult brain.

The functional role of cytokines in brain development

Taking into consideration the morphology of immature microglia and the increased production of cytokines within the developing brain described above, one might assume that the primary role of microglia within the developing brain is related to their role as brain macrophages, specifically that they are actively engaged in the phagocytosis of cellular debris of apoptotic cells as well as the induction of apoptosis in other cells (Bessis *et al.*, 2007; Marin-Teva *et al.*, 2004). However, recent work suggests that microglia, cytokines, and chemokines have a more complex role in the developing immune system.

In addition to phagocytosing dying cells and cellular debris, microglia have a critical role in the phagocytosis of spurious synapses throughout development (Stevens *et al.*, 2007; Schafer *et al.*, 2012). Synapse elimination is an important process of neural development and is critical for the formation of functional neural circuits. C1q, the initiating protein within the classical complement cascade of the immune system, localizes to synapses within the postnatal brain intended for elimination. Microglia expressing the complement receptor for this protein are subsequently activated for phagocytosis of these individual synapses (Schafer *et al.*, 2012). A large number of cytokines and other immune molecules, many of which are microglial-derived, have been characterized for their importance in many neurodevelopmental processes such as neurogenesis, neuronal and glial cell migration, proliferation, differentiation, and synaptic maturation and pruning. These include members of the gp130, bone morphogenetic protein (BMP), and transforming growth factor beta (TGF-β) super-families, as well as many traditionally defined "pro-inflammatory" cytokines (e.g., IL-1β, TNF-α) (Garay and McAllister, 2010; Deverman and Patterson, 2009). Chemokines also have a more ubiquitous function within the developing brain. For example, the chemokine (C-X-C motif) CXCL12 (SDF-1) and its exclusive receptor CXCR4 have a critical role in the migration of different neuronal populations to their final destination within brain regions such as the developing cerebellum, dentate gyrus, cortex, and hypothalamus (see Deverman and Patterson, 2009, for review). These data suggest that similar to their chemoattractant role within the immune system, chemokines may be produced and/or secreted by other cell types within the brain and as such guide the migration of neurons to their final destination within their respective functional circuits. We anticipate that future research will identify additional mechanisms by which immune molecules and microglia guide the normal development of the nervous system.

The Long-term Consequences of Early-Life Infection: Neuroimmune and Cognitive Dysfunction

Given the evidence presented above describing the important role of the immune system in normal brain development, it is likely no surprise that elevated levels of pro-inflammatory cytokines, caused by perinatal infection (bacterial or viral), have been linked with abnormal brain development and an increased risk of neurodevelopmental disorders in humans (Cai *et al.*, 2000; Meyer *et al.*, 2006; Pang, Cai, and Rhodes, 2003; Urakubo *et al.*, 2001). Bacterial infection represents the number-one cause of perinatal infection in newborns worldwide and is a significant cause and consequence of premature births (Osrin, Vergnano, and Costello, 2004; Skogstrand *et al.*, 2008). Human newborns are particularly impaired in their ability to mount an immune response against bacteria, and this results in increased infant mortality, especially within developing countries (Marshall-Clarke *et al.*, 2000; Osrin, Vergnano, and Costello, 2004). Viral infections, such as maternal influenza infection, result in increased cytokine production via the activation of the maternal immune system, the fetal immune system, and immune cells within the placenta. The increased synthesis of cytokines following maternal influenza infection has been linked to an increased risk of schizophrenia in offspring, as well as a host of other cognitive disorders (Brown *et al.*, 2004; Mortensen *et al.*, 1999).

Recent advances in maternal and perinatal medicine have greatly increased survival rates following perinatal infection, particularly among populations in developed countries. Despite this, it remains to be determined what the total impact of perinatal infection may be on the physiology and behavior of surviving individuals. In contrast to cellular or neural damage, one of the most common long-term consequences of perinatal infection or inflammation is *cognitive dysfunction* (Bauman, Filipek, and Kemper, 1997), which includes general deficits in learning, memory, and attention; however, the exact mechanisms underlying these deficits are unknown. In addition, neuropsychiatric conditions as diverse as Alzheimer's disease, autism, and depression are similarly associated with neuroimmune abnormalities, including exaggerated microglial activation and altered cytokine expression; yet the proposed etiology of these disorders, such as a single precipitous event or infection, has been either insufficient or may simply not be well understood. Thus, the early-life immune "history" of an individual may be the key to understanding the later-life risk of developing not only general cognitive deficits but also the risk of other neuropsychiatric disorders.

Developmental or "fetal programming" is an area of research that is based on the idea that experiences during the pre- or postnatal period may modulate or "program" the trajectory of a particular developmental processes, with the result that adult outcomes such as behavior are significantly and often permanently affected. This concept has been well-described with regards to the long-term consequences of early-life stress and resulting glucocorticoid exposure, maternal interactions, fetal growth, and metabolism (Champagne *et al.*, 2008; de Boo and Harding, 2006; Owen, Andrews, and Matthews, 2005). In contrast, the concept of perinatal programming of the immune system and the potential effects on brain and behavior in adulthood remains relatively unexplored, despite strong evidence that perinatal exposure to infectious agents has a number of influences on later life outcomes including disease susceptibility, and, as mentioned above, increased vulnerability to cognitive and/or neuropsychiatric disorders (Hornig *et al.*, 1999; Nelson and Willoughby, 2000; Shi *et al.*, 2009).

We hypothesize the developing brain is particularly sensitive to early life immune activation and the associated risk of later-life cognitive disorders because: 1) microglia are long-lived, such that previously activated microglia (e.g. microglia exposed to an early-life immune challenge) may remain within the brain into adulthood; 2) immature microglia within the developing brain are functionally and/or immunologically different than microglia within the adult brain, such that early-life immune activation can have greater consequences for neuroimmune function when compared to the adult brain; and 3) microglia and their inflammatory products are critical for normal cognitive function and behavior, such that *neuroimmune dysfunction results in cognitive dysfunction*. We present evidence within the following sections that directly support this hypothesis and describe techniques that can be used to explicitly test these general ideas for researchers interested in understanding the long-term consequences of early-life infection on later-life behavior.

A rodent model of early-life infection and later-life cognitive dysfunction

Infection of rat pups with a non-lethal dose of *Escherichia coli* (*E. coli*) on P4, a developmental time point in rodents that is similar to the third trimester of prenatal development in humans, produces a robust immune response within the periphery and the brain. Within the hippocampus, neonatal infection causes a prolonged (~ 48 hour) increase in cytokine expression, with a distinct increase in the expression of genes from the IL-1 family of cytokines. *E. coli* increases the expression of IL-1β, Caspase 1 (which cleaves IL-1β from its pro- to its active form), IL-18, and the IL-1 receptors 1 and 2 within the hippocampus (Bilbo *et al.*, 2005b; Schwarz and Bilbo, 2011). Cytokine receptors are distributed throughout the developing and adult brain and the hippocampus, in particular, has one of the highest densities of microglia and cytokine receptors within the brain, including receptors for IL-1β.

The hippocampus is a brain region critical for learning and memory, spatial navigation, and attention in adulthood. The hippocampus is particularly vulnerable to damage from events such as chronic/severe stress, epilepsy, stroke, hypoxia/ischemia, or cardiac arrest that occur during development or in adulthood (Fujioka *et al.*, 2000; Petito *et al.*, 1987; Salmenpera *et al.*, 1998; Sapolsky *et al.*, 1987). The developing hippocampus is similarly vulnerable to an early-life infection, as a single neonatal infection can affect cognitive processes such as learning and memory in adulthood. However, there are two potential mechanisms by which a neonatal infection might influence adult neural function and associated learning and memory. Early-life immune activation could permanently damage or disrupt the development of neural pathways important for learning and memory within the hippocampus, or alternatively early-life immune activation could re-program immune function thereby negatively affecting how the adult immune system responds to a subsequent immune challenge via either prolonged or exaggerated pro-inflammatory cytokine production or decreased anti-inflammatory regulation. In this case, abnormal levels of cytokines and chemokines would *indirectly* impair the neural processes important for learning and memory.

To distinguish between these two potential hypotheses, adult rats infected neonatally with *E. coli* were tested in a modified version of contextual fear-conditioning known as the context pre-exposure task, a simple yet robust method for assessing a rat's memory for a recently explored context (Rudy, Huff, and Matus-Amat, 2004). In this task, when a rat is placed into a specific context and *immediately* shocked, he displays little or no conditioned fear (freezing) to the context the next day. This absence of fear to the context is thought to occur because the rat does not have the opportunity to adequately sample the environment and thus store a representation of its features (a hippocampal-dependent process) prior to an immediate shock. If, however, a rat is pre-exposed to the context for several minutes the day before, an immediate shock the following day will produce substantial freezing on a subsequent test day. The benefit of this technique is that a representation of the context can be learned and thus stored a day prior to immediate shock and the memory test. Thus, an immune challenge given immediately after the context pre-exposure can affect learning without directly affecting the behavioral output during the memory test given days later.

Neonatally infected rats or controls received no injection, saline, or a low dose of lipopolysaccharide (LPS) (which by itself does not cause memory impairments) immediately following the context pre-exposure. If the adult LPS challenge causes an exaggerated or prolonged immune response in neonatally infected rats that would interfere with learning the context, then only rats that experience the combination of a neonatal infection and LPS after context pre-exposure would display impaired memory. However, if neonatal *E. coli* infection directly alters the development of neural pathways that support memory formation, one would find that neonatally infected rats should display impaired memory regardless of the adult immune challenge. The results of these experiments demonstrate that only rats that experience the *combination* of neonatal infection and subsequent LPS exposure display impaired memory for the explored context (Bilbo *et al.*, 2005a). In contrast, neonatally infected rats that do not receive an adult immune challenge at the time of context pre-exposure do not exhibit memory deficits, similar to controls. Interestingly, this treatment paradigm has no effect on conditioned fear to a tone that was paired with the shock (Bilbo *et al.*, 2006), indicating the long-term consequences of early-life infection on cognitive function are specific to hippocampal-dependent learning and memory. Taken together, these data support the hypothesis that neonatal immune activation increases the risk of cognitive deficits *indirectly*, via long-term programming of neuroimmune responses which subsequently interferes with learning and memory. In addition, these data suggest that the hippocampus is particularly sensitive to the effects of early-life infection.

Is there a sensitive period for the long-term cognitive effects of early-life infection?

While the model presented above indicates that neonatal infection can program neuroimmune function for the life of the rat, thereby affecting adult cognition, these data could alternatively be explained by a general sensitization of the neuroimmune system caused by a single *E. coli* infection, *regardless of age*. If the neonatal period is a particularly sensitive time-point for long-term programming of neuroimmune function and adult cognition, an infection given to developing rats at a later time point should yield no significant impairment on learning and memory in adulthood. In fact, treatment of juvenile rats (P30) with a non-lethal, though significantly larger (2.5×10^{-8} colony-forming units versus the 1×10^{-6} colony-forming units given to neonates) dose of *E. coli* produces a significant increase in cytokine expression within the periphery and brain at the time of the *E.* coli infection (Campisi *et al.*, 2003), but produces no long-term deficits in learning and memory into adulthood (Bilbo *et al.*, 2006). Thus, these data provide critical evidence that neonatal development is a particularly sensitive period for the long-term consequences of early-life infection on later-life neuroimmune function and associated cognitive dysfunction. These data also support the hypothesis that microglia are functionally and/or immunologically different during early brain development than microglia within the adult, or even juvenile/early adolescent brain.

What is the mechanism by which early-life infection can impact later-life cognitive function?

The evidence presented thus far indicate that a neonatal infection can reprogram the neuroimmune system such that a second immune challenge in adulthood results in an exaggerated immune response which interferes with the processes of learning and memory. An increasing body of literature indicates that immune molecules have a critical role in the molecular and cellular processes of learning and memory. For example, IL-1β is induced within the hippocampus in response to normal learning and is critical for maintaining long-term potentiation

(LTP), a cellular process of synaptic strengthening thought to underlie learning and memory (Ross *et al.*, 2003; Schneider *et al.*, 1998). Decreased levels of IL-1β or IL-1β activity in mice lacking the gene for IL-1β, or mice over-expressing the endogenous IL-1 receptor antagonist (IL1ra) exhibit markedly impaired HP-dependent learning and memory (Goshen *et al.*, 2007; Spulber, Bartfai, and Schultzberg, 2009). In contrast, exaggerated levels of IL-1β can similarly impair memory (Barrientos *et al.*, 2002). These data suggest that IL-1β is important for normal learning and memory, and that either low or exaggerated levels of this particular cytokine can impair learning and memory.

The neonatal infection model lends critical insight into the role of cytokines and microglial function in the processes of learning and memory, in addition to the mechanisms by which early-life immune activation can impair learning and memory. Treatment of neonatally infected rats with LPS produces an exaggerated IL-1β response within the hippocampus, which peaks approximately 2 hours after LPS treatment and returns to baseline 24 hours after LPS treatment (Bilbo *et al.*, 2005a). In contrast, control rats given LPS show a significant increase in IL-1β protein which peaks later, at around 4–8 hours post-LPS treatment. Thus, if LPS is given immediately after the context pre-exposure, the exaggerated IL-1β response within the hippocampus of neonatally infected rats' peaks *at the same time* that consolidation of the context memory is occurring, and therefore significantly interferes with the consolidation of the context memory (Figure 15.2). In control rats, the peak in IL-1β which results from the LPS treatment occurs after the consolidation of the context memory. In support of the hypothesis that exaggerated IL-1β synthesis interferes with memory consolidation, treatment of neonatally infected rats with an inhibitor of Caspase-1, the enzyme which synthesizes the active form of IL-1β, at the time of LPS administration completely prevents the memory impairment in neonatally infected rats (Bilbo *et al.*, 2005a), providing causal evidence that exaggerated IL-1β within the hippocampus of neonatally infected rats following context pre-exposure and LPS treatment can significantly interfere with learning and memory.

Analysis of brain-derived neurotrophic factor, BDNF, within the hippocampus at the time of learning has revealed significant insight into the potential mechanisms by which exaggerated IL-1β interferes with contextual memory formation. BDNF is well-characterized for its role in learning and memory, is a molecule necessary for inducing/maintaining the long-term potentiation of hippocampal circuits, and is up-regulated specifically within the hippocampus following contextual learning (Hall, Thomas, and Everitt, 2000). Following contextual fear-conditioning, BDNF expression is similarly elevated within the hippocampus of control and neonatally infected rats that were treated with saline at the time of context pre-exposure, consistent with its role in learning and memory and the data presented above, indicating that the mechanisms of learning are not globally disrupted in neonatally infected rats. In contrast, LPS treatment significantly decreases BDNF production in all hippocampal regions. Neonatally infected rats treated with LPS immediately after context pre-exposure exhibit the greatest decrease in BDNF within the CA1 of the hippocampus when compared to LPS treated controls, indicating that BDNF may never reach a threshold necessary for consolidating the representation of the context in neonatally infected rats (Bilbo *et al.*, 2008). In addition, this significant *decrease* in BDNF within the hippocampus of neonatally infected rats occurs shortly after the exaggerated *increase* in IL-1β production following LPS administration (Bilbo *et al.*, 2008) (Figure 15.2). Thus, over-production of IL-1β within the hippocampus caused by long-term programming of neuroimmune function by early-life infection can produce significant cognitive deficits, as well as significant alterations in the cellular mechanisms underlying normal learning and memory.

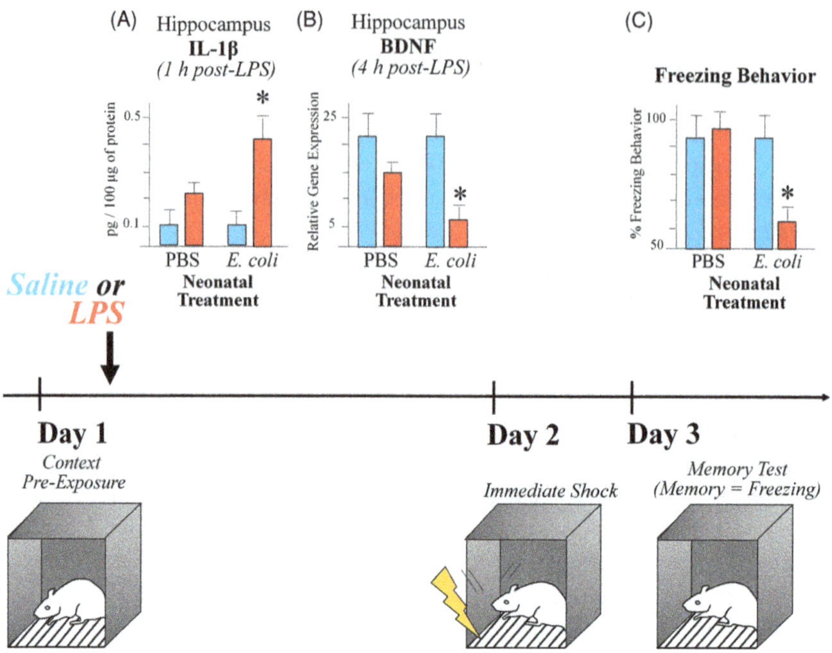

Figure 15.2 Neonatal infection produces long-term changes in neuroimmune function which directly impairs learning and memory in a context pre-exposure paradigm. On Day 1, rats are allowed to explore a novel context (context pre-exposure) for a few minutes before being injected with either saline or a low dose of lipopolysaccharide (LPS, 25 μg/kg). A. One hour (h) after LPS treatment, IL-1β protein is significantly increased within the hippocampus of neonatally infected rats. B. Four hours after LPS treatment, brain-derived neurotrophic factor (BDNF) is significantly decreased within the hippocampus, particularly in neonatally infected rats. BDNF is a critical mechanism by which new memories are formed within the hippocampus. Twenty-four hours after context pre-exposure, rats are placed back into the same context where they receive an immediate brief shock. This paradigm results in a fear of the context 24 hours later. C. Neonatally infected rats given LPS immediately after context pre-exposure display significant deficits in memory for the context, the result of increased IL-1β production within the hippocampus. From Bilbo *et al.*, 2005; 2008.

Interestingly, a slight variation of the previous experimental paradigm provides an entirely new perspective on the role of IL-1β in learning and memory and the long-term programming of neuroimmune function and cognition (Figure 15.3). Treatment of neonatally infected rats with LPS *24 hours prior* to simple contextual fear-conditioning produces a deficit in learning and memory similar to when neonatally infected rats are injected with LPS immediately *after* the context pre-exposure in the context pre-exposure task (Bilbo *et al.*, 2006). This impairment in learning and memory cannot be accounted for by an exaggerated LPS-induced immune response in neonatally infected rats because IL-1β is undetectable in both control and neonatally infected rats 24 hours after the LPS treatment (Bilbo *et al.*, 2005a). In contrast, microglia within the hippocampus of neonatally infected rats continue to show an activated profile, characterized by increased levels of the activation markers cluster of differentiation (CD) 11b and glial fibrillary acidic protein (GFAP), 24 hours after LPS administration (Bilbo *et al.*, 2005a) (Figure 15.3).

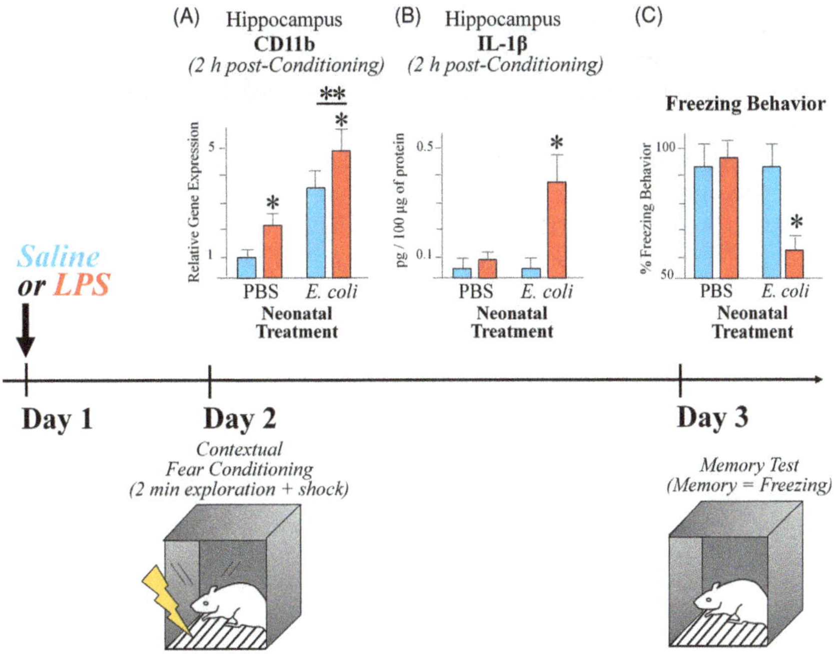

Figure 15.3 Neonatal infection produces long-term changes in neuroimmune function which directly impair learning and memory during a contextual fear-conditioning paradigm given 24 hours after an immune challenge. Treatment of control and neonatally infected rats with LPS (25 μg/kg) results in exaggerated glial activation within the hippocampus of neonatally infected rats 24 hours later. A. Specifically, CD11b expression within the hippocampus is significantly elevated in neonatally infected rats, and significantly more so after LPS treatment. B. Two hours after contextual fear-conditioning (2 minutes of exploration followed by a brief shock) results in detectable learning-induced IL-1β within the hippocampus of all rats. However, neonatally infected rats given an LPS challenge 24 hours prior have significantly elevated IL-1β levels, the result of exaggerated glial activation. C. Twenty-four hours after fear-conditioning, all rats show a memory for the context in which they received the shock except neonatally infected rats, who exhibit a marked memory deficit. From Williamson *et al.*, 2011.

Given these findings and data indicating that IL-1β is normally increased during processes of learning and memory (Schneider *et al.*, 1998) and necessary for learning and memory, one might hypothesize that neonatally infected rats have exaggerated IL-1β levels within the hippocampus *directly as a consequence of learning* which is subsequently interfering with memory selectively in these rats. In fact, IL-β is detected at low but physiological levels within the hippocampus 2 hours after contextual fear-conditioning even in control rats (Williamson *et al.*, 2011). In contrast, IL-1β is undetectable within the adjacent parietal cortex or prefrontal cortex following contextual fear-conditioning, confirming that IL-1β is significantly and selectively elevated within the hippocampus at the time of context learning. In addition, IL-1β is undetectable within the hippocampus following either exposure to the context (with no shock) or footshock alone, suggesting that IL-1β is only synthesized within the hippocampus during a learning experience. Twenty-six hours after LPS administration and 2 hours after fear-conditioning, IL-1β levels were significantly *exaggerated* within the hippocampus of neonatally infected rats, while IL-1β levels were not significantly increased above learning alone in control rats (Williamson *et al.*, 2011) (Figure 15.3). These data indicate that LPS given 24 hours prior to learning and memory causes a significant shift in microglial function in neonatally infected rats such that learning itself results in exaggerated IL-1β production which impairs learning and memory.

Consistent with this interpretation, rapid isolation and separation of microglia ($CD11b^+$ cells) and other neuronal cell types ($CD11b^-$) using fluorescence activated cell sorting (FACS) for analysis of IL-1β expression indicates that microglia are the sole source of IL-1β production at the time of learning, and similarly the sole source of exaggerated IL-1β in neonatally infected rats (Figure 15.4). Inhibiting microglia with minocycline either at the time of LPS treatment or at the time of learning can reverse the memory impairment in neonatally infected

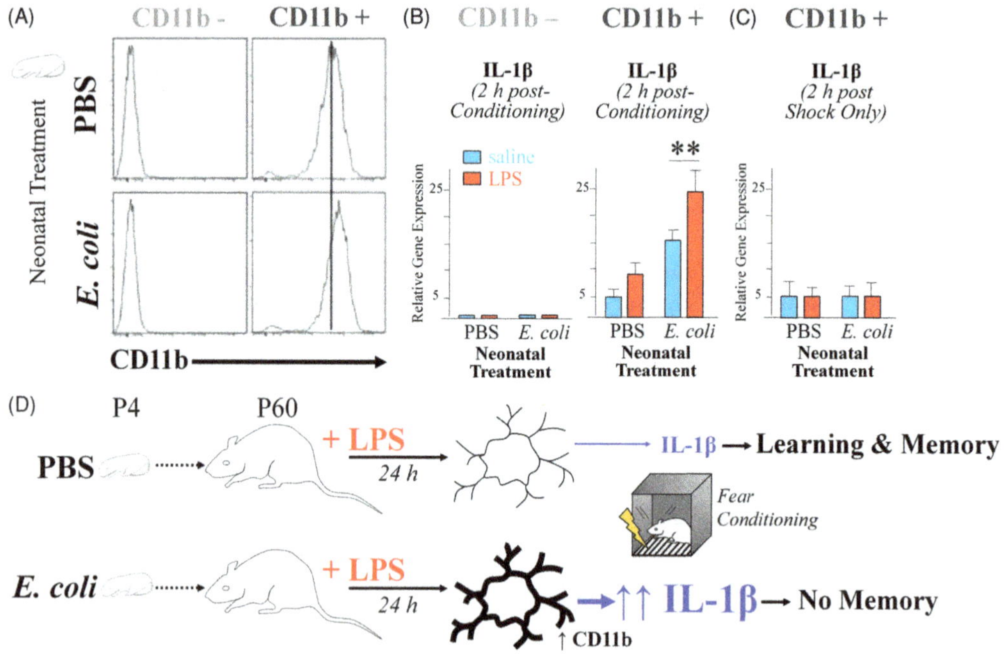

Figure 15.4 Learning-induced IL-1β is produced by microglia. A. Microglia (CD11b+ cells) isolated and separated from other neuronal cell types (CD11b- cells) using fluorescence activated cell separation (FACS) of hippocampal tissue from neonatally infected rats exhibit increased CD11b staining compared to microglia isolated from control rats (even in the absence of an LPS challenge). B. CD11b- cells (astrocytes, neurons, and oligodendrocytes) exhibit undetectable levels of IL-1β expression 24 hours after LPS treatment and 2 hours after context fear-conditioning, indicating that learning-induced IL-1β occurs specifically within microglia. Microglia (CD11b+ cells) express detectable levels of IL-1β 2 hours after context fear-conditioning and neonatally infected rats exhibit significantly exaggerated expression of IL-1β in microglia compared to control rats given the same treatment. C. Microglia (CD11b + cells) express low levels of IL-1β following LPS and a footshock alone (no context learning) given 2 hours prior to collection, but this does not differ as a consequence of neonatal treatment, indicating that a combination of LPS and *learning* is required to elicit the exaggerated response in neonatally infected rats. D. Neonatal programming of microglial function results in exaggerated CD11b expression on microglia and exaggerated IL-1β production following a learning experience (fear-conditioning) which directly impairs learning and memory. From Williamson *et al.*, 2011.

rats (Williamson *et al.*, 2011). These data directly indicate that: 1) Microglia have a critical role in learning and memory (via the production of IL-1β); 2) IL-1β is increased within the hippocampus during learning and necessary for memory formation; and 3) Neuroimmune dysfunction (exaggerated IL-1β) directly results in cognitive dysfunction (learning impairments). As a result, early-life programming of microglial function can significantly impact cognitive function for life via its effects on neuroimmune function.

The Long-Term Consequences of Early-Life Infection: Aging-related Glial Activation and Associated Cognitive Decline

One of the most novel and important conclusions from the previously described set of experiments is that early-life immune activation can significantly shift the developmental trajectory of microglia, thereby altering the function of these cells to subsequent challenges *for the life of the individual.* Normal aging is associated with increased glial activation and inflammation within the brain, characterized by increases in the expression of major histocompatibility (MHC) II on microglia and astrocytes and increased expression of pro-inflammatory cytokines, including IL-1β (see Lynch, 2010, for review). Given that neonatally infected rats are more vulnerable to exaggerated pro-inflammatory cytokine production following an LPS challenge in adulthood, one might similarly hypothesize that neonatally infected rats may also be more vulnerable to aging-related changes in glial function and neuroinflammation, and thus more vulnerable to associated cognitive decline. In fact, aged rats (16 months of age) infected neonatally with *E. coli* show significant cognitive deficits in an ambiguous-cue fear-conditioning task when compared to their age-matched controls. In contrast to the contextual fear-conditioning task, this version of fear-conditioning determines whether animals can distinguish between a light cue which *consistently* predicts a shock and a tone cue which only *occasionally* predicts a shock (and thus is "ambiguous") (Bilbo, 2010). This task is also a robust measure of learning and memory, yet can detect much more subtle deficits in learning and memory than contextual fear-conditioning. At two months of age, there were no significant differences between neonatally infected rats and control rats in their ability to correctly associate the light with the shock; however, at 16 months of age, neonatally infected rats froze equally to the light and the tone, an effect that was not seen in controls (Bilbo, 2010). These results indicate that only *aged* neonatally infected rats were inaccurate in acquiring the associative memory between the light and the shock, and instead generalized the fear-conditioning to both cues. Notably, neither treatment group received an LPS "second hit" at either 2 or 16 months of age.

In a second task to assess spatial hippocamapal-dependent learning and memory, the Morris water maze, both young and old rats (neonatally infected and controls) learned the location of a hidden/submerged platform in a large swimming pool at the same rate over the course of 24 training trials. However, during a probe trial given 24 hours after the final training session, 16 month old neonatally infected rats spent significantly less time searching in the target quadrant of the maze for the hidden platform than did their age-matched controls, suggesting they had forgotten the location of the hidden platform. A similar effect was seen 96 hours after the final training session (Bilbo, 2010). The results of this cognitive task indicate that while the older neonatally infected rats were able to learn the task correctly, they were unable to maintain this spatial representation of the task just 24 or 96 hours later (Bilbo, 2010). Thus, neonatal immune activation increases the risk for later-life cognitive dysfunction, such that neonatally infected rats fair far worse after the onset of aging; and aging, which is associated with a general increase in microglial activation and cytokine production, is acting as a "second hit" (similar to the LPS challenge described above) for these vulnerable rats.

The analysis of microglial activation markers (CD11b and MHC II) and astrocyte activation markers (GFAP) within the brains of neonatally infected and control rats support this interpretation. Aged rats have significantly higher levels of all three proteins within the hippocampus than their younger counterparts; however, neonatally infected rats have significantly elevated levels of CD11b within all subregions of the hippocampus and significantly elevated levels of GFAP within the dentate gyrus at 16 months of age when compared to their age-matched controls (Bilbo, 2010) (Figure 15.5). In conclusion, aging itself is similar to an immune challenge during which time microglia shift into a more reactive phenotype and function (Griffin *et al.*, 2006; Lynch, 2010; Nolan *et al.*, 2005).

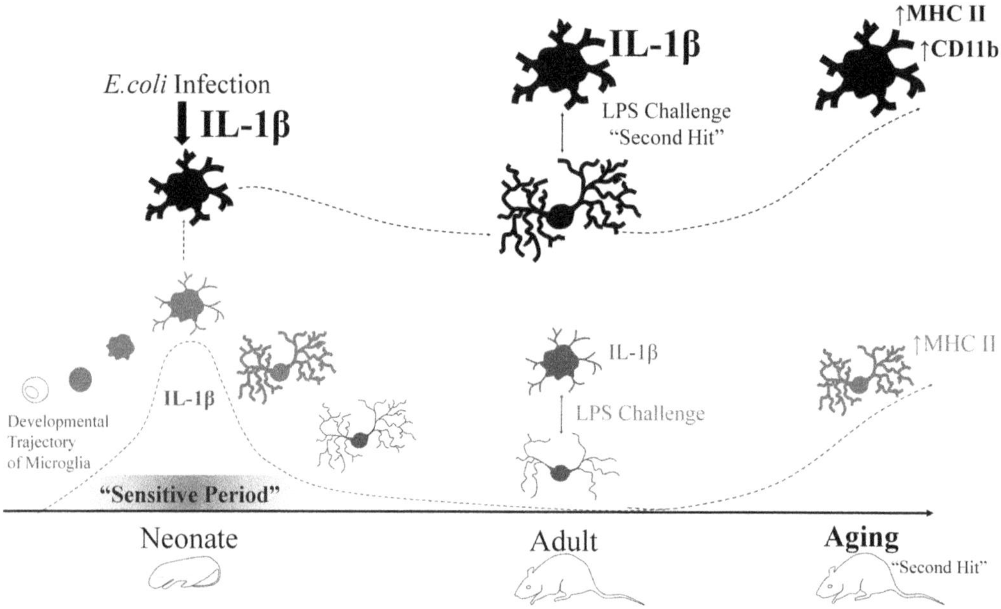

Figure 15.5 Neonatal infection alters the developmental trajectory and function of microglia within the brain for the life of the rodent. Microglia within the developing hippocampus express naturally elevated levels of IL-1β around birth and a distinctly different morphology, when compared to the adult hippocampus, which results in a particularly "sensitive period" for neonatal immune challenges (illustrated in gray). A neonatal *E. coli* infection significantly increases the expression of IL-1β at this time for approximately 48 hours, and significantly shifts the developmental trajectory of microglia, such that in adulthood microglia are "primed" to over-respond to subsequent immune challenges (illustrated in black). Specifically, an immune challenge (LPS) given in adulthood (a "second hit") results in the over-production of IL-1β from microglia which directly impairs learning and memory at that time. Aging is associated with steadily increasing microglial sensitization (including increased surface antigen expression, e.g. major histocompatibility complex (MHC) II), especially in advanced stages, and thus can be considered a "second hit". This process is exaggerated or accelerated in neonatally infected rats, as evidenced by increased expression of microglial activation markers, CD11b and MHC II, in middle age, and increased age-related cognitive decline. From Bilbo *et al.*, 2005; Bilbo, 2010.

Conclusions

Early-life programming of later-life neuroimmune function, caused by a single neonatal infection, is a vulnerability factor such that later-life immune challenges and microglial activation is exacerbated in these rats, with significant negative consequences for cognition. These effects of early-life infection are relatively subtle. Specifically, neonatally infected rats are *vulnerable*, not damaged. They are capable of learning cognitive tasks, and impairments are only revealed by a second immune challenge or increasing age, indicating that the neural circuitry necessary for learning and memory is intact. At the same time, the effects of early-life infection are profound. Specifically, a minor yet significant shift in microglial function has significant negative consequences for cognition. Finally, the effects of early-life infection are very long-lasting. The immediate immune response to a neonatal infection occurs over the course of a few days, after which point the infection is completely cleared. Despite this, neonatal immune activation that occurs during this narrow time-frame in development has long-term consequences on the developmental trajectory of microglia in the brain, significantly affecting microglial function for months and even years after the initial insult.

We propose that this model of early-life immune activation reveals novel insights into the mechanisms of cognitive dysfunction and the many neuropsychiatric disorders that display a strong immune dysregulation and a strong developmental component to their etiology. At birth, the neonatal immune system faces the critical challenge of transferring from a sterile environment to a world filled with pathogens, microbes, and toxins, where it must effectively defend the newborn. It is highly unlikely that one would go through life without ever getting sick or developing an infection. We are, instead, exposed to many immune challenges on a daily basis, some more than others; yet most of us live our lives without developing a neuropsychiatric disorder. Many of us live our lives in good health. This model of early-life infection reveals that it is likely the neuroimmune "history" and thus the early-life programming of neuroimmune function which makes an individual vulnerable to the development of cognitive disorders in adulthood. Thus the ultimate challenge for scientists will be to understand how the *combination* of early-life events and later-life events which impact the immune system may affect an individual's risk of developing cognitive dysfunction and/or neuropsychiatric disorders. In addition, future research should be aimed at understanding how early-life events which directly impact the immune system can produce long-term changes in neuroimmune function.

References

Ashwell, K. (1991). The distribution of microglia and cell death in the fetal rat forebrain. *Brain Research. Developmental Brain Research*, 58, 1–12.

Barrientos, R.M., Higgins, E.A., Sprunger, D.B., Watkins, L.R., Rudy, J.W., and Maier, S.F. (2002). Memory for context is impaired by a post context exposure injection of interleukin-1 beta into dorsal hippocampus. *Behavioural Brain Research*, 134, 291–298.

Bauman, M.L., Filipek, P.A., and Kemper, T.L. (1997). Early infantile autism. In Ronald, J. Bradley, R. Adron, Harris, Peter Jenner, and Jeremy D. Schmahmann (eds.), *International Review of Neurobiology*, Vol. 41 (pp. 367–386). San Diego: Academic Press.

Bessis, A., Bechade, C., Bernard, D., and Roumier, A. (2007). Microglial control of neuronal death and synaptic properties. *Glia*, 55, 233–238.

Bilbo, S.D. (2010). Early-life infection is a vulnerability factor for aging-related glial alterations and cognitive decline. *Neurobiology of Learning and Memory*, 94, 57–64.

Bilbo, S.D., Barrientos, R.M., Eads, A.S., Northcutt, A., Watkins, L.R., Rudy, J.W., et al. (2008). Early-life infection leads to altered BDNF and IL-1beta mRNA expression in rat hippocampus following learning in adulthood. *Brain, Behavior, and Immunity*, 22, 451–455.

Bilbo, S.D., Biedenkapp, J.C., Der-Avakian, A., Watkins, L.R., Rudy, J.W., and Maier, S.F. (2005a). Neonatal infection-induced memory impairment after lipopolysaccharide in adulthood is prevented via caspase-1 inhibition. *Journal of Neuroscience*, 25, 8000–8009.

Bilbo, S.D., Levkoff, L.H., Mahoney, J.H., Watkins, L.R., Rudy, J.W., and Maier, S.F. (2005b). Neonatal infection induces memory impairments following an immune challenge in adulthood. *Behavioral Neuroscience*, 119, 293–301.

Bilbo, S.D., Rudy, J.W., Watkins, L.R., and Maier, S.F. (2006). A behavioural characterization of neonatal infection-facilitated memory impairment in adult rats. *Behavioural Brain Research*, 169, 39–47.

Brown, A.S., Begg, M.D., Gravenstein, S., Schaefer, C.A., Wyatt, R.J., Bresnahan, M., Babulas, V.P., and Susser, E.S. (2004). Serologic evidence of prenatal influenza in the etiology of schizophrenia. *Archives of General Psychiatry*, 61, 774–780.

Cai, Z., Pan, Z.L., Pang, Y., Evans, O.B., and Rhodes, P.G. (2000). Cytokine induction in fetal rat brains and brain injury in neonatal rats after maternal lipopolysaccharide administration. *Pediatric Research*, 47, 64–72.

Campisi, J., Hansen, M.K., O'Connor, K.A., Biedenkapp, J.C., Watkins, L.R., Maier, S.F., and Fleshner, M. (2003). Circulating cytokines and endotoxin are not necessary for the activation of the sickness or corticosterone response produced by peripheral E. coli challenge. *Journal of Applied Physiology (Bethesda, Md.: 1985)*, 95, 1873–1882.

Champagne, D.L., Bagot, R.C., van Hasselt, F., Ramakers, G., Meaney, M.J., de Kloet, E.R., et al. (2008). Maternal care and hippocampal plasticity: evidence for experience-dependent structural plasticity, altered synaptic functioning, and differential responsiveness to glucocorticoids and stress. *Journal of Neuroscience*, 28, 6037–6045.

Chan, W.Y., Kohsaka, S., and Rezaie, P. (2007). The origin and cell lineage of microglia: new concepts. *Brain Research Reviews*, 53, 344–354.

Cowell, R.M., and Silverstein, F.S. (2003). Developmental changes in the expression of chemokine receptor CCR1 in the rat cerebellum. *Journal of Comparative Neurology*, 457, 7–23.

Cowell, R.M., Xu, H., Parent, J.M., and Silverstein, F.S. (2006). Microglial expression of chemokine receptor CCR5 during rat forebrain development and after perinatal hypoxia-ischemia. *Journal of Neuroimmunology*, 173, 155–165.

Cuadros, M.A., and Navascués, J. (1998). The origin and differentiation of microglial cells during development. *Progress in Neurobiology*, 56, 173–189.

de Boo, H.A., and Harding, J.E. (2006). The developmental origins of adult disease (Barker) hypothesis. *Australian and New Zealand Journal of Obstetrics and Gynaecology*, 46, 4–14.

Deverman, B.E., and Patterson, P.H. (2009). Cytokines and CNS development. *Neuron*, 64, 61–78.

Fujioka, M., Nishio, K., Miyamoto, S., Hiramatsu, K.I., Sakaki, T., Okuchi, K., et al. (2000). Hippocampal damage in the human brain after cardiac arrest. *Cerebrovascular Diseases (Basel, Switzerland)*, 10, 2–7.

Garay, P.A., and McAllister, A.K. (2010). Novel roles for immune molecules in neural development: Implications for neurodevelopmental disorders. *Frontiers in Synaptic Neuroscience*, 2, 136.

Ginhoux, F., Greter, M., Leboeuf, M., Nandi, S., See, P., Gokhan, S., et al. (2010). Fate mapping analysis reveals that adult microglia derive from primitive macrophages. *Science (New York, N.Y.)*, 330, 841–845.

Giulian, D., Young, D.G., Woodward, J., Brown, D.C., and Lachman, L.B. (1988). Interleukin-1 is an astroglial growth factor in the developing brain. *Journal of Neuroscience*, 8, 709–714.

Goshen, I., Kreisel, T., Ounallah-Saad, H., Renbaum, P., Zalzstein, Y., Ben-Hur, T., et al. (2007). A dual role for interleukin-1 in hippocampal-dependent memory processes. *Psychoneuroendocrinology*, 32, 1106–1115.

Griffin, R., Nally, R., Nolan, Y., McCartney, Y., Linden, J., and Lynch, M.A. (2006). The age-related attenuation in long-term potentiation is associated with microglial activation. *Journal of Neurochemistry*, 99, 1263–1272.

Hahn, Y.K., Vo, P., Fitting, S., Block, M.L., Hauser, K.F., and Knapp, P.E. (2010). Beta-chemokine production by neural and glial progenitor cells is enhanced by HIV-1 tat: effects on microglial migration. *Journal of Neurochemistry*, 114, 97–109.

Hall, J., Thomas, K.L., and Everitt, B.J. (2000). Rapid and selective induction of BDNF expression in the hippocampus during contextual learning. *Nature Neuroscience*, 3, 533–535.

Hornig, M., Weissenbock, H., Horscroft, N., and Lipkin, W.I. (1999). An infection-based model of neurodevelopmental damage. *Proceedings of the National Academy of Sciences of the United States of America*, 96, 12102–12107.

Lynch, M.A. (2010). Age-related neuroinflammatory changes negatively impact on neuronal function. *Frontiers in Aging Neuroscience*, 1, 6.

Marin-Teva, J.L., Dusart, I., Colin, C., Gervais, A., van Rooijen, N., and Mallat, M. (2004). Microglia promote the death of developing purkinje cells. *Neuron*, 41, 535–547.

Marshall-Clarke, S., Reen, D., Tasker, L., and Hassan, J. (2000). Neonatal immunity: how well has it grown up? *Immunology Today*, 21, 35–41.

McKimmie, C.S., and Graham, G.J. (2010). Astrocytes modulate the chemokine network in a pathogen-specific manner. *Biochemical and Biophysical Research Communications*, 394, 1006–1011.

Meyer, U., Feldon, J., Schedlowski, M., and Yee, B.K. (2006). Immunological stress at the maternal–foetal interface: a link between neurodevelopment and adult psychopathology. *Brain, Behavior, and Immunity*, 20, 378–388.

Mortensen, P.B., Pedersen, C.B., Westergaard, T., Wohlfahrt, J., Ewald, H., Mors, O., et al. (1999). Effects of family history and place and season of birth on the risk of schizophrenia. *New England Journal of Medicine*, 340, 603–608.

Nelson, K.B., and Willoughby, R.E. (2000). Infection, inflammation and the risk of cerebral palsy. *Current Opinion in Neurology*, 13, 133–149.

Nolan, Y., Maher, F.O., Martin, D.S., Clarke, R.M., Brady, M.T., Bolton, A.E., et al. (2005). Role of interleukin-4 in regulation of age-related inflammatory changes in the hippocampus. *Journal of Biological Chemistry*, 280, 9354–9362.

Osrin, D., Vergnano, S., and Costello, A. (2004). Serious bacterial infections in newborn infants in developing countries. *Current Opinion in Infectious Diseases*, 17, 217–224.

Owen, D., Andrews, M.H., and Matthews, S.G. (2005). Maternal adversity, glucocorticoids and programming of neuroendocrine function and behaviour. *Neuroscience and Biobehavioral Reviews*, 29, 209–226.

Pang, Y., Cai, Z., and Rhodes, P.G. (2003). Disturbance of oligodendrocyte development, hypomyelination and white matter injury in the neonatal rat brain after intracerebral injection of lipopolysaccharide. *Developmental Brain Research*, 140, 205–214.

Perry, V.H., Hume, D.A., and Gordon, S. (1985). Immunohistochemical localization of macrophages and microglia in the adult and developing mouse brain. *Neuroscience*, 15, 313–326.

Petito, C.K., Feldmann, E., Pulsinelli, W.A., and Plum, F. (1987). Delayed hippocampal damage in humans following cardiorespiratory arrest. *Neurology*, 37, 1281–1286.

Rezaie, P., Patel, K., and Male, D.K. (1999). Microglia in the human fetal spinal cord – patterns of distribution, morphology and phenotype. *Brain Research. Developmental Brain Research*, 115, 71–81.

Rezaie, P., Trillo-Pazos, G., Everall, I.P., and Male, D.K. (2002). Expression of beta-chemokines and chemokine receptors in human fetal astrocyte and microglial co-cultures: potential role of chemokines in the developing CNS. *Glia*, 37, 64–75.

Ross, F.M., Allan, S.M., Rothwell, N.J., and Verkhratsky, A. (2003). A dual role for interleukin-1 in LTP in mouse hippocampal slices. *Journal of Neuroimmunology*, 144, 61–67.

Rudy, J.W., Huff, N.C., and Matus-Amat, P. (2004). Understanding contextual fear conditioning: Insights from a two-process model. *Neuroscience and Biobehavioral Reviews*, 28, 675–685.

Salmenpera, T., Kalviainen, R., Partanen, K., and Pitkanen, A. (1998). Hippocampal damage caused by seizures in temporal lobe epilepsy. *Lancet*, 351, 35.

Sapolsky, R., Rivier, C., Yamamoto, G., Plotsky, P., and Vale, W. (1987). Interleukin-1 stimulates the secretion of hypothalamic corticotropin-releasing factor. *Science (New York, N.Y.)*, 238, 522–524.

Schafer, D.P., Lehrman, E.K., Kautzman, A.G., Koyama, R., Mardinly, A.R., Yamasaki, R., Ransohoff, R.M., Greenberg, M.E., Barres, B.A., Stevens, B. (2012). Microglia sculpt postnatal neural circuits in an activity and complement-dependent manner. *Neuron*, 74, 691–705.

Schneider, H., Pitossi, F., Balschun, D., Wagner, A., del Rey, A., and Besedovsky, H.O. (1998). A neuromodulatory role of interleukin-1beta in the hippocampus. *Proceedings of the National Academy of Sciences of the United States of America*, 95, 7778–7783.

Schwarz, J.M., and Bilbo, S.D. (2011). LPS elicits a much larger and broader inflammatory response than escherichia coli infection within the hippocampus of neonatal rats. *Neuroscience Letters*, 497, 110–115.

Shi, L., Smith, S.E.P., Malkova, N., Tse, D., Su, Y., and Patterson, P.H. (2009). Activation of the maternal immune system alters cerebellar development in the offspring. *Brain, Behavior, and Immunity*, 23, 116–123.

Skogstrand, K., Hougaard, D.M., Schendel, D.E., Bent, N.P., Svaerke, C., and Thorsen, P. (2008). Association of preterm birth with sustained postnatal inflammatory response. *Obstetrics and Gynecology*, 111, 1118–1128.

Spulber, S., Bartfai, T., and Schultzberg, M. (2009). IL-1/IL-1ra balance in the brain revisited – evidence from transgenic mouse models. *Brain, Behavior, and Immunity*, 23, 573–579.

Stevens, B., Allen, N.J., Vazquez, L.E., Howell, G.R., Christopherson, K.S., Nouri, N., et al. (2007). The classical complement cascade mediates CNS synapse elimination. *Cell*, 131, 1164–1178.

Urakubo, A., Jarskog, L.F., Lieberman, J.A., and Gilmore, J.H. (2001). Prenatal exposure to maternal infection alters cytokine expression in the placenta, amniotic fluid, and fetal brain. *Schizophrenia Research*, 47, 27–36.

Wang, C.-C., Wu, C.-H., Shieh, J.-Y., and Wen, C.-Y. (2002). Microglial distribution and apoptosis in fetal rat brain. *Developmental Brain Research*, 139, 337–342.

Williamson, L.L., Sholar, P.W., Mistry, R.M., Smith, S.H., and Bilbo, S.D. (2011). Microglia and memory: modulation by early-life infection. *Journal of Neuroscience*, 31, 15511–15521.

Xu, J., Kaur, C., and Ling, E.A. (1993). Variation with age in the labelling of amoeboid microglial cells in rats following intraperitoneal or intravenous injection of a fluorescent dye. *Journal of Anatomy*, 182, 55–63.

16

Aging and the Immune System

Ashley M. Fenn,[1] Angela W. Corona,[2] and Jonathan P. Godbout[1]

[1]*Department of Neuroscience, Ohio State University, Columbus, OH, USA*
[2]*Department of Neurosciences, Case Western Reserve University, Cleveland, OH, USA*

Introduction

Aging is an intrinsic and progressive physiological process that results in the gradual deterioration of physical, mental, and social capacities. In general, these deteriorations accelerate as reproductive vitality decreases. Aging significantly affects every major organ system in the body including the immune and central nervous systems. This is relevant to the field of psychoneuroimmunology because these age-associated changes significantly alter bidirectional communication between these two systems. Disruption in coordinated immune–brain communication prevents appropriate physiological, immunological, and behavioral responses to an infectious pathogen. This is significant because normal aging is associated with a higher risk of infection, prolonged recovery following infection, and a higher frequency of neurobehavioral complications concomitant with infection including depression and delirium. Therefore, these age-related deficits in immunity have a profound influence on health and lifespan.

Invading pathogens elicit a synchronized peripheral innate and adaptive immune response that is interpreted by the central nervous system (CNS). This interpretation leads to a reorganization of the host's priorities to shift energy distribution towards fighting infection and limiting the spread of disease. During the normal process of aging these coordinated responses are disrupted by reduced immune capacity in the periphery and heightened inflammatory potential in the CNS. The result is an inability to eliminate invading pathogens and induction of cognitive and behavioral complications.

Many of these immune, cognitive, and behavioral deficits following infection are recapitulated in rodent models of aging. For example, aged mice and rats that receive a peripheral immune challenge have exaggerated microglial activity associated with a maladaptive sickness response characterized by delayed and prolonged fever, increased lethargy, cognitive impairment, and induction of depression-like behavior. Therefore, the purpose of this chapter is to use clinical and experimental data to detail key age-associated deficits in both the peripheral and central immune systems. Moreover, we will discuss how these impairments may contribute to the increased frequency of neurobehavioral complications the elderly concomitant with peripheral infection.

The Wiley-Blackwell Handbook of Psychoneuroimmunology, First Edition. Edited by Alexander W. Kusnecov and Hymie Anisman.

Bidirectional Communication Between the Immune System and the Brain

CNS–immune bidirectional communication is important because the brain is responsible for the induction of key physiologic and behavioral components of the immune response (e.g., fever, sickness behavior, and immunomodulation) (Figure 16.1). This immune–brain communication is mediated by inflammatory cytokines and their corresponding secondary messengers. During a peripheral infection, activation of peripheral innate immune cells leads to secretion of inflammatory cytokines including interleukin (IL)-1β, IL-6, and tumor necrosis factor-α (TNF-α). These signaling molecules are then communicated across the blood–brain barrier (BBB) and activate microglia and astrocytes to produce the same inflammatory cytokines and secondary mediators, including prostaglandins and nitric oxide (NO). Microglial and astrocytic propagation of these inflammatory mediators is critical because cytokines do not readily diffuse through the CNS parenchyma and have a short half-life. Effective propagation allows for these signals to target neuronal substrates in diffuse brain regions and elicit a coordinated physiological and behavioral sickness response.

In order for the peripheral cytokine signal to reach the brain, cytokines must overcome the obstacle of the BBB. This is accomplished through several distinct pathways. First, cytokines in the blood can readily gain access into the brain by diffusion through a few, relatively porous regions of the BBB adjacent to the circumventricular organs (CVOs). In this manner, cytokines

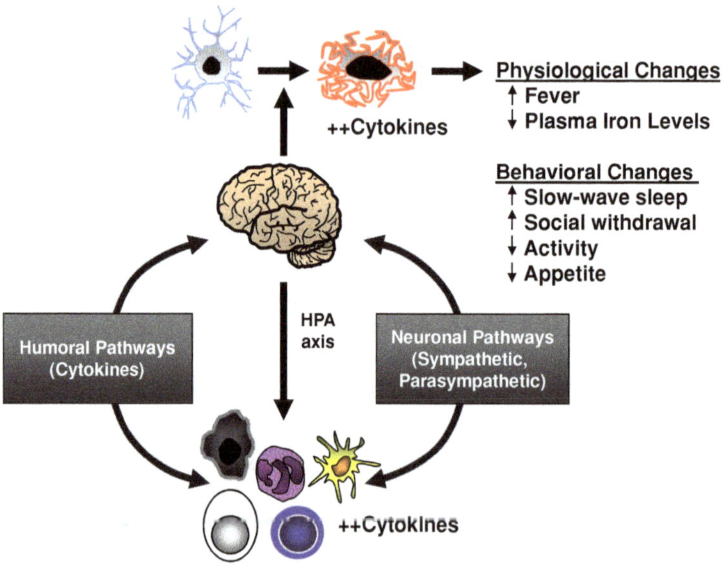

Figure 16.1 Sickness represents a reorganization of the host's priorities. Activation of the peripheral immune results in the release of cytokines that signal to the CNS through humoral and neuronal pathways. Once in the brain, these cytokines are propagated in part by activated microglia. Collectively, cytokines and their secondary mediators elicit the physiological and behavioral components of the sickness response that represent a reorganization of the host's priorities towards fighting infection. Furthermore, brain cytokines activate the HPA axis causing the release of immunomodulatory glucocorticoids in the periphery.

directly interact with microglia and astrocytes of the glial limitans. A second key pathway involves interactions between cytokines and endothelial cells of the brain. These endothelial cells have IL-1 receptors and transmit the cytokine signal into the brain by either transporting IL-1β to the abluminal side or by producing IL-1β *de novo*. A third pathway involves direct neural activation by cytokines in the periphery via the vagus nerve and catecholaminergic circuits of the sympathetic nervous system. The degree to which each pathway is activated depends on the stimulus, but all of these pathways likely contribute to immune–brain signaling.

Once this cytokine-mediated signal reaches the brain it is propagated by astrocytes, microglia, and perivascular macrophages to elicit the physiological and behavioral symptoms of sickness. The physiological responses are aimed at attenuating replication of pathogens (e.g., fever and reduced plasma iron concentrations) and relocating resources to the breakdown of carbohydrate, fat, and protein (hypothalamic–pituitary–adrenal (HPA) axis and acute-phase response). In addition, activation of the HPA axis results in the release of glucocorticoids, endogenous steroids that are important in immunomodulation. In general, glucocorticoids promote an adaptive immune response and provide a negative feedback loop to dampen innate immune activation. The behavioral responses primarily contribute to fever by preserving energy required for this metabolically demanding process. Examples include suppressing appetite, libido, and social interaction. In addition, social avoidance plays a key role in preventing the spread of disease. These physiological and behavioral aspects of the sickness response are evolutionarily conserved and exhibited by mammals, birds, reptiles, and invertebrates. Importantly, if these sickness responses are disrupted, including fever and appetite suppression, then survival of the host is negatively impacted.

In summary, this cytokine-meditated sickness response is transient, evolutionarily conserved, and beneficial to the host organism in fighting infection. Elevated or prolonged exposure of the brain to immune-induced inflammatory cytokines, however, can lead to maladaptive sickness responses including prolonged lethargy, disruption of sleep patterns, cognitive impairment, and depression-like behaviors. Each of these maladaptive responses significantly increases morbidity and mortality and is observed in the aged population (Godbout and Johnson, 2009).

Aging and the Peripheral Immune System

A hallmark of aging is the reduction in peripheral immune capacity, or immunosenescence. Immunosenescence reflects the reduction in the number of adaptive immune cells and impaired innate and adaptive immune cell function (Figure 16.2). Collectively, immunosenescence is associated with decreased antibody production, reduced cellular toxicity and, ultimately, impaired pathogen clearance and increased reactivation of latent viruses.

Aging and the innate immune system of the periphery

The innate immune system is comprised of monocytes (macrophages, dendritic cells) and granulocytes (neutrophils, eosinophils, basophils, natural killer cells). These innate cells are involved in the immediate reaction to viral and bacterial pathogens. Pathogens are recognized by the innate immune system using a diverse set of pathogen associated molecular pattern (PAMPs) receptors or Toll-Like receptors (TLRs). Activation of these receptors elicits a stereotyped inflammatory response that involves the release of a myriad of cytokines and chemokines.

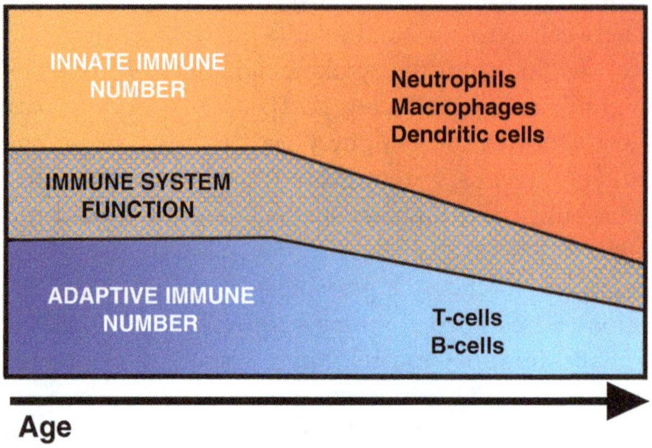

Figure 16.2 Immunosenescence with age. Aging is associated with a gradual increase in innate immune cell number and concomitant decrease in adaptive immune cell number. Cell number does not correspond with function, however, as both innate and adaptive immune function decreases with age.

Because innate immune cells represent the first line of defense against invading pathogens and are responsible for activating cells of the adaptive immune system (i.e., T-cells and B-cells), impaired function of these cells has significant consequences in an older population. For example, reduced functional capacity of neutrophils, macrophages, and dendritic cells with age is associated with increased susceptibility to bacterial, viral, and yeast infections.

Urinary tract infections (UTIs) caused by *Escherichia coli (E. coli)* are common in the elderly (over 65–80 years old), and increased incidence with age may be related to impaired function of neutrophils. Neutrophils are the most abundant immune cell within the body and represent 45–70% of the total white cell count. Neutrophils are important because they are the first innate cells to respond to a bacterial or yeast infection. These cells play a key role in phagocytosis and cytotoxic-mediated clearance of the pathogen. When neutrophils from older humans are challenged ex vivo with *E. coli* these cells have impaired phagocytosis associated with decreased CD16 expression (Butcher *et al.*, 2001) and reduced production of reactive oxygen species (Plackett *et al.*, 2004). Therefore, neutrophil-associated deficits with age may contribute to increased bacterial infection rates in the elderly.

Pneumonia is another example of a bacterial infection more prevalent in the elderly. Pneumonia is a major cause of death in the elderly and develops from a respiratory infection by the Gram-positive bacterium *Streptococcus pneumoniae*. The development of these infections is not only related to impaired phagocytosis and cytotoxic action of neutrophils, but also a shift in the cytokine profile produced by activated monocytes/macrophages. Macrophages represent two distinct populations of cells: those that actively circulate and traffic to tissue, and those that take residence in tissue. Circulating macrophages are typically more inflammatory than tissue-resident macrophages, and arrive at sites of inflammation shortly after neutrophils. In addition to their phagocytic and cytolytic actions, tissue-resident and trafficking macrophages also produce and secrete cytokines and chemokines to promote immune cell activation. Monocytes isolated from healthy elderly patients and stimulated ex vivo with lipopolysaccharide (LPS), a cell wall component of Gram-negative bacteria and a potent activator of the innate immune response, produce significantly fewer pro-inflammatory cytokines (i.e., IL-1β, TNF-α, and macrophage inflammatory protein (MIP)-1α) than monocytes isolated from adult controls

(Gon *et al.*, 1996). In support of these clinical findings, macrophages from aged C57BL/6 (20–22 month) mice stimulated with LPS produce less inflammatory cytokines and more of the anti-inflammatory cytokine IL-10 than adults (Chelvarajan *et al.*, 2006). This shift towards an anti-inflammatory activation profile is more permissive to the growth and survival of invading pathogens.

In addition to fighting infection, activation of resident inflammatory macrophages is required for effective wound healing. For instance, activated macrophages phagocytose dead tissue, secrete chemokines for inflammatory cell recruitment, and produce cytokines and other mediators to induce tissue repair, platelet aggregation, and scarring. Impaired macrophage phagocytosis and a more anti-inflammatory cytokine profile in the elderly results in increased susceptibility to the development of chronic wounds. People 60 years or older are at increased risk for the development of venous ulcers, which are chronic wounds associated with increased inflammation. In rodent models of dermal injury, macrophages from aged mice have reduced phagocytosis, limited chemokine production, and impaired recruitment of adaptive immune cells associated with delayed wound healing (Swift *et al.*, 2001). Furthermore, deficits in phagocytosis are coupled with impaired production of reactive oxygen species necessary for tissue repair including NO and hydrogen peroxide (Plowden *et al.*, 2004).

These impairments in cytokine production, phagocytosis, and cytolytic capacity may stem from impairments in recognition of pathogens and danger signals. Toll-like receptors (TLRs) are pathogen recognition receptors (PRRs) responsible for the recognition of PAMPs and subsequent activation of innate immune cells. For example, macrophages isolated from aged C57BL/6 mice have reduced expression of all TLRs investigated (Plowden *et al.*, 2004). Reduced TLR expression corresponds with decreased production and secretion of inflammatory cytokines, including TNF-α, following stimulation with specific TLR agonists.

Functional deficits in the innate immune system also contribute to increased viral infection as a result of impaired adaptive immunity. As professional antigen presenting cells (APCs), dendritic cells and macrophages coordinate a synchronized innate and adaptive response required for the effective clearance of viral infections. APCs present antigen and activate T-cells through major histocompatibility complex (MHC) II. Without stimulation with MHC II and co-stimulatory molecules, T-helper cells remain quiescent limiting the cytolytic activity of innate immune cells and preventing B-cell activation. Macrophages from aged mice have lower surface expression of MHC II compared to adult controls, and this corresponds to a weakened adaptive response with age (Plackett *et al.*, 2004). Reduced MHC II expression is also detected in dendritic cells of aged mice. Impaired MHC II expression on dendritic cells is further associated with reduced CD40 expression, a necessary signal for maintained T-cell-dendritic cell interaction (Pereira *et al.*, 2011). Taken together, reduced antigen presentation by both macrophages and dendritic cells results in a reduction in functional activation of the adaptive immune system.

Impairments in the cells of the innate immune system with age support the notion of immunosenescence. It is important to point out, however, that these impairments in innate immunity exist with age despite an increased number of innate immune cells (Figure 16.2). For example, aging is associated with a preferential shift towards myelopoiesis in the bone marrow at the expense of lymphopoiesis. In a mouse model of aging, there is a reduced proliferative capacity of bone marrow lymphocyte precursor cells and increased gene expression associated with myeloid progenitor cells (Beerman *et al.*, 2010). Thus, increased immune cell number does not equate to enhanced immunity. This notion is supported by work showing that macrophages in the chronic wounds of aged mice have decreased phagocytosis and cytotoxic function despite being 56% more abundant than macrophages in the wounds of adult mice (Swift *et al.*, 2001). Therefore, aging promotes an increased population of innate cells that are less functional. These effects are compounded by reduced adaptive stimulation by innate cells, reduced adaptive cell number, and reduced adaptive function following activation.

Aging and the adaptive immune system

The adaptive immune system is comprised of lymphocytes: T-cells, B-cells, and natural killer cells. Although natural killer cells derive from a lymphoid precursor cell, they act in concert with the innate immune system providing non-specific cytotoxic killing based on MHC I expression. T- and B-cells, however, are specialized in that each T- and B-cell receptor (TCR and BCR, respectively) will only bind to and respond to a single and unique epitope. Gene recombination of the TCR and BCR provides immense diversity, allowing for vertebrates to recognize hundreds of thousands of different pathogens. Furthermore, the specialization of the response and the development of memory T- and B-cells provide a directed attack against a pathogen and effective clearance by antibody targeting and cell-mediated cytotoxicity. Maintaining a diverse repertoire of naïve T- and B-cells is necessary to mount this directed attack against new and mutated pathogens. Because aging is associated with a reduced number of naïve T- and B-cells, impaired adaptive immune activation, and reduced antibody and cytotoxic function, older populations are at greater risk for viral infection and reactivation of latent viruses.

Annual viral influenza pandemics in temperate climates represent one of the leading causes of death for the elderly. Between 80 and 90% of influenza-related deaths occur in people aged 65 years or older. A combined effect of reduced number of naïve T-cells available to respond to new viral infections and reduced T-cell function may underlie the increased susceptibility of an older population. T-cells derive from bone marrow progenitor cells and travel to the thymus to mature and develop specialized TCRs. Relatively early in life the thymus begins to involute. Progressive involution of the thymus continues throughout development and no longer supports naïve T-cells by 40 years of age (Naylor *et al.*, 2005). This process is coupled with an age-associated shift in hematopoiesis away from lymphopoiesis resulting in a significant reduction in the number of naïve T-cells and B-cells in the aged.

Immunosenescence in the context of the adaptive immune system is also associated with impaired function. T-cells are subdivided into three main categories, $CD8^+$ cytotoxic T-cells, $CD4^+$ T-helper (T_H)1 cells, and $CD4^+$ T_H2 cells. Cytotoxic T-cells extracted from elderly human patients have reduced perforin expression and impaired cytotoxic killing of virally infected host cells (Stowe *et al.*, 2007). Latent viruses are particularly opportunistic in these conditions. According to the Center for Disease Control and Prevention, as many as 95% of people in the United States aged 35–40 years of age have contracted Epstein–Barr Virus (EBV) and 30–50% of women aged 40 have contracted cytomegalovirus (CMV), two incurable herpesvirus infections. With a healthy and functioning adaptive immune system these viruses remain latent and relatively innocuous. The severity and frequency of EBV and CMV reactivation, however, is increased in the elderly, corresponding to impaired cytotoxic T-cell activation and reduced cytolytic function (Stowe *et al.*, 2007).This adds to a state of chronic inflammation in the aged, with potential consequences including chronic fatigue syndrome and increased risk of cancer (Glaser *et al.*, 2005).

There are several subtypes of T_H cells, including T_H1 and T_H2, and both of these have impaired function with age. Whereas T_H1 cells promote macrophage activation with the release of inflammatory cytokines, T_H2 cells support B-cell activation and antibody class switching using cytokines associated with anti-inflammation and alternative activation. Normal aging is associated with a gradual skew towards a T_H1 phenotype. As with the age-associated increase in innate immune cells, an increase in T_H1 cell number does not correlate with enhanced immunity. In fact, T_H1 cells collected from influenza infected aged mice produce less IL-2 and IFN-γ (Han *et al.*, 2000), two inflammatory cytokines critical for maintained T-cell activation and macrophage-mediated cytotoxicity. Concomitant with an increase in the T_H1 skew with age is a decrease in T_H2 cell number. Clinical data indicate that the elderly have difficulties mounting effective antibody titers to viruses and viral vaccinations. Indeed, vaccination against the annual influenza virus only achieves about 17–53% efficacy in elderly patients compared to 70-90% in young adults. These deficits may also correspond with decreases in the number of circulating B-cells.

Relationship between immunosenescence and inflamm-aging

As described above, the peripheral immune system is profoundly affected by the normal aging process. Overall the population of innate and adaptive immune cells fail to mount an appropriate response to invading pathogens. An impaired response is related to reduced inflammatory capacity on a per cell basis. Nonetheless, aging is associated with increased risk of developing several inflammatory-mediated diseases. This generalized increase in inflammation with age has lead to the hypothesis of "inflamm-aging." At first glance immunosenescence and inflmam-aging seem to be in direct opposition, but closer examination demonstrates that the development of immunosenescence contributes to enhanced inflammatory load with age.

Immunosenescence results in a failure to effectively eliminate an invading pathogen and resolve infection. As a result, the elderly suffer from prolonged or persistent infections. This is because immune activation is decreased overall. Thus, chronic inflammatory processes are actually maintained with age. For example, advanced age is associated with higher levels of circulating IL-6, TNF-α, and acute-phase proteins (Krabbe *et al.*, 2004).

Increased peripheral inflammation also results in an impaired immune–brain response following infection. As discussed, a peripheral immune response elicits adaptive sickness behaviors that may last for a few hours to a few days. In the aged, however, a prolonged and eventually exaggerated peripheral response elicits an exaggerated and prolonged central response resulting in maladaptive sickness behaviors that may last for weeks. Adding insult to injury, an exaggerated central response to infection causes impaired brain–immune communication resulting in further peripheral immunosuppression, increased antigenic load, and a potentiation of this dyscoordinated response.

Aging and the Central Immune System

Coinciding with the aforementioned deficits in the peripheral immune system with age, the innate immune system within the CNS also changes with age. While the CNS is devoid of any resident adaptive immune cells, it does have an important innate immune system comprising CNS-resident microglia and astrocytes, and perivascular macrophages. These cells are critical for communication between the CNS and immune systems as they receive and propagate inflammatory signals initiated in the periphery. As described earlier, activation of these CNS immune cells results in the evolutionarily adaptive sickness response to help restrict, fight, and clear infectious pathogens. It is important that these innate responses within the brain are tightly regulated, because amplified or prolonged exposure to inflammatory mediators within the CNS can have unfavorable effects on neuronal function and plasticity.

Astrocytes and microglia are particularly sensitive to the effects of aging because their rate of turnover is low (Ginhoux *et al.*, 2010). In general, microglia and astrocytes have an increased inflammatory profile with age that also corresponds with a decrease in regulation (Figure 16.3). Microglia derive from a primitive macrophage in the embryonic yolk sac that migrate to the area of the brain early in embryogenesis (Ginhoux *et al.*, 2010). These cells make up approximately 10% of the CNS population and are present in both gray and white matter. Microglia are considered the primary immune cell of the CNS and are pivotal in the interpretation and propagation of inflammatory signals, and phagocytosis and clearance of Aβ. Astrocytes derive from glial restricted neuronal precursor cells. Depending on species, these cells comprise 40–50% of the cellular population of the brain. While astrocytes are not classically defined as immune cells, they express several TLRs and have the innate capacity to respond to inflammatory signals and secrete cytokines. Their primary role in the brain is to facilitate neuronal development, maintain brain structure, act as a sink for neuronal transmitters, and sustain synaptic health. In the absence of BBB breakdown these cells represent stable, long-lived, and self-sustaining populations.

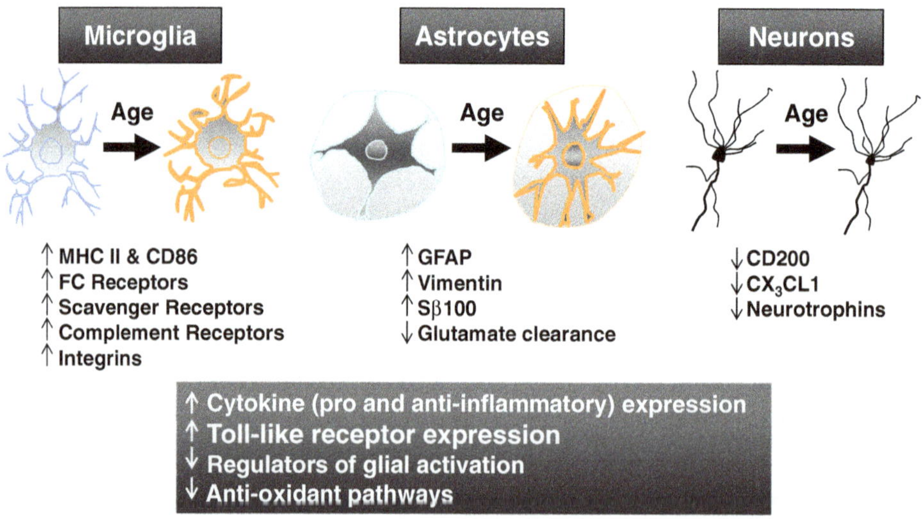

Figure 16.3 Aging results in morphological and functional changes in CNS cells. Microglia have an increased inflammatory profile with age and upregulate several markers associated with immune presentation and activation. These cells also become more hypertrophic with enlarged cell bodies and condensed processes. Astrocytes upregulate expression of several intermediate filaments and cytoskeletal elements associated with a more fibrous phenotype in advanced age. Functional impairments include reduced glutamate uptake resulting in increased toxicity. Aging is associated with reduced neuronal cell body size and reduced regulatory factor production including CD200 and fractalkine ligand (CX3CL1).

Aging is associated with a higher frequency of neurobehavioral complications concomitant with infection, including depression and delirium. Delirium is a significant issue that is diagnosed in approximately 30% of elderly patients admitted to the hospital. Depression is also prevalent in the older population, with an incidence of between 15 and 30% of the general elderly population (Godbout and Johnson, 2009). Importantly, the increased prevalence of these neurological and behavioral complications in the elderly typically coincide with a peripheral infection or illness. Along with increases in neurological and behavioral complications in advancing age there is an increase in the inflammatory status of brain microglia, as detected by positron emission tomography (PET). Following activation, microglia upregulate a receptor for peripheral benzodiazepine called PK11195 (or 1-(2-chlorophenyl)-N-methyl-N-(1-methyl-propyl)-3-isoquinoline carboxamide). PK11195 is normally lowly expressed in the human brain, associated with low levels of microglial activity. By labeling PK11195 with carbon-11, PET scans show that healthy aged individuals have a steady increase in the expression of PK11195, particularly in the temporal and thalamus regions (Cagnin *et al.*, 2001). In patients diagnosed with Alzheimer's or aged individuals with minor cognitive impairments, PK11195 expression is further increased in the temporal and thalamic regions and also noted in the entrorhinal and prefrontal cortices. This is important because the entrorhinal cortex of the hippocampus and the prefrontal cortex are involved in learning and memory and cognitive processing. Thus, exaggerated microglial activation in these CNS regions corresponds to a higher prevalence of age-related brain pathologies.

The extent to which reactive microglia directly contribute to the observed neurological and behavioral deficits in older humans is unknown. Nonetheless, studies using rodent models of aging support the hypothesis that amplified microglial reactivity with age causes a maladaptive sickness response. Along with humans, mice, rats, gerbils, dogs, and non-human primates have increased microglial-specific expression of several inflammatory markers associated with immunity, including MHC II, CD68, CD86, CD11b, and TLRs (Corona *et al.*, 2011). Of these, higher MHC II expression in the brain is conserved across several species. As mentioned previously, MHC II is involved in the process of antigen presentation. Because T-cells are rarely associated with the CNS, MHC II is normally expressed at very low levels in the brain. Increased MHC II expression is associated with a more "reactive" or "primed" microglial population. In support of this notion, microglia isolated from LPS-injected aged mice secrete elevated levels of inflammatory cytokines including IL-1β and IL-6. Importantly, it is the MHC II^+ microglia population responsible for this robust increase in IL-1β production (Henry *et al.*, 2009). Another key point is that increased MHC II expression and IL-1β production do not occur because of an increase in microglial population size with age. The number of microglia remains similar between adult and aged male mice.

Exaggerated IL-1β in the brain of aged rodents is critical because IL-1β expression is the primary cytokine implicated in the induction of the CNS sickness response. Amplified brain IL-1β can result in prolonged and maladaptive sickness behavior. This has been well documented in rodent models of aging. For example, peripheral injection of LPS causes exaggerated body weight loss, prolonged social avoidance, and protracted depressive-like complications in aged mice compared to adults (Godbout *et al.*, 2005). Moreover, infection with a replicating pathogen like *E. coli* results in a delayed and prolonged febrile response associated with increased *E. coli* antigenic load in aged rats (Barrientos *et al.*, 2010). These behaviors are associated with amplified and prolonged IL-1β and IL-6 expression in the brain and plasma, respectively. Importantly, these maladaptive sickness responses lead to more debilitating behavioral and cognitive challenges. Aged mice tested for depression-like behavior following the resolution of a prolonged sickness response show increased resignation compared to adults (Godbout *et al.*, 2008). Furthermore, aged rats infected with *E. coli* have impaired learning and memory in the Morris water maze, radial arm water maze, and contextual fear-conditioning (Barrientos *et al.*, 2010). A key point is that under normal conditions aged mice and rats do not cognitively or behaviorally differ from adults. In the absence of neurodegeneration, problems only manifest following a peripheral immune challenge. Thus, aging leads to glial "priming" and the secondary immune challenge is required to cause exaggerated neuroinflammatory responses and elicit maladaptive behavioral responses (Figure 16.4).

To parse out the contribution of peripheral immunosenescence in the induction of neurological and behavioral complications following immune activation, experiments using direct central immune challenges have been performed. Similar to peripheral challenges, central immune challenge (e.g., intracerebroventricular infusion of LPS or gp120) also promotes exaggerated microglial activity, IL-1β-associated neuroinflammation, and a maladaptive sickness response. Therefore, the inflammatory signals initiated in the periphery are amplified within the brain of older mice by microglia. In support of this idea, central infusion of IL-1 receptor antagonist (RA) just prior to a peripheral injection of LPS attenuated the exaggerated sickness response in older mice (Abraham and Johnson, 2009). Furthermore, central infusion of IL-1RA 24 h following a peripheral injection of *E. coli* protects against age-associated deficits in long-term memory (LTM) (Barrientos *et al.*, 2010). Brain specific IL-1RA treatment also prevents exaggerated LPS-associated IL-6 levels in the plasma of aged mice (Abraham and Johnson, 2009). This is relevant to humans because high plasma IL-6 is the most significant indicator of neurological disease. Elevated IL-6 is detected in older patients suffering from depression, delirium, and dementia (Yirmiya *et al.*, 2000).

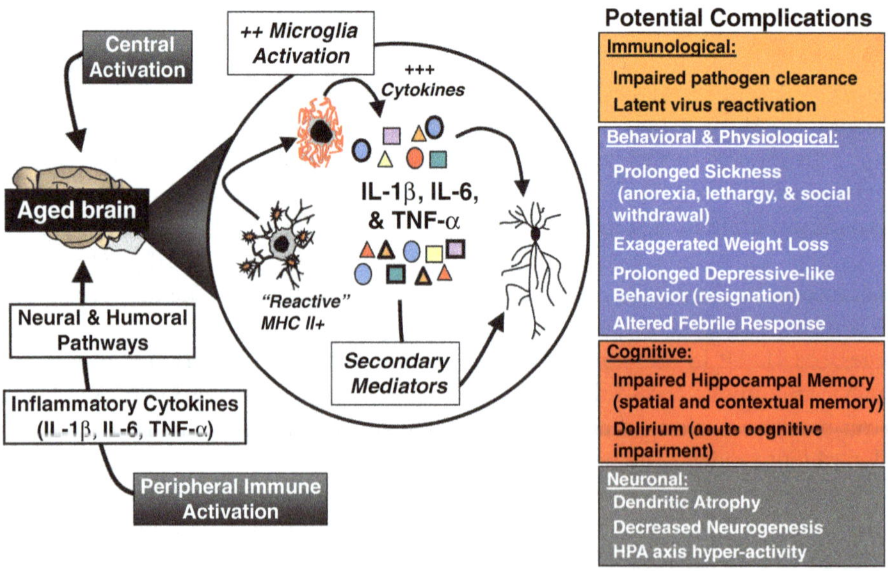

Figure 16.4 Immune activation in the aged is associated with maladaptive sickness responses. In rodent models of aging microglia become hyper-responsive to inflammatory signals from the periphery. They release exaggerated levels of cytokines for a longer duration impairing normal neuronal function and inducing several behavioral and cognitive complications.

Further support for microglial hyperactivity as the mechanism for increased delirium and cognitive impairment in the elderly is derived from mouse models of prion disease. Mad cow and Creutzfeldt–Jakob disease are two examples of prion disease in bovine and humans, respectively. Prion disease is incurable and involves the gradual deterioration of the nervous system coupled with exaggerated brain inflammation. In mouse models of prion disease microglia have a more primed and reactive phenotype weeks prior to onset of clinical symptoms. Therefore, analysis of microglial-associated cognitive deficits can be evaluated independent of neuronal pathology. When prion-infected mice received a peripheral injection of LPS prior to the onset of clinical symptoms, these mice had a hyperactive microglial response associated with exaggerated IL-1β production. This resulted in an acute state of delirium assessed by a decrease in working memory (Murray *et al.*, 2010).

Independent of neurological disease, it is unclear how microglia become primed with age. Nonetheless, recent experiments in rodent models of aging demonstrate that age-related increases in peripheral immune stimulation and oxidative stress, and the reduction of key regulatory systems in the CNS, may underlie priming in normal aging. Microglia are normally under strict paracrine regulation by neuronal and astrocyte products such as hormones and chemokines, and autocrine regulation by anti-inflammatory cytokines. In the aged, these regulatory systems decline, either in concentration or efficacy.

Neurons help regulate microglia through several mediators, including fractalkine ligand (CX_3CL1) and CD200. Within the brain, fractalkine and CD200 are expressed by neurons, while their receptors, fractalkine receptor (CX_3CR1) and CD200R, are exclusively expressed on microglia. Normally, fractalkine and CD200 are highly expressed in the brain and help maintain an anti-inflammatory environment. In the brains of aged rodents, however, both factors are reduced, coinciding with increased microglial activity (Lyons *et al.*, 2007a; Wynne *et al.*, 2010) (Figure 16.3). Furthermore, fractalkine receptor is dysregulated on aged microglia. Following immune activation, fractalkine receptor on the surface of microglia is reduced and associated with increased microglial activation. In adult mice, fractalkine receptor expression returns to baseline levels within 24 hours after the immune challenge. In aged mice, however, fractalkine receptor expression on microglia remains low, coupled with prolonged microglial activation and IL-1β mRNA expression (Wynne *et al.*, 2010). These data are consistent with studies using adult mice deficient in fractalkine receptor. For example, adult mice deficient in fractalkine receptor also have an amplified and prolonged microglial response associated with protracted depressive-like behavior after peripheral challenge with LPS (Corona *et al.*, 2010). CD200 deficits with age correspond with impaired long-term potentiation (LTP) in aged rats and increased microglial IL-1β production. Furthermore, amplified activation of aged microglia by Aβ stimulation can be abrogated with the addition of exogenous CD200 (Lyons *et al.*, 2007b). Deficits in CD200 in the aged brain suggest a role for dysregulated anti-inflammatory regulation of microglia. Specifically, reductions in IL-4 levels in the aged brain coincide with CD200 deficits. Furthermore, increasing IL-4 concentrations in the hippocampus of aged rats restores CD200 expression to adult levels and reverses age-associated deficits in LTP. A recent study indicates that the response to IL-4 is also impaired in microglia of aged mice. Following immune activation, microglia significantly upregulate their receptor for IL-4 (IL-4Rα). Aged microglia, however, fail to upregulate IL-4Rα following activation, and this coincides with prolonged microglial activation even in the presence of increased IL-4 (Fenn *et al.*, 2012).

In addition to IL-4, dysregulation of microglia by IL-10 represents another anti-inflammatory mechanism disrupted with age. Even though IL-10 levels are decreased within the brain of aged mice (Ye and Johnson, 2001), immune challenge induces exaggerated IL-10 production in concert with elevated IL-1β in aged microglia. Despite the concomitant elevation in IL-10 secretion, however, inflammatory processes are sustained in the aged brain (Henry *et al.*, 2009). This may indicate that reactive microglia of the age brain are refractory to anti-inflammatory feedback. Another important regulator of microglial activity is triggering receptor expressed on myeloid cells (TREM)-2. The ligand for TREM-2 is unknown, but stimulating the TREM-2 receptor counteracts TLR signaling and promotes microglial quiescence. People who have a genetic mutation that results in a loss of TREM-2 expression directly support a link between microglial dysregulation and cognitive impairment in humans. Deficient TREM-2 expression results in Nasu–Hakola disease and the development of bone cysts and presenile dementia. Importantly, Nasu–Hakola-associated dementia is connected with reduced microglial regulation and impaired homeostatic function, including phagocytosis (Garden and Moller, 2006).

Astrocyte-mediated regulation of microglia has received less attention. But it is important to mention that significant age-associated changes in astrocyte number and function is observed with age and may influence brain inflammation through microglial regulation, or directly through the production of cytokines or ATP. Astrocyte numbers significantly increase in the cellular layer of the cortex in aged humans in the absence of any neurological disease. Increased glial acidic fibrillary protein (GFAP) and vimentin expression in aged rodents is also noted indicating a more reactive astrocyte population (Cotrina and Nedergaard, 2002). The functional consequence of increased GFAP and vimentin staining or increased astrocyte number with age is unknown, but may be related to impaired microglial regulation and an increased inflammatory CNS environment with age. Further studies investigating the role of reactive astrocytes should be conducted to determine the level of contribution these cells play in microglial hyperactivity with age.

Microglial hyperactivity also has serious implications for brain–immune system communication. In addition to signals propagating from the periphery to the brain, signals from the brain can also feed back to modify peripheral immune function. IL-1β, in addition to regulating sickness responses, is also an important activator of the HPA axis. HPA axis stimulation results in the release of endogenous steroids, or glucocorticoids, from the adrenal gland. These typically provide a negative feedback loop to inhibit innate immune activation and promote adaptive function. Thus, exaggerated and prolonged IL-1β expression in the aged brain following an immune challenge chronically activates the HPA axis. Indeed cortisol, the human glucocorticoid, is chronically increased in the elderly corresponding to a dampening of the immune response. High levels of cortisol also correspond to increased prevalence of depression and cognitive impairment (Yirmiya *et al.*, 2000). Consequently, the cycle of impaired peripheral immune activation, pathogen persistence, hyperactivation of central microglia, and behavioral and cognitive complications is potentiated.

Microglial immunosenescence

It is important to highlight that age-associated changes in microglia have also been linked to immunosenescence. Microglial immunosenescence has largely been described in work investigating the role of microglia in Alzheimer's disease. As mentioned previously, Alzheimer's patients show exaggerated microglial activity in the entrorhinal and prefrontal cortices by PET scan. In transgenic mouse models of Alzheimer's disease, these primed and reactive microglia are also less efficient in phagocytosis and subsequent clearance of Aβ (Hanisch and Kettenmann, 2007). If the inflammatory capacity of microglia is reduced, then Aβ deposition significantly decreases. For example, transgenic mice that express Aβ plaques bred with mice deficient in iNOS are protected from early mortality and Aβ deposition (Hanisch and Kettenmann, 2007). Therefore, microglial priming and hyperactivity may be a component of microglial immunosenescence and microglia characterized as primed and more reactive with age are likely the same microglia characterized as immunosenescent and less phagocytic (Njie *et al.*, 2010).

Successful Versus Normal Aging

Aging can be subdivided into successful, normal, and neurodegenerative aging, and is influenced by genetics, the environment, and disease. Compelling evidence discussed in this chapter supports age-related changes in the peripheral and central immune systems that affect coordinated responses to infection significantly increasing morbidity and mortality. An important topic to discuss is the relationship between longevity and immune function. An example of longevity or perhaps "successful" aging can be found in studies of the centenarian population (i.e., individuals who are 100 years or older). Studies of centenarians show there is a strong association between retained immune system function and longevity. Whereas all aged individuals had reduced lymphopoiesis, only centenarians maintained immune function at levels comparable to adults (aged 19–36 years). In contrast, the majority of aged individuals (65–98 years) had both reduced lymphocyte cell number and reduced immune function (reduced cytotoxicity and T-cell proliferation). Therefore, a loss of immune function was associated with normal aging (Figure 16.5). In further support of this notion, aging alone was associated with a higher incidence of neurological disease or cognitive decline, conditions that were absent in the centenarian population (Sansoni *et al.*, 1993). Thus, maintained immune function corresponded with increased longevity and improved mental health. Studies investigating the connection between lifetime inflammatory exposure and longevity have also found significant correlations linking the two. An historical study correlating infant mortality rates and cohort longevity for populations in Sweden since 1751, France since 1806, England since 1841, and Switzerland since 1876 found that increased infant mortality rates corresponded with reduced cohort lifespan. Therefore, if more children born in 1841 died as a result of infection then children that survived tended to have shorter life-spans (Crimmins and Finch, 2006). Increased exposure to infections and other inflammatory events during childhood significantly reduced longevity in each population investigated. Less exposure to infections and illness also corresponded to reduced incident of heart disease, indicating that reducing inflammatory burden could potentially increase health and life-span.

Incidence of neurodegenerative disease with age can be considered "unsuccessful" aging (Figure 16.5). One of the most debilitating age-associated neurodegenerative diseases in the general population is Alzheimer's disease. As mentioned previously, markers of microglial activation are increased in the entorhinal and prefrontal cortices of Alzheimer's patients and individuals with mild cognitive impairment. Hence, rather than a site specific increased in microglial hyperactivity associated with normal aging, neurodegenerative aging may be related to a widespread increase in the microglial priming or hyperactivation. A widespread primed and hyperactive microglial population results in heightened neuroinflammation beyond that observed in normal aging and may lead to Aβ plaque formation. Indeed, limiting microglial

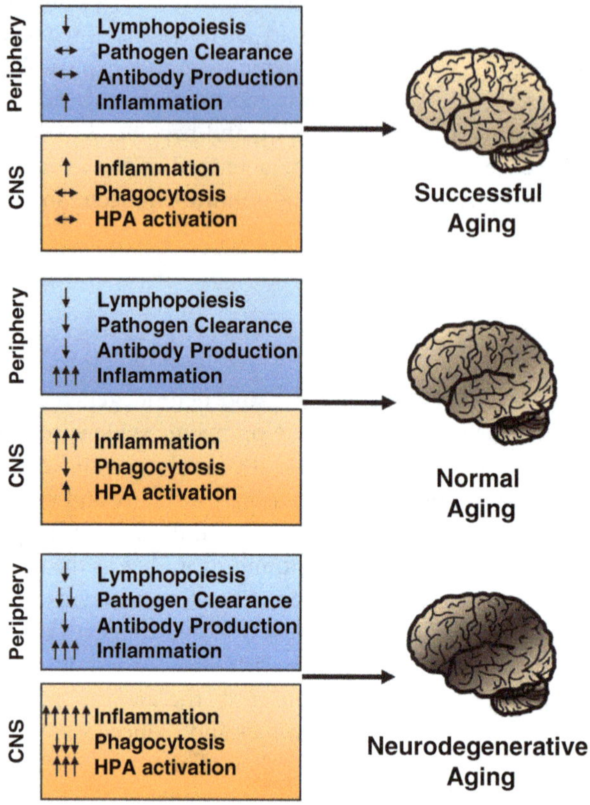

Figure 16.5 Immune function underlies successful, normal, and neurodegenerative aging. Aging is associated with reduced lymphopoiesis and increased inflammation. In successful aging, however, these changes are associated with maintained immune function. More commonly, these immune changes correspond with impaired function and heightened inflammation resulting in cognitive and behavioral complications associated with infection (normal aging). In neurodegenerative aging, immunosenescence is severe resulting in significant reductions in peripheral immune function and an exaggerated inflammatory response in the brain. Exaggerated neuroinflammation beyond that observed in normal aging is associated with neuronal toxicity (Aβ deposition) and death corresponding to precipitous neurodegeneration.

activation can attenuate Aβ plaque formation and ameliorate disease progression in mouse models of Alzheimer's disease. Microglial hyperactivity is also associated with impaired phagocytic function, reducing their ability to effectively clear Aβ. This may be compounded by the effects of immunosenescence in the periphery. Recent evidence indicates that infiltrating and inflammatory macrophages are required for the effective clearance of Aβ plaques (Simard *et al.*, 2006). Advanced age, however, is associated with impaired macrophage inflammatory function and reduced phagocytosis. Combined, an exaggeration of the primed microglial phenotype and increased peripheral immunosenescence may result in increased Aβ plaque deposition and the development of Alzheimer's disease. These effects could be genetically predetermined or an effect of traumatic life events. For example, post-mortem studies of athletes in contact sports (e.g., American football) suggest that these players have early-life Aβ plaque formation characteristic of impaired microglial homeostatic function. Furthermore, in rat models of early-life infection, accelerated microglial priming and hyperactivity is associated with infection-mediated learning and memory impairments in adults. Thus, increased immunosenescence, widespread microglial priming, and exaggerated neuroinflammation coincide with neurodegenerative aging.

Conclusion

Age-associated impairments within the peripheral and central immune systems result in a breakdown in coordinated bidirectional communication between the immune and central nervous systems. As a result, the elderly consistently suffer from higher rates of peripheral infection and neurological and behavioral complications associated with infection. Moreover, exaggerated changes in the immune system with age contribute to the development of neurodegenerative disease. Thus, ensuring maintained immune regulation and function with age may be necessary to retain health and achieve successful aging.

References

Abraham, J., and Johnson, R.W. (2009). Central inhibition of interleukin-1[beta] ameliorates sickness behavior in aged mice. *Brain, Behavior, and Immunity*, 23, 396–401.

Barrientos, R., Frank, M., Watkins, L., and Maier, S. (2010). Memory impairments in healthy aging: role of aging-induced microglial sensitization. *Aging and Disease*, 1, 212–231.

Beerman, I., Bhattacharya, D., Zandi, S., Sigvardsson, M., Weissman, I.L., Bryder, D., et al. (2010). Functionally distinct hematopoietic stem cells modulate hematopoietic lineage potential during aging by a mechanism of clonal expansion. *Proceedings of the National Academy of Sciences of the United States of America*, 107, 5465–5470.

Butcher, S.K., Chahal, H., Nayak, L., Sinclair, A., Henriquez, N.V., Sapey, E., et al. (2001). Senescence in innate immune responses: reduced neutrophil phagocytic capacity and CD16 expression in elderly humans. *Journal of Leukocyte Biology*, 70, 881–886.

Cagnin, A., Brooks, D.J., Kennedy, A.M., Gunn, R.N., Myers, R., Turkheimer, F.E., et al. (2001). In-vivo measurement of activated microglia in dementia. *Lancet*, 358, 461–467.

Chelvarajan, R.L., Liu, Y., Popa, D., Getchell, M.L., Getchell, T.V., Stromberg, A.J., et al. (2006). Molecular basis of age-associated cytokine dysregulation in LPS-stimulated macrophages. *Journal of Leukocyte Biology*, 79, 1314–1327.

Corona, A., Fenn, A., and Godbout, J. (2011). Cognitive and behavioral consequences of impaired immunoregulation in aging. *Journal of Neuroimmune Pharmacology*, 7, 7–23.

Corona, A., Huang, Y., O'Connor, J., Dantzer, R., Kelley, K., Popovich, P., et al. (2010). Fractalkine receptor (CX3CR1) deficiency sensitizes mice to the behavioral changes induced by lipopolysaccharide. *Journal of Neuroinflammation*, 7, 93.

Cotrina, M.L., and Nedergaard, M. (2002). Astrocytes in the aging brain. *Journal of Neuroscience Research*, 67, 1–10.

Crimmins, E.M., and Finch, C.E. (2006). Infection, inflammation, height, and longevity. *Proceedings of the National Academy of Sciences of the United States of America*, 103, 498–503.

Fenn, A.M., Henry, C.J., Huang, Y., Dugan, A., and Godbout, J.P. (2012). Lipopolysaccharide-induced interleukin (IL)-4 receptor-α expression and corresponding sensitivity to the M2 promoting effects of IL-4 are impaired in microglia of aged mice. *Brain, Behavior, and Immunity*, 26, 766–777.

Garden, G., and Moller, T. (2006). Microglia biology in health and disease. *Journal of Neuroimmune Pharmacology*, 1, 127–137.

Ginhoux, F., Greter, M., Leboeuf, M., Nandi, S., See, P., Gokhan, S., et al. (2010). Fate mapping analysis reveals that adult microglia derive from primitive macrophages. *Science*, 330, 841–845.

Glaser, R., Padgett, D.A., Litsky, M.L., Baiocchi, R.A., Yang, E.V., Chen, M., et al. (2005). Stress-associated changes in the steady-state expression of latent Epstein-Barr virus: implications for chronic fatigue syndrome and cancer. *Brain, Behavior, and Immunity*, 19, 91–103.

Godbout, J., Chen, J., Abraham, J., Richwine, A., Berg, B., Kelley, K., et al. (2005). Exaggerated neuroinflammation and sickness behavior in aged mice following activation of the peripheral innate immune system. *FASEB Journal*, 10, 1329–1331.

Godbout, J.P., and Johnson, R.W. (2009). Age and neuroinflammation: a lifetime of psychoneuroimmune consequences. *Immunology and Allergy Clinics*, 29, 321–337.

Godbout, J., Moreau, M., Lestage, J., Chen, J., Sparkman, N., O'Connor, J., et al. (2008). Aging exacerbates depressive-like behavior in mice in response to activation of the peripheral innate immune system. *Neuropsychopharmacology*, 33, 2341–2351.

Gon, Y., Hashimoto, S., Hayashi, S., Koura, T., Matsumoto, K., and Horie, T. (1996). Lower serum concentrations of cytokines in elderly patients with pneumonia and the impaired production of cytokines by peripheral blood monocytes in the elderly. *Clinical and Experimental Immunology*, 106, 120–126.

Han, S.N., Wu, D., Ha, W.K., Beharka, A., Smith, D.E., Bender, B.S., et al. (2000). Vitamin E supplementation increases T helper 1 cytokine production in old mice infected with influenza virus. *Immunology*, 100, 487–493.

Hanisch, U.-K., and Kettenmann, H. (2007). Microglia: active sensor and versatile effector cells in the normal and pathologic brain. *Nature Neuroscience*, 10, 1387–1394.

Henry, C., Huang, Y., Wynne, A.M., and Godbout, J.P. (2009). Peripheral lipopolysaccharide (LPS) challenge promotes microglial hyperactivity in aged mice that is associated with exaggerated induction of both pro-inflammatory IL-1[beta] and anti-inflammatory IL-10 cytokines. *Brain, Behavior, and Immunity*, 23, 309–317.

Krabbe, K.S., Pedersen, M., and Bruunsgaard, H. (2004). Inflammatory mediators in the elderly. *Experimental Gerontology*, 39, 687–699.

Lyons, A., Downer, E., Crotty, S., Nolan, Y., Mills, K., and Lynch, M. (2007a). CD200 ligand receptor interaction modulates microglial activation in vivo and in vitro: a role for IL-4. *Journal of Neuroscience*, 27, 8309–8313.

Lyons, A., Griffin, R.J., Costelloe, C.E., Clarke, R.M., and Lynch, M.A. (2007b). IL-4 attenuates the neuroinflammation induced by amyloid-β in vivo and in vitro. *Journal of Neurochemistry*, 101, 771–781.

Murray, C., Sanderson, D.J., Barkus, C., Deacon, R.M.J., Rawlins, J.N.P., Bannerman, D.M., et al. (2010). Systemic inflammation induces acute working memory deficits in the primed brain: relevance for delirium. *Neurobiology of Aging*, 33, 603–616.

Naylor, K., Li, G., Vallejo, A., Lee, W., Koetz, K., Bryl, E., et al. (2005). The Influence of age on T cell generation and TCR diversity. *Journal of Immunology*, 174, 7446–7452.

Njie, E.G., Boelen, E., Stassen, F.R., Steinbusch, H.W.M., Borchelt, D.R., and Streit, W.J. (2010). Ex vivo cultures of microglia from young and aged rodent brain reveal age-related changes in microglial function. *Neurobiology of Aging*, 33, 195.

Pereira, L.F., Duarte de Souza, A.P., Borges, T.J., and Bonorino, C. (2011). Impaired in vivo CD4+ T cell expansion and differentiation in aged mice is not solely due to T cell defects: decreased stimulation by aged dendritic cells. *Mechanisms of Ageing and Development*, 132, 187–194.

Plackett, T.P., Boehmer, E.D., Faunce, D.E., and Kovacs, E.J. (2004). Aging and innate immune cells. *Journal of Leukocyte Biology*, 76, 291–299.

Plowden, J., Renshaw-Hoelscher, M., Engleman, C., Katz, J., and Sambhara, S. (2004). Innate immunity in aging: impact on macrophage function. *Aging Cell*, 3, 161–167.

Sansoni, P., Cossarizza, A., Brianti, V., Fagnoni, F., Snelli, G., Monti, D., et al. (1993). Lymphocyte subsets and natural killer cell activity in healthy old people and centenarians. *Blood*, 82, 2767–2773.

Simard, A.R., Soulet, D., Gowing, G., Julien, J.-P., and Rivest, S. (2006). Bone marrow-derived microglia play a critical role in restricting senile plaque formation in Alzheimer's disease. *Neuron*, 49, 489–502.

Stowe, R.P., Kozlova, E.V., Yetman, D.L., Walling, D.M., Goodwin, J.S., and Glaser, R. (2007). Chronic herpesvirus reactivation occurs in aging. *Experimental Gerontology*, 42, 563–570.

Swift, M.E., Burns, A.L., Gray, K.L., and DiPietro, L.A. (2001). Age-related alterations in the inflammatory response to dermal injury. *Journal of Investigative Dermatology*, 117, 1027–1035.

Wynne, A., Henry, C., Huang, Y., Cleland, A., and Godbout, J. (2010). Protracted downregulation of CX3CR1 on microglia of aged mice after lipopolysaccharide challenge. *Brain, Behavior, and Immunity*, 24, 1190–1201.

Ye, S.M., and Johnson, R.W. (2001). An age-related decline in interleukin-10 may contribute to the increased expression of interleukin-6 in brain of aged mice. *Neuroimmunomodulation*, 9, 183–192.

Yirmiya, R., Pollak, Y., Morag, M., Reichenberg, A., Barak, O., Avitsur, R., et al. (2000). Illness, cytokines, and depression. *Annals of the New York Academy of Sciences*, 917, 478–487.

17

Peripheral Pro-inflammatory Cytokines and Cognitive Aging

The Role of Metabolic Risk

Alvin Lim and Anna Marsland

Department of Psychology, University of Pittsburgh, Pittsburgh, PA, USA

Introduction

Age-related cognitive decline is marked by gradual and progressive deterioration in function across multiple cognitive domains, including working and episodic memory, attention, processing speed, and executive function. On average, these declines begin in early adulthood and continue at a consistent rate across adulthood (Salthouse, 2004). Progressive declines in cognitive functions, such as working memory and executive function, negatively impact quality of life among many older adults and also predict future risk for Alzheimer's disease and other dementias, personal injury, hospitalization, and death (eg., Barbeger-Gateau *et al.*, 1999; Salthouse, 2004). To identify possible targets of early intervention, recent attention has focused on isolating mid-life risk factors that may contribute to the onset of pathological processes that ultimately result in dementia. In this regard, growing evidence shows that the metabolic syndrome (MetS), a clustering of risk factors including insulin resistance, dyslipidemia, central adiposity, and elevated blood pressure (BP) that covary and predict risk for cardiovascular and metabolic disease (Grundy *et al.*, 2004), is associated with increased risk for accelerated neurocognitive aging (e.g., Dik *et al.*, 2007; Elias *et al.*, 2003). Prevalence of MetS has increased considerably over time in parallel with population increases in obesity, and also increases with age to 45% among US individuals aged 60 and older (Ford, Giles, and Mokdad, 2004). Despite robust associations of MetS and its component factors with future cognitive risk (Yaffe, 2007), mechanistic understanding of how these processes are related remains poorly understood. Among epidemiologic investigations, strong covariation in components of the MetS raises the possibility that a common etiologic mechanism may account for observed relationships between the MetS and neurocognitive decline (Grundy *et al.*, 2004). In this regard, mounting evidence suggests that inflammation provides a common link between established components of the MetS (Marsland, McCaffery, Muldoon, and Manuck, 2010) and contributes to accelerated cognitive aging (Yaffe, 2007). In this chapter, evidence linking peripheral inflammation and its sources to human neurocognitive function will be examined, considering the possibility that age-related increases in inflammation and related metabolic

The Wiley-Blackwell Handbook of Psychoneuroimmunology, First Edition. Edited by Alexander W. Kusnecov and Hymie Anisman.

risk may contribute to the pathophysiology of accelerated neurocognitive aging, ultimately increasing risk for dementia in later life.

Peripheral Sources of Inflammation: The Role of Adiposity

The inflammatory response is a non-specific immune reaction that is initiated when monocytes and tissue-residing macrophages are activated by pathogens or tissue damage to release pro-inflammatory cytokines, such as interleukin (IL)-6, IL-1β, and tumor necrosis factor (TNF)-α. These cytokines act as a paracrine signal to recruit circulating leukocytes to areas of infection or injury, but can also enter general circulation, where they induce hepatic synthesis and release of acute phase proteins, such as C-reactive protein (CRP) (Black and Garbutt, 2002). While TNF-α and IL-1β both decay rapidly, IL-6 and CRP have longer half-lives and can be reliably detected in human plasma/serum. Thus, they are widely measured and circulating levels are assumed to reflect cumulative systemic inflammation at the time of the blood draw. However, caution should be taken in assuming that circulating inflammatory mediators provide a measure of immune-derived inflammatory processes, as many cells other than immune cells produce these signaling proteins, including adipocytes and endothelial cells (e.g., Mohamed-Ali *et al.*, 1997). Indeed, adipose tissue contributes towards circulating levels of inflammatory cytokines, with adipocytes producing 10–35% of circulating IL-6 (Mohamed-Ali *et al.*, 1997) and adiposity being positively associated with circulating levels of a number of inflammatory mediators (Park, Park, and Yu, 2004). In this regard, obesity (defined as BMI >30) reflects a chronic subclinical inflammatory condition (Lee and Pratley, 2005). Recently, central adiposity, described as adipose tissue surrounding the visceral abdominal organs, has been identified as a particularly potent source of circulating inflammatory mediators (Park, Park, and Yu, 2004). Regardless of source, systemic IL-6 increases during the normal aging process, is relatively stable over extended periods, and predicts risk for accelerated cognitive decline among elderly populations (Maggio, Guralnik, Longo, and Ferrucci, 2006).

Cytokines and Cognitive Function: Animal studies

In addition to playing a pivotal role in the organization of local inflammatory responses, peripheral cytokines also signal the central nervous system (CNS), mediating the cognitive, affective, and behavioral sickness symptoms that accompany infectious/inflammatory disease (Dantzer, 2004). These symptoms include elevations in negative mood, anhedonia, sleep, fatigue, and social withdrawal, along with reductions in cognitive function. Indeed, evidence shows that inflammatory cytokines modulate the cellular and molecular processes that subserve cognitive function (reviewed by McAfoose and Baune, 2009), and it is widely accepted that peripheral release of pro-inflammatory cytokines is responsible for the transient affective and cognitive declines that accompany acute illness (Dantzer and Kelley, 2007). Moreover, epidemiologic evidence suggests that age-related increases in systemic inflammation also contribute to concomitant cognitive declines (Weaver *et al.*, 2002; Yaffe *et al.*, 2003, 2004). By crossing periventricular blood–brain barriers, binding to receptors on endothelial cells in brain microvasculature, and/or activating vagal nerve sensory afferents, peripheral pro-inflammatory cytokines stimulate the production of central pro-inflammatory cytokines by microglial cells in discrete brain regions (McAfoose and Baune, 2009; Yirmiya and Goshen, 2011). Emerging evidence shows that this central inflammation negatively impacts specific cognitive functions (eg., Rosczyk, Sparkman, and Johnson, 2008).

To date, much of the evidence that pro-inflammatory cytokines in the periphery affect neurocognitive function derives from animal models. Within the central nervous system, receptors for pro-inflammatory cytokines are expressed on microglia (Poluektova *et al.*, 2005) and are concentrated in the hippocampus and prefrontal cortex (PFC) (Gadient and Otten, 1994). When stimulated by pro-inflammatory cytokines, microglia adopt an inflammatory phenotype characterized by the production of high levels of IL-1β, TNF-α and IL-6 (Pugh *et al.*, 1998). In the hippocampus, these increases in central cytokines interfere with long-term potentiation (LTP), neurogenesis, and synaptic plasticity (McAfoose and Baunne, 2009), resulting in impaired performance on hippocampal-dependent learning and memory tests (Heyser *et al.*, 1997; Weaver *et al.*, 2002). Conversely, pro-inflammatory receptor antagonists prevent inflammation-related disruption of hippocampal LTP (Ross, Allan, Rothwell, and Verkhratsky, 2003). When compared with wild type mice, IL-6 knockout mice show facilitated working memory and are refractory to peripheral endotoxin-induced impairments of spatial memory (eg., Pugh *et al.*, 1998). However, transgenic mice that overexpress central IL-6 show impairments in synaptic plasticity manifested by deficits in avoidance learning (Heyser *et al.*, 1997). Together, these animal findings suggest that increases in peripheral levels of pro-inflammatory cytokines are associated with activation of central hippocampal inflammatory mechanisms that negatively affect cognitive processes, including memory and learning.

Initial animal research focused on the effect of acute increases in peripheral cytokines secondary to exogenous administration or *in vivo* immune challenge; however, recent evidence suggests that more chronic conditions can "prime" or sensitize microglia to switch to an inflammatory phenotype, resulting in exaggerated central inflammatory responses to peripheral stimuli (Perry, Cunningham, and Holmes, 2007). For example, chronic stress can activate microglia, resulting in central inflammation that inhibits adult neurogenesis, synaptic plasticity, and LTP (Frank *et al.*, 2006; Monje, Toda, and Palmer, 2003) and disrupts learning and memory (e.g., Licastro *et al.*, 2000; Reichenberg *et al.*, 2001). Similarly, aging is associated with priming of microglia (Smith, Tyrrell, Coyle, and Higgins, 1998), increased levels of pro-inflammatory cytokines in the hippocampus and cerebral cortex (Schram *et al.*, 2007), amplified central inflammatory cytokine production, and concomitant deficits in spatial working memory following peripheral inflammation (Tilvis *et al.*, 2004). A pattern of increased microglial sensitivity has also been demonstrated to accompany human aging and to be exacerbated among individuals with Alzheimer's disease (AD) and dementia (Richwine *et al.*, 2005). Recent evidence suggests that even mild stress induces neuroinflammation and associated disruption of learning and memory in aged mice (Buchanan *et al.*, 2008). Thus, although research on the impact of systemic inflammation on chronic neurodegeneration is in its infancy, recent evidence suggests that microglia become primed with age to produce an exaggerated central inflammatory response to systemic inflammatory signals that could play a role in age-related cognitive decline.

Peripheral Cytokines and Cognitive Function: Human Evidence

In accordance with animal studies, there are several independent lines of research that support an association between peripheral inflammation and the modulation of cognitive function in humans. Studies of human dementia suggest that pro-inflammatory cytokines play a pathogenic role in several age-related diseases that involve impairments of cognitive function, including AD, vascular dementia (VD), and age-related cognitive decline. Generally, these syndromes have been associated with elevated expression of peripheral and central cytokines, including IL-6 and IL-1β (eg., McGeer and McGeer, 1995). For example, when compared with healthy controls, 222 individuals diagnosed with AD or VD showed elevated serum levels of TNF-α and IL-1β, and individuals with VD showed higher serum IL-6 (Zuliani *et al.*, 2007). Cross-sectional associations of this kind do not shed light on the direction of the observed effects. Indeed, it is plausible that raised peripheral cytokine levels are the consequence of central inflammatory processes, possibly resulting from the neurodegenerative process (Licastro *et al.*, 2000; Krabbe *et al.*, 2004). However, evidence that inflammation presages cognitive decline comes from longitudinal studies showing that individuals with heightened systemic inflammation are at increased risk for accelerated cognitive decline. For example, Engelhart and colleagues (2004) followed a sample of 916 dementia-free elderly (mean age at baseline = 72 years) for an 8-year period. Findings showed that higher baseline levels of IL-6, and to a lesser extent CRP, predicted probability of developing dementia (N =188) across this period. Similarly, Schmidt and colleagues (2002) followed a sample of 1,050 Japanese-Americans from mid-life for 25 years. They observed a 3-fold increased risk of incident dementia among men in the upper 3 quartiles of midlife CRP as compared to those in the lowest quartile. By adjusting for key demographic and health-related variables including age, gender, education, smoking status, and cardiovascular disease status, both of these studies suggest that elevated markers of peripheral inflammation may convey independent risk for future cognitive decline.

Individual differences in circulating levels of pro-inflammatory cytokines have also been associated with normative variation in cognitive function. Initial studies examining cognitive decline in the well-functioning elderly have shown that systemic levels of IL-6 and CRP covary inversely with global cognitive functioning (Teunissen *et al.*, 2003), with higher levels also predicting future cognitive decline (Teunissen *et al.*, 2003; Tilvis *et al.*, 2004; Weaver *et al.*, 2002; Yaffe *et al.*, 2003; but not Alley *et al.*, 2008; Dik *et al.*, 2005). For example, the Health, Aging, and Body Composition (Health ABC) Study followed 3,031 participants between the ages of 70 and 79 years (Yaffe *et al.*, 2003). Results showed that higher circulating levels of IL-6 and CRP were associated with poorer cognitive performance and greater cognitive decline over a 2-year period. Again, these associations persisted after adjustment for demographics including age, race, gender, and education, and lifestyle characteristics, including smoking, alcohol use, and BMI. Although a number of studies have demonstrated that higher levels of peripheral markers of inflammation predict future cognitive decline (Yaffe *et al.*, 2003; Yaffe *et al.*, 2004; Weaver *et al.*, 2002), not all findings are consistent (Alley *et al.*, 2008; Dik *et al.*, 2005). For example, an examination of 851 high functioning older adults (70–79 years) taking part in the MacArthur Study of Successful Aging revealed negative cross-sectional associations of systemic inflammation, as assessed by IL-6 and CRP, with cognitive function, but no significant prospective associations over a 3.5-year follow-up (Alley *et al.*, 2008). Reasons for discrepant findings are unclear, but may relate to differences in the nature of samples. Specifically, the MacArthur Successful Aging Study recruited a high functioning sample of individuals who fell in the top tertile for their age on measures of physical and cognitive function. In contrast, the Health ABC study recruited a more representative sample in regard to cognitive function. In sum, the weight of evidence supports an association of inflammation with increased risk of neurocognitive decline among representative elderly samples.

Interleukin-6 and Cognitive Performance Among Middle-Aged Community Volunteers

While the majority of studies focus on populations aged 65 and older, there is increasing recognition that trajectories of cognitive decline that presage dementia begin in mid-life (Kivipelto *et al.*, 2006; Schmidt *et al.*, 2002). Thus, in order to develop preventative interventions, modifiable risk factors that predict the subclinical neurocognitive deterioration that occurs during mid-life are needed. In this regard, research from our laboratory has shown an inverse association of plasma IL-6 with attention/working memory and executive function among cognitively-normal adults between the ages of 30 and 54 years (Marsland *et al.*, 2006). In this study, blood was drawn from 500 healthy community volunteers (51% male) to determine plasma levels of IL-6. Participants then completed a battery of neuropsychological tests. Based on the animal literature showing that peripheral pro-inflammatory cytokines interfere with memory formation in the hippocampus and possibly activity in the prefrontal cortex, we hypothesized that IL-6 levels would covary inversely with performance on cognitive tests that assess the functions of these regions, including verbal and nonverbal learning and memory, attention, and executive function. Memory and attention were assessed with the Wechsler Memory Scale – Third Edition (WMS-III; Wechsler, 1997). In addition, participants were administered two tests of executive function: the Trial Making Test (Reitan and Wolfson, 1985) and the Stroop Color-Word Test (Golden, 1978).

As hypothesized, our analyses revealed an inverse association of plasma IL-6 with performance on clusters of tests assessing attention/working memory, executive function, and auditory recognition memory after adjustment for age, gender, ethnicity, and years of education. This association was largely independent of blood pressure, antihypertensive treatment, sleep duration, alcohol use, physical activity, and BMI. Thus, our findings are consistent with studies of older adults that show inverse associations of IL-6 with cognitive function that are largely independent of established risk factors for subtle and clinical cognitive impairments, including hypertension, diabetes, smoking, and subclinical atherosclerosis (e.g., Elwood *et al.*, 1999). Our findings are displayed in Figures 17.1 and 17.2. For the figures, we divided the distribution of plasma IL-6 into tertiles (Low, Medium and High IL-6: means = 0.74, 1.32, and 3.35 pg/ml, respectively).

These findings raise the possibility that inflammation-related cognitive impairment begins well before the appearance of clinically-significant deficits and provide further support for the hypothesis that inflammation precedes, and may contribute to, neurocognitive decline. However, the direction of observed effects remains to be determined. Reverse causation remains a possibility, with poorer cognitive function earlier in life resulting in increases in systemic inflammation. This could be a direct effect or through associations of lifestyle or health behaviors. It is also possible that higher levels of peripheral IL-6 and poorer cognitive function are independently related to a third factor, such as subclinical neuroinflammatory conditions or cerebral vascular disease (Krabbe *et al.*, 2004; Licastro *et al.*, 2000). Longitudinal studies tracking individuals from mid-life are necessary to shed further light on the direction of these associations, exploring whether markers of systemic inflammation among mid-life individuals predict increased risk for future cognitive dysfunction.

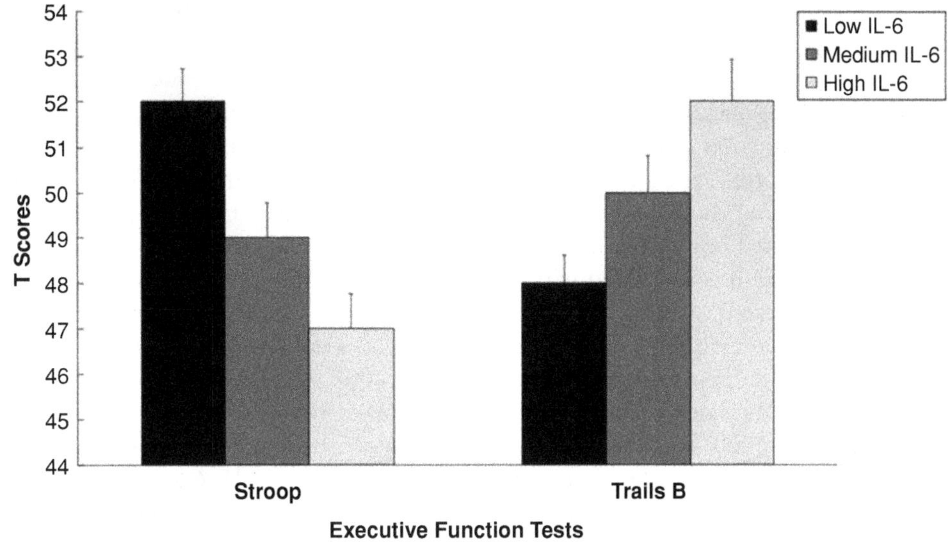

Figure 17.1 Mean performance on tests of executive function among Individuals with low, medium, and high plasma IL-6. Tests were the Trail Making Test and the Stroop Color-Word Test; higher scores reflect better performance on the Stroop task and worse performance on Trail Making. (Reprinted from Marsland *et al.*, 2006, with permission from Wolters Kluwer Health.)

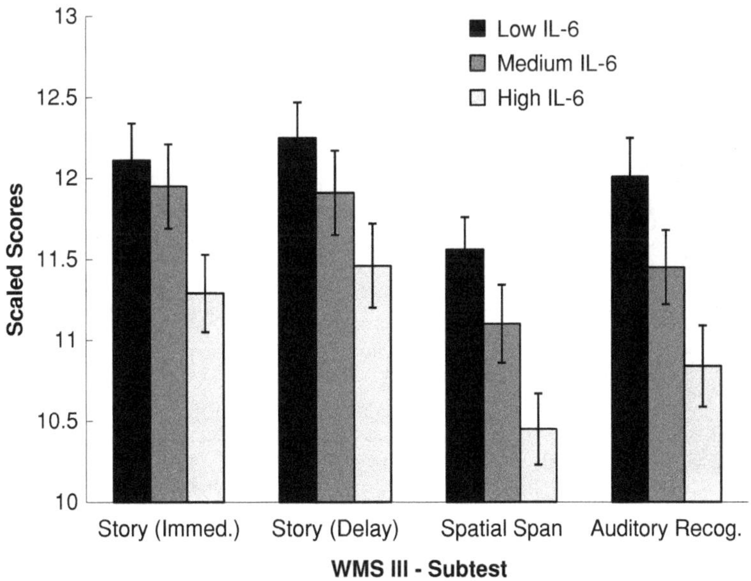

Figure 17.2 Mean performance on the Wechsler Memory III scales assessing auditory and visual attention/working memory among individuals with low, medium, and high plasma IL-6. (Reprinted from Marsland *et al.*, 2006, with permission from Wolters Kluwer Health.)

Inflammation and Specific Brain Regions: Hippocampus and Prefrontal Cortex

Converging evidence, including our own, suggests that aging is associated with alterations in the structure and function of regions of the brain where pro-inflammatory cytokines, such as IL-6, and their receptors are expressed most abundantly (Gadient and Otten, 1994; Schobitz *et al.*, 1994), including the hippocampus (Jack *et al.*, 2000) and PFC (Mattay *et al.*, 2006). We recently conducted one of the first neuroimaging studies to examine the possibility that peripheral inflammation is associated with hippocampal morphology. Decreased gray matter volume in the hippocampus has been associated with memory impairments (Van Petten, 2004); thus, we hypothesized that higher peripheral levels of IL-6 would correlate inversely with gray matter volume of the hippocampus (Marsland *et al.*, 2008). In this study, we employed a computational structural neuroimaging method, optimized voxel-based morphometry (Ashburner, and Friston, 2000) to assess hippocampal gray matter volume in a sample of 76 mid-life adults (aged 30–54 years) on whom we previously examined plasma IL-6 levels and cognitive function (Marsland *et al.*, 2006). Consistent with our hypothesis, higher plasma IL-6 was associated with lower hippocampal gray matter volume (see Figure 17.3). This relationship was independent of multiple demographic and health factors, including age, sex, race, years of education, percent body fat, blood pressure, smoking, physical activity, hours of sleep, alcohol use, and total gray matter volume.

This finding is consistent with animal evidence that peripheral activation of central inflammatory mechanisms results in hippocampal remodeling, particularly neurodegeneration (e.g., Monje, Toda, and Palmer, 2003). The hippocampus plays a key role in episodic memory

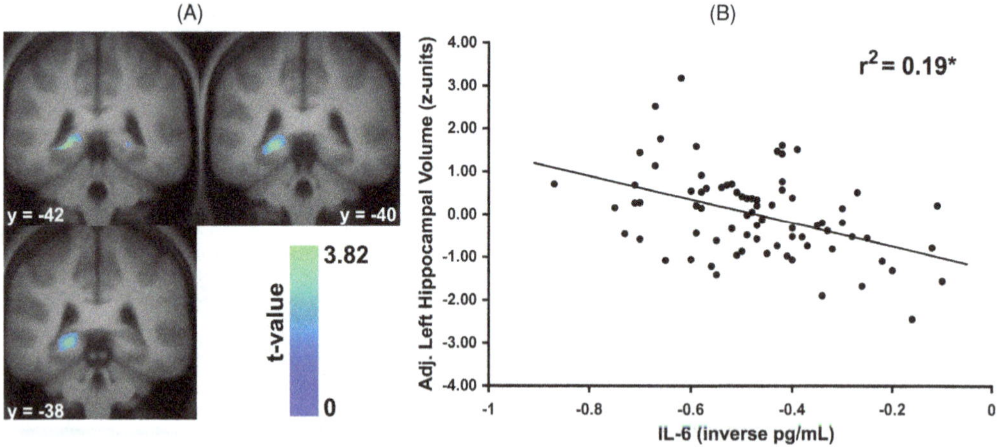

Figure 17.3 Higher levels of plasma IL-6 are associated with decreased gray matter volume in left, but not right, hippocampus at a family-wise error rate corrected level of significance. Panel A: Statistical parametric maps profiling clusters of the left and right hippocampus where higher IL-6 was associated with decreased gray matter volume after controlling for age, sex, race, and total gray matter volume. Panel B: Plotted along the *y*-axis are extracted left hippocampal gray matter volumes in standardized units adjusted for age, sex, race and total gray matter volume. Plotted along the *x*-axis are transformed plasma IL-6 values (less negative values indicate higher IL-6 levels). * $p < .01$. (Reprinted from Marsland *et al.*, 2008, with permission from Elsevier.)

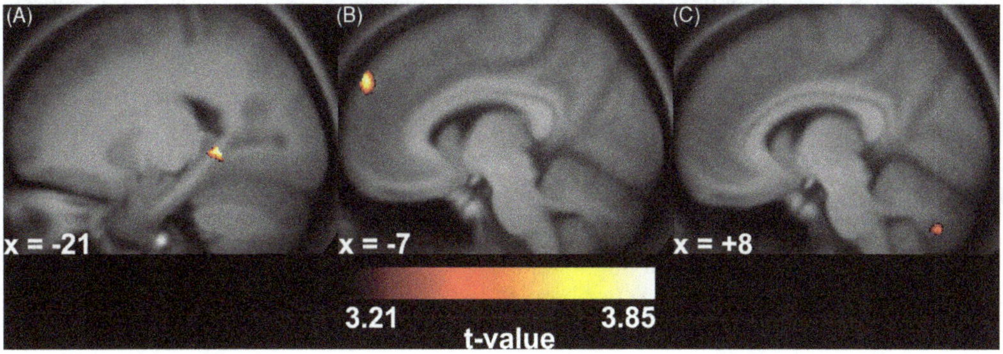

Figure 17.4 A whole brain regression analysis showed that higher leves of plasma IL-6 were associated with reduced gray matter volume in the left hippocampus (panel A), area 9 of the medial prefrontal cortex (panel B), and posterior cerebellum (panel C), after controlling for age, sex, race, and total gray matter volume. (Reprinted from Marsland *et al.*, 2008, with permission from Elsevier.)

encoding (e.g., Wagner *et al.*, 1998) and hippocampal atrophy is frequently associated with poorer memory function (Van Petten, 2004). Thus, it is possible that low-grade systemic inflammation relates to age-related declines in learning and memory via hippocampal pathways.

In addition to examining hippocampal gray matter volume, we conducted a whole brain analysis examining the associations of peripheral IL-6 with gray matter volumes throughout the brain. Interestingly this exploratory investigation revealed an inverse association of IL-6 with gray matter volume of the prefrontal cortex (see Figure 17.4). This is consistent with our earlier finding that plasma IL-6 covaried inversely with performance on tests of working memory and executive function that typically engage this brain region (Marsland *et al.*, 2006). Functional neuroimaging studies demonstrate that a network of brain regions are activated during the encoding of stimuli that will be subsequently remembered, including the hippocampus and prefrontal cortices (e.g., Wagner *et al.*, 1998; whereas, working memory and executive function are generally accepted to involve activation of the PFC (Tisserand and Jolles, 2003). Future exploration of the structure and function of these brain regions in inflammation-related cognitive decline is warranted.

Experimental Evidence that Inflammation Impacts Cognitive Function

More direct evidence that peripheral inflammation results in declines in cognitive function comes from experimental studies that examine the cognitive consequences of acute immune activation. In general, these studies involve the peripheral injection of an agent that generates a systemic inflammatory response, but is incapable of penetrating the blood–brain barrier. To date, several inflammatory agonists have been utilized in these studies, including endotoxins such as *Escherichia coli* and *Salmonella abortus equi* toxin, typhoid vaccine, interferon-alpha, and recombinant IL-6 (Capuron and Miller, 2004; Krabbe *et al.*, 2005; Reichenberg *et al.*, 2001; Spath-Schwalbe *et al.*, 1997). While the pharmacological agents and method of cognitive testing vary across studies, findings are consistent and show that peripheral activation of innate inflammatory mechanisms result in declines in cognitive function. For example, an early experimental study conducted by Reichenberg and colleagues (2001) employed a balanced double-blind crossover design and administered low-dose *Salmonella abortus equi* endotoxin and saline placebo to 20 male volunteers. When compared with cognitive function following the placebo condition, the dose of endotoxin resulted in impaired performance on immediate and delayed verbal recall tasks. Moreover, this effect was dependent on individual differences in the magnitude of endotoxin-stimulated increases in IL-6, with higher cytokine responses predicting greater impairments in performance. A similar experimental paradigm has been utilized by Brydon and colleagues (2008). Here, 16 male volunteers were randomized to receive either typhoid vaccination or placebo in a crossover-controlled design. Although no group differences in cognitive function were observed between the typhoid and placebo condition, within the typhoid vaccination group, magnitude of IL-6 response was negatively correlated to performance on the Stroop task, a measure of executive function (Golden, 1978). Similarly, Krabbe and colleagues (2005) administered low-dose *Escherichia coli* endotoxin to 12 males and showed an inverse association of IL-6 response with declarative memory performance. In a more direct examination of the impact of peripheral IL-6, Spath-Schwalbe *et al.* (1998) showed that, when compared with a placebo condition, peripheral administration of recombinant IL-6 was associated with a decrease in self-reported attentional capacity. Taken together, these experimental findings show that acute increases in peripheral inflammation, as assessed by circulating levels of IL-6, predict decreases in memory, attention, and executive function.

Further evidence that peripheral cytokines negatively impact cognitive processes comes from an examination of the effects of therapeutic cytokine administration during the treatment of some forms of cancer and chronic infection. Here, the peripheral administration of IFN-α, a cytokine that induces endogenous pro-inflammatory cytokine release, is associated with disturbances in cognitive function, including impairments in attention, psychomotor speed, and memory (Capuron and Miller, 2004). Furthermore, the magnitude of this cognitive impact is directly related to dose, with higher doses of IFN-α being related to greater declines in cognitive function (Pavol *et al.*, 1995).

More naturalistic studies also show that disturbances of attention, memory, and executive function accompany both acute and chronic inflammatory conditions among individuals with and without existing dementia (Bucks *et al.*, 2008). For example, a recent study conducted by Holmes and colleagues (2009) followed a sample of 275 subjects with mild to severe AD over a six-month period and recorded episodes of acute systemic infections (e.g., respiratory or genitourinary infection) and accidental trauma. Individuals who experienced infections/injury showed an increase in circulating levels of TNF-α and a concomitant two-fold increase in the rate of cognitive decline over the 6-month follow-up period when compared with their peers who remained healthy. In addition, baseline levels of TNF-α were positively associated with increases in the rate of cognitive decline over the 6-month period (Holmes *et al.*, 2009). Similar findings have been reported among samples without dementia. For example, Bucks and colleagues (2008) followed 80 healthy subjects and showed that when compared with healthy controls matched on age, gender and IQ, the 21 individuals who developed symptoms of upper respiratory tract infection showed significantly reduced speed of accessing stored memories and labeling facial emotions, although no effects of infection were found on episodic or working memory. Impairments of attention, memory and executive function have also been shown to accompany chronic inflammatory conditions (e.g., Kozora, Laudenslager, Lemieux, and West, 2001) among individuals with and without dementia, with greater infection-related declines in cognitive function observed among older than younger adults (Bucks *et al.*, 2008).

Peripheral Inflammation and Cognitive Function: Interim Summary

In summary, converging evidence shows that peripheral inflammation is associated with poorer working and episodic memory and executive function, with declines in cognitive function accompanying the peripheral administration of immune agonists, and the naturalistic occurrence of acute and chronic inflammatory disease. Further evidence shows that more stable age-related increases in markers of systemic inflammation, such as IL-6, also covary inversely with these cognitive functions and predict incident cognitive pathology in the elderly. Thus, levels of pro-inflammatory cytokines in peripheral circulation provide a marker of increased risk for accelerated cognitive decline, as well as for a number of other age-related disease processes. Accordingly, recent attention has begun to focus on factors that are associated with increases in levels of systemic inflammation during mid-life. Given existing evidence that the MetS and its core components – insulin resistance, dyslipidemia, central adiposity, and elevated blood pressure (BP) – covary with levels of systemic inflammation (Dandona *et al.*, 2005) and predict risk for accelerated and pathological neurocognitive aging (e.g., Dik *et al.*, 2007; Whitmer *et al.*, 2005; Yaffe *et al.*, 2004), recent interest has focused on inflammation as a possible mechanism for the cognitive covariates of MetS. In this regard, we have recently shown that plasma concentrations of CRP and IL-6 are positively associated with the common covariation of insulin resistance, dyslipidemia, adiposity, and BP, accounting for 55% of its variance and partially mediating the statistical aggregation of the component factors of MetS (Marsland, McCaffery, Muldoon, and Manuck, 2010). Statistical mediation was particularly strong for adiposity, raising the possibility that inflammatory processes stimulated by intra-abdominal adipose tissue contribute to the association of the core components of the metabolic syndrome and to risk for accelerated cognitive aging.

A number of studies have shown that inflammation contributes to cognitive risk beyond the risk associated with traditional cardiovascular risk factors, including education, hypertension, MetS, smoking, subclinical atherosclerosis and symptoms of CVD (e.g., Elwood *et al.*, 1999; Marsland *et al.*, 2006). For example, in the Health, Aging and Body Composition study, subjects with MetS and high levels of inflammatory markers (IL-6 and CRP) showed significantly higher rates of cognitive decline than subjects with the metabolic syndrome but lower levels of inflammatory markers (Schram *et al.*, 2007). These findings support the possibility that inflammation explains associations of the MetS with cognitive function (Craft, 2009). However, systemic inflammation covaries significantly with other cardiovascular risk factors in the prediction of cognitive aging, thus making it difficult to isolate its unique contribution. In this regard, recent evidence shows that a synergistic combination of traditional and inflammatory risk factors predicts greater risk for cognitive impairment than single risk factors (Roberts *et al.*, 2010). Thus, it is likely that composite risk profiles will be of more predictive value than any single marker of risk.

Adiposity and Risk for Dementia

One risk factor that is strongly related to peripheral levels of inflammation is visceral adiposity, a core component of MetS. Adipose tissue is a potent source of peripheral inflammatory mediators, and BMI is inversely associated with cognitive function independently of age (Cournot *et al.*, 2006) predicting temporal lobe and global brain atrophy, cognitive decline, and the incidence of dementia (Cournot *et al.*, 2006; Elias *et al.*, 2003; Gustafson *et al.* 2004). Indeed, a recent meta-analysis showed that individuals who are obese during midlife harbor a 1.35-fold increased risk for dementia during late-life as compared their non-obese counterparts (Anstey, Cherbuin, Budge, and Young, 2011). For example, one prospective study followed a sample of 10,136 midlife individuals (age 40–45) without dementia over an average of 36 years and showed that individuals who were obese in mid-life were 3 times more likely to develop AD than those who were not obese in midlife (Whitmer *et al.*, 2005). Interestingly, this increase in risk persisted after adjusting for multiple traditional risk factors including demographics; metabolic factors including hyperlipidaemia and hypertension; and cardiovascular disease. A similar pattern of results was reported in a prospective study of 2,798 elderly individuals (average age 74.7 years) without dementia who were followed for an average of 5.4 years (Fitzpatrick *et al.*, 2009). By utilizing data gathered during midlife health assessments, investigators showed that individuals who were obese in mid-life (BMI >30 at age 50) were at 40% greater risk for developing dementia in later life than their normal-weight counterparts (BMI 20–25), with findings withstanding adjustment for age, gender, and ethnicity (Fitzpatrick *et al.* 2009). Other studies also show that the prospective association of mid-life adiposity with risk for dementia is independent of hypertension and lipid profiles (Kivipelto *et al.*, 2006).

Indirect evidence that inflammation plays a role in the pathological cognitive decline that accompanies obesity comes from studies showing that dementia risk differs as a function of adipose tissue distribution. Central adiposity is a particularly potent source of circulating inflammatory mediators (Park, Park, and Yu, 2004) and is also a stronger predictor of dementia risk than other patterns of fat distribution. For example, Whitmer and colleagues (2008) followed 6,583 adults from mid-life for an average of 36 years and showed that midlife (age 40–45) sagittal abdominal diameter (SAD), a measure of central adiposity, predicted dementia incidence independently of BMI. Furthermore, among normal-weight individuals, those with high SAD were 89% more likely to develop dementia as compared with those with low SAD. This association persisted after adjustment for traditional metabolic risk factors, suggesting that central adiposity may play a specific role in the prediction of cognitive risk, possibly by increasing systemic levels of inflammation.

Obesity and Cognitive Function

Individual differences in obesity have also been associated with normative variation in cognitive function, including age-related cognitive decline. Here, consistent evidence shows an inverse association of BMI with neurocognitive test performance independently of age (e.g, Cournot *et al.*, 2006; Gustafson, 2004). For example, in an age-stratified (62, 52, 42, and 32 years at baseline) sample of 2,223 healthy individuals, Cournot *et al.* (2006) found negative cross-sectional associations of BMI with performance on a battery of neurocognitive tests, with this relationship persisting after adjustment for demographics, type-2 diabetes, and systolic blood pressure. Moreover, baseline BMI also predicted declines in cognitive performance over the course of a 5-year follow-up. A similar pattern of findings was observed in an analysis of 1,423 participants in the Framingham Heart Study, with an inverse association of obesity (defined as BMI >30) with future neurocognitive function (Elias *et al.*, 2003). Consistent with previous findings, this relationship persisted after adjustment for traditional cardiovascular risk factors, including blood pressure, smoking, type-II diabetes, and lipid levels, suggesting that BMI may predict risk for neurocognitive decline independently of other metabolic factors. Finally, in a sample of 781 individuals obtained from the Swedish Twin Cohort study, Dahl and colleagues

(2010) showed a negative association of midlife BMI (mean age 41.6 years) with rate of cognitive decline over an approximate 15 year follow-up during late-life. In sum, growing evidence links higher BMI to poorer cognitive function and accelerated preclinical cognitive decline.

Thus, parallel evidence shows that systemic inflammation and adiposity, in particular central adiposity, are inversely associated with cognitive function, accelerated cognitive aging, and risk for dementia. Given that adipose tissue is a metabolically active tissue that secretes inflammatory mediators, called adipocytokines, accounting for up to 35% of circulating levels of common inflammatory mediators including as IL-6 (Mohammed-Ali *et al.*, 1997), it is possible that inflammation derived from adipose tissue contributes to the neurodegenerative processes that accompany adiposity. Central adiposity is a core component of the MetS, raising the possibility that inflammatory processes stimulated by intra-abdominal adipose tissue contribute to the association of the MetS with accelerated cognitive aging. This possibility is supported by recent evidence showing that among individuals with the MetS, those with elevated levels of systemic inflammation have greater risk of cognitive decline than those without elevated inflammation. (Schram *et al.*, 2007; Yaffe *et al.*, 2007). Consistent with the findings of others (Khaodhiar, Ling, Blackburn, and Bistrian, 2004), we have shown that percent body fat is associated with higher plasma IL-6, poorer cognitive function, and lower hippocampal gray matter volume (Marsland *et al.*, 2006, 2008). However, observed relationships of IL-6 with cognitive function and hippocampal gray matter volume were partially independent of percent body fat, making it unlikely that adipose tissue is the sole source of the variability in IL-6 levels associated with cognitive function or hippocampal gray matter volume. However, our findings are consistent with the possibility that inverse relationships between BMI and cognitive function are secondary to inflammation (Marsland *et al.*, 2008).

Summary: Implications for Prevention, and Future Directions

Although some inconstancies have been reported, converging evidence suggests that systemic inflammation is a risk factor for poorer working and episodic memory and executive function, accelerated cognitive decline across mid-life, and incident cognitive pathology in the elderly. To date, the majority of studies in this literature, including our own, have considered MetS and its component factors as "nuisance" covariates in analyses, and have shown that inflammation contributes to cognitive risk beyond metabolic factors. However, considering MetS components as covariates likely underestimates the full effect of systemic inflammation on cognitive function. Indeed, recent evidence raises the possibility that inflammatory processes stimulated by intra-abdominal adipose tissue contribute to the association of the MetS with accelerated cognitive aging. Thus, a synergistic combination of metabolic and inflammatory risk factors is likely to predict greater risk for cognitive impairment than the independent influence of inflammation. In this regard, composite risk profiles assessed during mid-life may be of more predictive value than any single marker of risk. The presented findings suggest that further investigation is warranted to examine the contributions of metabolic and inflammatory factors in the prediction of cognitive risk.

The current findings have potential implications for the early detection and treatment of central adiposity and systemic inflammation. Although animal findings show that anti-inflammatory drugs can restore hippocampal neurogenesis in rats (Monje, Toda, and Palmer, 2003) and some epidemiologic evidence suggests that nonsteroidal anti-inflammatory drugs

(NSAIDS) may slow the progression of memory loss in patients with dementia (in t'Veld *et al.*, 2001) and decrease risk for AD (McGeer and McGeer, 1995), randomized clinical trials show no beneficial effect of NSAIDS in preventing cognitive decline in patients with dementia (Aisen *et al.*, 2003). It remains to be determined whether NSAIDS are beneficial if offered earlier in the disease process and/or at a younger age, such as mid-life, when peripheral levels of inflammatory markers increase and preclinical cognitive decline becomes evident. Initial evidence suggests that this may be the case, with a recent study showing that anti-inflammatory drug use protects against normal age-related declines in gray and white matter volume among cognitively normal older women (Walther *et al.*, 2011).

Given that adipose tissue is a key source of peripheral inflammatory mediators and higher BMI is associated with age-related cognitive declines, it is possible that interventions that reduce visceral fat mass will also protect cognitive function. To date, there is evidence that weight loss by dieting and exercise or by bariatric surgery is associated with reduced systemic inflammation, with lower circulating levels of IL-6 and CRP (Tziomalos *et al.*, 2010). However, it is unknown whether reductions in inflammation of this magnitude sufficiently convey protective effects in longitudinal cognitive decline.

There are a number of limitations of the current literature that warrant attention in future work. Many studies within this literature are cross-sectional, and debate continues regarding whether peripheral cytokine levels are the cause or consequence of brain inflammation (Licastro *et al.*, 2000). It is also possible that observed associations between peripheral cytokines, cognitive function, and brain structure are independently accounted for by a third, possibly genetic, factor. Another general limitation of the literature is the use of single assessments of inflammatory markers. Although evidence suggests that these markers are relatively stable over extended periods (e.g., Rao, Pieper, Currie, and Cohen, 1994), a more reliable indicator of chronic inflammation would be derived from multiple assessments over time. In the future, larger, longitudinal investigations are warranted beginning in early adulthood and employing serial assessments of low-grade systemic inflammation, cognitive function, and structural and functional brain images. In this work, it will be important to determine whether variation in inflammatory mediators among mid-life adults predicts cognitive decline and the onset of dementia. These studies will also need to examine the independent and combined contributions of closely related metabolic risk factors, such as central adiposity.

References

Aisen, P.S., Schafer, K.A., Grundman, M., Pfeiffer, E., Sano, M., Davis, K.L., et al. (2003). Effects of rofecoxib or naproxen vs placebo on Alzheimer disease progression: a randomized controlled trial. *Journal of the American Medical Association*, 289, 2819–2826.

Anstey, K.J., Cherbuin, N., Budge, M., and Young, J. (2011). Body mass index in midlife as a risk factor for dementia: A meta-analysis of prospective studies. *Obesity Reviews*, 12, 426–437.

Ashburner, J., and Friston, K.J. (2000). Voxel-based morphometry – the methods. *Neuroimage*, 11, 805–821.

Barbeger-Gateau, P., Fabrigoule, C., Helmer, C., Rouch, I., and Dartigues, J.F. (1999). Functional impairment in instrumental activities of daily living: an early clinical sign of dementia? *Journal of the American Geriatrics Society*, 47, 456–462.

Black, P.H., and Garbutt, L.D. (2002). Stress, inflammation, and cardiovascular disease. *Journal of Psychosomatic Research*, 52, 1–23.

Brydon, L., Walker, C., Wawrzyniak, A., Whitehead, D., Okamura, H., Yajima, J., et al. (2009). Synergistic effects of psychological and immune stressors on inflammatory cytokine and sickness responses in humans. *Brain, Behavior, and Immunity*, 23, 217–224.

Bucks, R.S., Gidron, Y., Harris, P., Teeling, J., Wesnes, K.A., and Perry, V.H. (2008). Selective effects of upper respiratory tract infection on cognition, mood and emotion processing: a prospective study. *Brain, Behavior, and Immunity*, 22, 399–407.

Capuron, L., and Miller, A.H. (2004). Cytokines and psychopathology: lessons learned from interferon-alpha. *Biological Psychiatry*, 56, 819–824.

Cournot, M., Marquié, J.C., Ansiau, D., Martinaud, C., Fonds, H., Ferrières, J., et al. (2006). Relation between body mass index and cognitive function in healthy middle-aged men and women. *Neurology*, 67, 1208–1214.

Craft, S. (2009). The role of metabolic disorders in Alzheimer disease and vascular dementia; two roads converged. *Archives of Neurology*, 66, 300–305.

Dahl, A., Hassing, L.B., Fransson, E., Berg, S., Gatz, M., Reynolds, C.A., et al. (2010). Being overweight in midlife is associated with lower cognitive ability and steeper cognitive decline in late life. *Journal of Gerontology: Biological Sciences*, 65, 57–62.

Dantzer, R. (2004). Cytokine-induced sickness behavior: a neuroimmune response to activation of innate immunity. *European Journal of Pharmacology*, 500, 399–411.

Dantzer, R., and Kelley, K.W. (2007). Twenty years of research on cytokine-induced sickness behavior. *Brain, Behavior, and Immunity*, 21, 153–160.

Dandona, P., Aljaada, A., Chaudhuri, A., Mohanty, P., and Garg, R. (2005). Metabolic syndrome: a comprehensive perspective based on interactions between obesity, diabetes, and inflammation. *Circulation*, 22, 1448–1454.

Dik, M.G., Jonker, C., Comijs, H.C., Deeg, D.J., Kok, A., Yaffe, K., et al. (2007). Contribution of metabolic syndrome components to cognition in older individuals. *Diabetes Care*, 30, 2655–2660.

Dik, M.G., Jonker, C., Hack, C.E., Smit, J.H., Comijs, H.C., and Eikelenboom, P. (2005). Serum inflammatory proteins and cognitive decline in older persons. *Neurology*, 64, 1371–1377.

Elias, M.F., Elias, P.K., Sullivan, L.M., Wolf, P.A., and D'Agostino, R.B. (2003). Lower cognitive function in the presence of obesity and hypertension: the Framingham heart study. *International Journal of Obesity and Related Metabolic Disorders: Journal of the International Association for the Study of Obesity*, 27, 260–268.

Elwood, P.C., Gallacher, J.E., Hopkinson, C.A., Pickering, J., Rabbitt, P., Stollery, B., et al. (1999). Smoking, drinking, and other life style factors and cognitive function in men in the Caerphilly cohort. *Journal of Epidemiology and Community Health*, 53, 9–14.

Engelhart, M.J., Geerlings, M.I., Meijer, J., Kiliaan, A., Ruitenberg, A., van Swieten, J.C., et al. (2004). Inflammatory proteins in plasma and the risk of dementia: the Rotterdam study. *Archives of Neurology*, 61, 668–672.

Fitzpatrick, A.L., Kuller, L.H., Lopez, O.L., Diehr, P., O'Meara, E.S., Longstreth, W.T., et al. (2009). Midlife and late-life obesity and the risk of dementia. *Archives of Neurology*, 66, 336–342.

Ford, E.S., Giles, W.H., and Mokdad, A.H. (2004). Increasing prevalence of the metabolic syndrome among US adults. *Diabetes Care*, 27, 2444–2449.

Frank, M.G., Baratta, M.V., Sprunger, D.B., Watkins, L.R., and Maier, S.F. (2006). Microglia serve as a neuroimmune substrate for stress-induced potentiation of CNS pro-inflammatory cytokine responses. *Brain, Behavior, and Immunity*, 21, 47–59.

Gadient, R.A., and Otten, U. (1994). Expression of interleukin-6 (IL-6) and interleukin-6 and interleukin-6 receptor (IL-6R) mRNA in rat brain during postnatal development. *Brain Research*, 637, 10–14.

Golden, J.C. (1978). *Stroop color and word test*. Chicago, IL: Stoelting.

Grundy, S.M., Brewer, B., Cleeman, J.I., Smith, S.C., and Lenfant, C. (2004). Definition of metabolic syndrome. *Circulation*, 109, 433–438.

Gustafson, D., Lissner, L., Bengtsson, C., Bjorkelund, C., and Skoog, I. (2004). A 24-year follow-up of body mass index and cerebral atrophy. *Neurology*, 63, 1876–1881.

Heyser, C.J., Masliah, E., Samimi, A., Campbell, I.L., and Gold, L.H. (1997). Progressive decline in avoidance learning paralleled by inflammatory neurodegeneration in transgenic mice expressing interleukin 6 in the brain. *Proceedings of the National Academy of Sciences of the United States of America*, 94, 1500–1505.

Holmes, C., Cunningham, C., Zotova, E., Woolford, J., Dean, C., Kerr, S., et al. (2009). Systemic inflammation and disease progression in Alzheimer disease. *Neurology*, 73, 768–774.

in 't Veld, B.A., Ruitenberg, A., Hofman, A., Launer, L.J., van Duijn, C.M., Stijnen, T., et al. (2001). Nonsteroidal antiinflammatory drugs and the risk of Alzheimer's disease. *New England Journal of Medicine*, 345, 1515–1521.

Jack, C.R., Jr., Petersen, R.C., Xu, Y., O'Brien, P.C., Smith, G.E., Ivnik, R.J., et al. (2000). Rates of hippocampal atrophy correlate with change in clinical status in aging and AD. *Neurology*, 55, 484–489.

Khaodhiar, L., Ling, P.R., Blackburn, G.L., and Bistrian, B.R. (2004). Serum levels of interleukin-6 and C-reactive protein correlate with body mass index across the broad range of obesity. *Journal of Parenteral and Enteral Nutrition*, 28, 410–415.

Kivipelto, M., Ngandu, T., Laatikainen, T., Winblad, B., Soininen, H., and Tuomilehto, J. (2006). Risk score for the prediction of dementia risk in 20 years among middle aged people: a longitudinal, population-based study. *Lancet Neurology*, 5, 735–741.

Kozora, E., Laudenslager, M., Lemieux, A., and West, S.G. (2001). Inflammatory and hormonal measures predict neuropsychological functioning in systemic lupus erythematosus and rheumatoid arthritis patients. *Journal of the International Neuropsychological Society*, 7, 745–754.

Krabbe, K.S., Reichenberg, A., Yirmiya, R., Smed, A., Pedersen, B.K., and Bruunsgaard, H. (2005). Low dose endotoxemia and human neuropsychological functions. *Brain, Behavior, and Immunity*, 19, 453–460.

Lee, Y.H., and Pratley, R.E. (2005). The evolving role of inflammation in obesity and the metabolic syndrome. *Current Diabetes Reports*, 5, 70–75.

Licastro, F., Pedrini, S., Caputo, L., Annoni, G., Davis, L.J., Ferri, C., et al. (2000). Increased plasma levels of interleukin-1, interleukin-6 and alpha-1-antichymotrypsin in patients with Alzheimer's disease: peripheral inflammation or signals from the brain? *Journal of Neuroimmunology*, 103, 97–102.

Maggio, M., Guralnik, J.M., Longo, D.L., and Ferrucci, L. (2006). Interleukin-6 in aging and chronic disease: a magnificent pathway. *Gerontology Series A-Biological Sciences and Medical Sciences*, 61, 575–584.

Marsland, A.L., Gianaros, P.J., Abramowitch, S.M., Manuck, S.B., and Hariri, A.R. (2008). Interleukin-6 covaries inversely with hippocampal grey matter volume in middle-aged adults. *Biological Psychiatry*, 64, 484–490.

Marsland, A.L., McCaffery, J.M., Muldoon, M.F., and Manuck, S.B. (2010). Systemic inflammation and the metabolic syndrome among middle-aged community volunteers. *Metabolism*, 59, 1801–1808.

Marsland, A.L., Petersen, K.L., Sathanoori, R., Muldoon, M.F., Neumann, S.A., Ryan, C., et al. (2006). Interleukin-6 covaries inversely with cognitive performance among middle-aged community volunteers. *Psychomatic Medicine*, 68, 895–903.

Mattay, V.S., Fera, F., Tessitore, A., Hariri, A.R., Berman, K.F., Das, S., et al. (2006). Neurophysiological correlates of age-related changes in working memory capacity. *Neuroscience Letters*, 392, 32–37.

McAfoose, J., and Baune, B.T. (2009). Evidence for a cytokine model of cognitive function. *Neuroscience and Biobehavioral Reviews*, 33, 355–366.

McGeer, P.L., and McGeer, E.G. (1995). The inflammatory response system of brain: implications for therapy of Alzheimer and other neurodegenerative diseases. *Brain Research Reviews*, 21, 195–218.

Mohamed-Ali, V., Goodrick, S., Rawesh, A., Katz, D.R., Miles, J.M., Yudkin, J.S., et al. (1997). Subcutaneous adipose tissue releases interleukin-6, but not tumor necrosis factor-alpha, in vivo. *Journal of Clinical Endocrinology and Metabolism*, 82, 4196–4200.

Monje, M.L., Toda, H., and Palmer, T. D. (2003). Inflammatory blockade restores adult hippocampal neurogenesis. *Science*, 302, 1760–1765.

Park, H.S., Park. J.Y., and Yu, R. (2004). Relationship of obesity and visceral adiposity with serum concentrations of CRP, TNF-α and IL-6. *Diabetes Research and Clinical Practice*, 69, 29–35.

Pavol, M.A., Meyers, C.A., Rexer, J.L., Valentine, A.D., Mattis, P.J., and Talpaz, M. (1995). Pattern of neurobehavioral deficits associated with interferon alpha therapy for leukemia. *Neurology*, 45, 947–950.

Perry, V.H., Cunningham, C., and Holmes, C. (2007). Systemic infections and inflammation affect chronic neurodegeneration. *Nature Reviews. Immunology*, 7, 161–167.

Poluektova, L., Meyer, V., Walters, L., Paez, X., and Gendelman, H.E. (2005). Macrophage-induced inflammation affects hippocampal plasticity and neuronal development in a murine model of HIV-1 encephalitis. *Glia*, 52, 344–353.

Pugh, C.R., Kumagawa, K., Fleshner, M., Watkins, L.R., Maier, S.F., and Rudy, J.W. (1998). Selective effects of peripheral lipopolysaccharide administration on contextual and auditory-cue fear conditioning. *Brain, Behavior, and Immunity*, 12, 212–229.

Rao, K.M., Pieper, C.S., Currie, M.S., and Cohen, H.J. (1994). Variability of plasma IL-6 and crosslinked fibrin dimers over time in community dwelling elderly subjects. *American Journal of Clinical Pathology*, 102, 802–805.

Reichenberg, A., Yirmiya, R., Schuld, A., Kraus, T., Haack, M., Morag, A., et al. (2001). Cytokine-associated emotional and cognitive disturbances in humans. *Archives of General Psychiatry*, 58, 445–452.

Reitan, R.M., and Wolfson, D. (1985). *The Halstead-Reitan Neuropsychological Test Battery*. Tucson, AZ: Neuropsychology Press.

Richwine, A.F., Godbout, J.P., Berg, B.M., Chen, J., Escobar, J., Millard, D.K., et al. (2005). Improved psychomotor performance in aged mice fed diet high in antioxidants is associated with reduced ex vivo brain interleukin-6 production. *Brain, Behavior, and Immunity*, 19, 512–520.

Roberts, R.O., Geda, Y.E., Knopman, D.S., Cha, R.H., Boeve, B.F., Ivnik, R.J., et al. (2010). Metabolic syndrome, inflammation, and nonamnestic mild cognitive impairment in older persons. *Alzheimer Disease and Associated Disorder*, 24, 11–18.

Rosczyk, H.A., Sparkman, N.L., and Johson, R.W. (2008). Neuroinflammation and cognitive function in aged mice following minor surgery. *Experimental Gerontology*, 43, 840–846.

Ross, F.M., Allan, S.M., Rothwell, N.J., and Verkhratsky, A. (2003). A dual role for interleukin-1 in LTP in mouse hippocampal slices. *Journal of Neuroimmunology*, 144, 61–67.

Salthouse, T.A. (2004). What and when of cognitive aging. *Current Directions in Psychological Science*, 13, 140–144.

Schmidt, R., Schmidt, H., Curb, J.D., Masaki, K., White, L.R., and Launer, L.J. (2002). Early inflammation and dementia: a 24-year follow-up of the Honolulu-Asia Aging Study. *Annuls of Neurology*, 52, 168–174.

Schram, M.T., Euser, S.M., de Craen, A.J., Witteman, J.C., Frölich, M., Hofman, A., et al. (2007). Systemic markers of inflammation and cognitive decline in old age. *Journal of the American Geriatrics Society*, 55, 708–716.

Smith, A.D., Tyrrell, D., Coyle, K., and Higgins, P. (1998). Effects of interferon alpha on performance in man: a preliminary report. *Psychopharmacology*, 96, 414–416.

Spath-Schwalbe, E., Hansen, K., Schmidt, F., Schrezenmeier, H., Marshall, L., Burger, K., et al. (1998). Acute effects of recombinant human interleukin-6 on endocrine and central nervous sleep functions in healthy men. *Journal of Clinical Endocrinology and Metabolism*, 83, 1573–1579.

Teunissen, C.E., van Boxtel, M.P.J., Bosma, H., Bosmans, H., Delanghe, J. De Bruijn, C., et al. (2003). Inflammation markers in relation to cognition in a healthy aging population. *Journal of Neuroimmunology*, 134, 142–150.

Tilvis, R.S., Kahonen-Vare, M.H., Jolkkonen, J., Valvanne, J., Pitkala, K.H., and Strandberg, T.E. (2004). Predictors of cognitive decline and mortality of aged people over a 10-year period. *Journals of Gerontology Series A. Biological Sciences and Medical Sciences*, 59, 268–274.

Tisserand, D.J., and Jolles, J. (2003). On the involvement of prefrontal networks in cognitive ageing. *Cortex*, 39, 1107f–1128.

Tziomalos, K., Dimitroula, H.V., Katsiki, N., Savopoulos, C., and Hatzitolios, A.I. (2010). Effects of lifestyle measures, antiobesity agents, and bariatric surgery on serological markers of inflammation in obese patients. *Mediators of Inflammation*, 2010, 364–357.

Van Petten, C. (2004). Relationship between hippocampal volume and memory ability in healthy individuals across the lifespan: review and meta-analysis. *Neuropsychologia*, 42, 1394–1413.

Wagner, A.D., Schacter, D.L., Rotte, M., Koutstaal, W., Maril, A., Dale, A.M., et al. (1998). Building memories: remembering and forgetting of verbal experiences as predicted by brain activity. *Science*, 281, 1188–1191.

Walther, K., Bendlin, B.B., Glisky, E.L., Trouard, T.P., Lisse, J.R., Posever, J.O., et al. (2011). Anti-inflammatory drugs reduce age-related decreases in brain volume in cognitively normal older adults. *Neurobiology of Aging*, 32, 495–505.

Weaver, J.D., Huang, M.H., Albert, M., Harris, T., Rowe, J.W., and Seeman, T.E (2002). Interleukin-6 and risk of cognitive decline: MacArthur Studies of Successful Aging. *Neurology*, 59, 371–378.

Whitmer, R.A., Gunderson, E.P., Barrett-Connor, E., Quesenberry, C.P., and Yaffe, K. (2005). Obesity in middle age and future risk of dementia: a 27 year longitudinal population based study. *British Medical Journal*, 330, 1360–1362.

Whitmer, R.A., Gustafson, D.R., Barrett-Connor, E., Haan, M.N., Gunderson, E.P., and Yaffe, K. (2008). Central obesity and increased risk of dementia more than three decades later. *Neurology*, 71, 1057–1064.

Yaffe, K. (2007). Metabolic syndrome and cognitive disorders: is the sum greater than its parts? *Alzheimer Disease and Associated Disorders*, 21, 167–171.

Yaffe, K., Kanaya, A., Lindquist, K., Simonsick, E.M., Harris, T., Shorr, R.I., et al. (2004). The metabolic syndrome, inflammation, and risk of cognitive decline. *Journal of the American Medical Association*, 292, 2237–2242.

Yaffe, K., Lindquist, K., Penninx, B.W., Simonsick, E.M., Pahor, M., Kritchevsky, S., et al. (2003). Inflammatory markers and cognition in well-functioning African-American and white elders. *Neurology*, 61, 76–80.

Yirmiya, R., and Goshen, I. (2011). Immune modulation of learning, memory, neural plasticity and neurogenesis. *Brain, Behavior, and Immunity*, 25, 181–213.

Zuliani, G., Ranzini, M., Guerra, G., Rossi, L., Munari, M.R., Zurlo, A., et al. (2007). Plasma cytokines profile in older subjects with late onset alzheimer's disease or vascular dementia. *Journal of Psychiatric Research*, 41, 686–693.

18

Immune Stimulation and Cognitive Function

Defining the Deficits and Avoiding the Pitfalls

Colm Cunningham

Trinity College Institute of Neuroscience and School of Biochemistry and Immunology, Trinity College Dublin, Dublin, Ireland

Introduction

It is now very well accepted that immune stimulation such as that occurring during infection leads to a constellation of CNS effects. Though many of these effects have in the past been dismissed as mere unpleasant side-effects of the immune system's battle to fight infection, they are now recognized to represent part of the organisms coordinated strategy to return the system to homeostasis as rapidly as possible. Thus, the sick animal reorganizes its priorities by minimizing energy expenditure and maximizing rest, in favor of mounting a fever response, mobilizing immune cell repertoires and clearing infection.

This reimagining of the sickness behavior response (Hart, 1988) rehabilitated this unpleasant syndrome as an evolutionarily conserved response that is advantageous and indeed necessary for the survival of the sick or injured individual. That is to say, the sickness behavior response is adaptive. The sick or injured animal will typically become hypoactive, will decrease its tendency to socially interact, will show suppression of appetite and often display taste aversion for substances that it may associate temporally with the onset of sickness, and this also leads to anorexia/weight loss. In addition there is an acute induction of the stress response, mediated by the hypothalamic–pituitary–adrenal axis (HPA), and a decreased motivation to engage in activities that were previously pleasurable to the individual (anhedonia). These depressive-like changes are consistent with the idea that the individual might want to minimize its exposure to further risks such as predation, consumption of food that may have contributed to its current sickness and indeed to limit its interaction with others in the "herd" to minimize the spread of infection. It is rather less intuitive that an inability to learn or to remember would be a normal component of this adaptive sickness behavior response. However, impairments in learning and memory have frequently been reported in animals experiencing acute sickness and these cognitive deficits are widely accepted as a part of the sickness behavior response. However, the very changes of behavior that define the sickness behavior response also interfere

The Wiley-Blackwell Handbook of Psychoneuroimmunology, First Edition. Edited by Alexander W. Kusnecov and Hymie Anisman.

in a very significant way in the processes that we exploit to assess the cognitive performance of rodents. Therefore good experimental design is essential if we are to avoid mistaking emotional, motivational, locomotor, or stress axis changes for cognitive impairments in these experiments. To state with confidence that a manipulation has interfered with learning or memory, it is essential to rule out the possibility that the observed changes could equally be explained by a change in motivation, locomotor speed, reward seeking, or stress and anxiety responses. These possibilities have often not been controlled for in studies of cognitive effects of immune stimulation, largely because the cognitive paradigms arising from the field of experimental psychology were simply not designed with a view to assessing animals experiencing sickness behavior.

In this chapter I will discuss studies of cognitive impairment during immune stimulation, dissect some of the confounding factors that may have affected interpretation of data arising from these studies, attempt to summarize what we can and can say with confidence and, finally, propose some useful ground rules for performing these types of studies while avoiding the major pitfalls. The entire literature on this subject cannot be covered in the format required for this chapter and thus we will take the approach of using a small number of "case studies" consisting of groups of two or three papers that have been influential in the field, some that are useful examples of where difficulties can arise and others that have gone to some lengths to avoid the confounding factors referred to above. A very substantial review of the interaction of immune system function with cognitive function and brain plasticity has recently been published (Yirmiya and Goshen, 2011) and we have previously published a detailed critical dissection of the impact of bacterial endotoxin (LPS) and the pro-inflammatory cytokine interleukin-1β (IL-1β) on aspects of cognitive function (Cunningham and Sanderson, 2008).These reviews are recommended for more fully referenced discussions of the studies and issues raised here.

Case 1: When Sweet Turns Sour: The Problems of Appetitive Tasks

In one of the earliest studies of LPS and IL-1β altering cognitive function (Aubert, Vega, Dantzer, and Goodall, 1995) rats were placed in an operant box in which a lever was presented. Pressing of this lever would lead to its retraction and the presentation of a food reward two seconds later. In the absence of the lever being pressed, retraction of the lever occurred and food reward was presented in any case, but only after 15 seconds. Animals quickly learn to press the lever and their latency to do so indicates how quickly they learn the association between lever-pressing and food reward. When animals were challenged with LPS (250 μg/kg), directly after a single training session in this task, latency to press the lever remained considerably higher than control-treated animals for 12 days. In further experiments, in the same study, IL-1β increased latency in a similar way, this time for a period of 4 days. The authors concluded that LPS-treated animals failed to make an association between the lever and food reward because LPS had interfered with their associative learning, while those treated with IL-1β were also impaired but eventually formed an association after 4 days. However, it is well known that animals develop taste aversion to normally palatable foods when these are paired with an aversive stimulus such as IL-1β (Tazi, Dantzer, Crestani, and Le Moal, 1988). In this case, the pairing of the lever press-induced reward of condensed milk with the context (the operant box) was apparently not consolidated, but this is most likely to be because these animals instead associated the operant box and the food reward with the sickness they experienced soon after they consumed the food rewards from this box. The consequence of making this association would be that the animals continue to avoid lever pressing since the food "reward" actually has a significant association with sickness. The most compelling evidence that taste aversion rather than failure to learn is the correct interpretation lies in the fact that animals never shorten their latency across the entire 12-day experiment even though LPS effects would have subsided by 24 hours. That is to say, if LPS affected learning, then by day 2, or day 3 at the latest, they would then have begun to make this association. Though the authors' conclusion was that there was a failure to learn, rather it is highly likely that they did learn: they made a very strong association between the food reward and sickness and thus the latency remained high until the end of the experiment. Since the IL-1β treatment would be less aversive than the LPS treatment the association between this and the sickness is probably eventually overcome (i.e., in 4 days) by the palatable food reward.

Our own experience of food-rewarded tasks during sickness is interesting for similar reasons. We trained animals on a T-maze alternation task in which animals initially visited the only open arm of a T-maze and consumed a reward of sweetened condensed milk there. They were then replaced in the maze, with both arms available, and had to alternate their performance (i.e. choose the arm they had not visited the first time) in order to receive another food reward. Alternation demonstrates good working-memory performance, since the animal must remember where it has just visited in order to guide where it will next visit. We trained animals to good, and stable, performance (80–90% alternation) on this task and then challenged them with LPS (100-200 μg/kg) 3 hours before testing them for 10 trials on this task. At 3 hours post-LPS the animals had begun to experience acute sickness. However, having successfully consumed this sweetened condensed milk for 7 days of training, as well as prior consumption in their home cages, the mice actually continued to alternate their performance and even consumed some of the milk. Their working memory remained intact at 80–90%. Thus, LPS did not affect their working memory, and we later verified this with a water-motivated working-memory task (Murray *et al.*, 2012). What was striking was that on the following day, after sickness had subsided, when they were replaced in the maze these animals now showed a profound aversion to the milk. That is to say, they either did not move at all in the maze, or they alternated but did not approach the condensed milk at any point (Cunningham, unpublished data). Thus if food "rewards" are paired with aversive stimuli such as LPS, then these stimuli become associated with the sickness and rapidly change from having rewarding to aversive associations for the animal. It thus becomes obvious that we have to interpret the findings of such experiments accordingly. In the case of Aubert *et al.*, my conclusion would be that LPS did not impair their learning. Instead they learned that when they consume the food they become sick, so the appropriate response, for survival, is to avoid the food reward, which is exactly what they did. Given this very serious confound, it seems unwise to assess inflammation-induced effects on cognitive function using food-rewarded tasks.

Avoiding the pitfalls

- Food-rewarded tasks are inherently ill-suited to the investigation of effects of immune stimulation on learning and memory.

Case 2: Malaise in the Water Maze: Locomotor Speed, Motivation and Stress

Many studies of inflammatory effects on learning and memory have been carried out in the Morris Water Maze, which was first developed in 1982 (Morris, Garrud, Rawlins, and O'Keefe, 1982), to demonstrate that the hippocampus had a role in visuospatial learning and memory. In this task one assesses animals' ability to use visuospatial cues to locate, and swim to, a platform hidden 1 cm below the surface of the water in a circular water-filled tank. The most commonly quoted parameter is the *latency*, or time taken to find the platform, although in most animals this is correlated very closely with the distance travelled to find the platform. Based on the latency of responses, several investigators reported learning and memory impairments after infection or inflammation. However, when this maze is used to assess learning in animals experiencing sickness there are a number of additional measures that must be made in order to avoid confounding factors, such as decreased swimming speed, decreased motivation, and alternative stress-induced swimming patterns. Therefore, one also needs to assess, using video-tracking, the *distance travelled* and the *route taken* to find the platform. Finally, after all of the training blocks have been completed, or at some predetermined intermediate time, one can perform a *probe trial* in order to assess whether the animal can use the visuospatial cues in the room to assess where the platform should be. In a probe trial, the hidden platform is actually removed and one measures the amount of time the animal swims proximal to where the platform had been during training. These data are usually presented as time spent in each of the four quadrants of the circular maze.

Thus latency, distance travelled, route taken and proportion of time in the correct quadrant in a probe trial are all necessary parameters to judge with confidence whether a treated animal can find the hidden platform, whether it does so differently to control animals and whether it uses visuospatial cues or uses some other strategy to achieve this. A number of studies of learning and memory after immune stimulation have assessed less than this full complement of parameters and, as a result, have left some lingering uncertainty about precisely what sort of effect was measured. It is important to realize that in raising these possibilities, I do not necessarily imply that conclusions of those papers are not correct, but that in some cases they have been insufficiently tested and controlled for and therefore *might not* be correct. More importantly, the aim is to point out that in future studies, we should avoid the same pitfalls.

One of the earliest and most often cited studies in this field showed that IL-1β (100 ng/mouse i.p.) or a suspension containing *Legionella pneumophila* (8×10^6 bacteria/mouse i.p.) both induced longer latencies to find the hidden platform in the MWM (Gibertini, Newton, Friedman, and Klein, 1995). Animals were given three blocks of three trials on each of two consecutive days and those given IL-1β were treated on both days, while the *Legionella* suspension was administered only once but infection persisted throughout the two days of testing. The treated animals showed considerably longer latencies to find the platform on day 2 with respect to controls, suggesting impaired learning of the location of the platform. These data look quite robust, but given the sickness that IL-1β animals, and particularly the *Legionella pneumophila* animals, would be experiencing it would be important to see whether swim speed, distance travelled and route travelled also show marked differences. The importance of this is emphasized by follow up studies from the same authors (Gibertini, 1998) in which a number of interesting features were revealed. Firstly, they found that IL-1β treatment affected latency to find the platform only when the water was at 23 °C (as it was in their 1995 study). When the water temperature was lowered to 18 °C, the mice were perfectly capable of finding the platform at the same rate as the vehicle-treated animals. This indicates that motivation to solve the maze is the major component that dictates the strategy of the mouse when placed in the maze and makes clear that IL-1β-treated mice can learn equally well in this maze if they have the motivation to do so. Secondly, the authors found an apparent dissociation between performance during training and in the probe trial: the training phase indicated clear learning but the probe trial indicated that mice spent equal times in all quadrants, which is consistent with a failure to learn. But this apparent failure is also very informative: the video-tracking data showed evidence of a thigmotaxic strategy in the sick animals. Thigmotaxis is the tendency for an animal to remain near to the wall of mazes and is a well-described rodent response to anxiogenic situations (Simon, Dupuis, and Costentin, 1994). Being placed in a brightly lit, novel, open field that is filled with water is undoubtedly one such anxiogenic situation: swimming is stressful for mice and they will often avoid the anxiogenic center of an open area, even in dry mazes. Thus, it is clear, that in a pool of 1m diameter, with a platform 10–15 cm from the wall, that an animal could find the platform without ever crossing the center of the maze and in doing so could significantly decrease its stress levels. Thus in the example above, the mice have learned to solve the maze, as seen by decreasing latency, but have learned to do so without using the visuospatial cues in the room, but rather have learned to swim close to the wall until they find the platform, and this is consistent with the probe trial strategy of spending equal time in each quadrant. Thirdly, the authors also reported that IL-1β at higher doses (1000 ng/mouse) actually facilitated learning in the MWM. As we will see later, many divergent effects of immune stimulation have been explained by a putative U-shaped curve, but this usually predicts that cytokines such as IL-1 are necessary at low doses to facilitate learning but are disruptive at high doses. This Gibertini study shows that at 100 ng/mouse (with appropriate motivation – water at 18 °C) IL-1β does not affect learning and at 1000 ng/mouse it facilitates more rapid learning. Remarkably, this informative 1998 Gibertini study is cited at only one-third of the frequency of the 1995 study.

This example is used to make the point that if we do not provide sufficient motivation then the sick rodent may appear to show learning impairments when in fact it is merely less motivated to solve the maze. In addition it shows us that a stressed mouse may find an alternative strategy to solve the maze, and if we do not assess the full range of parameters (i.e. distance and route travelled *as well as* latency) then we may fail to observe these features and make incorrect conclusions. Since this Gibertini study was published there have been further studies that have reported thigmotaxis (Song *et al.*, 2004; Sparkman *et al.*, 2005b) and others that show increased latency even to a visible platform (Sparkman *et al.*, 2005a), but many studies continue to rely on latency as the main measure. The tendency towards thigmotaxis means that even latency, distance travelled and swim speed combined may be insufficient to distinguish between a genuine learning impairment and an alternative stress-minimizing strategy. Other groups have also used latency to a visible platform as an additional control to show that when they can see the platform sick animals can reach it as quickly as control animals. Comparable performance to controls on this measure means that even sick mice are prepared to cross the center of the maze when the target is visible, but it does not address the possibility that when it is not visible the mouse might initially take a less anxiogenic route and once this is found to work, the animal is likely to persist with it. All of which to say, all of these controls add to the confidence in the result, but the route taken remains a necessary control to inform the strategy the animals used to find the platform. Having read the MWM literature in detail we have not found evidence for latency, distance, route travelled and probe trials all being impaired in animals treated with LPS or IL-1β (see Table 18.1).

Table 18.1 Summary of Studies of Spatial Reference Memory in the Morris Water Maze after Treatment with LPS, Bacteria, or IL-1β

Reference	*Species*	*Treatment*	*Dose*	*Route of admin*	*Timing (before testing)*	*Latency to find platform*	*Distance (path length)*	*Route taken*	*Probe or retention (r) trial*
Oitzl (1993)	Rat	IL-1β	100 ng	i.c.v.	60 min	↑(day 2, trial 1)	N.D.	N.D.	N.D.
	Rat	IL-6	100 ng	i.c.v.	60 min	No effect	N.D.	N.D.	N.D.
	Rat	IL-1β	100 ng	i.c.v.	0 min	No effect	N.D.	N.D.	N.D.
Gibertini(1995)	Mouse	Legionella	8×10^6	i.p.	24 hours	↑	↑	N.D.	No+ preference
	Mouse	IL-1β	100 ng	i.p.	2 hours	↑	No effect	N.D.	N.D.
Gibertini (1998) spaced protocol	Mouse	IL-1β	100 ng	i.p.	2 hours	N.D.	No effect	↑ Thigmotaxis	No preference
	Mouse	IL-1β	1000 ng	i.p.	2 hours	N.D.	↓	N.D.	N.D.
massed protocol	Mouse	IL-1β	100 ng	i.p.	2 hours	23 °C ↑ 18 °C No effect	N.D.	N.D.	N.D.
Arai (2001)	Mouse	LPS	400–800 μg/kg	i.p.	6 hours	↑	N.D.	N.D.	No* impairment
Shaw (2001) Fixed start location	Rat	LPS	100μg/kg	i.p.	4 hours	No effect	↓ (day 1–3)	Path analyses suggest deficit	No^ difference
Yirmiya (2002)	Rat	IL-1β	10 ng	i.c.v.	Immediately after training	No effect	N.D.	N.D.	N.D.
	Rat	IL-1 ra	100 ng	i.c.v.	Immediately after training	↑	N.D.	N.D.	N.D.
Song (2004)	Rat	IL-1β	15 ng	i.c.v.	Immediately after training	↑	N.D.	↑ Thigmotaxis	No preference
Sparkman (2005a)	Mouse	LPS	250 μg/kg	i.p.	4 hours	↑	No effect d1 Modest ↑d3	N.D	No **(r)** impairment
Sparkman (2005b)	Mouse	LPS	250 μg/kg	i.p.	4 hours	↑	No effect	Thigmotaxis shown	No **(r)** impairment
Thomson (2006)	Rat	IL-1β	2 μg/kg	i.p.	1 and 24 hours	No effect	N.D.	N.D.	No impairment

All data refer to hidden platform versions of the MWM and all papers are fully referenced and discussed in Cunningham and Sanderson, 2008. N.D.: not determined in this study. No effect: LPS/IL-1β did not impair animals on this measure. Arrows indicate increase (↑) or decrease (↓). In probe trials (in which the hidden platform has been removed): + no preference (the data is shown, or described in text, and animals spend only 25% of distance travelled in target quadrant). * no impairment (the data is shown and treated animals show a clear preference for the target quadrant). ^ no difference – the limited probe data shows no difference between treated and control groups. Probe trials have been performed at variable times post-training as discussed in the text. Retention trials **(r)** are performed, like probe trials, at the end of training but retain the hidden platform.

Table adapted from Cunningham and Sanderson (2008) *Brain, Behavior and Immunity*, courtesy of Elsevier.

Avoiding the pitfalls

- Latency, distance travelled, route travelled and % time spent in all four quadrants are necessary parameters if we are to distinguish cognitive impairment from motivational, locomotor or stress-minimizing strategies in the Morris Water Maze.

Case 3 Do It Again: Hypersensitivity, Tolerance and State-Dependent Learning

Another highly cited study of LPS effects on learning was performed with an unusual experimental design (Shaw, Commins, and O'Mara, 2001). These authors challenged rats with LPS once or on each of five consecutive days and examined their learning in the MWM. This study is remarkable for two reasons:

1. A little prior knowledge of inflammation biology tells us that the biological response to LPS is probably different on each successive day of treatment. We know that there are both hypersensitive and hyposensitive or tolerant responses to systemic LPS after prior exposure, and these depend on the time-interval between first and successive changes (Greer and Rietschel, 1978). If one wants to examine what effect a treatment has on learning and memory it is obviously preferable that this treatment has a stable and constant effect across the period examined.
2. Despite the considerable dosing with LPS, the animals show remarkably efficient learning, which is barely different to vehicle-treated animals at any point. LPS-treated animals showed equivalent, or perhaps even better learning than controls on day one, equivalent memory of this on day two and continued on a similar trajectory of learning across the five days. A difference in latency is reported on the fourth day after a single challenge with LPS, but this is not matched by a difference in distance travelled at the same time point so it is difficult to be convinced that there is a learning deficit that has been induced by LPS. Interestingly, the daily LPS-treated group do not show this latency difference at 4 days, which raises the issue of state-dependent differences. State-dependent learning will be discussed further below.

The unusual strategy of testing learning with five consecutive days of LPS treatment would not merit special mention had it not been adopted by successive research groups, such that the 5 × LPS strategy appears several times in the literature. Another MWM study with five daily LPS challenges versus a single LPS treatment demonstrated the principle of early hypersensitivity followed by tolerance, in that swim speeds were significantly lower on the second day of LPS treatment than on the first, and these confounded measurements of latency to find the platform: the authors showed that the daily LPS group were also slower to find a visible platform (Sparkman *et al.*, 2005a) demonstrating a locomotor rather than a learning deficit. If anything, what these studies really demonstrate is that the Morris Water Maze is not very appropriate for assessing the impact of acute inflammation on learning and memory because most protocols for the MWM require consecutive days of testing in order to achieve clear learning and memory. Since the temporal window of immune activation with LPS treatment at moderate doses is from 1 hour to approximately 8 hours, tests where the entire process of learning can be achieved during this period and the memory of what has been learned can also be tested in this period would be ideal (as well as testing recall at some later time after sickness has passed).

An interesting feature of both the Shaw and Sparkman studies is that LPS had no impact on the first day's learning nor on the second day's retrieval of this memory and further improvement of performance. However, both showed some indication of later divergence between controls and LPS, albeit mild. One can only speculate as to why a late deficit might occur, but one possible explanation is that there is some "state-dependent" learning occurring in the early days, during peak sickness. Typically a number of contextual stimuli may constitute relevant cues during a learning experience. Contextual stimuli are typically external but the internal state of the animal may also be a contextual cue. Therefore, learning episodes may be "state-dependent" in that internal state cues may also form part of the association with the outcome. In the current discussion, the feeling of sickness may form part of the context or "state" in which learning occurred. The context in which learning occurs plays a key role in the subsequent retrieval of memories. One well-known example of this is with learning that occurs during alcohol intoxication. It is known that subsequent retrieval is poor if tested when sober, but this impairment is not apparent if the subject is once again intoxicated (Goodwin *et al.*, 1969). Thus, the absence of the internal "state" of sickness during re-testing may influence the ability of the individual to remember what was learned while feeling sick. Therefore, in an ideal testing design the manipulation of interest (sickness) must be present at both the training and the test of learning to ensure that changes in the state cannot be used to explain any observed effects on learning. In order to understand how inflammation may interfere with memory function it is important that we can delineate, even in a case where immune stimulation may have had an amnesic effect, whether the this reflects a failure to retrieve memory due to the state-dependency of that memory (Miller and Springer, 1973) or a failure to encode a memory in the first place. Even though this presents difficulties for experimental design, it is possible to confirm or refute this possibility with one additional experiment: testing in the presence of the same sickness as that present when learning took place. In the Shaw and Sparkman studies described above, the animals that have emerged from sickness show a slight impairment on day 4 (Shaw) or day 3 (Sparkman), which is absent on the following day, while those who receive LPS every day never show differences from saline-treated animals.

One study in which "state-dependent effects" offer a possible interpretation of the findings is in one of the earliest studies in this area (Oitzl, Van Oers, Schobitz, and De Kloet, 1993). In this study the authors injected rats with IL-1β (100 ng i.c.v.) and placed them in the MWM for three trials on each of two days. On the first day, in which the animals experienced the acute effects of IL-1β, there was no difference in latency between IL-1β and vehicle-treated animals. However on day 2, on the first trial, animals who had been treated with IL-1β the previous day showed clearly longer latencies to find the platform. On the second trial of the second day, their performance was equivalent to, or slightly better than, controls. This may be explained by a failure to remember what had been apparently learned on the first day. However, the rapid improvement on trial 2 on the second day suggested that they had not failed to encode the previous day's information. It is possible that the subjective feelings caused by IL-1β formed part of the context of learning on day one and in its absence, on day 2, the task was somewhat different, but upon recognition that this was indeed the same maze, but performed under different internal "state" the previous day's learning was rapidly expressed. We cannot state that the findings of Oitzl and colleagues are the result of state-dependent learning. However, neither can we state that they are not. It is possible that those animals that successfully learned in the presence of LPS were, for the duration of the first trial on the second day, confused in its absence. But if this is to be ruled out, it needs to be tested. Notwithstanding what we have previously said about multiple challenges with immune stimulants, it would be of interest to know whether another group, treated with IL-1β i.c.v also on the second day would have been impaired compared to controls.

Avoiding the pitfalls

- State-dependence of observed deficits should be tested in each new task, which may necessitate a second challenge with the same stimulus. However, repeated challenges with immune stimuli will produce altered inflammatory responses and these need to be characterized if they are to be used.

Case 4 : It's Been Emotional: Aversive Tasks and Non-monotonic Dose Relationships

One task that has been widely used in the assessment of immune effects on learning and memory has been contextual fear-conditioning (CFC). The first of these studies (Pugh *et al.*, 1998) showed that LPS impaired consolidation of memory for context. In this task, as used in the Pugh study, juvenile rats were placed in a box (context A) which they explored. While in this context they received two mild electric shocks (the unconditioned stimulus), paired with a tone (the conditioned stimulus). Immediately on removal the animals were challenged i.p with LPS (0.125 mg/kg or 0.5 mg/kg). 24 hours later the animals were replaced in context A and their memory of this context (and the shock they received there) can be assessed by examining the amount of time the animal spends "freezing" (the conditioned response): a learned stress response as opposed to a simple lack of movement. In addition the animal was then placed in context B, which was distinct from context A, and the tone was presented again. Once again the freezing response can be measured, and by using these measures one can separately assess their memory of the tone and of the context. The authors reported that LPS at 0.125 mg/kg, but not at 0.5 mg/kg, disrupted CFC but did not affect auditory fear-conditioning and concluded that systemic inflammation could induce a hippocampal selective memory deficit in juvenile animals. They replicated this finding, albeit at the much higher dose of 1 mg/kg in adult rats. CFC is classically described as hippocampal-dependent, while auditory fear-conditioning is thought not to be (Kim and Fanselow, 1992) and it is typically seen as a two-stage process: the encoding of a memory for the context and the association of the foot-shock with the context in which it was received. The authors did several useful experiments to show that if the animals were pre-exposed to the context, in the absence of foot-shock, then LPS administered postconditioning no longer impaired memory (i.e. the freezing response was the same in LPS and vehicle-treated animals). Furthermore, if LPS was administered after the pre-exposure instead of after conditioning, the initial encoding of the context was once again impaired. These data combine to provide good evidence that inflammation, and specifically IL-1β, applied directly after a conditioning stimulus can impair memory for spatial context.

CFC has probably been the task that has most consistently demonstrated effects of inflammation on memory function. Other groups have replicated both the LPS-induced deficit and the differential effect at different doses (Thomson and Sutherland, 2005). These authors found significant deficits at 2 μg/kg but not at 4 μg/kg (these LPS doses were chosen on basis of matching by endotoxin units to the Pugh studies, rather than by mass). A similar dose-dependency of effects on CFC revealed an interesting aspect of the interaction between inflammatory mediators and memory function. Goshen and colleagues showed that while IL-1β, injected directly into the ventricles of the brain, could impair CFC, its natural receptor antagonist IL-1ra could also achieve the same effect (Goshen *et al.*, 2007). Many authors had proposed U-shaped curves to explain biphasic responses to different concentrations of mediators, but these authors actually showed that 10 ng of IL-1β impaired learning, 1 ng of IL-1β improved learning and 100 μg of IL-1ra, which should block endogenous levels of IL-1β, also impaired learning, thus constructing something finally resembling an inverse U-shaped curve. While these data give credence to the notion that these dose relationships exist, it does not explain the biphasic effect of LPS in CFC, in which lower doses of LPS apparently produce impairments while higher doses do not. Indeed in the original Pugh paper, LPS in adults did not impair at 0.5 mg/kg or at 2 mg/kg, but did impair at 1 mg/kg. This relationship is now inverted with respect to the IL-1β effects reported by Goshen; why LPS and IL-1β might have U-shaped curves of opposite directionality is not intuitive. Furthermore, IL-1β, applied intra-hippocampally, produced working memory deficits in a runway task that were straightforwardly dose-dependent, albeit in an appetitive task (Matsumoto, Yoshida, Watanabe, and Yamamoto, 2001). These issues are fundamental to understanding how immune stimulation might impact on memory, and it is important that they are addressed, since CFC has become widely used in the neuroinflammatory area. In focusing on effects that only appear at specific doses (and not at higher *or* lower doses) we run the risk of oversimplifying a set of processes that are likely to be rather complex. Given that the task measures a response to a specific type of aversive stimulus (foot shock) and that LPS is itself a rather aversive stimulus, it is important to ask whether LPS, applied directly after exposure to the context, is alone sufficient to induce freezing on re-exposure to the context. LPS is used as a conditioning stimulus in many other types of experiment and its ability to induce conditioned taste-aversion is well described. One might think intuitively that if both foot-shock and LPS independently produce freezing then the combination of these factors might produce an exaggerated freezing response. However, it is possible for a large unconditioned stimulus to support a less-potentiated fear response (Walker and Davis, 1997), and in the CFC experimental design favored by many there may be, in effect, two unconditioned stimuli (shock and inflammatory stimulation). Therefore, it is necessary to test whether inflammogens used in the CFC paradigm produce freezing to context even when the context has not been paired with a foot-shock. The CFC paradigm has become popular for the rapid, robust and enduring memory it produces, with no prior-training required, thus mechanistic data can be relatively quickly gathered. It is also attractive in studies of immune stimulation because the animals are not sick when exploring the context, thus avoiding some of the confounders referred to above. However, given the caveats mentioned here it is important that the field does not rely solely on this task to delineate the mechanisms by which inflammation interacts with memory.

Avoiding the pitfalls

- Multiple doses of immunogens should be tested in contextual fear-conditioning to adequately encompass non-monotonic dose relationships. The impact of immune stimulation on freezing, in the absence of footshock should be examined to determine whether sickness itself acts an unconditioned stimulus.

Reconciling Mice with Men and Old Observations with New Ones

It is clear that one can find deficits in a number of cognitive tasks after immune stimulation, but it is also apparent that some of these impairments can be explained by performance deficits, motivational and locomotor differences, and alternative, stress-minimizing strategies. When all of these features have been controlled for, for example in the MWM, it is apparent that one has to look very closely to find even mild learning deficits, and several studies report no deficits. When one assesses the latency, the distance travelled, the route taken and the probe trials, there is limited evidence that LPS or IL-1β significantly impair learning or memory in the MWM (Table 18.1, Figure 18.1). More recent studies with other inflammogens have provided further interesting data: In a study of simulated mycoplasma infection (using fibroblast-stimulating lipopeptide 1) it was shown that animals displayed marked sickness across 3 days, but demonstrated intact learning of the location of a visible platform between 18 hours and 4 days (Swanepoel *et al.*, 2011). In animals challenged with the Gram-positive bacterial superantigen Staphylococcal enterotoxin A, it is apparent that learning of the location of the hidden platform is not different to control animals, but when retested one month later, without further injections, SEA-treated animals showed better relearning of this maze with respect to control animals (Woodruff *et al.*, 2011), suggesting that they may have encoded more, rather than less, about the maze environment while experiencing the effects of elevated systemic cytokines such as TNF-α.

Conversely, aversive tasks involving footshock and measuring fear responses consistently find inflammation-induced deficits with non-monotonic dose relationships. A nice example of this disparity between contextual fear conditioning and spatial navigation tasks is in a model of very robust and long-lasting hippocampal IL-1β expression. These animals show impaired fear-conditioning but remarkably little evidence of spatial learning deficits in the MWM, despite very marked chronic IL-1β expression and CNS inflammation (Hein *et al.*, 2010). Since both of these tasks are demonstrably hippocampal-dependent, one has to ask why they might be so differentially sensitive. Animals in which sickness has been experimentally induced fail to consolidate the memory of an association between an electric shock and the visuospatial context in which it was presented, but their memory for visuospatial cues seen from the MWM is reasonably intact when the outcome is escape from water.

However, it is also true that when the visuospatial tasks are made more difficult by daily rearrangement of escape position/hidden platforms, such that animals must "forget" the previous day's location in order to solve today's task, LPS can induce impairments (Sparkman *et al.*, 2006). These impairments may be described as working-memory deficits, in that animals failed to integrate new, trial-specific, information with existing memories to complete the task. How this might differ from alternation working-memory tasks in which we do not find LPS-induced deficits in young healthy animals (Murray *et al.*, 2012) is not clear. However, it is of interest that Sparkman *et al.*, reported that their working-memory deficits were dependent upon IL-6 expression. There are older experiments showing that IL-6 can impede memory consolidation, leading to the hypothesis that IL-6 is important in "forgetting" (Balschun *et al.*, 2004). This may be a necessary function in working-memory tasks, since integration of trial-specific information is necessary for completion of the task and extinction of information from previous trials may be a necessary component of this.

As discussed earlier, most aspects of sickness behavior have an intuitive benefit for the recovery and or survival of the organism. From an adaptive point of view, it is not clear how an acute cognitive deficit might benefit the organism. Furthermore, if short-lived and fully

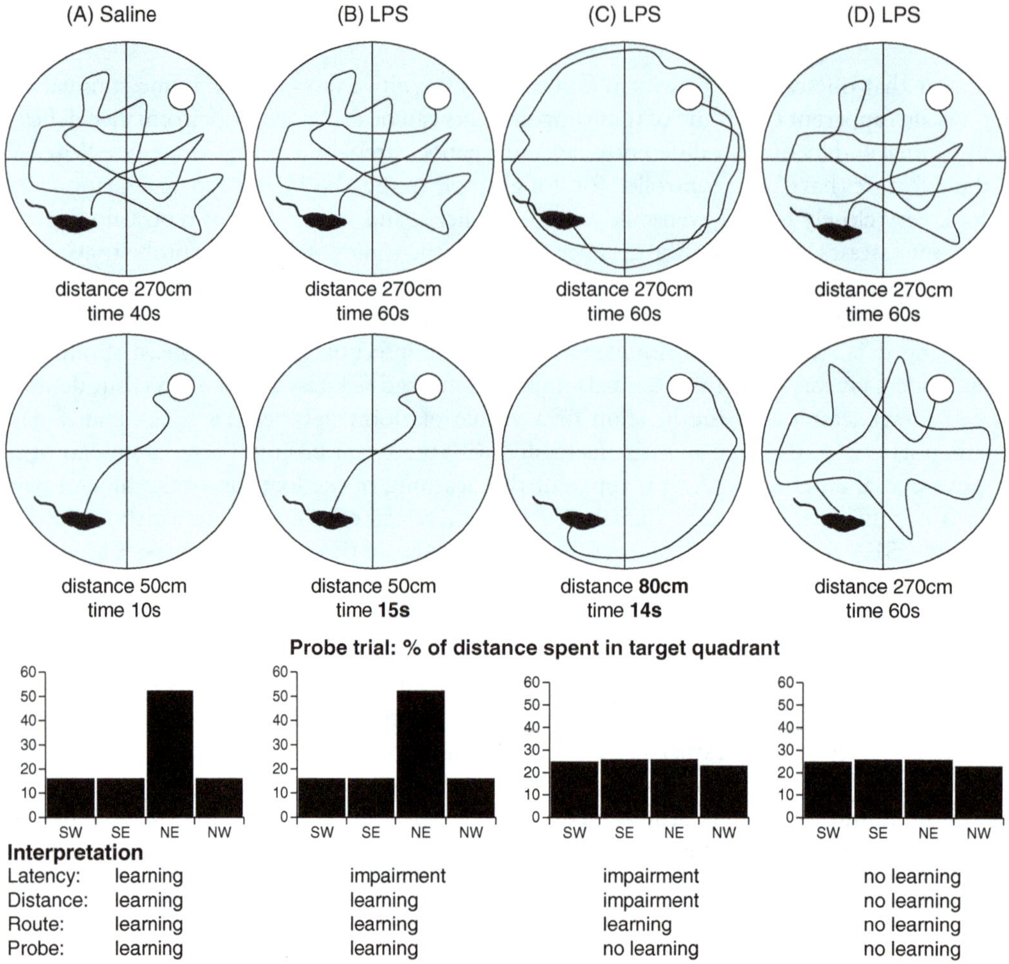

Figure 18.1 Theoretical illustrations of Morris Water Maze strategies. When *latency* is the only measure of performance in the MWM, the improvement between trials 1 and 2 (directly below) would be interpreted as successful learning in A with impairments in B and C, and no learning whatsoever in D. If *distance* is considered, B now shows equivalent learning to A, C appears somewhat impaired, and D shows no evidence of learning. If the *route* is examined it is obvious that A and B are using spatial cues to move directly towards the platform while neither C nor D use these spatial cues. Nonetheless, C shows clear learning by a non-spatial strategy (thigmotaxis). Examination of the *probe trial* data that would have resulted from the removal of the hidden platform, reveals that only A and B know where the platform is relative to spatial cues while C and D are indistinguishable in they both visit all quadrants equally. Only examination of all four of these parameters give the full picture of how the animals behave in the maze. Most studies have used only latency. Those using distance, route and/or probe trials have shown evidence for strategies B and C. No studies, to our knowledge, have shown evidence for D (see Table 18.1 for details). Figure adapted from Cunningham and Sanderson (2008) *Brain, Behavior and Immunity*, courtesy of Elsevier.

reversible inflammation and infection cause cognitive deficits then these should be readily apparent in the human population. It is now abundantly clear that sepsis produces robust acute and long-term cognitive impairments, but what of the sort of sickness episodes that the psychoneuroimmunology field has been interested in? There have been a number of studies with human volunteers on the effects of experimental endotoxemia. Healthy young volunteers have been administered 0.2–2 ng LPS/kg body weight and various emotional, attentional and cognitive parameters have been assessed and correlated with pro-inflammatory cytokines, cortisol or other hormones/neurotransmitters. These studies are compared in Table 18.2. Though immediate and delayed recall in declarative memory tasks have been reported to be impaired in humans administered 0.8 ng/kg (Reichenberg *et al.*, 2001), the general trend in these studies is that attention, working memory, and other measures of cognitive function are not significantly impaired, even with 2 ng/kg LPS (van den Boogaard *et al.*, 2010). The TNF-α, IL-6 and cortisol levels observed in the two more recent studies (Grigoleit *et al.*, 2010; van den Boogaard *et al.*, 2010) match or exceed the levels in those from the original Reichenberg study but fail to find cognitive deficits. A full discussion of the human literature is beyond the scope of this chapter and I mention it here only to make the point that there is not a consistently described cognitive impairment in humans administered endotoxin analogous to the conclusions made in the rodent studies that have been the focus of this chapter.

Thus, while there are some reports of cognitive impairment, in both humans and animals they are matched by reports of intact performance despite robust sickness behavior and/or elevated cytokines. Therefore, further data are required to confirm or reject the idea that mild to moderate systemic inflammation interferes significantly with cognitive function in humans. This does not contradict earlier data that chemotherapy with inflammatory cytokines such as IL-2 and IFNα can affect memory function, but it is important to be specific in what one reports, and to be cautious about generalizing from effects of specific cytokines, under specific dosing regimes, to espousing a more general dogma that systemic inflammation interferes significantly with cognitive function. Cognitive impairment is increasingly listed among the features of sickness behavior, but in light of these findings it is difficult to argue that this its inclusion is correct in the case of sickness behavior in healthy young individuals. It may be the case that certain features of memory function are affected during sickness, at certain doses/severities of illness, but it is relatively clear that it is not a feature that appears with the consistency of the classical descriptors of sickness behavior, and thus may not be a core feature of sickness behavior.

Systemic Inflammation Induces Cognitive Dysfunction in Susceptible Populations

There are, however, situations in which acute inflammation can have profound effects on human cognitive function and these can have serious consequences. In the elderly, and particularly in those with existing cognitive impairment, inflammation caused by infection, injury, and surgery can produce profound cognitive impairment. The extreme end of this spectrum is delirium. Delirium is an acute-onset and typically transient impairment in multiple cognitive domains. Though attentional dysfunction is now seen as the core component, episodes comprise severely affected short-term and working memory, disorientation, confusion, and clouded

Table 18.2 Volunteer Studies of Human Endotoxemia and Cognitive Function

Study	*LPS*	*Subjects*	*TNF-α pg/ml plasma*	*IL-6 pg/ml plasma*	*Cortisol fold induction*	*Temp °C*	*Effects reported*
Reichenberg *et al.*, 2001	*Salmonella equi abort.* 0.8 ng/kg	20 male (crossover)	100	100	1.6 fold	+ 0.5 °C	Declarative memory (immediate and delayed recall) impairments. No deficits in attention or executive function or reaction time.
Cohen *et al.*, 2003	*Salmonella equi abort* 0.8 ng/kg	10 male	"	"	"	"	Subset of above group: improved working memory performance.
Krabbe *et al.*, 2005	*E. coli* 0.2 ng/kg	12 male (crossover)	4	5	No increase	No change	No significant cognitive impairment in any domain.
Grigoleit *et al.*, 2010	*E. coli* 0.4 ng/kg	24 male	95	140	2.5 fold	>+0.5 °C	No impairment of memory performance, attention or executive function.
van den Boogaard *et al.*, 2010	*E. coli* 2 ng/kg	25 male (15 LPS, 10 vehicle)	800	1000	2 fold	+1.5 °C	No cognitive impairment. Increased alertness correlated with increased cortisol and alpha power on EEG.

consciousness, and may encompass altered perception, hallucinations, and delusions. Though defined by its transient nature, delirium is now recognized to have significant long-term effects: episodes of delirium accelerate cognitive decline, increase the likelihood of dementia, and shorten time to permanent institutionalization and death (Witlox *et al.*, 2010). Therefore, studying how inflammation interacts with and affects cognitive circuitry remains extremely important both for the understanding of the acute episode and its long-term consequences, and there is little doubt that experiments performed in young healthy animals have a role to play in understanding the mechanisms by which inflammatory mediators may alter cognitive function. However, it is undeniable that if we wish to understand why inflammatory insults that have little cognitive effect in the young healthy population can produce profound derangement of function in elderly or demented patients, it is necessary to perform similar experiments in aged rodents and in those with prior disease. All of the same confounding factors that I have previously discussed also apply to experiments in older or diseased rodents. Indeed, since research into exaggerated cognitive impairments in the aged and diseased rodent arose partly from the observation of exaggerated sickness behavior responses in these animals (Combrinck, Perry, and Cunningham, 2002; Godbout *et al.*, 2005), attention to these confounding factors becomes more important than ever.

In the contextual fear-conditioning paradigm, infection with *E. coli* was found to affect long-term but not short-term anterograde memory for context in aged animals but was without effect in young adult rats (Barrientos *et al.*, 2006), and this was associated with exaggerated CNS IL-1β responses to infection as suggested by the prior demonstration of microglial priming (Combrinck, Perry, and Cunningham, 2002; Cunningham *et al.*, 2005). Kohman and colleagues showed, using active avoidance experiments, that LPS induced a more marked failure to avoid the context in which foot shock was administered in aged mice compared to younger ones (Kohman, Tarr, Byler, and Boehm, 2007). Likewise, in a radial arm working memory task, LPS (0.33 mg/kg) induced acute deficits in old mice (Chen *et al.*, 2008). Notably, LPS did not produce impairments in young animals in this task, which has similar requirements to the task previously used by these authors to report deficits induced by LPS in young mice (Sparkman *et al.*, 2006). With a specific focus on prior neurodegeneration as a susceptibility factor, animals with prior neurodegenerative disease, encompassing significant synaptic loss in the hippocampus, showed impaired learning of a Y-maze visuospatial reference memory task when treated with LPS, compared to normal animals given the same challenges (Cunningham *et al.*, 2009). These animals also showed acute and transient working memory deficits in a T-maze alternation task in response to systemic LPS (100 μg/kg) when neither this dose nor 200 μg/kg had any effect in normal animals on this task (Murray *et al.*, 2012). The inflammatory underpinning of these deficits is being actively investigated in a number of these laboratories, but the trends emerging suggest roles for IL-1β, TNF-α, PGE2 and corticosterone. If these pathways are consistently implicated it is essential that we are collectively diligent in providing all possible controls to rule out the confounders that have been discussed above.

Avoiding the pitfalls

- Aged rodents and those with prior neurodegenerative disease show exaggerated sickness responses to systemic inflammatory stimulation and thus those confounding factors described above are even more prevalent than in younger animals.

Concluding Remarks

It has been an important aim of this chapter to emphasize good experimental design in assessing the impact of inflammation on cognitive function. That inflammation impairs learning and memory has become dogma in the field. Despite the well known features of sickness behavior and their ability to confound tests of learning and memory, both experimental design and expectations in new studies are frequently guided by those studies that have previously been published. Such an approach may potentially lead to self-perpetuating replication of findings rather than an increased understanding of the nature and mechanisms of the impairments. Obviously, we need to focus on elucidating the nature of the impairments, and careful attention to experimental design will be of benefit in this regard. It bears repeating that to state with confidence that a manipulation has interfered with learning or memory it is necessary to rule out the possibility that the observed changes could equally be explained by a change in motivation, locomotor speed, reward-seeking, or stress and anxiety responses. Undoubtedly there are some impairments induced by some inflammatory stimuli at some doses, but robust cognitive impairment during infection or experimental inflammation is by no means universally observed. However, unlike inflammation in young healthy individuals, the elderly and demented suffer very serious consequences even after relatively mild inflammatory stimuli and there is a real imperative to understand these processes in these older, more frail populations. Clearly defining the deficits, and avoiding the pitfalls discussed here, are important responsibilities for researchers in this field if we are to correctly identify the molecular pathways to cognitive dysfunction and to offer therapeutic solutions for those who experience these dreadful episodes.

Acknowledgements

The author would like to thank Stephen Maren and David Sanderson for helpful discussions and comments. Work in the author's laboratory is supported by the Wellcome Trust.

References

Aubert, A., Vega, C., Dantzer, R., and Goodall, G. (1995). Pyrogens specifically disrupt the acquisition of a task involving cognitive processing in the rat. *Brain, Behavior, and Immunity*, 9, 129–148.

Balschun, D., Wetzel, W., Del Rey, A., Pitossi, F., Schneider, H., Zuschratter, W., et al. (2004). Interleukin-6: a cytokine to forget. *FASEB Journal*, 18, 1788–1790.

Barrientos, R.M., Higgins, E.A., Biedenkapp, J.C., Sprunger, D.B., Wright-Hardesty, K.J., Watkins, L.R., et al. (2006). Peripheral infection and aging interact to impair hippocampal memory consolidation. *Neurobiology of Aging*, 27, 723–732.

Chen, J., Buchanan, J.B., Sparkman, N.L., Godbout, J.P., Freund, G.G., and Johnson, R.W. (2008). Neuroinflammation and disruption in working memory in aged mice after acute stimulation of the peripheral innate immune system. *Brain, Behavior, and Immunity*, 22, 301–311.

Combrinck, M.I., Perry, V.H., and Cunningham, C. (2002). Peripheral infection evokes exaggerated sickness behaviour in pre-clinical murine prion disease. *Neuroscience*, 112, 7–11.

Cunningham, C., Campion, S., Lunnon, K., Murray, C.L., Woods, J.F., Deacon, R.M., et al. (2009). Systemic inflammation induces acute behavioral and cognitive changes and accelerates neurodegenerative disease. *Biological Psychiatry*, 65, 304–312.

Cunningham, C., and Sanderson, D.J. (2008). Malaise in the water maze: untangling the effects of LPS and IL-1beta on learning and memory. *Brain, Behavior, and Immunity*, 22, 1117–1127.

Cunningham, C., Wilcockson, D.C., Campion, S., Lunnon, K., and Perry, V.H. (2005). Central and systemic endotoxin challenges exacerbate the local inflammatory response and increase neuronal death during chronic neurodegeneration. *Journal of Neuroscience*, 25, 9275–9284.

Gibertini, M. (1998). Cytokines and cognitive behavior. *Neuroimmunomodulation*, 5, 160–165.

Gibertini, M., Newton, C., Friedman, H., and Klein, T.W. (1995). Spatial learning impairment in mice infected with Legionella pneumophila or administered exogenous interleukin-1-beta. *Brain, Behavior, and Immunity*, 9, 113–128.

Godbout, J.P., Chen, J., Abraham, J., Richwine, A.F., Berg, B.M., Kelley, K.W., et al. (2005). Exaggerated neuroinflammation and sickness behavior in aged mice following activation of the peripheral innate immune system. *FASEB Journal*, 19, 1329–1331.

Goodwin, D.W., Powell, B., Bremer, D., Hoine, H., and Stern, J. (1969). Alcohol and recall: state-dependent effects in man. *Science*, 163, 1358–1360.

Goshen, I., Kreisel, T., Ounallah-Saad, H., Renbaum, P., Zalzstein, Y., Ben-Hur, T., et al. (2007). A dual role for interleukin-1 in hippocampal-dependent memory processes. *Psychoneuroendocrinology*, 32, 1106–1115.

Greer, G.G., and Rietschel, E.T. (1978). Lipid A-induced tolerance and hyperreactivity to hypothermia in mice. *Infection and Immunity*, 19, 357–368.

Grigoleit, J.S., Oberbeck, J.R., Lichte, P., Kobbe, P., Wolf, O.T., Montag, T., et al. (2010). Lipopolysaccharide-induced experimental immune activation does not impair memory functions in humans. *Neurobiology of Learning and Memory*, 94, 561–567.

Hart, B.L. (1988). Biological basis of the behavior of sick animals. *Neuroscience and Biobehavioral Reviews*, 12, 123–137.

Hein, A.M., Stasko, M.R., Matousek, S.B., Scott-Mckean, J.J., Maier, S.F., Olschowka, J.A., et al. (2010). Sustained hippocampal IL-1beta overexpression impairs contextual and spatial memory in transgenic mice. *Brain, Behavior, and Immunity*, 24, 243–253.

Kim, J.J., and Fanselow, M.S. (1992). Modality-specific retrograde amnesia of fear. *Science*, 256, 675–677.

Kohman, R.A., Tarr, A.J., Byler, S.L., and Boehm, G.W. (2007). Age increases vulnerability to bacterial endotoxin-induced behavioral decrements. *Physiology and Behavior*, 91, 561–565.

Matsumoto, Y., Yoshida, M., Watanabe, S., and Yamamoto, T. (2001). Involvement of cholinergic and glutamatergic functions in working memory impairment induced by interleukin-1beta in rats. *European Journal of Pharmacology*, 430, 283–288.

Miller, R.R., and Springer, A.D. (1973). Amnesia, consolidation, and retrieval. *Psychological Review*, 80, 69–79.

Morris, R.G., Garrud, P., Rawlins, J.N., and O'Keefe, J. (1982). Place navigation impaired in rats with hippocampal lesions. *Nature*, 297, 681–683.

Murray, C., Sanderson, D.J., Barkus, C., Deacon, R.M., Rawlins, J.N., Bannerman, D.M., et al. (2012). Systemic inflammation induces acute working memory deficits in the primed brain: relevance for delirium. *Neurobiology of Aging*, 33, 603–616.

Oitzl, M.S., Van Oers, H., Schobitz, B., and De Kloet, E.R. (1993). Interleukin-1 beta, but not interleukin-6, impairs spatial navigation learning. *Brain Research*, 613, 160–163.

Pugh, C.R., Kumagawa, K., Fleshner, M., Watkins, L.R., Maier, S.F., and Rudy, J.W. (1998). Selective effects of peripheral lipopolysaccharide administration on contextual and auditory-cue fear conditioning. *Brain, Behavior, and Immunity*, 12, 212–229.

Reichenberg, A., Yirmiya, R., Schuld, A., Kraus, T., Haack, M., Morag, A., et al. (2001). Cytokine-associated emotional and cognitive disturbances in humans. *Archives of General Psychiatry*, 58, 445–452.

Shaw, K.N., Commins, S., and O'Mara, S.M. (2001). Lipopolysaccharide causes deficits in spatial learning in the watermaze but not in BDNF expression in the rat dentate gyrus. *Behavioural Brain Research*, 124, 47–54.

Simon, P., Dupuis, R., and Costentin, J. (1994). Thigmotaxis as an index of anxiety in mice. Influence of dopaminergic transmissions. *Behavioural Brain Research*, 61, 59–64.

Song, C., Phillips, A.G., Leonard, B.E., and Horrobin, D.F. (2004). Ethyl-eicosapentaenoic acid ingestion prevents corticosterone-mediated memory impairment induced by central administration of interleukin-1beta in rats. *Molecular Psychiatry*, 9, 630–638.

Sparkman, N.L., Buchanan, J.B., Heyen, J.R., Chen, J., Beverly, J.L., and Johnson, R.W. (2006). Interleukin-6 facilitates lipopolysaccharide-induced disruption in working memory and expression of other proinflammatory cytokines in hippocampal neuronal cell layers. *Journal of Neuroscience*, 26, 10709–10716.

Sparkman, N.L., Kohman, R.A., Scott, V.J., and Boehm, G.W. (2005a). Bacterial endotoxin-induced behavioral alterations in two variations of the Morris water maze. *Physiology and Behavior*, 86, 244–251.

Sparkman, N.L., Martin, L.A., Calvert, W.S., and Boehm, G.W. (2005b). Effects of intraperitoneal lipopolysaccharide on Morris maze performance in year-old and 2-month-old female C57BL/6J mice. *Behavioural Brain Research*, 159, 145–151.

Swanepoel, T., Harvey, B.H., Harden, L.M., Laburn, H.P., and Mitchell, D. (2011). Dissociation between learning and memory impairment and other sickness behaviours during simulated Mycoplasma infection in rats. *Brain, Behavior, and Immunity*, 25, 1607–1616.

Tazi, A., Dantzer, R., Crestani, F., and Le Moal, M. (1988). Interleukin-1 induces conditioned taste aversion in rats: a possible explanation for its pituitary-adrenal stimulating activity. *Brain Research*, 473, 369–371.

Thomson, L.M., and Sutherland, R.J. (2005). Systemic administration of lipopolysaccharide and interleukin-1beta have different effects on memory consolidation. *Brain Research Bulletin*, 67, 24–29.

Van Den Boogaard, M., Ramakers, B.P., Van Alfen, N., Van Der Werf, S.P., Fick, W.F., Hoedemaekers, C.W., et al. (2010). Endotoxemia-induced inflammation and the effect on the human brain. *Critical Care (London)*, 14, R81.

Walker, D.L., and Davis, M. (1997). Involvement of the dorsal periaqueductal gray in the loss of fear-potentiated startle accompanying high footshock training. *Behavioral Neuroscience*, 111, 692–702.

Witlox, J., Eurelings, L.S., De Jonghe, J.F., Kalisvaart, K.J., Eikelenboom, P., and Van Gool, W.A. (2010). Delirium in elderly patients and the risk of postdischarge mortality, institutionalization, and dementia: a meta-analysis. *Journal of the American Medical Association*, 304, 443–451.

Woodruff, R.T., Schorpp, K.M., Lawrenczyk, A.J., Chakraborty, T., and Kusnecov, A.W. (2011). Effects of acute and repeated administration of Staphylococcal enterotoxin A on Morris water maze learning, corticosterone and hippocampal IL-1beta and TNFalpha. *Brain, Behavior, and Immunity*, 25, 938–946.

Yirmiya, R., and Goshen, I. (2011). Immune modulation of learning, memory, neural plasticity and neurogenesis. *Brain, Behavior, and Immunity*, 25, 181–213.

19

The Role of NF-κB in Behavioral and Neural Plasticity

Elyse M. Mallimo and Alexander W. Kusnecov

Department of Psychology, Behavioral Neuroscience Program, Rutgers, The State University of New Jersey, New Brunswick, NJ, USA

Overview

It has become increasingly clear that pro-inflammatory cytokines exert diverse effects on Central Nervous System (CNS) function. Cytokines such as interleukin-1 beta (IL-1β) and tumor necrosis factor alpha (TNF-α) are necessary for activation of the hypothalamic–pituitary–adrenal (HPA) axis and can alter a range of basic motivational and cognitive behaviors (Rossi-George *et al.*, 2005). Furthermore, cytokines can exert either beneficial or detrimental effects on learning and memory (Yirmiya and Goshen, 2011). Indeed, the list of behavioral effects, and the range of cytokines known to be implicated in neurobiological and behavioral alterations, has grown, although many of the seminal, and consistently more powerful effects are restricted to IL-1 and TNF. What is particularly pertinent, however, is that these, and other cytokines, such as interleukin-6 (IL-6), orchestrate their biological effects via common intracellular transcriptional mechanisms that are now recognized to be relevant in CNS function. A primary focus in recent years is the transcription factor (TF) nuclear factor of the immunoglobulin (Ig) kappa (κ) light chain, or NF-κB, which was first identified in B-lymphocytes (Sen and Baltimore, 1986), and found to be critical to immune system development and regulation of inflammatory cytokine expression. Moreover, evidence has implicated NF-κB in stress, food intake, and neuroplasticity. Consequently, this chapter will provide an overview of NF-κB, and consider its role as a pivotal mechanism mediating, as well orchestrating, changes in adaptational behavior. To this extent, we have chosen to focus our attention on learning and memory paradigms, where much of the behavioral evidence has been gathered.

Nuclear Factor κB: A Critical Regulator of Immune Function

It is beyond the scope of this chapter to review the enormous and highly complex literature that exists on NF-κB. A brief overview will suffice, and the reader is referred to detailed discussions of NF-κB and the immune system that have served as the basis of our understanding of NF-κB in the CNS (Bonizzi and Karin, 2004; Hayden, West, and Ghosh, 2006; Sun, 2011). For the unfamiliar, it is easy to get lost among the many different combinations and alternative

The Wiley-Blackwell Handbook of Psychoneuroimmunology, First Edition. Edited by Alexander W. Kusnecov and Hymie Anisman.

states of NF-κB in its restrained and activated states. What becomes apparent is that any discussion of NF-κB requires certain qualifications, as it may not always be the "same" NF-κB that is recruited (or inhibited) within different cells, tissues, or physiological conditions. Therefore, it is hoped that this section serves to clarify matters, rather than confuse the reader regarding the many facets of NF-κB machinery. One should also note that while it is referred to in the singular, NF-κB is actually a family of proteins, consisting of five different subunits that function as homodimers or heterodimers. Furthermore, the unique ways in which these protein subunits combine can confer NF-κB with the ability to induce, as well as, repress, gene transcription. For example, rel proteins (Rel-A or p65, Rel-B, and c-Rel or just Rel) contain a transactivation domain (TAD) and are capable of inducing gene transcription. However, p50/p105 (NF-κB1) and p52/p100 (NF-κB2) lack transactivation domains, which results in their activation and formation into homodimers (i.e., p50/p50 or p52/p52) or heterodimers (i.e., p50/p52) conferring transcriptional *repressor* function and prevention of gene expression (Barger *et al.*, 2005).

Finally, it should be noted that for the remainder of this chapter, p65 and RelA are used interchangeably, since some studies have used one or the other term. Moreover, use of the term NF-κB may refer to a particular combination of subunits (e.g., p50 and p65; p50/p65) or to the transcription factor in general. Therefore, NF-κB should be interpreted in a context-dependent manner. For clarification purposes, Table 19.1 summarizes many of the components of the two major pathways for activation of NF-κB.

The classical or canonical pathway

All members of the NF-κB family of transcription factors share a Rel homology domain (RHD) that permits dimerization and association with inhibitory kappa B (IκB) proteins (these include IkBα, IκBβ, IκBε, IκBγ, BCL-3, p100 and p105 (Barger *et al.*, 2005)). In most cell types IκB proteins mask a nuclear localization sequence (NLS) present in the RHD, which serves to sequester inactive or latent dimers in the cytoplasm. In response to activating stimuli (e.g., cytokines), the IκB kinase (IKK) initiates a signaling cascade that culminates in the destruction of IκB and liberation of NF-κB. Figure 19.1 shows the sequential activation of NF-κB via the classical or "canonical" pathway, which includes p50, p65 and c-Rel containing-dimers. These are held latent by one of the IκB proteins, but most commonly IκBα. Upon activation, the gamma (γ) subunit of IKK (IKKγ; also known as NEMO or NF-κB essential modulator), contacts inactive dimers of additional IKK subunits (IKKα and IKKβ) through its catalytic core, which results in IκBα phosphorylation by IKKβ and tags it for ubiquitination and proteasomal degradation. This degradation of IκBα exposes the nuclear localization signal (NLS) on the IKK complex, and directs translocation of NF-κB (now said to be "activated") to the nucleus (Figure 19.1).

The canonical pathway of NF-κB is commonly engaged in innate immunity, regulating the expression of inflammatory cytokines (Grigoriadis *et al.*, 1996; Bonizzi and Karin, 2004), chemokines (Newton *et al.*, 2007), enzymes (Hayden, West, and Ghosh, 2006) and cell adhesion molecules (Rafiee *et al.*, 2010) (see Figure 19.1). For example, conditional mutations in the c-Rel subunit altered expression of pro-inflammatory cytokines, elevating LPS-stimulated concentrations of IL-6 three-fold when compared to normal macrophages (c-Rel$^{+/+}$), but reducing TNF-α concentrations in response to *Listeria monocytogenes*, a Gram-positive bacterium (Grigoriadis *et al.*, 1996). This demonstrates that c-Rel can either positively or negatively regulate the expression of cytokines during an innate immune response.

Table 19.1 Components of the NF-κB System

Component	*Function*	*Alternative name(s)*
Canonical/Classical Pathway		
Subunits		
p65	Protein subunit, regulates mRNA transcription	Rel-A
p50	Protein subunit, regulates mRNA transcription, derived from larger precursor protein, p105	NF-κB1; refers to the gene from which it is transcribed
c-Rel	Protein subunit, regulates mRNA transcription	Rel
Inhibitory kappa B Proteins (IκB)		
IκBα	Sequesters NF-κB in the cytoplasm, removes activated dimers from DNA and shuttles them back to the cytoplasm	
IκBβ	Sequesters NF-κB in the cytoplasm	
IκBε	Sequesters NF-κB in the cytoplasm	
IκBγ	Sequesters NF-κB in the cytoplasm	
p105	The precursor to the p50 subunit	
IκB Kinase Complex (IKK)		
IKKγ	Tethers together the catalytic subunits of the IKK complex, brings inactive dimers in contact with catalytic subunits	NF-κB essential modulator (NEMO)
IKKα	Catalytic subunit of IKK complex, phosphorylates protein subunits	
IKKβ	Catalytic subunits of IKK complex, phosphorylates IκB protein	
Non-Canonical/Alternative Pathway		
Subunits		
p52	Protein subunit, regulates mRNA transcription, derived from larger precursor protein, p100	NF-κB2; refers to the gene from which it is transcribed
Rel-B	Protein subunit, regulates mRNA transcription	
Inhibitory Proteins		
p100	Sequesters Rel-B subunits in the cytoplasm, is the precursor to the p52 subunit	
Bcl-3	Inhibitory protein present in the nucleus, binds both Rel-B and p52 subunits, and as a heterodimer (p52/Bcl-3) Bcl-3 converts p52 into a transcriptional activator	
IκB Kinase Complex (IKK)		
IKKα	Phosphorylates p100	

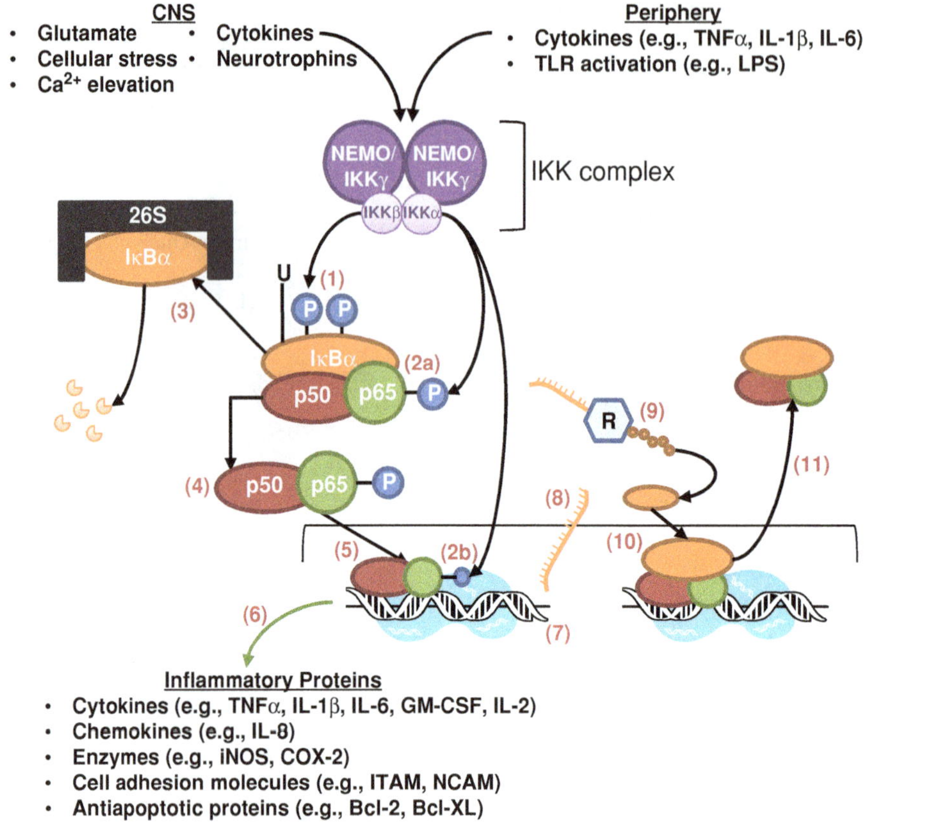

Figure 19.1 Canonical or classical pathway for activation of NF-κB. In response to activating stimuli, the β-subunit of the IKK complex (IKKβ) phosphorylates the IκBα inhibitory protein, tagging it for ubiquitination (1). By contrast, the α-subunit of the IKK complex (IKKα) phosphorylates key serine residues along p65 either before (2a) or after (2b) its dissociation from IκBα. The IκBα protein is subsequently degraded by the 26S proteasome (3). Activated p50/p65 heterodimers then dissociate from IκBα (4) and translocate to the cell nucleus (5). In the nucleus, p50/p65 initiates the transcription of inflammatory proteins (6). Moreover, NF-κB initiates transcription of the *IκBα* gene (7). Once transcribed and processed, mature IκBα mRNA then exits the nucleus (8). In the cytoplasm ribosomes translate IκBα mRNA into protein (9). Newly synthesized IκBα protein then re-enters the nucleus and binds to activated NF-κB dimers (10). Unlike other IκB proteins, IκBα contains a nuclear export signal (NES) that directs the IκBα: p50/p65 complex back to the cytoplasm (11). In this way, IκBα negatively regulates the activity of NF-κB. Note: some components of the classical pathway *are not shown* in this figure; the NF-κB subunit c-Rel and other IκB proteins (IκBα, IκBβ, IκBε and IκBγ). Additionally, while c-Rel, p50 and p65 can form homo- or heterodimers, for the sake of simplicity only the p50/p65 heterodimer is illustrated in this figure. Abbreviations used: NEMO/IKKγ, NF-κB essential modulator/IKKγ; P, phosphorylation; 26S, 26S proteasome; U, ubiquitination; R, ribosome. Green arrow, initiation of gene expression.

Cytokines are also well recognized *inducers* of NF-κB (Figure 19.1), which in turn alters the expression of other inflammatory proteins (Newton *et al.*, 2007; Rafiee *et al.*, 2010). For instance, IL-1β and TNF-α form part of a feedforward loop with NF-κB, amplifying their own expression via NF-κB activation (Bonizzi and Karin, 2004). Additionally, inhibition of IKK prevents expression of IL-1 and TNF-α stimulated cell adhesion molecules, such as intracellular adhesion molecule (ICAM), as well as the chemokine IL-8 (CXCL8) (Newton *et al.*, 2007; Rafiee *et al.*, 2010). All these molecules are key constituents in leukocyte trafficking and local migration within sites of infection, promoting cell–cell interactions between infiltrating leukocytes and vascular endothelial cells. This underscores the role of NF-κB in the regulation of innate immunity.

The canonical pathway is also involved in the development of adaptive immunity (Ghosh *et al.*, 1993; Kontgen *et al.*, 1995; Snapper *et al.*, 1996; Doi *et al.*, 1997; Horwitz *et al.*, 1997; Grundstrom, Anderson, Scheipers, and Sundstedt, 2004). For example, NF-κB differentially regulates the expression of IL-2, a cytokine that prompts the proliferation and differentiation of naïve T-cells into effector cells (Ghosh *et al.*, 1993; Kontgen *et al.*, 1995; Grundstrom, Anderson, Scheipers, and Sundstedt, 2004). In unstimulated, naïve T-cells p50/p50 homodimers exhibit strong DNA binding activity at the IL-2 promoter, suggesting that basal IL-2 expression is negatively regulated by NF-κB (Grundstrom, Anderson, Scheipers, and Sundstedt, 2004). By contrast, T-cell stimulation induces the nuclear accumulation of Rel-A and c-Rel, suggesting that one or both of these subunits initiate the transcription of IL-2 (Ghosh *et al.*, 1993). In line with this idea, c-Rel$^{-/-}$ T cells exhibit deficits in their capacity to produce IL-2 and do not proliferate or differentiate in response to mitogenic stimuli (Kontgen *et al.*, 1995). Likewise, p50 and Rel-A subunits are necessary for antigen-induced B-cell proliferation (Snapper *et al.*, 1996; Horwitz *et al.*, 1997) and both c-Rel$^{-/-}$ mice and doubly deficient (p50$^{-/-}$/p65$^{-/-}$) B-cells exhibit deficits in antibody class switching (Doi *et al.*, 1997; Horwitz *et al.*, 1997).

Finally, activation of the canonical pathway regulates apoptosis, or programmed cell death (Ouaaz *et al.*, 2002; Wan and DeGregori, 2003). For example, p50/c-Rel heterodimers protect dendritic cells (DC) from apoptosis by inducing the expression of the anti-apoptotic gene, *BCL-XL* (Ouaaz *et al.*, 2002). Similarly, Rel-A is necessary for the survival of stimulated T-lymphocytes (Wan and DeGregori, 2003).

The alternative or non-canonical pathway

In contrast to the canonical pathway, activation of the non-canonical or alternative pathway (see Figure 19.2) is NEMO-independent and does not require IKKβ. This is because cytoplasmic p100, the full-length precursor of the p52 subunit, functions as an IκB protein (Sun, 2011). In response to various activating stimuli, homodimers of IKKα are either autophosphorylated or phosphorylated by the kinase, NIK (NF-κB inducing kinase), which also promotes binding of IKKα to p100. Subsequent to these modifications, IKKα phosphorylates the inhibitory protein at two C-terminal residues (Ser 866 and Ser 870) cleaving it into its mature form, p52 (Sun, 2011). Dissociated heterodimers (p52/Rel-B) then translocate to the cell nucleus and initiate gene expression (see Figure 19.2).

Activation of the non-canonical pathway is primarily concerned with the development of lymphoid organs, particularly the spleen (Bonizzi and Karin, 2004). Transgenic NF-κB deficient mice (p52$^{-/-}$ or Rel-B$^{-/-}$) show deficits in the formation of the marginal zones (MZ) of

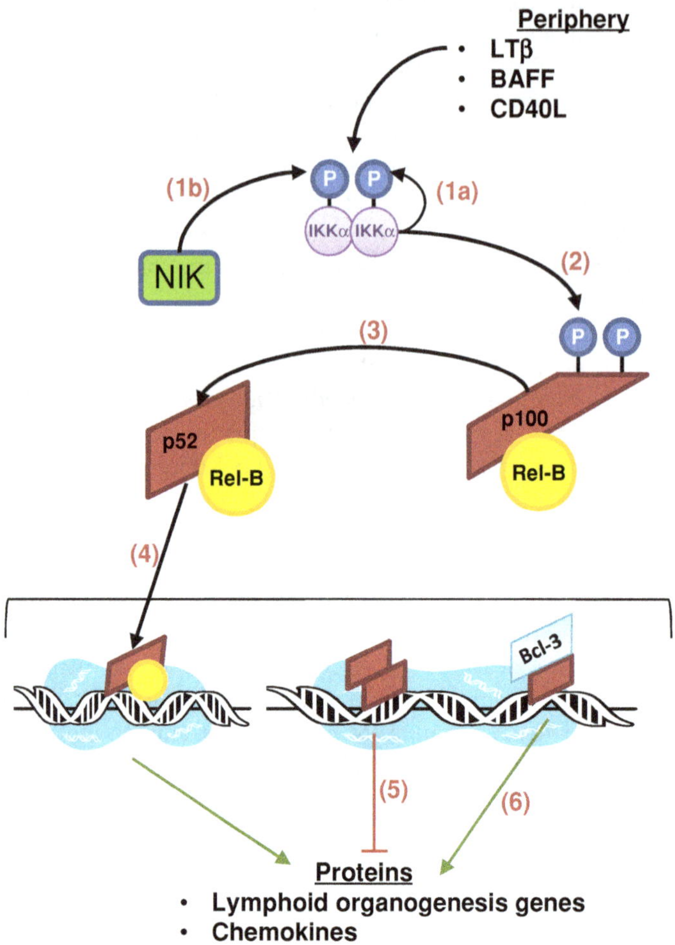

Figure 19.2 Non-canonical or alternative pathway for activation of NF-κB. In response to activating stimuli (lymphotoxin β, LTβ; B-cell activating factor, BAFF; or CD40L) homodimers of the alpha subunit of the IKK complex (IKKα) are autophosphorylated (1a), or phosphorylated by the NF-κB inducing kinase (NIK) (1b). IKKα then phosphorylates the inhibitory IκB protein, p100 (2). Once phosphorylated p100 is cleaved into its mature form, p52 (3) and p52/Rel-B heterodimers translocate to the nucleus (4). Inside the nucleus, p52/Rel-B heterodimers initiate the transcription of chemokines and proteins that are concerned with the development of secondary lymphoid tissues, like the spleen. Normally, homodimers of p52 function as transcriptional repressors (5). However, when bound to Bcl-3, p52/Bcl-3 heterodimers are converted into transcriptional activators (6). Finally, in the alternative pathway Rel-B does not homodimerize with itself. Abbreviations used: P, phosphorylation. Green arrows, initiation of gene expression; Red line, repression of gene expression.

the spleen (Weih, Yilmaz, and Weih, 2001), a region surrounding the lymphocyte-rich white pulp of the spleen, and that contains a heterogeneity of cells, including resident macrophages and transient populations of lymphocytes. For example, in Rel-B$^{-/-}$ mice there are fewer MZ macrophages than in normal wild-type mice, with macrophages being randomly distributed outside of the MZ, rather than forming a characteristic ring-like structure around the white pulp (Weih, Yilmaz, and Weih, 2001). Similarly, targeted deletion of the p52 subunit completely abolished the expression of the metallophilic sub-class of macrophages in the spleen (Franzoso *et al.*, 1997).

These findings suggest that p52 and Rel-B, respectively, are necessary for establishing resident splenic macrophages. Moreover, these cellular deficits result in impaired adaptive immune responses (Sha, Liou, Tuomanen, and Baltimore, 1995; Weih, Yilmaz, and Weih, 2001). For example, Rel-$B^{-/-}$ and $p52^{-/-}$ mice had significantly reduced secretion of IgG1 antibody following immunization with keyhole limpet hemocyanin (KLH), a T-cell dependent antigen (Ag) (Weih, Warr, Yang, and Bravo, 1997; Caamano *et al.*, 1998). Additionally, Rel-$B^{-/-}$ mice lack a specialized population of B cells in the MZ of the spleen that respond to antigen without help from activated T-cells (Guinamard, Okigaki, Schlessinger, and Ravetch, 2000). The latter finding is consistent with other evidence that NF-κB knockout mice had significantly reduced IgG3 antibody production following immunization with T-cell independent antigens (Weih, Warr, Yang, and Bravo, 1997; Caamano *et al.*, 1998).

In summary, the NF-κB system is a highly complex mechanism for ensuring both signal transduction and gene regulation by cytokines and other molecules. As such it is a pivotal process that can drive cellular responses in varying directions dictated by local functional needs. Within the immune system it is important for development of lymphoid architecture and function, and in the fully developed immune system, it ensures a balance of pro- and anti-inflammatory immune responses. The presence of classic and alternative modes of activation, and the presence of elements that can serve repressor functions, also suggests that activation of NF-κB is not always pro-inflammatory.

NF-κB in the Central Nervous System (CNS)

General overview

The bulk of our understanding about NF-κB is grounded in immunology. However, over the past two decades there has been increased interest in what functions NF-κB might exert in the CNS. Indeed, the neuromodulatory effects of NF-κB have been thoroughly reviewed by others (Mattson and Meffert, 2006), and therefore the purpose of this section is to offer only a brief overview of this information before considering the role of NF-κB in cognitive behavior.

The growing accumulation of shared molecules in the brain and immune system has included a number of cytokines (viz. IL-1, TNF, IL-6) that are significant regulators of NF-κB, and so it should not be surprising that inducible forms of NF-κB have been found in neurons, astrocytes, and microglia. Moreover, the most widely expressed and closely studied forms of brain NF-κB are p50, p65 and c-Rel, implicating classical or canonical signaling as the predominant pathway for NF-κB activation. To be sure, NF-κB is responsive to a number of neural elements, including glutamatergic agonists (Guerrini, Blasi, and Denis-Donini, 1995; Kaltschmidt, Kaltschmidt, and Baeuerle, 1995) and neurotrophic factors (Foehr *et al.*, 2000; Russo *et al.*, 2009). Importantly, given that NF-κB controls the transcription of many different CNS genes (Mattson and Meffert, 2006), higher-order elements of brain function, such as learning and memory, motivation and emotional regulation, are likely to be affected by its activation. These questions have begun to be addressed, as will be made clear below.

At a more fundamental level, NF-κB can exert a neuroprotective role, controlling the expression of anti-apoptotic proteins (Tamatani *et al.*, 1999), antioxidants (Mattson *et al.*, 1997) and growth factors (Foehr *et al.*, 2000; Russo *et al.*, 2009) thereby promoting retention of neuronal viability under neurotoxic conditions, especially in the hippocampus and basal forebrain (Qiu *et al.*, 2001). However, alterations in the subunit composition of activated dimers of NF-κB can facilitate apoptosis. For instance, application of IL-1β to cultured cerebellar and hippocampal neurons did not elicit toxicity unless c-Rel was inhibited, suggesting that endogenous c-Rel maintains neuronal survival (Pizzi *et al.*, 2002). Similarly, the p50 subunit of NF-κB is highly expressed in the nucleus of surviving, but not degenerating neurons (Kassed *et al.*, 2002). Confirmation that such upregulation was necessary for survival was provided in p50-deficient ($p50^{-/-}$) mice, who showed dramatically augmented degeneration of granule cells in the dentate gyrus (DG) of the hippocampus in response to a systemic injection of the neurotoxicant trimethyltin hydroxide (TMT) (Kassed *et al.*, 2002).

It has also been shown that preactivation of NF-κB can protect hippocampal neurons from subsequent exposure to oxidative stress (Mattson *et al.*, 1997). Normally, free oxygen radicals are converted to hydrogen peroxide (H_20_2) by the antioxidant enzyme, manganese superoxide dismutase (Mn-SOD) and subsequently detoxified by other enzymes. However, during periods of oxidative stress (e.g., ferrous iron (Fe^{2+}) exposure) oxygen radicals (0_2^{-}) react with nitric oxide (NO) to produce reactive oxygen species (ROS) like peroxynitrite. Significant accumulation of peroxynitrite can induce membrane lipid peroxidation, or degradation of the cell membrane and ultimately cell death. Interestingly, exposure of cultured hippocampal neurons to Fe^{2+} resulted in minimal apoptosis, increased Mn-SOD and decreased peroxynitrite if neurons were pre-exposed to TNF-α, a well-recognized inducer of NF-κB (Mattson *et al.*, 1997). However, this protective effect of TNF-α was disrupted if cells were incubated with a κB decoy DNA[1] sequence that prevented NF-κB activity (Mattson *et al.*, 1997). Similarly, the pro-survival effects of NF-κB were linked to the transcription of anti-apoptotic genes, such as *Bcl-2* and *Bcl-XL*, which are induced by TNF-α (Tamatani *et al.*, 1999).

To conclude this section, one is left with little doubt that NF-κB is recruited under circumstances in which neurons and other local cells are subjected to metabolic and/or neurotoxic distress. Under such conditions, NF-κB seems to be involved in promoting neural resilience. However, the absence of significant elements of the NF-κB assembly proteins (e.g., c-rel and p50) can impair neuron survival. Nonetheless, whether modulation of these particular elements of NF-κB underlies deficiencies in resistance to degenerative and other neurological diseases remains to be fully determined.

Brain NF-κB and Behavior

This section considers evidence for the role of NF-κB and related molecules in adaptational behavior. In particular, the focus will be on learning and memory, although a range of other behaviors have been examined. A summary of the various behavioral effects (as well as "non-effects," as the case may be) of NF-κB manipulation using a variety of different techniques is summarized in Tables 19.2–19.4. More detailed discussion of many of these studies is provided below in the context of using learning and memory paradigms.

The use of IL-1β and TNF-α in the aforementioned studies demonstrates that brain NF-κB mediates cytokine-dependent signaling. Indeed, exposure to IL-1β and TNF-α induced IκBα

[1] κB decoy DNA is a double-stranded oligonucleotide sequence expressing a κB consensus site. Decoy DNA inhibits NF-κB-dependent transcription by binding to activated subunits thus preventing DNA binding.

Table 19.2 The Effects of NF-κB Blockade on Amygdalar and Hippocampal-dependent Associative Fear Learning

Subunit	*Subjects*	*Technique*	*Cognitive test*	*Effects*	*Reference*
All	Male rats	Protease Inhibitors, site specific (LA or BLA) prior to training	FPS	Impaired long-term fear memory; ↓startle potentiation	Yeh *et al.*, 2002
All	Male mice	IKK inhibitor, i.c.v.; post training κB decoy DNA, i.c.v.; pre training	PA	Impaired LTM but not acquisition of PA; ↓latency to step through	Freudenthal *et al.*, 2005
All	Male & female mice	Super-repressor (GFAP-IκBα-dn), restricted to astrocytes of Ctx and HC	TFC CFC	*Females* Impaired acquisition of TFC and LTM for context only; ↓freezing to context *Males* No effect	Bracchi-Ricard *et al.*, 2008
c-Rel	Male & female mice	Subunit-specific knockout, widespread	TFC CFC	**Modest training (1X, CS-US pairing)** No effect on acquisition of TFC Impaired LTM for context only; ↓ freezing to context **Robust training (3X, CS-US pairing)** No effect on acquisition or LTM	Ahn *et al.*, 2008
c-Rel	Male mice	Subunit-specific knockout, widespread	PA	Impaired LTM but not acquisition of PA ↓Latency to step through	O'Riordan *et al.*, 2006

Abbreviations and symbols used: LA, lateral amygdala; BLA, basolateral amygdala; i.c.v., intracerebroventricular; Ctx, cortex; HC, hippocampus; IKK, IκB kinase; FPS, fear potentiated startle; PA, passive avoidance; TFC, tone fear conditioning; CFC, contextual fear conditioning; LTM, long-term memory; ↑, increased; ↓, decreased; 1X, a single CS-US pairing; 3X, three CS-US pairings.

Table 19.3 The Effects of NF-κB Blockade on Hippocampal-dependent and Hippocampal-independent Spatial Learning

Subunit	*Subjects*	*Technique*	*Cognitive test*	*Effects*	*Reference*
All	Male mice	Super-repressor (IκBα-SR), robustly expressed in GABAergic interneurons of the Ctx, HC, med, hyp and PC	MWM RAM (Spatial)	**MWM** Enhanced spatial learning and long-term reference memory; ↓Escape latency ↑Memory for target quadrant **RAM** Enhanced spatial learning; ↓Number of errors	O'Mahony *et al.*, 2006
All	Male mice	Super-repressor (IκBα-AA), robustly expressed in glutamatergic neurons of the forebrain	MWM	Impaired spatial learning and long-term reference memory; ↑Escape latency ↓Memory for target quadrant	Kaltschmidt *et al.*, 2006
p50	Male mice	Subunit-specific knockout, widespread	MWM Barnes Maze (Hidden)	**MWM** Enhanced spatial learning and long-term reference memory; ↓Escape latency ↑Memory for target quadrant **Barnes maze (Hidden)** No effect	Lehmann *et al.*, 2010
p65	Male mice	Subunit-specific knockout, widespread, concomitant TNFR knockout	RAM (Cued and spatial)	**RAM (Spatial)** Impaired acquisition of task; ↑Number of within and between trial errors ↓Percentage of correct arm choices **RAM (Cued)** No effect	Meffert *et al.*, 2003

All	Male & female mice	Super-repressor (GFAP-IκBα-dn), restricted to astrocytes of Ctx and HC	Barnes maze (Hidden & Cued)	**Barnes maze (Hidden)** *Females* Impaired spatial learning and reference memory ↑Latency to find goal box ↓Latency to first correct nose poke ↓Time spent investigating goal box *Males* No effect **Barnes maze (Cued)** *Females* Impaired working memory ↑Latency to find goal box *Males* No effect	Bracchi-Ricard *et al.*, 2008

Abbreviations and symbols used: Ctx, cortex; HC, hippocampus; med, medulla; hyp, hypothalamus; PC, purkinje cells of cerebellum; TNFR, TNF-α receptor; MWM, Morris Water Maze; RAM, Radial Arm Maze; ↑, increased; ↓, decreased.

Table 19.4 The Effects of NF-κB Blockade on Non-spatial Contextual Memory

Subunit	*Subjects*	*Technique*	*Cognitive test*	*Effects*	*Reference*
All	Male mice	Super-repressor (IκBα-SR), robustly expressed in GABAergic interneurons of the Ctx, HC, med, hyp and PC	Object Recognition (LTM)	No effect	O'Mahony *et al.*, 2006
All	Male mice	Super-repressor (IκBα-AA), robustly expressed in glutamatergic neurons of the forebrain	Object Recognition (STM)	No effect	Kaltschmidt *et al.*, 2006
c-Rel	Male and female mice	Subunit-specific knockout, widespread	Object Recognition (LTM)	Impaired object recognition memory; ↓ Time spent investigating a novel object	Ahn *et al.*, 2008

Abbreviations and symbols used: Ctx, cortex; HC, hippocampus; med, medulla; hyp, hypothalamus; PC, purkinje cells of cerebellum; LTM, long-term memory; STM, short-term memory; ↓, decreased.

degradation and stimulated nuclear translocation of NF-κB in cultured astrocytes, effects that were abolished in the presence of the NF-κB inhibitor, pyrrolidine dithiocarbamate (PDTC) (Marcus, Karackattu, Fleegal, and Sumners, 2003). Interestingly, *in vivo* studies show that brain NF-κB is also responsive to immune–brain signaling (Nadjar et al., 2005a, b). For example, intracerebroventricular (i.c.v.) administration of an NF-κB inhibitor, NEMO binding domain (NBD)[2] peptide, inhibited recombinant rat IL-1β (rrIL-1β)-induced expression of cyclooxygenase-2 (COX-2) in endothelial-like cells of the medial septal nucleus (MSN) (Nadjar *et al.*, 2005b). The COX-2 enzyme is activated by inflammatory proteins, such as IL-1β, and is involved in the synthesis of prostaglandins (PGs). In the brain, PGs are responsible for inducing a fever response and for stimulating the hypothalamic-pituitary-adrenal (HPA) axis. Additionally, central administration of NBD attenuated IL-1β-induced anorexia, suggesting that NF-κB also mediates the behavioral effects of peripheral immune stimuli (Nadjar *et al.*, 2005a). Consistent with this, i.c.v. administration of NBD abrogated the expression of *c-Fos*, an immediate early gene (IEG), in limbic and brain-stem regions associated with anxiety, fear and anorexia (Nadjar *et al.*, 2005a). Therefore, these results demonstrate that recruitment of NF-κB in the brain can serve to engage neural substrates of behavioral adaptation to stressors and other cognitive stimuli.

A growing body of evidence suggests that NF-κB is also critical for normal, cognitive function. Studies using invertebrate species have demonstrated that activation of NF-κB is required for the formation of long-term contextual memory (Merlo, Freudenthal, and Romano, 2002; Merlo and Romano, 2007), suggesting that the role of NF-κB in learning and memory-related processes is evolutionarily conserved. However, rodent studies have generated complex and conflicting findings that make it difficult to determine the exact contribution(s) of NF-κB to cognitive function (Yeh *et al.*, 2002; Meffert *et al.*, 2003; Freudenthal *et al.*, 2005; Kaltschmidt *et al.*, 2006; O'Mahony *et al.*, 2006; Ahn *et al.*, 2008; Bracchi-Ricard *et al.*, 2008; Lehmann, Brachman, Listwak, and Herkenham, 2010). Additionally, NF-κB has also been implicated in the molecular mechanisms underpinning the consolidation of long-term memory (LTM) in mammals (Kaltschmidt, Kaltschmidt, and Baeuerle, 1993; Meberg, Kinney, Valcourt, and Routtenberg, 1996; Albensi and Mattson, 2000; Yeh *et al.*, 2002; Meffert *et al.*, 2003; Kaltschmidt *et al.*, 2006; O'Mahony *et al.*, 2006; O'Riordan *et al.*, 2006; Ahn *et al.*, 2008; Bracchi-Ricard *et al.*, 2008; Russo *et al.*, 2009; O'Sullivan *et al.*, 2010). Therefore, in an attempt to shed further light on the role of NF-κB in memory-related processes, the remainder of this paper will review behavioral and molecular evidence that NF-κB is necessary for the consolidation of long-term memory.

Invertebrate Studies

The context-signal memory paradigm

Evidence linking NF-κB to the formation of long-term memory was first described in the context-signal memory paradigm of the crab, *Chasmagnathus* (Freudenthal *et al.*, 1998; Freudenthal and Romano, 2000; Merlo, Freudenthal, and Romano, 2002; Merlo and Romano, 2007). In this model, a crab is presented with a danger stimulus (i.e., an opaque figure passing

[2] NEMO binding domain (NBD) peptide inhibits activation of canonical NF-κB by disrupting the association of IKKβ with NEMO.

overhead, which in learning terminology is the conditioning stimulus or CS). This initially elicits a strong escape response, but which with repeated presentations produces a decline in escape responding. Under certain circumstances (Freudenthal and Romano, 2000), this is referred to as long-term habituation (LTH), and also can be considered an instance of long-term memory (LTM). Specifically, LTM is induced by spaced training protocols that consist of at least 15 or more trials, each separated by an inter-trial interval (ITI) of 100+ seconds (Freudenthal and Romano, 2000). Under these training conditions the crab forms an association between the eliciting stimulus and the context in which it is presented. When the crab is returned to the training context 24 hours later, presentation of the opaque figure will evoke a weak escape response. Conversely, presentation of the danger stimulus outside of the original training context elicits strong escape responding (Hermitte, Pedreira, Tomsic, and Maldonado, 1999). This context-dependent form of LTH appears at both the first trial and all subsequent trials of retention testing and persists for at least one week (Pedreira, Dimant, and Maldonado, 1996). Most importantly, like other types of LTM, context-dependent LTH requires new protein synthesis (Pedreira, Dimant, and Maldonado, 1996).

Given that the consolidation of LTM is dependent on protein synthesis, and that NF-κB regulates gene expression, Freudenthal *et al.* (1998) tested whether the development of LTM was associated with changes in NF-κB activity. As expected, neither exposure to the test apparatus nor the CS induced LTH, and only crabs that received spaced training showed evidence of retention 24 hours later (Freudenthal *et al.*, 1998). More importantly, a electrophoretic mobility shift assay (EMSA) performed with nuclear extracts indicated that spaced training (which produces LTH, and formation of LTM) significantly enhanced neural, but not thoracic[3], NF-κB DNA-binding activity above that observed in active and passive controls (Freudenthal *et al.*, 1998). These findings demonstrate that memory-specific activation of NF-κB is restricted to the brain and suggest that enhanced NF-κB activity is specifically related to LTM consolidation.

However, the changes in κB-like DNA-binding activity reported by Freudenthal *et al.* (1998) were correlational and do not provide direct evidence that activation of the transcription factor is *necessary* for LTM consolidation. To pursue this hypothesis, pre-training blockade of the NF-κB pathway using the IKK inhibitor, sulfasalazine (SSZ), significantly impaired LTH during a retention test performed 48 hours after cessation of training (Merlo, Freudenthal, and Romano, 2002; Merlo and Romano, 2007). This could not be accounted for by performance deficits during training, indicating that activation of NF-κB during spaced training is necessary for consolidation but not acquisition of LTH. Moreover, crabs administered SSZ 5 hours *after* training did not express LTH during retention testing. The latter finding, in particular, strengthens the argument that activation of NF-κB is necessary for the consolidation of LTM. However, it should be noted that while sulfasalazine can prevent phosphorylation of IκB proteins, it can also inhibit cyclooxygenases that promote production of prostaglandins (PG) (Merlo, Freudenthal, and Romano, 2002). This possibility was ruled out by showing that the PG synthesis inhibitor indomethacin had no effect on the acquisition or retention of LTH, thereby reinforcing the interpretation that activation of NF-κB specifically is required for LTM formation (Merlo, Freudenthal, and Romano, 2002).

[3] The thoracic ganglion controls the execution of motor responses, such as escape responding. In the present study no difference in thoracic, nuclear NF-κB activity was observed between trained and control groups (Freudenthal *et al.*, 1998). This finding demonstrates that memory-specific-activation of NF-κB is restricted to the brain, and that execution of the escape response itself does not influence neural NF-κB DNA-binding activity.

Similarly, inhibition of the ubiquitin–proteasome system (UPS) impaired the development of LTH (Merlo and Romano, 2007). Unlike IKK inhibitors, which prevent the phosphorylation of IκB proteins, proteasome inhibitors block activation of NF-κB by preventing the *degradation* of IκB proteins. On the one hand, inhibition of 26S proteasome activity is an effective means of inhibiting NF-κB activity, although it is not specific to the NF-κB system because UPS inhibitors prevent the degradation of many other proteins. Therefore, the possibility that the UPS functions in removing other inhibitory constraints, or that it is necessary for the normal degradation of other cellular proteins, during memory consolidation cannot be ruled out(Merlo and Romano, 2007). Nonetheless, the UPS inhibitor, MG-132, specifically impaired the consolidation of LTM (Merlo and Romano, 2007). Therefore, together with the previous NF-κB inhibition studies (Freudenthal *et al.*, 1998; Freudenthal and Romano, 2000; Merlo, Freudenthal, and Romano, 2002), these experiments using invertebrate models of learning suggest that activation of NF-κB is not only correlated with associative learning but also necessary for the consolidation of LTM.

Studies in Mammals

Associative fear memory

Conditioned fear The role of NF-κB in the formation of associative fear memory was first investigated using fear-potentiated startle (FPS) (Yeh *et al.*, 2002). In this paradigm a previously neutral, conditional stimulus (CS; e.g., a light) is explicitly paired with the presentation of an aversive, unconditional stimulus (US; e.g., foot-shock). Following repeated CS–US presentations, an association between the two stimuli is formed such that the light comes to predict the occurrence of foot-shock. Twenty-four hours later, the startle response to an acoustic stimulus (e.g., a short burst of white noise) is measured in the absence (CS−) and presence (CS+) of the CS on alternating trials. The magnitude of startle potentiation ([startle response on CS+ trial/startle response on CS− trial] × 100) is then taken as an index of learned fear, where values greater than 100% represent strong fear memory and values equal to or less than 100% indicate weak fear memory.

Yeh *et al.* (2002) demonstrated that fear-training was associated with increased NF-κB (p50/p65) activity in the lateral (LA) and basolateral (LA) nuclei of the amygdala. Specifically, 2–6 hours after training, p50/p65 DNA-binding (as measured by electrophoretic mobility) was significantly elevated in conditioned rats only. In contrast, rats that received an equal number of CS and US presentations during training, but in an explicitly *unpaired* fashion (pseudo-conditioned rats), exhibited levels of κB DNA-binding activity similar to that observed in naïve controls. Moreover, fear training generated a rapid (10-minute) increase in IKK activity that persisted for up to 30 minutes. Importantly, these training-specific changes in NF-κB were restricted to regions of the amygdala that are associated with the formation of fear memory.

In this same study, pre-training infusions (30 min prior) of NF-κB inhibitors impaired the development of a FPS response. For instance, intra-LA or BLA infusions of the protease inhibitors N^{α}-p-tosyl-L-lysine chloromethyl ketone (TLCK) or N-tosyl-L-phenylalanine chloromethyl ketone (TPCK) significantly attenuated the magnitude of FPS. Moreover, pretreatment with TLCK blocked the conditioning-induced (DNA) binding of NF-κB (Yeh *et al.*, 2002). Protease inhibitors, such as TLCK and TPCK, prevent NF-κB activation by inhibiting the activity of the 26S proteasome, and consequently the degradation of IκBα inhibitory proteins. However, it should be noted that the 26S proteasome mediates the degradation of many other proteins besides IκBα. Consequently, it could not be determined whether blockade of NF-κB, *specifically*, impaired the formation of fear memory.

Accordingly, Yeh *et al.* (2002) tested whether direct inhibitors of NF-κB similarly disrupted FPS. Specifically, rats were administered either an inhibitor of IKK (thalidomide) or a double-stranded (p50/p65) κB decoy DNA (Yeh *et al.*, 2002). Intra-amygdaloid infusions of thalidomide into the lateral or basolateral amygdala were given 30 minutes prior to training. In a separate group of rats κB decoy DNA was infused into the amygdala at both 2 and 24 hours prior to fear conditioning. The results showed that either form of NF-κB inhibition attenuated significantly fear-potentiated startle. Indeed, given the success of the κB decoy DNA treatment, these findings suggest that activation of NF-κB specifically, and p50/p65 containing dimers in particular, may be *required* for aversive memory consolidation (Yeh *et al.*, 2002). However, by blocking NF-κB activity *prior* to training it was not resolved whether the absence of a potentiated startle reflex was due to impaired acquisition, rather than impaired consolidation, of the CS–US association.

In contrast, Ahn *et al.* (2008) compared amygdala-dependent and hippocampal-dependent fear conditioning paradigms using widespread, subunit-specific, knockout of c-Rel. Amygdala-dependent conditioned-fear learning is specific to discrete cues associated with footshock (e.g., a light or tone linked to the aversive US), whereas hippocampal-dependent learning relies largely on the context in which shock is delivered (e.g., the apparatus or chamber in which the animal is housed when the aversive stimulus is presented). Normal wild-type (c-Rel$^{+/+}$) and c-Rel-deficient (c-Rel$^{-/-}$) mice were trained using a modest conditioned fear paradigm in which animals were subjected to a single CS (white noise)–US (foot-shock) pairing (Ahn *et al.*, 2008). Twenty-four hours later mice were tested for retention of fear memory as measured by freezing (% time spent freezing) in a new context. Irrespective of genotype, mice exhibited high levels of conditioned freezing behavior (≈35%–45%) to the noise CS, suggesting that activation of c-Rel may not be necessary for the formation of amygdala-dependent fear memory.

On the other hand, c-Rel$^{-/-}$ mice spent significantly less time freezing than wild-type mice when re-exposed to the original conditioning context 24 hours after training. Interestingly, activation of c-Rel may support the consolidation of long-term, contextual fear memory as c-Rel$^{-/-}$ mice did not show any deficits in freezing behavior when tested within an hour of CS–US training. Furthermore, in wild-type mice, contextual fear conditioning was associated with increased nuclear localization of c-Rel in the CA1 and dentate gyrus of the hippocampus (Ahn *et al.*, 2008).

Setting aside the obvious differences in species and use of non-discrete deletions of c-Rel in the brain, the foregoing reports by Yeh *et al.* (2002) and Ahn *et al.* (2008) raise the question that NF-κB subunits may be differentially involved in the formation of amygdala and hippocampal-dependent fear memory. That is p50/p65 and c-Rel containing subunits may be critical for consolidating amygdala and hippocampal-dependent fear memories, respectively (Ahn *et al.*, 2008). On the other hand, as discussed below, the contribution of NF-κB to the formation of associative fear memory is further complicated by the finding that conditional suppression of NF-κB spares both cued *and* contextual fear memory in male mice.

It was stated earlier that NF-κB dimers are normally held latent in the cytoplasm, bound to inhibitory proteins (e.g., IκBα), but in response to activating stimuli become phosphorylated at serine residues, Ser 32 and Ser 36, in the N-terminus. This phosphorylation of Ser 32 and Ser 36 tags IκBα for ubiquitination and degradation by the 26S proteasome, producing NF-κB dissociation from the inhibitory protein complex and translocation to the nucleus (see Figure 19.1). In a recent study, Bracchi-Ricard *et al.* (2008) generated transgenic mice overexpressing a truncated form of IκBα that lacks both Ser 32 and Ser 36 residues. Moreover, the expression of this transgene was under the control of the astroglial-specific GFAP promoter. Therefore, in the presence of the transgene (GFAP-IκBα-dn) activation of NF-κB was inhibited specifically in astrocytes. Nevertheless, male GFAP-IκBα-dn and wild-type mice acquired a conditioned-fear response at similar rates and showed equivalent retention of long-term cued or contextual fear memory (Bracchi-Ricard *et al.*, 2008). In the same study, female mice with conditional suppression of astroglial NF-κB showed impaired acquisition of conditioned fear and retrieval of contextual fear memory.

Given the methodological differences between the Ahn *et al.* (2008) study, and the immediately foregoing study by Bracchi *et al.* (2008), it is difficult to make any direct comparisons that might explain their opposite results. Specifically, Ahn *et al.* (2008) generated mice that were deficient throughout the entire CNS and periphery for a specific subunit (c-Rel) of NF-κB. In contrast, the GFAP-IκBα-dn super-repressor transgene prevented the activation of *all* NF-κB subunits, but only in astrocytes (Bracchi-Ricard *et al.*, 2008). Moreover, in both cases it is unknown whether the function of other subunits or signal transduction systems was affected by the absence of endogenous NF-κB. However, it was determined that neither c-Rel deficient mice (Ahn *et al.*, 2008) nor GFAP-IκBα-dn mice (Bracchi-Ricard *et al.*, 2008) demonstrated any gross structural abnormalities or alterations in cellular morphology. All things considered, it is possible that, at least for male mice, NF-κB-dependent signaling in astrocytes is not required for associative-fear learning.

Alternatively, the disparate findings regarding the role of NF-κB in contextual fear memory also raise the importance of how differences in training parameters could contribute to a lack of differentiation in the learning capabilities of different mouse genotypes. Specifically, GFAP-IκBα-dn mice were trained using two CS (white noise)–US (foot-shock) pairings (Bracchi-Ricard *et al.*, 2008) whereas c-Rel$^{-/-}$ mice were trained on a “modest” fear conditioning protocol comprised of only a single CS (white noise) – US (foot-shock) trial (Ahn et al., 2008). Additionally, the intensity and duration of the US differed between the two studies (e.g., 1.5 mA, 2-second foot-shock vs 0.5 mA, 1-second foot-shock). In light of such differences it is possible that the male GFAP-IκBα-dn mice showed normal fear memory because training was sufficient to overcome any type of learning deficit induced by the transgene. In line with this idea is the fact that c-Rel$^{-/-}$ mice, trained using a more “robust” conditioned fear paradigm (three CS–US pairings), exhibited normal levels of freezing behavior (relative to wild-type mice) upon re-exposure to the training context (Ahn *et al.*, 2008). Similarly, it was shown that CaMKII T286A mutants (Irvine, Vernon, and Giese, 2005) and transgenic Alzheimer's disease model mice (Dineley *et al.*, 2002) can overcome learning and memory deficits with additional training.

Finally, comment should be made regarding the sex differences that were observed for Bracchi-Ricard *et al.* (2008). Whereas Ahn *et al.* (2008) used both male and female mice, they did not differentiate freezing behavior on the basis of sex, making it impossible to determine whether their observed deficits in contextual memory were largely, or entirely, attributable to female subjects. Sex differences in peripheral NF-κB expression have been documented (Zhao and Eghbali-Webb, 2002) and other instances of sexual dimorphism in signal transduction have been identified (Kudo *et al.*, 2004). For example, the transcription factor cAMP-response element binding protein (CREB) was differentially activated in female versus male CA1 hippocampal neurons and these gender differences were correlated with sex differences in contextual fear conditioning (Kudo *et al.*). Therefore, such findings raise the question of whether inherent reliance on certain transcription factors to mediate learning effects is dependent on sex-related physiological factors. However, this important question has yet to be resolved in relation to immune-related modulation of learning and memory.

Inhibitory avoidance Evidence implicating NF-κB in the consolidation of aversive memory was provided by *post-training* inhibition of NF-κB. This resulted in disrupted recall of a passive avoidance task that involved measurement of step-down latencies into a compartment previously associated with footshock (Freudenthal *et al.*, 2005). Specifically, immediate but not delayed (3-hour or 24-hour) post-training i.c.v. infusion of the IKK inhibitor, sulfasalazine (SSZ), in rats resulted in significantly shorter latencies to re-enter the compartment, when compared to saline-infused controls. Additionally, pre-training administration of (p50/p65) κB decoy DNA significantly impaired the formation of long-term passive avoidance memory, but spared performance during training.

Inhibitory avoidance memory represents a type of aversive (contextual) memory that is in part dependent on the hippocampus (Izquierdo *et al.*, 1997). Accordingly, hippocampal κB DNA binding was measured at several time points after training (Freudenthal *et al.*, 2005). Results revealed a significant decrease (below that of naïve controls) in p50/p65 DNA binding 15 minutes after training followed by a significant increase in DNA binding activity at 45 minutes (Freudenthal *et al.*, 2005). However, these post-conditioning fluctuations in p50/p65 did not differ between trained (shocked; SH) and untrained (unshocked; USH) animals, suggesting that the observed changes in NF-κB were not specific to associations being formed between the CS and US (Freudenthal *et al.*, 2005). Rather, the activity of the p50/p65 dimers could support other aspects of inhibitory avoidance learning, such as encoding of contextual information in extra-hippocampal regions (Freudenthal *et al.*, 2005).

Spatial learning and memory

The Morris Water Maze (MWM), Radial Arm Maze (RAM) and Barnes Maze There have been few studies that have evaluated the role of NF-κB in spatial cognition (Meffert *et al.*, 2003; Kaltschmidt *et al.*, 2006; O'Mahony *et al.*, 2006; Bracchi-Ricard, *et al.*, 2008; Lehmann, Brachman, Listwak, and Herkenham, 2010). Testing for spatial learning and memory typically requires animals to use distinct cues in a given context to enable the location of food (e.g., RAM and the Barnes maze) and opportunities for escape (e.g., MWM). In one study transgenic mice were generated that expressed a non-phosphorylatable, and therefore non-degradable, form of IκBα in GABAergic neurons in the cerebellum, cortex, thalamus and midbrain (O'Mahony *et al.*, 2006). This transgene, termed the IκBα super repressor (IκBα-SR), was cloned downstream of a tetracycline transactivator (tTA)-responsive promoter (Tet-O). Animals that positively expressed the IκBα transgene were then crossed with mice bearing a tTA transgene, driven by a prion promoter-enhancer (Prp). In this way, expression of IκBα-SR could be regulated by oral administration of doxycycline (DOX), a tetracycline analogue that readily crosses the blood–brain barrier (BBB). In the *absence* of DOX, bigenic mice robustly expressed the IκBα-SR transgene (tTA/IκBα-SR$^+$) and activation of NF-κB was suppressed. However, in the *presence* of DOX, transcription of the super repressor was completely inhibited allowing for normal NF-κB activity (O'Mahony *et al.*, 2006).

Using this model O'Mahony *et al.* (2006) determined that tTA/IκBα-SR$^+$ mice exhibited superior spatial learning in both the Morris water maze (MWM) and radial arm maze (RAM) tasks. For instance, in the MWM, where mice have to swim and locate an escape platform, the tTA/IκBα-SR$^+$ mice located both the visible and hidden platforms in significantly less time than non-transgenic and single transgenic (IκBα-SR) controls, or the bigenic tTA/IκBα-SR$^+$ mice maintained on a DOX diet from one month of age onward (rendering them tTA/IκBα-SR$^-$ and therefore able to display NF-κB activity). By day 3of training, all mice showed a strong memory for the platform location, whereas tTA/IκBα-SR$^+$ mice exhibited a significant preference for the target quadrant (where the hidden platform was located) after only 1 day of training (O'Mahony et al., 2006). Similarly, in the radial arm maze tTA/IκBα-SR$^+$ mice exhibited significantly shorter latencies (relative to the above controls) to complete the maze and retrieve all food pellets. Moreover, mutant mice made significantly fewer errors (re-entries into previously visited arms) than tTA/IκBα-SR$^-$ or control mice (O'Mahony *et al.*, 2006). These results suggest that an inhibition of NF-κB activation (which occurred in tTA/IκBα-SR$^+$ mice) supported better spatial learning and memory formation.

However, in direct opposition to these observations, Kaltschmidt *et al.* (2006) demonstrated that suppression of NF-κB disrupted performance in the MWM. In this study, the authors generated a double-transgenic mouse model such that the inducible expression of an IκBα super repressor transgene (IκBα-AA) was driven by a tetracycline, tTA transgene cloned downstream of the calcium/calmodulin dependent Kinase II (CAMKIIα) promoter. Thus, IκBα-AA was predominantly expressed in excitatory neurons of the forebrain (Kaltschmidt *et al.*, 2006). Relative to various transgenic controls[4] (IκBα-AA and IκBα + DOX) and DOX-treated bigenic mice[5] (tTA/IκBα-AA + DOX), mice that lacked the ability to show NF-κB activation (the tTA/IκBα-AA double-transgenic mice), exhibited impaired learning, the results showing higher escape latencies across all days of hidden platform training (Kaltschmidt *et al.*, 2006). Moreover, during a probe test (conducted 5 days after the last training session) to determine memory for platform location, tTA/IκBα-AA double-transgenic mice traveled a significantly shorter distance and spent significantly less time in the target quadrant than single-transgenic controls (Kaltschmidt *et al.*, 2006). These effects were not due to any visual or motor deficits.

How then, can conditional inhibition of NF-κB both improve (O'Mahony *et al.*, 2006) and impair (Kaltschmidt *et al.*, 2006) spatial cognition? Notwithstanding significant differences between the models, with respect to promoter activity and the brain regions involved, it is tempting to speculate that conflicting observations reflect cell-type specific functions of NF-κB (Kaltschmidt *et al.*, 2006; O'Mahony *et al.*, 2006). For instance, conditional suppression of NF-κB in GABAergic interneurons could have enhanced memory formation by diminishing inhibitory tone and enhancing excitatory transmission (O'Mahony *et al.*, 2006). Consistent with this idea, the expression of mRNA and protein for GAD65 (the rate-limiting enzyme necessary to make the inhibitory neurotransmitter GABA), was dramatically reduced in

[4] Single-transgenic controls (IκBα-AA) refer to mice expressing the IκBα transgene but *not* the tetracycline, trans-activator (tTA) transgene. Therefore, IκBα-AA mice exhibit normal NF-κB activity, as the mutant gene cannot be expressed.

[5] In contrast to single-transgenic mice, double-transgenic mice express both the mutant IκBα gene and the trans-activator gene. Therefore, endogenous NF-κB cannot dissociate from the IκBα protein. However, in the presence of DOX, the transactivator transgene product cannot bind to the IκBα-AA promoter. Thus, DOX restores normal NF-κB activity.

hippocampal extracts obtained from NF-κB deficient tTA/IκBα-SR$^+$ mice (O'Mahony *et al.*, 2006). Reduction of GAD65 would decrease the production of GABA and disrupt the balance between excitatory and inhibitory transmission. Therefore, it could be hypothesized that inhibition of NF-κB, in GABAergic cells, may have augmented the activity of glutamatergic neurons and enhanced memory consolidation (O'Mahony *et al.*, 2006).

To account for the observation that blockade of NF-κB in excitatory neurons impaired spatial learning and memory (Kaltschmidt *et al.*, 2006), electrophysiological measures of synaptic plasticity were performed in the hippocampal Schaffer CA3-CA1 pathway. Specifically, this involved induction of long-term potentiation (LTP), which is considered to be a neurophysiological index of learning and memory formation (Lynch, 2004). It was observed that LTP was significantly reduced in tTA/IκBα-AA double transgenic mice (Kaltschmidt *et al.*, 2006), suggesting that conditional suppression of NF-κB in excitatory neurons could have induced memory deficits by disrupting forms of synaptic plasticity that are dependent on protein synthesis. This was supported by reduced hippocampal mRNA expression of the catalytic subunit of cyclic AMP (cAMP)-dependent protein kinase A and impaired phosphorylation of the transcription factor, CREB (Kaltschmidt *et al.*, 2006). Given that phosphorylated CREB is a critical step in the molecular processes thought to support the conversion of short-term memory to long-term memory (Abel *et al.*, 1997), these findings lend credence to the poor spatial learning of NF-κB deficient mice.

As if the above studies using conditional knockout technology were not sufficiently problematic to resolve, other studies using subunit-specific, knockout mice have generated similarly conflicting results (Meffert *et al.*, 2003; Lehmann, Brachman, Listwak, and Herkenham, 2010). For instance, on a five-day MWM task, p50$^{-/-}$ mice displayed faster learning and memory formation than their wild-type counterparts (Lehmann, Brachman, Listwak, and Herkenham, 2010). Whereas in mice with a concomitant ablation of the p65 and TNF-α receptor (TNFR) gene,[6] acquisition of spatial learning in an 8-arm, radial arm maze (RAM) was impaired (Meffert *et al.*, 2003).

Perhaps these disparities reflect differential involvement of NF-κB subunits in a task-dependent manner. For instance, although p50$^{-/-}$ mice exhibited superior learning in the MWM, their learning in the Barnes maze showed normal acquisition and retention (Lehmann, Brachman, Listwak, and Herkenham, 2010). While the Barnes maze and MWM both assess spatial learning, the former is considered less aversive. Therefore, it could be hypothesized that endogenous p50 influences learning under stressful conditions. Consistent with this hypothesis, endogenous p50 modulates the hypothalamic–pituitary–adrenal (HPA) axis response to stress, and deletion of p50 produced an anxiogenic phenotype in standard tests of anxiety-like behavior, such as the open field and elevated plus maze (Lehmann, Brachman, Listwak, and Herkenham, 2010). Indeed, when corticosterone elevations were blocked in p50$^{-/-}$ mice, MWM learning was no longer observed to be different from wild-type controls (Lehmann, Brachman, Listwak, and Herkenham, 2010). While this is consistent with the long-held view that glucocorticoids may be necessary (at moderate levels) to promote learning, these data also suggest that central NF-κB, and p50 in particular, may be necessary to ensure that glucocorticoid facilitation of learning is optimal.

[6] It should be noted that concomitant ablation of both the p65 and TNFR gene was necessary because deletion of p65 by itself is lethal at the embryonic stage (Beg and Sha 1995). However, simultaneous deletion of the TNFR gene rescues lethality (Rosenfield, Prichard et al. 2000).

Non-spatial, contextual memory

The object-recognition task Perhaps not surprisingly, given the complexity of findings discussed so far, the role of NF-κB in non-spatial memory tasks is no less ambiguous. The object recognition task involves an initial familiarization with an object that subsequently (e.g., 24 hours later) is presented again with a novel object that an animal has not previously encountered. Memory for the previously encountered object is measured as a ratio of the percent time spent with the novel object (i.e. animals orient to and explore a less familiar object). This task is hippocampal-dependent, although O'Mahony *et al.* (2006) reported no modification of object memory through conditional suppression of NF-κB activity. Similarly, conditional suppression of NF-κB in glutamatergic cells spared the formation of short-term object recognition (Kaltschmidt *et al.*, 2006). In stark contrast, genetic ablation of the c-Rel subunit produced deficits in long-term object recognition (Ahn *et al.*, 2008). Mice were first habituated (days 1–3) to an open field apparatus containing Lego blocks. Twenty-four hours later (day 4), two identical objects made from the familiar Legos were placed into the open field and mice were allowed to explore the objects for 10 minutes. On day 5, one of the familiar objects was replaced with a novel object and long-term object memory was assessed by measuring the time spent exploring each object. It was demonstrated that c-Rel$^{-/-}$ mice spent significantly less time exploring the novel object than their wild-type counterparts (c-Rel$^{+/+}$), suggesting that endogenous c-Rel participates in the formation of long-term, non-spatial, contextual memory (Ahn *et al.*, 2008).

It should be noted, however, that exploratory behavior per se is altered by NF-κB manipulation. For example, mutant tTA/IκBα-SR$^+$ (that have suppressed NF-κB activity) exhibited enhanced exploratory behavior in both the elevated plus maze and open field tests (O'Mahony *et al.*, 2006), which contrasts with the finding that p50$^{-/-}$ mice show inhibited exploration (Lehmann, Brachman, Listwak, and Herkenham, 2010). This is likely to be due to selective differences in what precisely is lost within the NF-κB complex of regulatory and transcriptional elements, and in the case of the tTA/IκBα-SR$^+$ mice, may be due to their known hyperactive phenotype (O'Mahony *et al.*, 2006; Ahn *et al.*, 2008). This could have masked any memory deficits produced by conditional suppression of NF-κB. Moreover, with respect to the findings of Kaltschmidt *et al.* (2006), who conditionally inhibited NF-κB in excitatory neurons, only short-term memory was assessed in the object recognition task, whereas long-term object memory was tested in c-Rel$^{-/-}$ mice (Ahn *et al.*, 2008). Consequently, it is not known whether NF-κB-mediated transcription in glutamatergic neurons is involved in the formation of long-term, object recognition memory.

Section summary

Overall, and although at times perplexing, given the differing approaches to interfering with NF-κB activation and/or activity, the literature to date does provide evidence for the involvement of NF-κB in memory formation. In the crab, NF-κB appears to support the consolidation of long-term contextual memory (Freudenthal *et al.*, 1998; Freudenthal and Romano, 2000; Merlo, Freudenthal, and Romano, 2002; Merlo and Romano, 2007), although as just reviewed, in the rodent it may play a broader role in many different types of memory. Specifically, NF-κB participates in the formation of associative fear memory, hippocampal-dependent spatial memory and non-spatial, contextual memory, as tested using object recognition. Moreover, rodent studies also suggest that NF-κB is necessary for the acquisition of new information

(Kaltschmidt *et al.*, 2006; O'Mahony *et al.*, 2006; Bracchi-Ricard *et al.*, 2008; (Lehmann, Brachman, Listwak, and Herkenham, 2010).

It is apparent, however, that we lack a firm prediction regarding how NF-κB is engaged during learning events, and what are the downstream events that might follow NF-κB activation. Some progress in this regard has been made, as exemplified by the changes in CREB that were reported subsequent to spatial learning. However, the literature at present is still quite small, making comparisons between contradictory effects based on differing technical procedures (and involving different NF-κB targets) largely speculative. What is particularly interesting is the suggestion that NF-κB effects on learning may be specific to its modulation in neurons. Whether this is something that directly and/or indirectly relies on glial cells, remains to be determined, although evidence exists for the role of astrocytes and microglial cells in learning and memory (Yirmiya and Goshen, 2011). Only further experimentation and selective manipulation of NF-κB in different brain regions and cell types will provide additional answers.

Molecular Evidence for NF-κB in the Consolidation of Long-Term Memory

Synaptic plasticity

Recent findings have implicated NF-κB in long-term potentiation (Albensi and Mattson, 2000; Kaltschmidt, *et al.*, 2006; O'Mahony *et al.*, 2006; O'Riordan *et al.*, 2006; Ahn *et al.*, 2008; Bracchi-Ricard *et al.*, 2008). Long term potentiation (LTP) was first described over forty years ago (Bliss and Lomo, 1973) and is characterized by an enduring increase in synaptic strength. In the hippocampus, a brain region critically involved in memory acquisition (Bannerman *et al.*, 2004), LTP is induced by the simultaneous stimulation of a presynaptic neuron and adequate depolarization of a postsynaptic cell (Lynch, 2004).

This property of associativity ensures that LTP remains input specific, occurring at stimulated synapses only. Moreover, strong depolarization of the postsynaptic cell paired with presynaptic glutamate release results in the activation of postsynaptic, *N*-methyl *D*-aspartate (NMDAr) receptors and calcium (Ca^{2+}) influx. Ultimately, the opening of NMDAr and Ca^{2+} triggers an intracellular cascade of events that produces long-term changes in the postsynaptic cell. These features (input specificity, associativity), coupled with the fact that LTP is rapidly induced and may persist for up to several weeks, are also typical of learning and memory. It is for these reasons that LTP remains the most intensively studied form of synaptic plasticity and is believed to be a physical representation for the formation of new memories.

Notably, stimuli that induce LTP also activate NF-κB. For instance, *in vitro* high-frequency stimulation (HFS) of the perforant path[7] significantly increased p65 and p50 mRNA expression in granule cells of the dentate gyrus (DG) (Meberg, Kinney, Valcourt, and Routtenberg, 1996), and induced nuclear κB-DNA binding in hippocampal extracts (Freudenthal, Romano, and Routtenberg, 2004). Similarly, in amygdala slices, tetanic stimulation or application of forskolin induced p65/p50 and p50/p50 DNA binding as well as IκBα degradation (Yeh *et al.*, 2002). Finally, *in vivo*, significantly greater p65 immunostaining was detected in the

[7] Axons emanating from the entorhinal cortex and terminating onto granule cells of the dentate gyrus.

dentate gyrus, CA3 and CA1 areas of the hippocampus 15 minutes after HFS than after low-frequency stimulation (LFS) of the perforant path (Freudenthal, Romano, and Routtenberg, 2004). Although some p65 immunostaining was evident following low-frequency electrical stimulation, it should be noted that in this particular assay, cytoplasmic expression was not differentiated from that of nuclear staining (Freudenthal, Romano, and Routtenberg, 2004). Therefore, following LFS some NF-κB may be liberated from IκB proteins without translocation to the nucleus (Freudenthal, Romano, and Routtenberg, 2004). Moreover, in light of the fact that LFS does not induce LTP, and that HFS only induced nuclear p65 DNA-binding (Freudenthal, Romano, and Routtenberg, 2004) these results can be taken as evidence for stimulus-specific, NF-κB activation.

Inhibition of NF-κB has been shown to disrupt the formation of LTP and prevented the formation of long-term depression (LTD), another form of synaptic plasticity characterized by long-term *decreases* in synaptic strength (Albensi and Mattson, 2000; Freudenthal, Romano, and Routtenberg, 2004). More specifically, conditional suppression of NF-κB in glutamatergic cells impaired the late, but not the early, phase of LTP following theta burst stimulation (TBS) of Schaffer collateral axons[8] (Kaltschmidt *et al.*, 2006). Similarly, pretreatment of hippocampal slices with double-stranded, κB decoy DNA reduced the magnitude of LTP, and prevented the formation of LTD (Albensi and Mattson, 2000). Besides non-specific inhibition of NF-κB, subunit-specific knockout has also impaired synaptic plasticity *in vivo*, where c-Rel$^{-/-}$ mice exhibited deficits in LTP in the hippocampus (O'Riordan *et al.*, 2006; Ahn *et al.*, 2008). Since LTP persists for up to several hours *in vitro* and for weeks *in vivo*, it is notable that both LTP and LTD require mRNA transcription and new protein synthesis (Bannerman *et al.*, 2004). That blockade of endogenous NF-κB selectively inhibited protein synthesis-dependent forms of synaptic plasticity is in good agreement with behavioral evidence that NF-κB supports the consolidation of short-term into long-term memory (Yeh *et al.*, 2002; Freudenthal *et al.*, 2005; Ahn *et al.*, 2008).

How then does NF-κB sustain activity-dependent changes in synapse efficiency? One suggestion is that it serves as a signal transducer converting input from distal processes into long-term transcriptional changes (Meberg, Kinney, Valcourt, and Routtenberg, 1996; Meffert *et al.*, 2003). Consistent with this, NF-κB exhibits a unique, subcellular localization throughout the CNS, with latent dimers (p50, p65 or c-Rel containing dimers) in neurons being restricted to proximal and distal dendrites and the pre-synaptic terminal. In response to glutamatergic stimulation of hippocampal neurons these latent dimers are activated and translocate to the nucleus, with p65 redistribution from the cytoplasm to the nucleus occurring gradually (Wellmann, Kaltschmidt, and Kaltschmidt, 2001; Meffert *et al.*, 2003). Within the nucleus activated NF-κB could then induce the expression of plasticity-associated genes, such as neuronal cell adhesion molecule (NCAM) (Simpson and Morris, 2000), a transmembrane glycoprotein expressed on the surface of neurons and certain immune cells, and important for brain development (Dityatev, Bukalo, and Schachner, 2008). However, in the developed brain, NCAM is increased in dendritic spines in response to a variety of stimuli, including the induction of LTP (Schuster, Krug, Hassan, and Schachner, 1998), with the increase in NCAM requiring de novo synthesis through possible transcriptional regulation by NF-κB binding to the NCAM promoter region (Simpson and Morris, 2000).

[8] Axons emanating from area CA3 of the hippocampus and terminating onto pyrimadal cells of area CA1; CA3-CA1 pathway.

In addition to NCAM, NF-κB may regulate the expression of other structure-related genes. Putative NF-κB binding motifs have been identified along the promoter regions of the Slit and Trk-like family member 1 (Slitrk1) and T-lymphoma and metastisis 1 (Tiam1) genes (O'Sullivan *et al.*, 2010). Both Slitrk1 and Tiam1 are expressed in the hippocampus and have been implicated in neuronal growth (Aruga and Mikoshiba, 2003; Matsuo, Terao, Nabeshima, and Hoshino, 2003). Interestingly, learning-specific upregulation of these genes was observed in the DG of the hippocampus after passive avoidance training, and this was associated with robust nuclear localization of p65 (O'Sullivan *et al.*, 2010).

Since mammalian LTP and learning are associated with postsynaptic, structural modifications, such as increased dendritic spine density or altered synaptic clustering, NF-κB may promote the consolidation of memory by initiating, or sustaining, some type of activity-dependent cellular plasticity. Blockade of NF-κB *in vitro* and *in vivo* inhibited neurite outgrowth (O'Sullivan *et al.*, 2010), prevented nerve growth factor (NGF)-induced differentiation of PC-12 cells, and the formation of dendritic spines in hippocampal neurons (Russo *et al.*, 2009). In addition to other evidence for the regulation of brain derived neurotrophic factor (BDNF), these findings provide potential molecular pathways through which endogenous NF-κB could support long-term changes in neuronal function and the formation of new memories (Simpson and Morris, 2000; Russo *et al.*, 2009; O'Sullivan *et al.*, 2010).

Conclusions and Future Directions

An accumulation of behavioral and molecular evidence points to a role for NF-κB in learning and memory related processes. Rodent studies (summarized in Tables 19.2–19.4) offer little evidence to suggest that NF-κB is exclusively required for the consolidation of memory, but likely plays a broader role. What that may be is difficult to surmise, as the present set of empirical investigations have generated complex and conflicting results. In particular, blockade of NF-κB through various means has both impaired and enhanced cognitive function.

One possible explanation for inconsistencies within the rodent literature could be related to subunit specificity. Consistent with this, targeted deletion of p65 impaired spatial navigation in the radial arm maze (Meffert *et al.* 2003) yet genetic ablation of p50 facilitated learning and enhanced long-term memory in the MWM (Lehmann, Brachman, Listwak, and Herkenham, 2010). Such observations suggest that p65 and p50, respectively, promote and hinder normal spatial learning. This hypothesis would be consistent with the selective functions of NF-κB in the immune system (Franzoso *et al.*, 1997; Weih, Yilmaz, and Weih, 2001; Pizzi *et al.*, 2002). For instance, in the spleen, p52 and Rel-B are differentially responsible for the formation of different types of macrophage populations (Franzoso *et al.*, 1997; Weih, Yilmaz, and Weih, 2001). Similarly, in the CNS c-Rel protects neurons from apoptosis induced by glutamate whereas p65 actually mediates the toxic effects of glutamate-induced cytotoxicity (Pizzi *et al.*, 2002). Such subunit specificity and/or reliance is likely to emerge in future studies addressing NF-κB and cognitive processes.

Acknowledgements

This work was supported by a grant from the National Institutes for Health: NIEHS P30 ES05022.

References

Abel, T., Nguyen, P.V., Barad, M., Deuel, T.A., Kandel, E.R., and Bourtchouladze, R. (1997). Genetic demonstration of a role for PKA in the late phase of LTP and in hippocampus-based long-term memory. *Cell*, 88, 615–626.

Ahn, H.J., Hernandez, C.M., Levenson, J.M., Lubin, F.D., Liou, H.C., and Sweatt, J.D. (2008). c-Rel, an NF-kappaB family transcription factor, is required for hippocampal long-term synaptic plasticity and memory formation. *Learning and Memory*, 15, 539–549.

Albensi, B.C., and Mattson, M.P. (2000). Evidence for the involvement of TNF and NF-kappaB in hippocampal synaptic plasticity. *Synapse*, 35, 151–159.

Aruga, J., and Mikoshiba, K. (2003). Identification and characterization of Slitrk, a novel neuronal transmembrane protein family controlling neurite outgrowth. *Molecular and Cellular Neuroscience*, 24, 117–129.

Bannerman, D.M., Rawlins, J.N., McHugh, S.B., Deacon, R.M., Yee, B.K., Bast, T., et al. (2004). Regional dissociations within the hippocampus – memory and anxiety. *Neuroscience and Biobehavioral Reviews*, 28, 273–283.

Barger, S.W., Moerman, A.M., Mao, X. (2005). Molecular mechanisms of cytokine-induced neuroprotection: NFkappaB and neuroplasticity. *Current Pharmaceutical Design*, 11, 985–998.

Bliss, T.V., and Lomo, T. (1973). Long-lasting potentiation of synaptic transmission in the dentate area of the anaesthetized rabbit following stimulation of the perforant path. *Journal of Physiology*, 232, 331–356.

Bonizzi, G., and Karin, M. (2004). The two NF-kappaB activation pathways and their role in innate and adaptive immunity. *Trends in Immunology*, 25, 280–288.

Bracchi-Ricard, V., Brambilla, R., Levenson, J., Hu, W.H., Bramwell, A., Sweatt, J.D., et al. (2008). Astroglial nuclear factor-kappaB regulates learning and memory and synaptic plasticity in female mice. *Journal of Neurochemistry*, 104, 611–623.

Caamaño, J.H., Rizzo, C.A., Durham, S.K., Barton, D.S., Raventós-Suárez, C., Snapper, C.M., et al. (1998). Nuclear factor (NF)-kappa B2 (p100/p52) is required for normal splenic microarchitecture and B cell-mediated immune responses. *Journal of Experimental Medicine*, 187, 185–196.

Dineley, K.T., Xia, X., Bui, D., Sweatt, J.D., and Zheng, H. (2002). Accelerated plaque accumulation, associative learning deficits, and up-regulation of alpha 7 nicotinic receptor protein in transgenic mice co-expressing mutant human presenilin 1 and amyloid precursor proteins. *Journal of Biological Chemistry*, 277, 22768–22780.

Dityatev, A., Bukalo, O., and Schachner, M. (2008). Modulation of synaptic transmission and plasticity by cell adhesion and repulsion molecules. *Neuron Glia Biology*, 4, 197–209.

Doi, T.S., Takahashi, T., Taguchi, O., Azuma, T., and Obata, Y. (1997). NF-kappa B RelA-deficient lymphocytes: normal development of T cells and B cells, impaired production of IgA and IgG1 and reduced proliferative responses. *Journal of Experimental Medicine*, 185, 953–961.

Foehr, E.D., Lin, X., O'Mahoney, A., Geleziunas, R., Bradshaw, R.A., and Greene, W.C. (2000). NF-kappa B signaling promotes both cell survival and neurite process formation in nerve growth factor-stimulated PC12 cells. *Journal of Neuroscience*, 20, 7556–7563.

Franzoso, G., Carlson, L., Scharton-Kersten, T., Shores, E.W., Epstein, S., Grinberg, A., et al. (1997). Critical roles for the Bcl-3 oncoprotein in T cell-mediated immunity, splenic microarchitecture, and germinal center reactions. *Immunity*, 6, 479–490.

Freudenthal, R., Boccia, M.M., Acosta, G.B., Blake, M.G., Merlo, E., Baratti, C.M., et al. (2005). NF-kappaB transcription factor is required for inhibitory avoidance long-term memory in mice. *European Journal of Neuroscience*, 21, 2845–2852.

Freudenthal, R., Locatelli, F., Hermitte, G., Maldonado, H., Lafourcade, C., Delorenzi, A., et al. (1998). Kappa-B like DNA-binding activity is enhanced after spaced training that induces long-term memory in the crab Chasmagnathus. *Neuroscience Letters*, 242, 143–146.

Freudenthal, R., and Romano, A. (2000). Participation of Rel/NF-kappaB transcription factors in long-term memory in the crab Chasmagnathus. *Brain Research*, 855, 274–281.

Freudenthal, R., Romano, A., and Routtenberg, A. (2004). Transcription factor NF-kappaB activation after in vivo perforant path LTP in mouse hippocampus. *Hippocampus*, 14, 677–683.

Ghosh, P., Tan, T.H., Rice, N.R., Sica, A., and Young, H.A. (1993). The interleukin 2 CD28-responsive complex contains at least three members of the NF kappa B family: c-Rel, p50, and p65. *Proceedings of the National Academy of Sciences of the United States of America*, 90, 1696–1700.

Grigoriadis, G., Zhan, Y., Grumont, R.J., Metcalf, D., Handman, E., Cheers, C., et al. (1996). The Rel subunit of NF-kappaB-like transcription factors is a positive and negative regulator of macrophage gene expression: distinct roles for Rel in different macrophage populations. *EMBO Journal*, 15, 7099–7107.

Grundstrom, S., Anderson, P., Scheipers, P., and Sundstedt, A. (2004). Bcl-3 and NFkappaB p50-p50 homodimers act as transcriptional repressors in tolerant CD4+ T cells. *Journal of Biological Chemistry*, 279, 8460–8468.

Guerrini, L., F. Blasi, F., and Denis-Donini, S. (1995). Synaptic activation of NF-kappa B by glutamate in cerebellar granule neurons in vitro. *Proceedings of the National Academy of Sciences of the United States of America*, 92, 9077–9081.

Guinamard, R., Okigaki, M., Schlessinger, J., and Ravetch, J.V. (2000). Absence of marginal zone B cells in Pyk-2-deficient mice defines their role in the humoral response. *Nature Immunology*, 1, 31–36.

Hayden, M.S., West, A.P., and Ghosh, S. (2006). NF-kappaB and the immune response. *Oncogene*, 25, 6758–6780.

Hermitte, G., Pedreira, M.E., Tomsic, D., and Maldonado, H. (1999). Context shift and protein synthesis inhibition disrupt long-term habituation after spaced, but not massed, training in the crab Chasmagnathus. *Neurobiology of Learning and Memory*, 71, 34–49.

Horwitz, B.H., Scott, M.L., Cherry, S.R., Bronson, R.T., and Baltimore, D. (1997). Failure of lymphopoiesis after adoptive transfer of NF-kappaB-deficient fetal liver cells. *Immunity*, 6, 765–772.

Irvine, E.E., Vernon, J., and Giese, K.P. (2005). AlphaCaMKII autophosphorylation contributes to rapid learning but is not necessary for memory. *Nature Neuroscience*, 8, 411–412.

Izquierdo, I., Quillfeldt, J.A., Zanatta, M.S., Quevedo, J., Schaeffer, E., Schmitz, P.K., et al. (1997). Sequential role of hippocampus and amygdala, entorhinal cortex and parietal cortex in formation and retrieval of memory for inhibitory avoidance in rats. *European Journal of Neuroscience*, 9, 786–793.

Kaltschmidt, B., Ndiaye, D., Korte, M., Pothion, S., Arbibe, L., Prüllage, M., et al. (2006). NF-kappaB regulates spatial memory formation and synaptic plasticity through protein kinase A/CREB signaling. *Molecular and Cellular Biology*, 26, 2936–2946.

Kaltschmidt, C., Kaltschmidt, B., and Baeuerle, P.A. (1993). Brain synapses contain inducible forms of the transcription factor NF-kappa B. *Mechanisms of Development*, 43, 135–147.

Kaltschmidt, C., Kaltschmidt, B., and Baeuerle, P.A. (1995). Stimulation of ionotropic glutamate receptors activates transcription factor NF-kappa B in primary neurons. *Proceedings of the National Academy of Sciences of the United States of America*, 92, 9618–9622.

Kassed, C.A., Willing, A.E., Garbuzova-Davis, S., Sanberg, P.R., and Pennypacker, K.R. (2002). Lack of NF-kappaB p50 exacerbates degeneration of hippocampal neurons after chemical exposure and impairs learning. *Experimental Neurology*, 176, 277–288.

Köntgen, F., Grumont, R.J., Strasser, A., Metcalf, D., L:i, R., Tarlinton, D., et al. (1995). Mice lacking the c-rel proto-oncogene exhibit defects in lymphocyte proliferation, humoral immunity, and interleukin-2 expression. *Genes and Development*, 9, 1965–1977.

Kudo, K., Qiao, C.X., Kanba, S., and Arita, J., (2004). A selective increase in phosphorylation of cyclic AMP response element-binding protein in hippocampal CA1 region of male, but not female, rats following contextual fear and passive avoidance conditioning. *Brain Research*, 1024, 233–243.

Lehmann, M.L., Brachman, R.A., Listwak, S.J., and Herkenham, M. (2010). NF-kappaB activity affects learning in aversive tasks: possible actions via modulation of the stress axis. *Brain, Behavior, and Immunity*, 24, 1008–1017.

Lynch, M.A. (2004). Long-term potentiation and memory. *Physiological Reviews*, 84, 87–136.

Marcus, J.S., Karackattu, S.L., Fleegal, M.A., and Sumners, C. (2003). Cytokine-stimulated inducible nitric oxide synthase expression in astroglia: role of Erk mitogen-activated protein kinase and NF-kappaB. *Glia*, 41, 152–160.

Matsuo, N., Terao, M., Nabeshima, Y., and Hoshino, M. (2003). Roles of STEF/Tiam1, guanine nucleotide exchange factors for Rac1, in regulation of growth cone morphology. *Molecular and Cellular Neurosciences*, 24, 69–81.

Mattson, M.P., Goodman, Y., Luo, H., Fu, W., and Furukawa, K. (1997). Activation of NF-kappaB protects hippocampal neurons against oxidative stress-induced apoptosis: evidence for induction of manganese superoxide dismutase and suppression of peroxynitrite production and protein tyrosine nitration. *Journal of Neuroscience Research*, 49, 681–697.

Mattson, M.P., and Meffert, M.K. (2006). Roles for NF-kappaB in nerve cell survival, plasticity, and disease. *Cell Death and Differentiation*, 13, 852–860.

Meberg, P.J., Kinney, W.R., Valcourt, E.G., and Routtenberg, A. (1996). Gene expression of the transcription factor NF-kappa B in hippocampus: regulation by synaptic activity. *Brain Research. Molecular Brain Research*, 38, 179–190.

Meffert, M.K., Chang, J.M., Wiltgen, B.J., Fanselow, M.F., and Baltimore, D. (2003). NF-kappa B functions in synaptic signaling and behavior. *Nature Neuroscience*, 6, 1072–1078.

Merlo, E., Freudenthal, R., and Romano, A. (2002). The IkappaB kinase inhibitor sulfasalazine impairs long-term memory in the crab Chasmagnathus. *Neuroscience*, 112, 161–172.

Merlo, E., and Romano, A. (2007). Long-term memory consolidation depends on proteasome activity in the crab Chasmagnathus. *Neuroscience*, 147, 46–52.

Nadjar, A., Bluthé, R.M., May, M.J., Dantzer, R., and Parnet, P. (2005a). Inactivation of the cerebral NFkappaB pathway inhibits interleukin-1beta-induced sickness behavior and c-Fos expression in various brain nuclei. *Neuropsychopharmacology*, 30, 1492–1499.

Nadjar, A., Tridon, V., May, M.J., Ghosh, S., Dantzer, R., Amédée, T., et al. (2005b). NFkappaB activates in vivo the synthesis of inducible Cox-2 in the brain. *Journal of Cerebral Blood Flow and Metabolism*, 25, 1047–1059.

Newton, R., Holden, N.S., Catley, M.C., Oyelusi, W., Leigh, R., Proud, D., et al. (2007). Repression of inflammatory gene expression in human pulmonary epithelial cells by small-molecule IkappaB kinase inhibitors. *Journal of Pharmacology and Experimental Therapeutics*, 321, 734–742.

O'Mahony, A., Raber, J., Montano, M., Foehr, E., Han, V., Lu, S.M., et al. (2006). NF-kappaB/Rel regulates inhibitory and excitatory neuronal function and synaptic plasticity. *Molecular and Cellular Biology*, 26, 7283–7298.

O'Riordan, K.J., Huang, I.C., Pizzi, M., Spano, P., Boroni, F., Egli, R., et al. (2006). Regulation of nuclear factor kappaB in the hippocampus by group I metabotropic glutamate receptors. *Journal of Neuroscience*, 26, 4870–4879.

O'Sullivan, N.C., Croydon, L., McGettigan, P.A., Pickering, M., and Murphy, K.J. (2010). Hippocampal region-specific regulation of NF-kappaB may contribute to learning-associated synaptic reorganisation. *Brain Research Bulletin*, 81, 385–390.

Ouaaz, F., Arron, J., Zheng, Y., Choi, Y., and Beg, A.A. (2002). Dendritic cell development and survival require distinct NF-kappaB subunits. *Immunity*, 16, 257–270.

Pedreira, M.E., Dimant, B., and Maldonado, H. (1996). Inhibitors of protein and RNA synthesis block context memory and long-term habituation in the crab Chasmagnathus. *Pharmacology, Biochemistry, and Behavior*, 54, 611–617.

Pizzi, M., Goffi, F., Boroni, F., Benarese, M., Perkins, S.E., Liou, H.C., et al. (2002). Opposing roles for NF-kappa B/Rel factors p65 and c-Rel in the modulation of neuron survival elicited by glutamate and interleukin-1beta. *Journal of Biological Chemistry*, 277, 20717–20723.

Qiu, J., Grafe, M.R., Schmura, S.M., Glasgow, J.N., Kent, T.A., Rassin, D.K., et al. (2001). Differential NF-kappa B regulation of bcl-x gene expression in hippocampus and basal forebrain in response to hypoxia. *Journal of Neuroscience Research*, 64, 223–234.

Rafiee, P., Stein, D.J., Nelson, V.M., Otterson, M.F., Shaker, R., and Binion, D.G. (2010). Thalidomide inhibits inflammatory and angiogenic activation of human intestinal microvascular endothelial cells (HIMEC). *American Journal of Physiology. Gastrointestinal and Liver Physiology*, 298, G167–176.

Rossi-George, A., Urbach, D., Colas, D., Goldfarb, B., and Kusnecov, A.W. (2005). Neuronal, endocrine, and anorexic responses to the T-cell superantigen staphylococcal enterotoxin A: dependence on tumor necrosis factor-alpha. *Journal of Neuroscience*, 25, 5314–5322.

Russo, S.J., Wilkinson, M.B., Mazei-Robison, M.S., Dietz, D.M., Maze, I., Krishnan, V., et al. (2009). Nuclear factor kappa B signaling regulates neuronal morphology and cocaine reward. *Journal of Neuroscience*, 29, 3529–3537.

Schuster, T., Krug, M., Hassan, H., and Schachner, M. (1998). Increase in proportion of hippocampal spine synapses expressing neural cell adhesion molecule NCAM180 following long-term potentiation. *Journal of Neurobiology*, 37, 359–372.

Sen, R., and Baltimore, D. (1986). Inducibility of kappa immunoglobulin enhancer-binding protein Nf-kappa B by a posttranslational mechanism. *Cell*, 47, 921–928.

Sha, W.C., Liou, H.C., Tuomanen, E.I., and Baltimore, D. (1995). Targeted disruption of the p50 subunit of NF-kappa B leads to multifocal defects in immune responses. *Cell*, 80, 321–330.

Simpson, C.S., and Morris, B.J. (2000). Regulation of neuronal cell adhesion molecule expression by NF-kappa B. *Journal of Biological Chemistry*, 275, 16879–16884.

Snapper, C.M., Zelazowski, P., Rosas, S.R., Kehry, M.R., Tian, M., Baltimore, D., et al. (1996). B cells from p50/NF-kappa B knockout mice have selective defects in proliferation, differentiation, germ-line CH transcription, and Ig class switching. *Journal of Immunology*, 156, 183–191.

Sun, S.C. (2011). Non-canonical NF-kappaB signaling pathway. *Cell Research*, 21, 71–85.

Tamatani, M., Che, Y.H., Matsuzaki, H., Ogawa, S., Okado, H., Miyake, S., et al. (1999). Tumor necrosis factor induces Bcl-2 and Bcl-x expression through NFkappaB activation in primary hippocampal neurons. *Journal of Biological Chemistry*, 274, 8531–8538.

Wan, Y.Y., and DeGregori, J. (2003). The survival of antigen-stimulated T cells requires NFkappaB-mediated inhibition of p73 expression. *Immunity*, 18, 331–342.

Weih, D.S., Yilmaz, Z.B., and Weih, F. (2001). Essential role of RelB in germinal center and marginal zone formation and proper expression of homing chemokines. *Journal of Immunology*, 167, 1909–1919.

Weih, F., Warr, G., Yang, H., and Bravo, R. (1997). Multifocal defects in immune responses in RelB-deficient mice. *Journal of Immunology*, 158, 5211–5218.

Wellmann, H., Kaltschmidt, B., and Kaltschmidt, C. (2001). Retrograde transport of transcription factor NF-kappa B in living neurons. *Journal of Biological Chemistry*, 276, 11821–11829.

Yeh, S.H., Lin, C.H., Lee, C.F., and Gean, P.W. (2002). A requirement of nuclear factor-kappaB activation in fear-potentiated startle. *Journal of Biological Chemistry*, 277, 46720–46729.

Yirmiya, R., and Goshen, I. (2011). Immune modulation of learning, memory, neural plasticity and neurogenesis. *Brain, Behavior, and Immunity*, 25, 181–213.

Zhao, X., and Eghbali-Webb, M. (2002). Gender-related differences in basal and hypoxia-induced activation of signal transduction pathways controlling cell cycle progression and apoptosis, in cardiac fibroblasts. *Endocrine*, 18, 137–145.

20

Inflammatory Roads to Neurodegeneration

A Focus on Parkinson's and Alzheimer's Disease

Shawn Hayley and Darcy Litteljohn

Department of Neuroscience, Carleton University, Ottawa, Ontario, Canada

Neuroinflammation across the Lifespan

Affecting more than 40 million people worldwide, a number that is expected to triple over the next half-century, Alzheimer's disease (AD) and Parkinson's disease (PD) are the most common age-related neurodegenerative disorders. In both conditions, select neuronal populations undergo progressive degeneration over the span of several years or even decades. It has become increasingly more apparent that multi-neurotransmitter dysfunction arising from pathological changes at several distinct brain regions contributes to the clinical phenotypes of AD and PD. Unfortunately, treatment of these diseases has remained almost exclusively symptomatic, with no known clinically available treatments that actually halt or even significantly slow down the primary neurodegenerative process. One of the most promising areas of ongoing research concerns the potential contributory role of immuno-inflammatory processes in these and other neurological illnesses. Indeed, converging lines of evidence, while not wholly incontrovertible, appear to implicate chronic activation of the inflammatory immune system in both PD and AD.

In the classic sense, inflammation refers to the host response against a pathogen or foreign agent that is characterized by several obvious clinical features, including fever, pain, edema, and redness. The inflammatory response is mediated by a variety of peripheral immune cells, most notably circulating neutrophils, macrophages, dendritic cells, and natural killer cells (which are collectively referred to as leukocytes). Activation of these cells following insult or challenge can occur rapidly, resulting in their mobilization and trafficking to various areas of the body. Once at a site of injury or infection, leukocytes can secrete various factors that cause blood vessels to dilate and become leaky, and induce the production of inflammatory messenger proteins, namely cytokines, which can act to limit the spread of infection and further mobilize other immune cells (e.g., B- and T-lymphocytes).

The brain has its own specialized immunocompetent cells, called microglia, which are essentially analogues of peripheral macrophages. Microglia are the primary cells involved in coordinating neuroinflammatory processes and, in effect, constitute the first line of defense against

The Wiley-Blackwell Handbook of Psychoneuroimmunology, First Edition. Edited by Alexander W. Kusnecov and Hymie Anisman.

pathogenic or other environmental threats to the brain. Although microglia can act independently from any peripheral immune input, they are also responsive to infiltrating immune cells. Indeed, circulating T-lymphocytes are known to routinely enter the cerebrospinal fluid (CSF), albeit in limited concentrations, and may penetrate the brain parenchyma where they come into close contact with local glial cells. In such cases, microglia express major histocompatibility complex (MHC) and associated molecules that allow for direct cell-to-cell synaptic interactions with receptors on invading T-lymphocytes. This can result in the priming of both the microglial and lymphocyte cell, and the orchestration of antigen-specific immune responses.

Beyond participating in coordinated multi-cell immune responses, microglia themselves can mediate rapid brain-based innate inflammatory responses in a manner similar to peripheral macrophages. Like their peripheral counterparts, microglia can release a host of inflammatory and oxidative molecules in defense against pathogens or other foreign insults. Although these defense mechanisms are absolutely essential for the protection of delicate post-mitotic neurons against microbial (and other, e.g., physical, xenobiotic) challenges, excessive or protracted release of oxidative factors from chronic "overactive" microglia can damage or even kill otherwise healthy neighboring neurons. In fact, enhanced microglial reactivity has routinely been detected in postmortem brain samples from individuals with AD and PD, as well as several other neurodegenerative conditions, such as multiple sclerosis and amyotrophic lateral sclerosis.

Activated microglia are also present in the "healthy" aging brain and are suspected to contribute to fairly low-grade neuronal loss together with accompanying subtle signs of cognitive decline (Schuitemaker *et al.*, 2010). Indeed, the increased microglial reactivity that occurs during the course of normal aging is associated with a small but steady loss of neurons in parallel with deficits in normally protective anti-oxidant and immunological defenses. Such losses are not uniform across the brain, and some brain regions appear to be affected more than others. For instance, the dopamine (DA)-producing neurons of the substantia nigra pars compacta (SNc) region of the midbrain, as well as certain neural populations within the basal forebrain and hippocampus are believed to be especially sensitive to the ravages of time. It should come as no surprise, then, that the SNc and hippocampus are among the brain regions hardest hit in PD and AD, respectively.

Critical to any discussion of age-related neuronal changes is the role of the blood–brain barrier (BBB), whose primary components are brain capillary endothelial cells tubularly arrayed in "tight junctions." Essentially, the BBB monitors exchanges between the brain and periphery, and prevents a range of potentially harmful substances (e.g., environmental toxins) from gaining access to the brain. Of course, the BBB also protects the brain from highly reactive endogenous peripheral immune factors, which would otherwise accumulate in the brain at potentially dangerous levels.

Although little is known about the effects of normal aging on the BBB, some studies have reported that the BBB becomes more permeable with advanced age, and that the integrity of this structure may be further disrupted in PD and AD patients (relative to normal aging). For instance, the xenobiotic transporter, P-glycoprotein, is significantly down-regulated in specific brain regions of aged humans, and polymorphism in the transporter's gene has been identified in PD patients (Westerlund *et al.*, 2009). It is also noteworthy that chronic neuroinflammation induced by bacterial toxins diminished the integrity of the BBB by disrupting P-glycoprotein functioning (Salkeni, Lynch, Otamis-Price, and Banks, 2009). Given the transporter's vital role in removing toxic substrates from the brain, any disruptions in P-glycoprotein could lead to the buildup of toxic material. Ultimately, a dysfunctional BBB transport system would be expected to magnify the central accumulation of exogenous (e.g., pesticides, heavy metals, microorganisms) and endogenous toxins (e.g., truncated or mutated β-amyloid and α-synuclein fragments), many of which have been implicated in neurological illness.

Microglia as mediators of neuroinflammation

The reactivity state of microglia varies along a spectrum ranging from resting to hyperactive and is under the strict control of several regulatory proteins. For the most part, microglia normally act as sentinels within the brain, slowly proliferating and removing any debris by phagocytosis and acting to maintain a homeostatic microenvironment. However, in response to environmental or pathogenic insults, microglia rapidly undergo a series of morphological changes, typically changing from a highly ramified state with many thin fiber projections to a more rounded and compacted state with a thickening of processes. In the most extreme cases, microglia become totally amoeboid in appearance and are indistinguishable from peripheral macrophages. Once in such a state, these cells upregulate several oxidative enzymes (e.g., inducible nitric oxide synthase (iNOS), nicotinamide adenine dinucleotide phosphate-oxidase (NADPH oxidase)) that contribute to the formation of neurotoxic free radicals, such as superoxide and peroxynitrite.

Despite the fact that microglia, as already mentioned, undergo functional changes with "normal" aging (heightened activation and reduced proliferative ability), the degree of activation in age-dependent neurodegenerative diseases appears to be substantially different. For instance, in the case of the two most common neurodegenerative conditions, AD and PD, microglial cells often undergo extreme morphological changes and adopt a potentially deleterious phenotype. As shown by recent imaging studies, microglial activation appears to occur in the early stages of neurodegeneration, thus supporting a primary role of these cells in pathology. Yet, it is known that heat-shock proteins and ATP released from damaged or dying neurons also activate microglia, a process (called "reactive microgliosis") that essentially serves to reinforce and further amplify the neuroinflammatory response (see Figure 20.1).

The principal signaling factors controlling microglial function and reactivity state are the pro- and anti-inflammatory cytokines. These soluble, low molecular weight glycoproteins are produced mainly by circulating immune cells, and to a lesser degree by glial cells in the case of injury or infection. In fact, microglia themselves can produce cytokines de novo within the brain. Cytokine receptors are located abundantly at the BBB and on microglia and astrocytes, and some receptors are even expressed on neurons following severe challenges. As the name suggests, pro-inflammatory cytokines, most notably TNF-α, IL-1β, IL-6 and IFN-γ, tend to promote an inflammatory microglial phenotypic state, whereas anti-inflammatory cytokines such as IL-4 and IL-10 generally diminish microglial reactivity and dampen the oxidative stress response elaborated by these cells.

The general picture that has emerged over the past decade or so has been one in which pro-inflammatory cytokines were painted as deleterious factors within the brain. This certainly is supported by the considerable data revealing a strong relationship between TNF-α, IL-1β and IFN-γ (and their impact on microglial reactivity) and the incidence of neural damage in several brain regions. Conversely, anti-inflammatory agents (e.g., minocycline, non-steroidal anti-inflammatory drugs; NSAIDs) or genetic silencing of specific cytokines, have generally been reported to impart neuroprotective consequences across a range of animal models of disease (Rogers, 2008; Litteljohn *et al.*, 2011). Yet, it is naïve to simply suggest that all

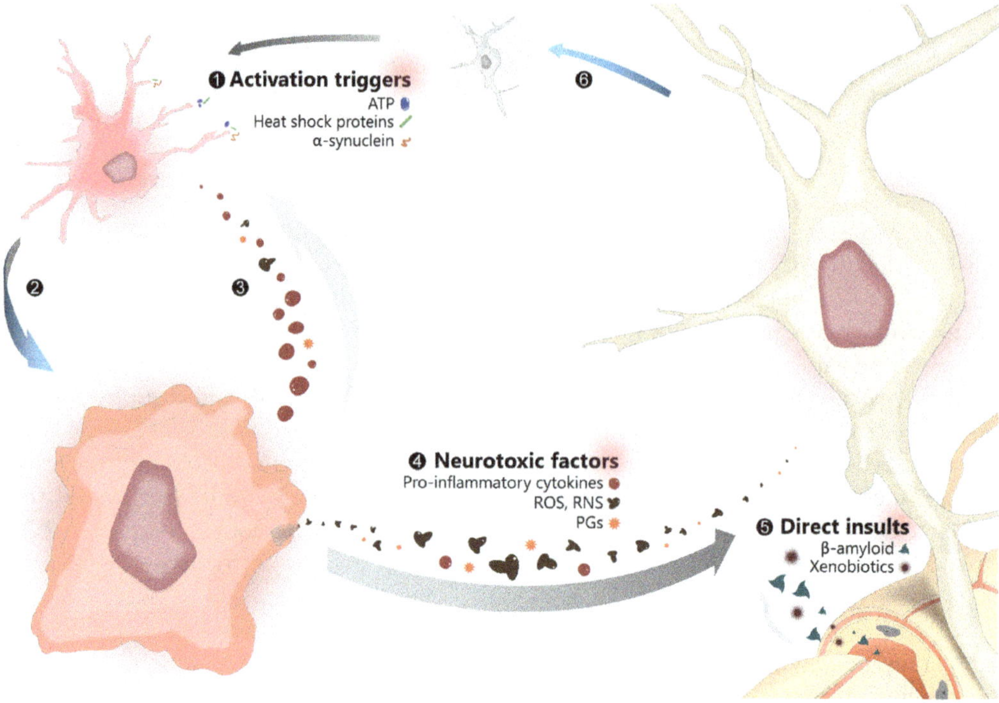

Figure 20.1 Schematic of our model depicting how microglia contribute to neurodegeneration in AD and PD. Black/gray arrows indicate relationships between cells, while blue arrows demarcate cellular transitions (over time). Following toxin exposure or genetic abnormalities: (1) intra-cellular accumulation of α-synuclein, as well as extracellular release of ATP and heat-shock proteins from damaged neurons can (2) trigger microglial activation (morphologically characterized by a switch to an amoeboid-like shape) leading to the liberation of potentially toxic factors, including pro-inflammatory cytokines, prostaglandins, and reactive oxygen and nitrogen species (ROS, RNS). Such pro-oxidant and pro-inflammatory factors can (3) feedback to further amplify the microglial response, and (4) directly damage neurons. Furthermore, (5) extracellular β-amyloid and xenobiotic toxins can directly affect and impair neuron functioning, further leading to (6) release of glial activation triggers.

pro-inflammatory cytokine effects within the brain are uniformly deleterious. It may be that relatively low endogenous cytokine levels act in a protective capacity to buffer against damage related to death processes, whereas high levels of these factors contribute to neuronal damage. Indeed, low levels of cytokines can provoke the release of potentially beneficial trophic factors (BDNF, GDNF) and free-radical scavengers, but elevated levels can activate oxidative–inflammatory cascades or even induce apoptotic cell death. In effect, the concentration as well as timing of cytokine exposure likely determines whether primarily protective or deleterious consequences arise from these immunotransmitters.

Parkinson's and Alzheimer's: The role of inflammatory factors

Parkinson's disease is a complex multi-faceted disorder whose origins can be traced to early pathological changes in aminergic brainstem nuclei (as well as the anterior olfactory bulb and certain cranial nerves), eventually spreading "up and outwards" to encompass large swaths of the more evolutionarily recent midbrain and neocortex. The neural component that has received the most attention is the degeneration of DA neurons within the SNc, resulting in the diminished monoamine release at downstream striatal neural terminals. Abnormal α-synuclein-containing neuronal inclusions called Lewy bodies are typically widely disseminated throughout the PD brain, most notably within midbrain nuclei, but also in the locus coeruleus, olfactory tract, hypothalamus, amygdala, and cortex (Braak *et al.*, 2003). In fact, Lewy body pathology in both brain and gut (i.e., enteric nervous system) is considered one of the earliest-occurring landmarks of PD.

The most frequently observed and severe clinical manifestations are motor symptoms, which are attributable primarily to midbrain DA neuron loss and include rigidity, resting tremor and bradykinesia (a slowing of movement). However, the long-held conceptualization of PD as a "purely motor" condition has given way to the realization that non-motor symptoms, including olfactory, gastrointestinal and sleep disturbances, as well as depression and other psychological and emotional problems (e.g., anxiety, apathy), are the norm and not the exception.

Parkinson's thus appears to be a highly heterogeneous phenotypic disorder with corresponding heterogeneity regarding etiological origins. Whereas autosomal dominant/recessive early-onset familial forms of PD appear to be at one end of the spectrum, purely environmental "toxic exposure" cases (e.g., pesticides, manganese poisoning) may represent the extreme other end. The bulk of "idiopathic" PD cases fall in the middle and will likely involve a mix of genetic and environmental influences. For instance, although mutations in the leucine-rich repeat kinase 2 (LRRK2) gene were initially thought to promote PD in a strictly autosomal dominant manner, incomplete or reduced penetrance (where penetrance refers to the proportion of gene carriers that actually express the phenotype) has been noted for several different inherited LRRK2 mutations (i.e., not all individuals with mutant alleles develop PD). Moreover, among PD patients carrying mutation(s) of the LRRK2 gene, several studies reported a variable age at onset, as well as variable clinical and pathological manifestations (a phenomenon referred to as "variable expressivity") (Taylor, Mata, and Farrer, 2006). The fact that LRRK2 mutations show incomplete penetrance and variable expressivity underscores the importance of environmental events (e.g., toxin exposures), acting on a backdrop of genetic or epigenetic influences, in triggering and shaping the evolution of the disease.

Although the precise normal function of LRRK2 remains undefined, recent studies showed that the kinase is expressed in several different immune cells (e.g., macrophages, T- and B-lymphocytes) and becomes markedly up-regulated following bacterial or viral challenge, as well as by direct exposure to pro-inflammatory cytokines (e.g., Hakimi *et al.*, 2011). It was subsequently proposed that LRRK2 might normally function as a pattern-recognition receptor for invading pathogens and endogenous stress signals (e.g., from damaged and dying cells) (Hakimi *et al.*, 2011). This is particularly interesting, as LRRK2 mutations confer susceptibility not only to PD, but also the inflammatory immune diseases, leprosy and Crohn's disease. Thus, LRRK2 mutations could conceivably influence normal immune cell trafficking and responding to environmental or infectious insults, potentially affecting communication across the neuro–immune interface.

Unlike PD, AD is characterized primarily by severe cognitive impairment, which normally presents as debilitating memory loss and marked deterioration of intellectual functioning. A definite AD diagnosis is only made after postmortem histopathological examination, although refinements of clinical rating scales and recent advances in AD biomarker research (e.g., genetic screens, functional brain scans) offer hope for improved diagnostic accuracy and reliability. The disease is associated with severe atrophy and neuronal loss in a range of cortical and subcortical regions known to be important for learning and memory, particularly the hippocampus, entorhinal cortex, and forebrain cholinergic areas. Other histopathological features include the accumulation of highly insoluble paired helical filaments, called neurofibrillary tangles. These abnormal intracellular aggregates contain a hyperphosphorylated form of the tau protein. Similarly, extracellular neuritic or the so-called "senile" plaques, which comprise a dense core of the truncated from of the peptide, β-amyloid, are believed to result from abnormal proteolytic cleavage of the amyloid prescursor protein.

In addition to the primary motor and cognitive symptoms that have become virtually synonymous with PD and AD, respectively, neuropsychiatric disturbances are now viewed as important features of both disorders (as well as other neurological illnesses such as stroke and amyotrophic lateral sclerosis). Depression is particularly common, with ~50% of PD patients and 25–40% of AD patients presenting with clinically significant symptoms. Importantly, the presence of anxiety and depressive symptoms among individuals with mild cognitive impairment increased the probability that they would later develop AD, and augmented the severity of cognitive decline (Palmer *et al.*, 2007). In the case of PD, retrospective analyses indicated that depressive symptoms predated motor pathology and hence PD diagnosis, suggesting that the depression did not stem (at least in a subset of patients) directly from the stress or disability of the primary diagnosis. Rather, accumulating evidence is beginning to link degeneration and/or dysfunction of widespread neural systems (e.g., the locus coruleus NE system in the case of PD), likely involving cytokine/microglial inflammatory cascades, with the development of co-morbid neuropsychiatric symptoms in both AD and PD.

Although accumulated psychological stressor exposure has clearly been implicated in depressive pathology, the ability of environmental toxins, immune agents and other non-psychological "systemic"-type stressors to also influence emotional functioning is beginning to be recognized. This is particularly germane to the case of AD and PD, where environmental factors (likely in conjunction with genetic vulnerability) have long been considered important contributors to neurodegeneration. For instance, besides their damaging actions on midbrain motor regulatory neurons, pesticides and several other environmental toxins (e.g., heavy metals) have been linked to anxiety- and- depressive-like behavioral outcomes (Hayley, 2010). In this regard, we and others have reported that the commonly used herbicide, paraquat, when administered systemically to mice or rats, can induce both motor and anxiety-like behavioral symptoms, along with neurotransmitter and oxidative changes in stressor-sensitive brain regions, including the locus coruleus, prefrontal cortex, hippocampus (reviewed in Litteljohn *et al.*, 2011). Paraquat was also found to reduce hippocamapal expression of the pro-neuroplastic neurotrophin, brain-derived neurotrophic factor (BDNF), and the anti-apoptotic factor, B-cell lymphoma 2 (Bcl-2) (Mangano *et al.*, 2011), suggesting that the pesticide might negatively affect hippocampal-dependent cognitive processes, as occurs with AD.

Microglia, cytokines and neurodegeneration

Alzheimer's and Parkinson's disease, despite having completely different primary clinical phenotypes (i.e., motor vs. cognitive pathology), share some common co-morbid features (e.g., depression) and a prominent neuroinflammatory component. In the case of PD, elevated levels of the pro-inflammatory cytokines, IL-1β, IL-2, IL-6, TNF-α and IFN-γ, were detected in postmortem brain as well as in the blood and/or CSF (Litteljohn *et al.*, 2011). Similarly, IL-1β, IL-6, IFN-γ and TNF-α were elevated in AD, and several groups have reported negative correlations between some of these cytokines and the protective growth factors, BDNF and insulin-like growth factor-1 (IGF-1) (Rogers, 2008). Perhaps even more importantly, significant correlations were noted between the levels of some of these cytokines and the severity of clinical symptoms (e.g., Reale *et al.*, 2009).

Recent findings have suggested that polymorphisms within genes encoding several different cytokines might contribute to AD and PD. For instance, polymorphism of the pro-inflammatory IL-18 cytokine gene was associated with a faster rate of cognitive decline in AD patients, as well as heightened risk of developing PD in a Han Chinese population (Bossù *et al.*, 2007; Xu *et al.*, 2011). Yet, the fact that polymorphism in the promoter region of the gene coding for the anti-inflammatory cytokine, IL-10, was also found to predict increased risk of AD in an Italian sample (Bagnoli *et al.*, 2007) suggests that the influence of pro- vs anti-inflammatory changes likely varies across differing populations. Moreover, it should also be considered that while some of these mutations comprise or lead to a "loss of function," others are a "gain of function." In fact, certain polymorphic variants of pro-inflammatory cytokine genes (e.g., IL-1α) may actually confer protection against AD or PD. In the end, cytokine gene polymorphism would be expected to result in some modification of neuro–immune communication, which in turn could impact disease state.

Indirect clinical evidence concerning inflammatory processes in AD comes from early studies showing that arthritic patients receiving anti-inflammatory drugs had a reduced risk of developing AD. Yet, more recent retrospective analyses and even clinical trials indicated minimal or non-existent effects of NSAIDs in AD (Heneka, O'Banion, Terwel, and Kummer, 2010). Similarly, while a few scattered reports suggested that NSAID anti-inflammatory drugs were associated with a lessened risk of developing PD, such outcomes seem to have been generally difficult to replicate. In effect, these relatively broad-spectrum anti-inflammatory agents seem to being having very modest brain effects in the context of both AD and PD; and these effects likely are strongly dependent upon the timing of drug exposure. In this regard, NSAIDs and other anti-inflammatory drugs might be most useful when used relatively early in the disease process or as a preventative strategy. Of course, as will be discussed in the final section of this chapter, developing more specific-acting immune regulatory agents (as opposed to the typical broad spectrum drugs) could greatly enhance beneficial outcomes. It is also important to consider the possibility of using inflammatory biomarkers to stratify an individual's risk of developing AD or PD, which would, in theory, allow for the initiation of prophylactic treatment.

Despite the shortcomings in translating anti-inflammatory strategies into viable clinical treatments, pre-clinical animal models have gone a long way in identifying key neuroinflammatory mechanisms involved in AD and PD. A common thread in virtually all animal models of the two diseases (from transgenic to toxin-based) has been the involvement (often requisite) of microglia and specific cytokines in many aspects of neural and behavioral pathology. Indeed, 1-methyl-4-phenyl-1,2,3,6-tetrahydropyridine (MPTP), 6-hydroxydopamine (6-OHDA), rotenone and paraquat, which are probably the most common and well-studied toxins used to model PD, have all been demonstrated to induce microglial activation in rodents and/or non-human primates (Hayley, 2010). In fact, even humans who inadvertently ingested MPTP displayed long-term (years after exposure) and apparently irreversible microglial activation that accompanied midbrain DA neuronal loss. Similarly, prominent microglial activation, which is most apparent clustering around abnormal senile plaques, is routinely observed in transgenic animals over-expressing AD-associated genes such as the presenilins and APP (Heneka, O'Banion, Terwel, and Kummer, 2010).

It appears that pro-inflammatory cytokines can interact with one another or with endogenous β-amyloid to influence glial-associated neurodegenerative developments in AD. In particular, IL-1β, IL-6 and TNF-α are upregulated in amyloid plaque-associated microglia (most of which are in an activated phagocytic state) and have been implicated in the deposition of β-amyloid in neuritic plaques as well as the development of neurofibrillary tangles (Yamamoto *et al.*, 2007; Heneka, O'Banion, Terwel, and Kummer, 2010). Moreover, TNF-α, IL-1β and IFN-γ synergistically enhanced the glial release of the potentially neurotoxic free radical, nitric oxide; an effect that was further amplified by addition of soluble β-amyloid fragments (Chiarini, Dal Pra, Whitfield, and Armato, 2006). Not only are cytokines associated with the presence of neuritic plaques, they may also contribute to plaque maturation (i.e., driving the evolution of plaques into their more mature dense core forms). This is an important point, since the density of mature core neuritic plaques but not the earlier, less mature, diffuse forms correlate well with cognitive decline in AD patients (Ding, Dimayuga, and Keller, 2007).

Toxin-based animal models of PD have similarly demonstrated the pathological importance of cytokines and their neuroinflammatory cascades. Indeed, MPTP, 6-OHDA, rotenone and paraquat all enhanced regional brain (e.g., SNc, striatum) and circulating levels of many pro-inflammatory cytokines, most notably TNF-α, IFN-γ and IL-1β (Litteljohn *et al.*, 2011). The fact that cytokine changes preceded toxin-induced DA neuronal loss suggests a primary role of these immunotransmitters in the neurodegenerative process. Several studies have also reported toxin-associated increases of anti-inflammatory cytokines, such as IL-10 and IL-4 (e.g., Yasuda *et al.*, 2008), although these alterations might have reflected a compensatory response to escalating neuroinflammation and neuronal damage.

Using pharmacological blockage and gene-knockout (and more recently gene-knockdown) strategies, it was demonstrated that animals lacking certain pro-inflammatory cytokines (or their receptors) could be made resistant to the neuronal and behavioral pathology ordinarily induced by DA toxins. Our work showed that mice deficient in IFN-γ or the pro-apoptotic cytokine, Fas, were protected against dopaminergic neurotoxicity induced by MPTP and paraquat; an effect that coincided with a reduction in activated microglia and the diminished expression of oxidative factors (e.g., NADPH oxidase, iNOS). Attesting to the importance of inflammatory factors in clinical outcomes, these knockout mice, as well as those lacking the prostaglandin synthetic inflammatory enzyme, COX-2, also had attenuated behavioral responses to PD toxins (e.g., motor, anxiety/depression-like symptoms) (reviewed in Litteljohn *et al.*, 2011).

In addition to directing microglial-dependent inflammatory and oxidative responses, a growing body of evidence suggests that cytokines may influence the progression of AD and PD by interfering with growth factor production (critical for the proper maintenance of neurons). For example, IL-1β inhibited BDNF signaling in cultured neurons by blocking the functioning of critical pro-growth enzymatic pathways, including the MAP kinase, ERK, which normally promotes beneficial neuroplastic responses to cellular stress (Tong *et al.*, 2008). Moreover, BDNF and its upstream transcription factor, CREB, are reduced in postmortem AD and PD brain, as well as in transgenic models of the disease (Caccamo *et al.*, 2010). The fact that circulating BDNF levels, which stem from both peripheral immune and cerebral sources, were also changed and correlated with motor impairment in PD raises the possibility that the growth factor might offer hope as a biomarker (Scalzo *et al.*, 2010). Consistent with this notion, our own work revealed that paraquat markedly diminished BDNF at early but not late stages of a chronic pesticide exposure paradigm in mice; knocking out the expression of IFN-γ (via genetic ablation of the cytokine) normalized this effect (Mangano *et al.*, 2012). Overall, the emerging picture would tend to suggest that deficiencies of BDNF signaling might impart some enhanced vulnerability of neurons to the impact of either environmental stresses or endogenous inflammatory events.

Neuroinflammation as a "double-edged sword"

Although we tend to focus on the negative effects of cytokines in relation to neurodegenerative diseases, one should not discount the evidence suggesting that cytokines may have protective or reparative functions under select conditions. In the case of AD for instance, pretreatment of neuronal cultures with TNF-α reduced β-amyloid-induced hippocampal neuronal death and tau hyperphosphorylation (Orellana, Quintanilla, and Maccioni, 2007). However, TNF-α together with IL-1β and other pro-inflammatory cytokines enhanced β-amyloid accumulation and augmented its neurodegenerative effects (Chiarini, Dal Pra, Whitfield, and Armato, 2006). These seemingly contradictory findings point to the often overlooked, but important issue of duality of functioning of TNF-α and other cytokines. For TNF-α, the dual role is, in part, related to the divergent effects of its two receptors, TNF-Rl and TNF-R2. Whereas TNF-Rl has pro-death effects that are mediated by its intracellular death domain and associated apoptotic caspases, TNF-R2 mainly has pro-survival and proliferative functions. Further, the degree of activation of microglial cells may influence the neurodegenerative effects of TNF-α. Indeed, this cytokine had neurotoxic effects in neuronal cultures exposed to β-amyloid in the presence of microglia, but not in those treated with the glial suppressor, Ara-C (e.g., Orellana, Quintanilla, and Maccioni, 2007). These findings suggest that the TNF-α-exposed glia may be releasing toxic factors that counteract any effects that the cytokine may have on neuroprotective pathways.

While this chapter is devoted primarily to the contributions of microglia and cytokines to neurodegeneration in AD and PD, it warrants mentioning that astrocytes are also strongly associated with neurological illness. Indeed, an excessive accumulation of these glial cells is well documented in AD and, to a lesser extent, PD, as well as many of their animal models. The extent of astroglial proliferation was found to correlate positively with AD lesions (neuritic plaques and neurofibrillary tangles), and was higher among carriers of the apolipoprotein E (ApoE) ε4 risk allele (compared to AD patients without the ApoE ε4 allele) (Overmyer *et al.*, 1999). Mobilized astrocytes, like microglia, can adopt a potentially deleterious phenotype in response to a range of environmental insults (e.g., trauma, infection, toxin). Once activated, astrocytes are capable of releasing oxidative radicals, complement proteins, and cytokines (both pro- and anti-inflammatory species), in addition to neurotrophic factors. In fact, β-amyloid accumulation in astrocytes was shown to provoke neuronal death in an *in vitro* model of AD; and, like microglia, this neurotoxicity was linked to the generation of ROS by astrocytes (via NADPH oxidase) (Abramov and Duchen, 2005).

Their potentially deleterious effects notwithstanding, astrocytes are normally key homeostatic regulators of brain function, acting to buffer excess ions and neurotransmitters (e.g., potassium, glutamate), and to remove potentially damaging free radicals and toxins. Other important housekeeping functions that fall under the purview of these cells include: providing structural support to neurons (especially at synapses), contributing to the integrity of the BBB, and producing a variety of prosurvival trophic factors. Indeed, the neurotrophin, GDNF, which has neuroprotective effects in both AD and PD animal models, is produced primarily by astrocytes. It should not be surprising, then, that a loss of normally protective astrocyte functioning has, in many instances, been linked with neurodegeneration. In this regard, defective glutamate recycling, reduced glutathione (a potent anti-oxidant) availability and altered energy metabolism have all garnered significant attention as potential astrocytic purveyors of neuronal loss in AD (Fuller, Münch, and Steele, 2009). The hypothesis was even ventured that widespread atrophy of astrocytes occurring at very early stages of AD might, in effect, drive the development of synaptic dysfunction and subtle cognitive decline- and therefore act as a harbinger of disease progression (Rodríguez, Olabarria, Chvatal, and Verkhratsky, 2009). Similarly, in PD, deposition of α-synuclein in astrocytes was revealed to cause marked dysfunction of these cells, resulting in the recruitment of microglia and the subsequent killing of DA neurons through oxidative stress (Halliday and Stevens, 2011). Hence, the precise role ("good vs bad") of these cells in the neurodegenerative process has proven rather difficult to nail down, and like the case of microglia (and the cytokines they produce), probably varies over the course of the illness.

Environmental triggers and neurodegeneration: Sensitized neuroinflammatory response?

Several compelling lines of evidence support a provocative role of pesticides and other environmental toxicants in PD. In particular, numerous epidemiological studies have uncovered an increased incidence of PD associated with occupational and rural pesticide exposure, with rotenone (an organic insecticide) and paraquat (a chemical herbicide still widely used throughout the world) being most prominent in this regard (Hayley, 2010). Animal studies have confirmed that paraquat and rotenone can induce PD-like pathology in rodents and non-human primates. For instance, systemic exposure to paraquat and, to a lesser extent, rotenone provoked a dose-dependent loss of SNc DA neurons and Lewy-body pathology, coupled with behavioral aspects of PD in rodents (Litteljohn *et al.*, 2011).

Pesticides can adversely affect neuronal survival by impairing neuronal mitochondrial functioning, as well as "overstimulating" microglial cells. Systemic infection may also interact with pesticides to induce exaggerated neuroinflammatory events. In fact, we previously suggested that exposure to pathogens might have especially marked neuronal consequences when encountered in the context of concomitant chemical toxin, traumatic head injury or even psychological stressor exposure. In this regard, the bacterial endotoxin, LPS, synergistically augmented neuronal death in cultured DA neurons also exposed to rotenone (Gao, Hong, Zhang, and Liu, 2003). Using *in vivo* experiments, our own lab has similarly shown that a low dose of LPS enhanced the neurotoxic effects of the herbicide, paraquat, such that a substantial number of DA-producing neurons were destroyed (i.e., more than was observed with paraquat alone) and PD-like behavioral symptoms emerged (Mangano and Hayley, 2009). Importantly, this study and others clearly implicated enhanced activity of the NADPH oxidase enzyme in microglia and the consequent production of the superoxide radical in the sensitizing effects of LPS. For instance, LPS sensitized the neurodegenerative impact of paraquat when administered at times prior to paraquat exposure, which coincided with maximal morphological and chemical changes in microglia (suggestive of a highly activated state). Conversely, genetic knockout of NADPH oxidase or treatment with the broad-spectrum anti-inflammatory drug, minocycline, prevented the sensitized neurodegenerative effect (Purisai *et al.*, 2007).

Environmental or inflammatory toxins might promote a sensitization across the lifespan, such that exposure to an immune or chemical toxin at one point in life enhances vulnerability to the behavioral and neurodestructive effects of challenges encountered months or even years later. In particular, during early life stages when neuronal migration and synaptic pruning are abundant, neurons are especially sensitive to environmental perturbations. Correspondingly, essential biological detoxification systems and the normally protective BBB have not yet fully developed in utero or during the perinatal period.

The most compelling evidence for early-life sensitization effects comes from studies showing that prenatal LPS exposure had long-term effects on the inflammatory and endocrine systems (e.g., cytokine and corticoid elevations), and rendered rodents especially vulnerable to the behavioral consequences of stressors and toxins encountered in adulthood. In fact, prenatal LPS exposure induced a relatively permanent elevation of TNF-α within the brain, coupled with augmented loss of midbrain DA neurons upon exposure to the pesticide, rotenone, in adulthood (Ling *et al.*, 2004). This might be especially relevant to the human condition, wherein bacterial vaginosis, a common infection during pregnancy, has been linked to the development of neurological disorders and with enhanced levels of IL-1β, IL-6, and TNF-α in adulthood. Consistent with these findings, our contention has been that early immunogenic exposure may provoke mild neuroinflammation that, over time, renders neurons vulnerable to the effects of normally low-grade insults later in life. It may also be that early toxin exposure causes modest neuronal damage that only becomes "unmasked" upon later multiple toxin exposures, resulting in some threshold of neuronal vulnerability eventually being breached.

Future Directions and Therapeutic Strategies for Neurodegeneration

It is a particularly exciting time for neurodegenerative research, given the many recent technological breakthroughs involving diverse methods ranging from stem cell therapies to transgenic mouse preparations to biomarker discoveries. The convergence of these different approaches to the better understanding of the diseases and the tailoring of novel treatment strategies will be fundamental for the translation of basic research findings into the clinical arena. Indeed, an enormous problem has been the lack of success in translating basic animal experimental outcomes into viable treatments for human populations. This, in part, likely stems from failures to model adequately the complexity of human disease in lower species, as well as shortcomings in outcome measures. While the former point revolves around the issue of species differences and "appropriateness" of existing animal models, the later point speaks to the importance of using multiple reliable endpoints (both biological and behavioral) that actually map onto the relevant clinical analogues. Fortunately, recent technological advancements have fueled substantial progress in detecting subtle cellular and molecular changes in human disease and corresponding animal models, and genetic strategies have given rise to the possibility of carefully manipulating discrete nodes within pathways to neuropathology.

Multi-tiered approach to neurodegeneration

Although this review is focused upon neuroinflammatory mechanisms, it is important to consider these in the context of a highly complex milieu of other simultaneous biological mediators that undoubtedly contribute to disease status. For instance, parallel changes in MAP kinase, cell cycle and autophagic pathways are believed to be active over the course of PD and AD, and these factors might even play different roles depending upon the particular stage of disease.

Another complication arises from the fact that these molecular pathways are activated not only by inflammatory stimuli, but a host of other environmental stressors, as well as endogenous perturbations in the neuronal microenvironment. Considering the diverse origins and mechanisms of brain pathology, it makes the most sense to ultimately adopt a multi-tiered combinatorial treatment strategy. In this regard, we believe that pharmacological or genetic means of targeting specific inflammatory factors would be a useful adjunct or add-on therapy together with similar approaches aimed at quieting overactive oxidative and pro-apoptotic pathways.

Besides treating the complex pathways to primary disease (e.g., motor or cognitive pathology), it is also critical to manage co-morbid features of neurological illness. Not only would such approaches importantly improve the quality of life in PD and AD patients, but also might enhance the overall level of functioning. This is illustrated by the case of PD patients with a high degree of depressive co-morbidity, who perform more poorly on motor tasks and tests of executive cognitive functioning than their non-depressed PD counterparts. Moreover, recent evidence (although quite scant) has indicated that antidepressant treatments might actually improve cognitive functioning in AD, suggesting that the co-morbid elements might adversely impact the primary illness. Indeed, chronic restraint/isolation stress, which "overactivates" the hypothalamic–pituitary–adrenal (HPA) axis, and is often used to induce a "depression-like" syndrome in rodents, was found to exacerbate AD pathology (e.g., tau hyperphosphorylation, β-amyloid accumulation, neuronal death) in a transgenic model of AD. Importantly, HPA axis dampening by antagonism of corticotropin-releasing factor receptor type-1, which is a promising new target for anti-depressant therapy, completely prevented these effects (Carroll *et al.*, 2011). In effect, concomitant disturbances in depressive and motor or cognitive neural circuits could conceivably reinforce symptomatology, suggesting once again the possibility of some overlap in (immuno-) neural mechanisms.

When considering the neuroinflammatory underpinnings of neurodegenerative disease it is important to bear in mind the "double-edged sword" role that inflammatory glia and cytokines, as mentioned earlier, normally play. Thus, any anti-inflammatory treatment approaches should necessarily carefully consider potential negative complications that might arise from a down-regulation of normally protective aspects of immunity. This could help explain why broad-spectrum anti-inflammatory agents, such as the NSAIDs, have had very limited success in treating PD and AD in the few clinical trials that have been undertaken. Such general anti-inflammatory approaches might suppress potentially beneficial inflammatory immune effects, such as the cellular scavenging and ionic buffering capabilities of glial cells, in addition to the potentially negative consequences. Indeed, a little "controlled" inflammation might actually help to spur on neurotrophic factor production and neuronal reparative processes. The question then remains, how do we limit the "bad" while promoting "good" inflammation? Also, how much is good and what is the timing for such positive inflammation and neural recovery?

Specifically regarding the issue of timing in the treatment of neurodegenerative disease, the fact that substantial neuronal pathology has already occurred – and several inflammatory cascades presumably long been active – by the time even a preliminary diagnosis has been reached poses a particularly confounding problem. Indeed, it is estimated that 50–80% of midbrain SNc dopamine neurons are lost in PD patients by the time they begin to display motor deficits. Similarly, the onset of significant memory disturbances in AD is believed to occur following substantial neuritic plaque and neurofibrillary tangle accumulation, coupled with a loss of hippocampal and temporal cortex neurons. Moreover, the fact that imaging studies revealed prominent microglial activation (more than what is seen in normal aging) in cortical and subcortical brain regions in both AD and PD patients at very early stages of disease suggests that inflammation might be an early pathogenic event. In effect, the fairly advanced stage of disease at the time of diagnosis might make it very difficult to halt the already "ramped-up" neurodegenerative and neuroinflammatory cascades. In this regard, finding reliable biomarkers for early disease detection would be invaluable. This is certainly the case where specific profiles of soluble inflammatory proteins (that are reflective of early disease brain changes) could be particularly useful. What is more, given the already substantial neuronal loss, it is of considerable importance to develop strategies to promote neuronal recovery processes, as well as stabilizing the surviving neuronal populations.

Neurotrophic strategies for treating neurodegeneration

One exciting new avenue for treating neurodegenerative disease involves administration (either through genetic or pharmacological methods) of trophic factors to: 1) either attenuate the disease process; or 2) promote compensatory recovery pathways. The animal literature is quite clear on the beneficial effects of several trophic factors, most notably nerve growth factor (NGF), BDNF and GDNF, in a variety of models of disease. For instance, central infusion of GDNF had neuroprotective effects in virtually all animal models of PD and not only attenuated the destructive effects of toxin exposure, but also promoted motor recovery. In fact, the positive effects of GDNF persisted months after trophic support was terminated (Rangasamy, Soderstrom, Bakay, and Kordower, 2010).

Due to the success of GDNF in rodent and non-human primate models of PD, this growth factor has been used in several clinical trials. Indeed, direct infusion of GDNF into the human putamen induced significant improvements in motor symptoms as early as three months after commencing the treatment (Slevin *et al.*, 2005). However, a randomized placebo-controlled study was unsuccessful at replicating these beneficial effects, possibly related to the fact that a few patients developed antibodies against GDNF. Also of concern was that some patients appeared to be more vulnerable to opportunistic infections.

While no clinical trials have been conducted on the feasibility or efficacy of GDNF for the treatment of AD, the past couple of decades have witnessed a growing interest in NGF as a possible disease-modifying therapy in AD. Interestingly, a recent study also showed that existing acetylcholinesterase inhibitors that are currently used clinically to provide marginal benefits to AD patients up-regulated the NGF and BDNF receptors, tyrosine receptor kinase A and B, respectively (Autio *et al.*, 2011). Yet, like GDNF, NGF and BDNF do not substantially cross the BBB, and it has become apparent that injecting NGF directly into the cerebral ventricles causes significant side effects in both animals and humans (Mandel, 2010).

Given the inconclusive beneficial actions and side effects associated with direct-brain GDNF and NGF delivery, several new techniques are presently being developed to get around the fact that neither trophic factor crosses the BBB (thus permitting systemic administration of neurotrophins). These include newer generation viral vectors that temporarily disrupt the BBB, implantation of trophic factor secreting neural progenitor cells, as well as encapsulating or breaking the trophic factor into small bioactive fragments. Neurotrophic factor inducers such as the orally active drug, Cogane (PYM50028), are also receiving recent attention. Indeed, Cogane, which has been shown to cross the BBB and increase brain concentrations of BDNF and GDNF, is currently being clinically tested for the treatment of early stage PD.

Finding novel neurotrophic factors that can cross the BBB and have minimal side-effects is of tremendous importance. In this regard, our own work has focused on using the hematopoietic cytokine, granulocyte-macrophage colony-stimulating factor (GM-CSF), which has well-documented trophic actions and has been shown to accumulate in reasonable levels within the brain. As the name suggests, this cytokine acts to rapidly mobilize and stimulate the proliferation and maturation of myeloid progenitors, which are the precursors of neutrophils, monocytes, macrophages, and eosinophils. Accordingly, GM-CSF is sometimes administered to cancer patients to re-populate the compromised leukocyte population resulting from chemotherapy or transplantation.

In addition to its effects on immune cells, GM-CSF has recently been shown to have potent growth factor-like properties within the brain. In fact, GM-CSF induced axonal regeneration and promoted functional recovery from traumatic spinal cord injury, and reduced infarct volume and improved neurological function following ischemia (Schäbitz *et al.*, 2008). Paralleling these findings, our own work recently indicated that either intraperitoneal or intracerebroventricular administration of GM-CSF blocked the impact of LPS and paraquat upon midbrain DA neurons, and attenuated the microglial response and BDNF reduction associated with these toxins (Mangano *et al.*, 2011). It remains to be determined whether GM-CSF might have more success than GDNF in translating into the clinical arena for treating neurodegeneration; at the very least, GM-CSF is an important option to consider given that it is currently approved for other clinical uses.

Protective immunity: Priming immunity for brain repair

The situation concerning the aging brain is not completely dismal as recent studies suggest that a certain degree of plasticity of the brain persists across the lifespan, and that novel means of encouraging positive immune responses could foster beneficial neuroplasticity. In this regard, exciting recent work by Schwartz and colleagues has suggested that immune cells can greatly influence several aspects of neuroplasticity, most notably hippocamapal neurogenesis and BDNF expression. In contrast to the usually deleterious effects of autoimmunity (as in the case of multiple sclerosis), this group of researchers has reported that "weak" autoimmune responses can protect the brain against various stressors and can have neuroprotective consequences (Schwartz and Shechter, 2010). It was also posited that immunization procedures that promote brain-directed T-cell responses might even play a prominent role in facilitating spatial learning, as well as imparting anti-anxiety and anti-depressant effects (Lewitus *et al.*, 2009). Such "protective autoimmunity" is suggested to stem from brain-directed T-cells causing a shift in the functioning of microglia and macrophages, as well as astrocytes, to a more neuroprotective phenotype. Similarly, protective vaccination strategies are believed to facilitate the mobilization of peripheral macrophages with reparative functions. This might be particularly important for fostering the removal and cleanup of abnormal extracellular debris and protein deposits, such as the widespread plaques observed in AD brains.

An important development in recent years has been the use of immunization strategies aimed at removing pathological β-amyloid-bearing neuritic plaques in AD patients. This approach has produced very promising effects in animal models, essentially resulting in a substantial lessening of plaque load and concomitant amelioration of many clinical signs of impairment. In parallel with the reduction of β-amyloid plaques, immunization of transgenic AD mice also reduced TNF-α levels, while elevating concentrations of the anti-inflammatory cytokine,

IL-10, and the trophic factor, IGF-1 (Butovsky *et al.*, 2006). Although there were some early limited successes in human clinical trials, these have not been fruitful in the long run. In fact, many complications related to immune toxicity (some possibly stemming from the immune adjuvant used) have generally slowed the translation into the clinic. Nevertheless, more recent attempts have been made to circumvent such problems by fine-tuning specific aspects of the immune response engendered by immunization with β-amyloid peptides. Interestingly, recent reports have even suggested that cytokines with trophic properties, such as macrophage colony-stimulating factor, might further help with the breakdown of β-amyloid plaques, suggesting the possibility of combined cytokine–immunization procedures for maximal benefit.

Although less attention has focused on the possibility of using vaccination strategies for neurological conditions other than AD, a few emerging studies have suggested that such approaches might be useful for PD, as well as acute cerebral injuries, most notably spinal cord injury. Indeed, immunization of mice with the drug, copaxone, which is a random collection of four amino acids found in myelin basic protein and is already clinically used to treat multiple sclerosis, reduced microglial activation and protected midbrain dopamine neurons following MPTP toxin treatment. This protection was associated with increased infiltration of T-lymphocytes and a concomitant elevation of the trophic factor, GDNF (Benner *et al.*, 2004). Hence, a brain region specific T-cell response likely contributed to this outcome. Yet, a more recent study questions the necessity of immunization with specific brain antigens since administration of an adjuvant (immune boosting agent that often contains attenuated bacterial components; in this case, either complete Freund's adjuvant or Bacillus Calmette–Guerin adjuvant) alone was just as effective in reducing microglial activation and preserving striatal dopamine terminals as brain region specific antigens (tyrosine hydroxylase or copaxone) (Yong *et al.*, 2011). Thus, it might be that mobilization of a wide range of immune responses could have beneficial central nervous system consequences in the context of certain neuronal challenges (e.g., some toxins).

Studies using spinal cord injury animal models have provided compelling data indicating that the neuroprotective effects of vaccines could stem from monocytes derived from peripheral bone marrow (which eventually migrate to various tissues to become macrophages; in fact, brain microglia originate from these cells). These studies have generally found that immunization of rodents subjected to spinal cord injury induces the migration of bone marrow monocytes and reduces the degree of spinal neuron injury, while fostering neuroplasticity and recovery processes (Ziv *et al.*, 2006). Importantly, conditional genetic ablation of a specific subset of monocytes (those expressing the CD11c surface marker; often referred to as having dendritic cell-like properties) augmented the damage provoked by spinal cord injury, but this effect was absent when ablation occurred by the second week after spinal cord injury (Shechter *et al.*, 2009). Thus, once again, timing of the immune response is critical in shaping its neuronal consequences. The fact that the infiltrating CD11c$^+$ monocytes expressed the anti-inflammatory cytokine, IL-10, and were associated with reduced activity of local microglia indicates that their mode of action within the spinal cord might involve a downregulation of the local inflammatory state.

Summary

It appears clear that cytokines and glial cells are important players in neurodegenerative conditions. Finding novel means of controlling deleterious neuroinflammatory processes, while at the same time harnessing the benefits of proneuroplastic and trophic immune factors presents a formidable challenge for modern therapeutics. Similarly, the potential utility of using the circulating profile of immune cells and their soluble factors (e.g., cytokines) as potential biomarkers of brain disease is a particularly appealing emerging enterprise.

Acknowledgements

This work was supported by funds awarded to S.H. and D.L. from the Canadian Institutes of Health Research (CIHR). S.H. is a Canada Research Chair in behavioral neuroscience. Many thanks to Neville Ko for help with the figure.

References

Abramov, A.Y., and Duchen, M.R. (2005). The role of an astrocytic NADPH oxidase in the neurotoxicity of amyloid beta peptides. *Philosophical Transactions of the Royal Society B: Biological Sciences*, 360, 2309–2314.

Autio, H., Mätlik, K., Rantamäki, T., Lindemann, L., Hoener, M.C., Chao, M., et al. (2011). Acetylcholinesterase inhibitors rapidly activate Trk neurotrophin receptors in the mouse hippocampus. *Neuropharmacology*, 61, 1291–1296.

Bagnoli, S., Cellini, E., Tedde, A., Nacmias, B., Piacentini, S., Bessi, V., et al. (2007). Association of IL10 promoter polymorphism in Italian Alzheimer's disease. *Neuroscience Letters*, 418, 262–265.

Benner, E.J., Mosley, R.L., Destache, C.J., Lewis, T.B., Jackson-Lewis, V., Gorantla, S., et al. (2004). Therapeutic immunization protects dopaminergic neurons in a mouse model of Parkinson's disease. *Proceedings of the National Academy of Sciences of the United States of America*, 101, 9435–9440.

Bossù, P., Ciaramella, A., Moro, M.L., Bellincampi, L., Bernardini, S., Federici, G., et al. (2007). Interleukin 18 gene polymorphisms predict risk and outcome of Alzheimer's disease. *Journal of Neurology, Neurosurgery and Psychiatry*, 78, 807–811.

Braak, H., Del Tredici, K., Rüb, U., de Vos, R.A., Jansen Steur, E.N., and Braak, E. (2003). Staging of brain pathology related to sporadic Parkinson's disease. *Neurobiology of Aging*, 24, 197–211.

Butovsky, O., Koronyo-Hamaoui, M., Kunis, G., Ophir, E., Landa, G., Cohen, H., et al. (2006). Glatiramer acetate fights against Alzheimer's disease by inducing dendritic-like microglia expressing insulin-like growth factor 1. *Proceedings of the National Academy of Sciences of the United States of America*, 103, 11784–11789.

Caccamo, A., Maldonado, M.A., Bokov, A.F., Majumder, S., and Oddo, S. (2010). CBP gene transfer increases BDNF levels and ameliorates learning and memory deficits in a mouse model of Alzheimer's disease. *Proceedings of the National Academy of Sciences of the United States of America*, 107, 22687–22692.

Carroll, J.C., Iba, M., Bangasser, D.A., Valentino, R.J., James, M.J., Brunden, K.R., et al. (2011). Chronic stress exacerbates tau pathology, neurodegeneration, and cognitive performance through a corticotropin-releasing factor receptor-dependent mechanism in a transgenic mouse model of tauopathy. *Journal of Neuroscience*, 31, 14436–14449.

Chiarini, A., Dal Pra, I., Whitfield, J.F., and Armato, U. (2006). The killing of neurons by beta-amyloid peptides, prions, and pro-inflammatory cytokines. *Italian Journal of Anatomy and Embryology*, 111, 221–246.

Ding, Q., Dimayuga, E., and Keller, J.N. (2007). Oxidative damage, protein synthesis, and protein degradation in Alzheimer's disease. *Current Alzheimer Research*, 4, 73–79.

Fuller, S., Münch, G., and Steele, M. (2009). Activated astrocytes: a therapeutic target in Alzheimer's disease? *Expert Review of Neurotherapeutics*, 9, 1585–1594.

Gao, H.M., Hong, J.S., Zhang, W., and Liu, B. (2003). Synergistic dopaminergic neurotoxicity of the pesticide rotenone and inflammogen lipopolysaccharide: relevance to the etiology of Parkinson's disease. *Journal of Neuroscience*, 23, 1228–1236.

Hakimi, M., Selvanantham, T., Swinton, E., Padmore, R.F., Tong, Y., Kabbach, G., et al. (2011). Parkinson's disease-linked LRRK2 is expressed in circulating and tissue immune cells and upregulated following recognition of microbial structures. *Journal of Neural Transmission*, 118, 795–808.

Halliday, G.M., and Stevens, C.H. (2011). Glia: initiators and progressors of pathology in Parkinson's disease. *Movement Disorders*, 26, 6–17.

Hayley, S. (2010). A comment on the role of environmental factors in Parkinson's disease. *Canadian Journal of Neurological Sciences*, 37, 555–556.

Heneka, M.T., O'Banion, M.K., Terwel, D., and Kummer, M.P. (2010). Neuroinflammatory processes in Alzheimer's disease. *Journal of Neural Transmission*, 117, 919–947.

Lewitus, G.M., Wilf-Yarkoni, A., Ziv, Y., Shabat-Simon, M., Gersner, R., Zangen, A., et al. (2009). Vaccination as a novel approach for treating depressive behavior. *Biological Psychiatry*, 65, 283–288.

Ling, Z., Chang, Q.A., Tong, C.W., Leurgans, S.E., Lipton, J.W., and Carvey, P.M. (2004). Rotenone potentiates dopamine neuron loss in animals exposed to lipopolysaccharide prenatally. *Experimental Neurology*, 190, 373–383.

Litteljohn, D., Mangano, E., Clarke, M., Bobyn, J., Moloney, K., and Hayley, S. (2011). Inflammatory mechanisms of neurodegeneration in toxin-based models of Parkinson's disease. *Parkinson's Disease*, 2011, 18 pp.

Mandel, R.J. (2010). CERE-110, an adeno-associated virus-based gene delivery vector expressing human nerve growth factor for the treatment of Alzheimer's disease. *Current Opinion in Molecular Therapeutics*, 12, 240–247.

Mangano, E.N., and Hayley, S. (2009). Inflammatory priming of the substantia nigra influences the impact of later paraquat exposure: neuroimmune sensitization of neurodegeneration. *Neurobiology of Aging*, 30, 1361–1378.

Mangano, E.N., Peters, S., Litteljohn, D., So, R., Bethune, C., Bobyn, J., et al. (2011). Granulocyte macrophage-colony stimulating factor protects against substantia nigra dopaminergic cell loss in an environmental toxin model of Parkinson's disease. *Neurobiology of Disease*, 43, 99–112.

Mangano, E.N., Litteljohn, D., So, R., Nelson, E., Peters, S., Bethune, C., et al. (2012). Interferon-γ plays a role in paraquat-induced neurodegeneration involving oxidative and proinflammatory pathways. *Neurobiology of Aging*, 33, 1411–1426.

Orellana, D.I., Quintanilla, R.A., and Maccioni, R.B. (2007). Neuroprotective effect of TNFalpha against the beta-amyloid neurotoxicity mediated by CDK5 kinase. *Biochimica et Biophysica Acta*, 1773, 254–263.

Overmyer, M., Helisalmi, S., Soininen, H., Laakso, M., Riekkinen, P. Sr., and Alafuzoff, I. (1999). Astrogliosis and the ApoE genotype. An immunohistochemical study of postmortem human brain tissue. *Dementia and Geriatric Cognitive Disorders*, 10, 252–257.

Palmer, K., Berger, A.K., Monastero, R., Winblad, B., Bäckman, L., and Fratiglioni, L. (2007). Predictors of progression from mild cognitive impairment to Alzheimer disease. *Neurology*, 68, 1596–1602.

Purisai, M.G., McCormack, A.L., Cumine, S., Li, J., Isla, M.Z., and Di Monte, D.A. (2007). Microglial activation as a priming event leading to paraquat-induced dopaminergic cell degeneration. *Neurobiology of Disease*, 25, 392–400.

Rangasamy, S.B., Soderstrom, K., Bakay, R.A., and Kordower, J.H. (2010). Neurotrophic factor therapy for Parkinson's disease. *Progress in Brain Research*, 184, 237–264.

Reale, M., Iarlori, C., Thomas, A., Gambi, D., Perfetti, B., Di Nicola, M., et al. (2009). Peripheral cytokines profile in Parkinson's disease. *Brain, Behavior, and Immunity*, 23, 55–63.

Rodríguez, J.J., Olabarria, M., Chvatal, A., and Verkhratsky, A. (2009). Astroglia in dementia and Alzheimer's disease. *Cell Death and Differentiation*, 16, 378–385.

Rogers, J. (2008). The inflammatory response in Alzheimer's disease. *Journal of Periodontology*, 79, 1535–1543.

Salkeni, M.A., Lynch, J.L., Otamis-Price, T., and Banks, W.A. (2009). Lipopolysaccharide impairs blood-brain barrier P-glycoprotein function in mice through prostaglandin- and nitric oxide-independent pathways. *Journal of Neuroimmune Pharmacology*, 4, 276–282.

Scalzo, P., Kümmer, A., Bretas, T.L., Cardoso, F., and Teixeira, A.L. (2010). Serum levels of brain-derived neurotrophic factor correlate with motor impairment in Parkinson's disease. *Journal of Neurology*, 257, 540–545.

Schäbitz, W.R., Krüger, C., Pitzer, C., Weber, D., Laage, R., Gassler, N., et al. (2008). A neuroprotective function for the hematopoietic protein granulocyte-macrophage colony stimulating factor (GM-CSF). *Journal of Cerebral Blood Flow and Metabolism*, 28, 29–43.

Schuitemaker, A., van der Doef, T.F., Boellaard, R., van der Flier, W.M., Yaqub, M., Windhorst, A.D., et al. (2010). Microglial activation in healthy aging. *Neurobiology of Aging*, 33, 1067–1072.

Schwartz, M., and Shechter, R. (2010). Systemic inflammatory cells fight off neurodegenerative disease. *Nature Reviews Neurology*, 6, 405–410.

Shechter, R., London, A., Varol, C., Raposo, C., Cusimano, M., Yovel, G., et al. (2009). Infiltrating blood-derived macrophages are vital cells playing an anti-inflammatory role in recovery from spinal cord injury in mice. *Public Library of Science Medicine*, 6:e1000113.

Slevin, J.T., Gerhardt, G.A., Smith, C.D., Gash, D.M., Kryscio, R., and Young, B. (2005). Improvement of bilateral motor functions in patients with Parkinson disease through the unilateral intraputaminal infusion of glial cell line-derived neurotrophic factor. *Journal of Neurosurgery*, 102, 216–222.

Taylor, J.P., Mata, I.F., and Farrer, M.J. (2006). LRRK2: a common pathway for parkinsonism, pathogenesis and prevention? *Trends in Molecular Medicine*, 12, 76–82.

Tong, L., Balazs, R., Soiampornkul, R., Thangnipon, W., and Cotman, C.W. (2008). Interleukin-1 beta impairs brain derived neurotrophic factor-induced signal transduction. *Neurobiology of Aging*, 29, 1380–1393.

Westerlund, M., Belin, A.C., Anvret, A., Håkansson, A., Nissbrandt, H., Lind, C., et al. (2009). Association of a polymorphism in the ABCB1 gene with Parkinson's disease. *Parkinsonism and Related Disorders*, 15, 422–424.

Xu, X., Li, D., He, Q., Gao, J., Chen, B., and Xie, A. (2011). Interleukin-18 promoter polymorphisms and risk of Parkinson's disease in a Han Chinese population. *Brain Research*, 1381, 90–94.

Yamamoto, M., Kiyota, T., Horiba, M., Buescher, J.L., Walsh, S.M., Gendelman, H.E., et al. (2007). Interferon-gamma and tumor necrosis factor-alpha regulate amyloid-beta plaque deposition and beta-secretase expression in Swedish mutant APP transgenic mice. *American Journal of Pathology*, 170, 680–692.

Yasuda, Y., Shimoda, T., Uno, K., Tateishi, N., Furuya, S., Yagi, K., et al. (2008). The effects of MPTP on the activation of microglia/astrocytes and cytokine/chemokine levels in different mice strains. *Journal of Neuroimmunology*, 204, 43–51.

Yong, J., Lacan, G., Dang, H., Hsieh, T., Middleton, B., Wasserfall, C., et al. (2011). BCG vaccine-induced neuroprotection in a mouse model of Parkinson's disease. *Public Library of Science One*, 6:e16610.

Ziv, Y., Avidan, H., Pluchino, S., Martino, G., and Schwartz, M. (2006). Synergy between immune cells and adult neural stem/progenitor cells promotes functional recovery from spinal cord injury. *Proceedings of the National Academy of Sciences of the United States of America*, 103, 13174–13179.

21

The Psychotic Face of the Immune System

Inflammation and Schizophrenia

Urs Meyer

Physiology and Behaviour Laboratory, Swiss Federal Institute of Technology (ETH), Zurich, Switzerland.

Introduction

Schizophrenia is a severe psychotic disorder characterized by a wide spectrum of behavioral and cognitive dysfunctions that can readily undermine basic human processes of perception and judgment. The disorder includes distinct but typically coexisting symptoms referred to as positive, negative, and cognitive symptoms (Tandon, Nasrallah, and Keshavan, 2009). Positive symptoms are pathological features that are absent in healthy individuals, but emerge as a result of psychotic disease. These comprise visual and/or auditory hallucinations, paranoia, delusions, and major thought-disorders. Negative symptoms refer to features that are normally present, but are decreased or even fully absent in schizophrenic patients. This symptom class includes deficits in social interaction and/or recognition, apathy, lack of motivation and/or pleasure, poverty of speech, and behavioral perseveration. Finally, cognitive symptoms typically include disturbances in executive functions, working memory impairment, and inability to sustain attention.

Schizophrenia affects approximately 1% of the population worldwide (Tandon, Keshavan, and Nasrallah, 2008). The onset of full-blown schizophrenic disease is typically in late adolescence or early adulthood. Despite extensive research and remarkable advances in the neurobiological, neurochemical, and genetic aspects of this disabling mental illness (van Os and Kapur, 2009), the underlying etiological processes remain a challenge for clinicians and basic researchers alike. Since its initial formulation in the late 1980s (Weinberger 1987), the neurodevelopmental hypothesis of schizophrenia has been one of the most enduring theoretical accounts of the disorder's etiology, and has since received converging support from various research fields, including epidemiology, neuroimaging, and postmortem analysis (Fatemi and Folsom, 2009). In essence, this hypothesis suggests that the etiology of schizophrenia involves changes in early fetal and/or neonatal brain development long before the illness is clinically manifest. Recent brain-imaging studies have led to an essential refinement of the neurodevelopmental hypothesis of schizophrenia by underscoring the relevance of progressive brain

The Wiley-Blackwell Handbook of Psychoneuroimmunology, First Edition. Edited by Alexander W. Kusnecov and Hymie Anisman.

changes that occur during the early stages of the disease, i.e., before and/or during the transition to full-blown psychosis in late adolescence or early adulthood (Wood *et al.*, 2008). It thus appears that brain changes in schizophrenia may be more dynamic than previously assumed, and it further seems that an interaction between early neurodevelopmental disturbances and pathological events occurring during postnatal brain maturation are necessary to trigger the onset of full-blown schizophrenic disease.

In addition to the clinical features that primarily relate to central nervous system (CNS) dysfunctions (van Os and Kapur, 2009), schizophrenic disease has also been linked to numerous disturbances in basic physiological and metabolic functions, including insulin resistance, type-2 diabetes, obesity, and cardiovascular disease (Meyer and Stahl, 2009). Furthermore, accumulating evidence suggest that this disorder is also associated with altered immune functions (Müller and Schwarz, 2010). One emerging aspect of immune change in schizophrenia relates to activated inflammatory processes (Meyer, Schwarz, and Müller, 2011). This chapter summarizes evidence for an activated inflammatory response system in schizophrenia and discusses its impact on behavioral and neuronal functions, disease progression, symptomatic pharmacotherapy, and preventive interventions.

Inflammatory Signs in Schizophrenia

Peripheral inflammation

It has repeatedly been noted that patients with schizophrenia display signs of an activated inflammatory response system in peripheral tissue and/or organs (for a recent review see Meyer, Schwarz, and Müller, 2011). Most of the existing evidence for this notion has been yielded by serologic studies documenting elevated serum/plasma levels or *in vitro* production of specific pro-inflammatory factors, including C-reactive protein (CRP), prostaglandin E2 (PGE_2), and numerous pro-inflammatory cytokines such as interleukin (IL)-1β, IL-6, IL-8, and tumor necrosis factor (TNF)-α (reviewed in Meyer, Schwarz, and Müller, 2011). Peripheral inflammatory responses in schizophrenia further appear to comprise abnormal numbers of circulating monocytes, which notably are one of the main sources of pro-inflammatory molecule production and secretion. For example, several studies have found significant increases in the absolute and/or relative counts of monocytes and total white blood cells in schizophrenic patients relative to unaffected controls (Drexhage *et al.*, 2010). In addition, functional changes in T helper 1 (T_H1) cell activity have been correlated with increased pro-inflammatory signaling in patients with schizophrenia (Drexhage *et al.*, 2011).

Inflammation-related abnormalities in schizophrenia may not only be restricted to altered pro-inflammatory activity, but may further include altered anti-inflammatory signaling. Indeed, accumulating evidence indicates that in schizophrenia, increased pro-inflammatory activity concurs with enhanced anti-inflammatory peripheral responses (for a recent review see Meyer, 2011). Among the most consistent findings in this context are elevated peripheral levels and/or *in vitro* production of soluble IL-1 receptor antagonist (sIL-1RA) and soluble IL-2 receptor (sIL-2R). sIL-1RA binds to IL-1 receptors in competition with IL-1α/β, but in contrast to the latter, it fails to activate intracellular signaling cascades. Likewise, sIL-2R is shed from the cellular surface of activated immune cells and efficiently blocks the biological activity of IL-2 by preventing its binding to the membrane-anchored and signal-transducing IL-2 receptor complex. sIL-1RA and sIL-2R can thus both efficiently block pro-inflammatory effects typically associated with IL-1 and IL-2 signaling, respectively (reviewed in Meyer, 2011). Changes in the anti-inflammatory response systems of schizophrenic patients may further involve peripheral elevations in soluble TNF receptor (sTNFR), IL-10, and transforming growth factor (TGF)-β, all of which are known to exert potent anti-inflammatory and/or immunosuppressive functions (Meyer, 2011).

In support of the notion that schizophrenia is associated with both enhanced pro-inflammatory and anti-inflammatory activity, several studies assessing within-subjects cytokine changes report a concomitant up-regulation of pro- and anti-inflammatory cytokines in the serum/plasma of affected individuals (e.g., Kim *et al.*, 2004). A recent study by Drexhage *et al.* (2011) further shows that this concurrent enhancement of pro- and anti-inflammatory activity can be readily extended to the level of peripheral immune cells. More specifically, it has been noted that schizophrenic patients not only show higher percentages of pro-inflammatory monocytes, activated $CD3^+CD25^+$ Tcells and pro-inflammatory T_H17 cells, but they also display higher amounts of anti-inflammatory $CD4^+CD25highFoxP3^+$ regulatory T-cells and $IL\text{-}4^+$ lymphocytes (Drexhage *el al.*, 2011).

The relative potency of schizophrenic patients to mount enhanced anti-inflammatory responses may readily be favorable in as much as this would provide an efficient way to counteract and restrict on-going pro-inflammatory processes, thereby preventing the development of progressive and potentially detrimental effects of chronic inflammation (Meyer, 2011). Indeed, it should be recognized that despite the presence of elevated pro-inflammatory responses, the severity of such responses seems relatively modest in schizophrenia as compared to pathologies that are characterized by marked chronic inflammation, such as rheumatoid arthritis or atherosclerosis (Serhan and Savill, 2005). The inflammatory response in schizophrenia may thus be best referred to as "low-grade inflammation" (Meyer, 2011).

Central inflammation

A great deal of interest has been centered upon the role of microglia in attempts to elucidate inflammatory processes in the CNS of schizophrenic patients (Monji, Kato, and Kanba, 2009). Microglia are the resident macrophages of the CNS, which constantly scavenge the CNS for damaged neurons, plaques, and infectious agents (Ransohoff and Perry, 2009). Microglia appear to play crucial roles in both neuronal protection and pathology, and are often referred to as a "double-edged sword" (Block, Zecca, and Hong, 2007). On the one hand, they secrete neurotrophic factors pivotal for cellular repair, and recruit immune cells into the brain for clearance of infection or cellular debris. On the other hand, chronic or exaggerated microglial activation has been linked to (progressive) neurodegenerative processes (Block, Zecca, and Hong, 2007).

Initial post-mortem immunohistochemical investigations in schizophrenia have provided inconsistent findings with regards to microglia abnormalities in this disorder: Whereas some studies report increased microglia cell densities in the brains of schizophrenic patients, others do not find significant microglia changes in affected individuals (reviewed in Schnieder and Dwork, 2011). More recent approaches have used positron emission tomography (PET) to study the role of microglia in schizophrenia. These studies have confirmed enhanced microglia activation especially in temporolimbic gray matter of schizophrenic patients (Doorduin *et al.*, 2009), suggesting that the disorder may indeed be associated with significant microglia over-activation. However, there is an ongoing debate as to whether such microglia abnormalities may be attributable to medication effects rather than genuine neuroinflammatory processes inherent to schizophrenic disease (Bernstein, Steiner, and Bogerts, 2009). This issue awaits further validation by investigations of possible microglia abnormalities in drug-naïve (or minimally medicated) first-episode patients.

Several research groups have also explored the potential role of abnormal astrocyte functions in schizophrenia. As reviewed in detail elsewhere (Rothermundt, Ahn, and Jörgens, 2009), one well-replicated finding is the increase in serum and/or cerebrospinal fluid (CSF) levels of S100B (Rothermundt, Ahn, and Jörgens, 2009), a protein of the S-100 protein family that is involved in variety of neuronal and glial signaling mechanisms. In the CNS, S100B is primarily produced by activated astrocytes, so that elevated central levels of this protein likely reflect astrocyte overactivation (Rothermundt, Ahn, and Jörgens, 2009). It is important to note that in schizophrenic patients, S100B overexpression takes place in the absence of astrogliosis (Bernstein, Steiner, and Bogerts, 2009). This suggests that the nature of such overexpression is related to altered astrocyte activity rather than density. The lack of overt astrogliosis is in line with the neurodevelopmental hypothesis of schizophrenia, suggesting that the majority of the histological and neuroanatomical changes is unlikely to be the result of marked neurodegeneration, but rather may reflect (progressive) changes in brain development and/or maturation (Weinberger, 1987; Fatemi and Folsom, 2009).

Increased CSF levels of pro-inflammatory cytokines such as IL-1β and IL-6 as well as upregulated cyclooxygenase (COX) expression have also been described in schizophrenic patients, providing additional support for the hypothesis of activated central inflammatory responses in affected individuals (reviewed in Meyer, Schwarz, and Müller, 2011). Some reports further suggest that schizophrenia is associated with reduced potency to mount anti-inflammatory and immunosuppressive responses in the CNS, as supported by findings of reduced gene and/or protein expression of sIL-1RA and TGF-β receptor (reviewed in Meyer, Schwarz, and Müller, 2011). Consistent with this impression, Müller *et al.* (1997) demonstrated that the levels of the soluble IL-6 receptor (sIL-6R) are increased in the CSF of schizophrenic patients. In contrast to other soluble cytokine receptors such as sIL-1RA or sIL-2R, sIL-6R does not inhibit IL-6 signaling, but instead enhances IL-6 functions by acting as an agonist in combination with IL-6 (reviewed in Meyer, 2011). Taken together, there seems to be a relative shift towards enhanced pro-inflammatory and blunted anti-inflammatory activity with regards to secreted inflammatory factors in the CNS of schizophrenic patients. This pattern readily contrasts the immunological profile described in the periphery, where enhanced pro-inflammatory activity appears to concur with increased release of anti-inflammatory and/or immunosuppressive factors (Meyer, Schwarz, and Müller, 2011).

Behavioral and Neuronal Effects of Enhanced Pro-inflammatory Signaling

Effects related to emotions, affect and social functions

Pro-inflammatory cytokines such as IL-1β, IL-6 and TNF-α are known to modulate various brain functions (Anisman, Kokkinidis, and Merali, 2002). One well-established finding is that enhanced peripheral and/or central pro-inflammatory cytokine signaling markedly impairs affective, emotional and social functions, as exemplified in the course of viral or bacterial infections and subsequent emergence of sickness behavior (Dantzer *et al.*, 2008). Experimental work in animals shows that peripheral and/or central administration of pro-inflammatory cytokine releasing agents robustly induces anhedonic behavior and social impairments (Anisman, Kokkinidis, and Merali, 2002; Dantzer *et al.*, 2008), both of which have been consistently linked to the negative symptoms of schizophrenia (Tandon, Nasrallah, and Keshavan, 2009). Furthermore, peripheral inflammation involving enhanced release of IL-6 has been associated with two other hallmark features of negative symptoms, namely deficiency in sustained attention (Holden *et al.*, 2008) and psychomotor retardation (Brydon *et al.*, 2008).

One of the emerging neuroimmunological mechanisms linking enhanced pro-inflammatory activity with the induction of affective, emotional and social impairment may involve alterations in the central tryptophan metabolism (Müller and Schwarz, 2010). Tryptophan is an essential amino acid required for the biosynthesis of serotonin. As discussed in detail elsewhere (Meyer, Schwarz, and Müller, 2011), enhanced pro-inflammatory actions in the CNS lead to increased tryptophan degradation into kynurenine by indoleamine 2,3-dioxygenase (IDO), thereby reducing the bioavailability of tryptophan for serotonin synthesis (Figure 21.1). Hence, increased pro-inflammatory actions in the CNS can critically contribute to central serotonin deficiency. Besides its involvement in depressive illness (Anisman, Kokkinidis, Merali, 2002; Dantzer *et al.*, 2008), serotonin insufficiency has also been suggested to play an important role in the pathogenesis of negative symptoms of schizophrenia (Abi-Dargham *et al.*, 1997).

Effects related to cognitive functions

The impact of activated inflammatory response systems in schizophrenia may well be extended to disease-relevant cognitive impairments. Indeed, there is a growing body of evidence highlighting a positive correlation between the severity of cognitive deficits and enhanced levels of inflammatory markers in schizophrenic patients, including IL-1β, IL-6, TNF-α, CRP, and S100B (reviewed in Meyer, Schwarz, and Müller, 2011). The specificity of the cognitive effects induced by inflammatory processes in schizophrenia remains to be further elucidated. However, experimental studies in animals and correlative investigations in non-schizophrenic individuals suggest that the spectrum of inflammation-mediated cognitive impairments may primarily affect domains of executive functions, sustained attention and working memory (Meyer, Schwarz, and Müller, 2011), all of which have been implicated in schizophrenia (Tandon, Nasrallah, and Keshavan, 2009). Molecular investigations in experimental rodent models have also confirmed that pro-inflammatory cytokines can exert appreciable influences on various forms of synaptic plasticity, the latter of which provides an important neuronal substrate for multiple aspects of learning and memory (Bauer, Kerr, and Patterson, 2007). It is therefore feasible that altered pro-inflammatory activity may exert its cognitive effects by modulating synaptic architecture and functions (McAfoose and Baune, 2009).

An alternative (but not mutually exclusive) neuronal mechanism by which enhanced pro-inflammatory activity could affect cognitive functions may again be related to changes in the central kynurenine pathway (Figure 21.1). More specifically, imbalances in the (local) astrocyte/microglia cytokine milieu together with enhanced astrocyte functions can result in altered expression and/or activation of catalytic enzymes involved in this pathway, eventually resulting in enhanced production of kynurenic acid (KYNA) (Müller and Schwarz, 2010; Wonodi and Schwarcz, 2010). KYNA is a potent endogenous *N*-methyl-D-aspartate (NMDA) receptor antagonist acting at the glycine site of the receptor (Wonodi and Schwarcz, 2010).

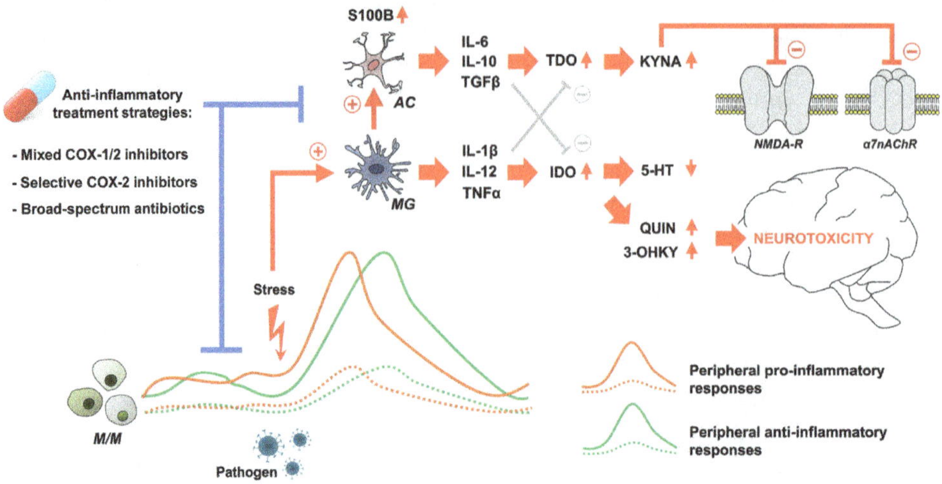

Figure 21.1 Simplified schematic representation of the characteristics and neuronal consequences of activated inflammatory responses in schizophrenia. Abnormal expression of inflammatory genes in monocytes/macrophages (M/M) facilitates the development of peripheral low-grade inflammation in patients with schizophrenia (represented by solid orange and green lines) as compared to healthy subjects (represented by dashed orange and green lines). Such peripheral low-grade inflammation seems to be characterized by fluctuations in abnormal pro- and anti-inflammatory activity, whereby enhanced pro-inflammatory activity (orange lines) typically precedes the onset of increased anti-inflammatory activity (green lines). In schizophrenia, inflammatory responses may follow processes of sensitization and thus may react more vigorously to the presence of specific environmental factors such as physical or psychological stress, or pathogen contact. Stress and/or pathogen exposure in psychosis-prone subjects may lead to an over-activation of microglia (MG) cells, which in turn promote functional activation of astrocytes (AST). Abnormally enhanced astrocyte activity is accompanied by up-regulated S100B expression. In addition, activated astrocytes release a set of cytokines (primarily IL-6, IL-10, and TGF-β) that stimulate the production of kynurenic acid (KYNA) by facilitating the enzymatic activity of tryptophan 2,3-dioxygenase (TDO) in astrocytes. KYNA blocks signaling at the NMDA receptor (NMDA-R) and α7 nicotinic acetylcholine receptor (α7nAChR). On the other hand, activated MG secrete a set of pro-inflammatory cytokines (primarily IL-1β, IL-12, and TNF-α) that stimulate the enzymatic activity of indoleamine 2,3-dioxygenase (IDO), which in turn weakens the biosynthesis of serotonin (5-HT) and promotes the production of quinolinic acid (QUIN) and 3-hydroxykynurenine (3-OHKY). QUIN and 3-OHKY are neurotoxic and may therefore contribute to inflammation-mediated neurotoxicity. Note that there is a mutual inhibitory effect of IDO and TDO, so that their enzymatic activities are critically determined by the prevailing cytokine milieu. Anti-inflammatory add-on therapy may provide a promising pharmacological approach to block the neuronal and behavioral effects of enhanced pro-inflammatory signaling in schizophrenia, and to improve psychopathological and neuropathological syndromes associated with the disorder. Currently used anti-inflammatory treatment strategies in schizophrenia are based on administration of mixed COX-1/2 inhibitors (acetylsalicylic acid = aspirin), selective COX-2 inhibitors (celecoxib), and broad-spectrum antibiotics (minocycline).

Impaired glutamatergic signaling at NMDA receptors has frequently been associated with schizophrenia in general, and with the emergence of disease-relevant cognitive symptoms in particular (Javitt, 2007). Moreover, enhanced production of KYNA and associated changes in the central kynurenine pathway have been consistently documented in schizophrenic patients (reviewed in Müller and Schwarz, 2010; Wonodi and Schwarcz, 2010). Experimental work in animals further shows that enhancement of KYNA disrupts a variety of schizophrenia-relevant cognitive functions (Chess, Simoni, Alling, and Bucci, 2007). Taken together, there is emerging evidence to support a model in which enhanced pro-inflammatory activity can lead to cognitive disturbances via inflammation-mediated modulation of the central kynurenine pathway and subsequent impairments in NMDA receptor-mediated signaling (Figure 21.1).

Besides its impact on NMDA receptor signaling, KYNA also potently inhibits cholinergic neurotransmission by blocking nicotinic acetylcholine receptors (nAChR), especially α7 nAChRs (Wonodi and Schwarcz, 2010). Such cholinergic effects are primarily induced at relatively low concentrations of KYNA (Wonodi and Schwarcz, 2010). In keeping with the suggested contribution of impaired nAChR signaling to cognitive symptoms of schizophrenia (Martin and Freedman, 2007), inhibition of nAChR by KYNA overproduction may provide an additional neuroimmunological link between activated central inflammatory responses and emergence of cognitive impairments in this disorder (Figure 21.1).

Effects related to positive psychotic symptoms

Enhanced pro-inflammatory signaling could also play a role in the emergence of positive symptoms. Of special interest in this context are the stimulatory effects of pro-inflammatory cytokines on dopamine and noradrenalin synthesis and release (Dunn, 2006). Increased dopamine and noradrenalin activity (especially in mesolimbic structures) have been repeatedly implicated in the emergence of positive psychotic symptoms through neuropsychological mechanisms that affect the salience of internal and/or external representations and induce states of hypervigilance, respectively (Yamamoto and Hornykiewicz, 2004; Howes and Kapur, 2009). Hence, there would be a feasible theoretical framework implicating a potential role of enhanced pro-inflammatory activity in the emergence of positive symptoms of schizophrenia. However, with the exception of a limited number of studies, the majority of investigations does not find a strict positive correlation between the severity of positive symptoms of schizophrenia and enhanced levels of prototypical pro-inflammatory cytokines such as IL-1β, IL-6 and TNF-α (reviewed in Meyer, 2011; Meyer, Schwarz, and Müller, 2011). A conclusion as to whether or not enhanced pro-inflammatory activity may play an essential role in the precipitation of positive symptoms thus seems premature at present. Further research is clearly warranted to address this issue in more detail.

Immunomodulatory Effects of Antipsychotic Drugs, Anti-inflammatory Treatment Strategies, and Disease Progression

Numerous antipsychotic drugs (APDs) are known to exert modulatory effects on immune functions in general, and on peripheral cytokine networks in particular (Drzyzga, Obuchowicz, Marcinowska, and Herman, 2006). Emerging evidence suggests that APDs potently enhance anti-inflammatory activity as indexed by the augmentation of peripheral production of IL-10, sIL-1RA, sIL-2R, and by the concomitant reduction of pro-inflammatory markers such as IL-1β, IL-6 sIL-6R, and TNF-α (Drzyzga, Obuchowicz, Marcinowska, and Herman, 2006). It has been suggested that the relative capacity of APDs to normalize pro-inflammatory immune changes may be an important contributing factor determining the clinical efficacy of APDs in the symptomatological treatment of psychotic symptoms (Müller and Schwarz, 2010).

Table 21.1 Anti-inflammatory Treatment Strategies in Schizophrenia

Drug	*Class*	*Main anti-inflammatory actions*	*Clinical trial*	*Effect in schizophrenia*
Acetylsalicylic acid(Aspirin)	Mixed COX-1/2 inhibitor	• irreversibly inactivates COX-1 and attenuates the enzymatic activity of COX-2 • blocks nuclear factor-kappa B (NF-κB) signaling • inhibits the production of prostanoids (prostaglandins, prostacyclin, and thromboxanes) and pro-inflammatory cytokines	Laan *et al.*, 2010	(+)
Celecoxib	Selective COX-2 inhibitor	• selectively blocks the enzymatic activity of COX-2 at sites of inflammation • inhibits nuclear factor-kappa B (NF-κB) signaling • inhibits the production of prostanoids (prostaglandins, prostacyclin, and thromboxanes) and pro-inflammatory cytokines	Müller *et al.*, 2002 Müller *et al.*, 2005 Müller *et al.*, 2010 Akhondzadeh *et al.*, 2007 Rapaport *et al.*, 2005	(+) (+) (+) (+) (-)
Minocycline	Tetracycline broad-spectrum antibiotic	• bacteriostatic effects limiting the growth of bacteria • inhibition of matrix metaloproteinase-9 • inhibits the production of pro-inflammatory cytokines and activation of peripheral as well as central immunocompetent cells, including T-cells, macrophages, and microglia	Miyaoka *et al.*, 2008 Levkovitz *et al.*, 2010	(+) (+)

The table outlines the different treatment strategies used in clinical trials of anti-inflammatory add-on therapy in schizophrenia. The main cellular and molecular targets of each class of anti-inflammatory drugs are also summarized.

Symbol (+) denotes the number of clinical trials showing superior beneficial treatment effects of combined anti-inflammatory and antipsychotic drug administration relative to antipsychotic drug administration alone; symbol (−) denotes the number of clinical trials showing no superior treatment effects of combined anti-inflammatory and antipsychotic drug administration relative to antipsychotic drug administration alone.

Consistent with this hypothesis, it has been show that schizophrenic patients who are resistant to APD-induced behavioral improvement display persistently high IL-6 levels, and that such immune abnormalities in treatment-resistant schizophrenic patients cannot be restored by APDs either (reviewed in Meyer, 2011; Meyer, Schwarz, and Müller, 2011).

In view of the apparent involvement of inflammatory processes, the use of compounds with primary anti-inflammatory properties has received increasing attention in the pharmacotherapy of schizophrenia (Figure 21.1). Importantly, recent clinical trials of anti-inflammatory add-on therapy in schizophrenia have provided promising results by showing superior beneficial treatment effects when standard APDs were co-administered with anti-inflammatory compounds, as compared with treatment outcomes using APDs alone. As summarized in Table 21.1, two main classes of anti-inflammatory drugs have been tested as adjunctive medication in schizophrenia, namely the tetracycline antibiotic minocycline (Miyaoka *et al.*, 2008; Levkovitz *et al.*, 2010) and non-steroidal anti-inflammatory drugs (NSAIDs), including the mixed COX-1/2 inhibitor acetylsalicylic acid (Laan *et al.*, 2010) and the selective COX-2 inhibitor celecoxib (Müller *et al.*, 2002; Müller, Riedel, Schwarz, and Engel, 2005; Müller *et al.*, 2010; Rapaport *et al.*, 2005; Akhondzadeh *et al.*, 2007).

Intriguing findings have recently been provided by Müller *et al.* (2010), who evaluated the potential beneficial effects of anti-inflammatory add-on therapy in the early-phase relative to late-phase of schizophrenic disease: In randomized, double-blind, placebo-controlled clinical trials using the COX-2 inhibitor celecoxib given in conjunction with atypical APDs, the authors highlighted that such anti-inflammatory add-on therapy has superior beneficial treatment effects especially when initiated in the early-phase of schizophrenia, as opposed to later chronic stages (Müller *et al.*, 2010; Müller and Schwarz, 2010). These novel findings raise the possibility that the nature and/or severity of activated inflammatory responses in schizophrenia may critically change as a function of disease progression, so that primary anti-inflammatory strategies may be particularly efficient when targeting those immune abnormalities that are characteristic of the early stage of schizophrenia. There is no doubt that our understanding of the precise immune signature in the early phase of schizophrenia is far from complete. However, from the findings provided by Müller *et al.* (2010), one may speculate on a model in which enhanced pro-inflammatory activity may be particularly prominent in the early-phase of schizophrenic disease. This impression would be compatible with the (limited amount of) data indicating that enhanced pro-inflammatory activity precedes altered anti-inflammatory activity in schizophrenia, so that the former is readily noticeable in drug-naïve first-episode schizophrenic patients (reviewed in Meyer, Schwarz, and Müller, 2011).

It is also of note that patients with schizophrenia frequently report phases of stress in the proximity of or during the transition to full-blown psychosis (Phillips *et al.*, 2006), and exposure to physical or psychological stressors is well known to enhance the production and release of pro-inflammatory cytokines such as IL-1β, IL-6, TNF-α (García-Bueno, Caso, and Leza, 2008). Psychosocial and/or physical stress in the early-phase of schizophrenic disease may therefore readily contribute to the enhancement of pro-inflammatory activity. Whatever the precise source of enhanced pro-inflammatory activity, the presence of such immune imbalances in the early-phase of schizophrenia may explain as to why anti-inflammatory strategies (at least those which are based on COX-2 inhibition) may be particularly efficient in improving schizophrenic symptoms when implemented at early stages of the disease (Figure 21.2).

Increased inflammatory signaling in the early stages of schizophrenia may also be relevant for the progressive reduction in gray matter volume that occurs in the proximity of or during of the onset of full-blown psychosis (Wood *et al.*, 2008). Such volume reduction seems

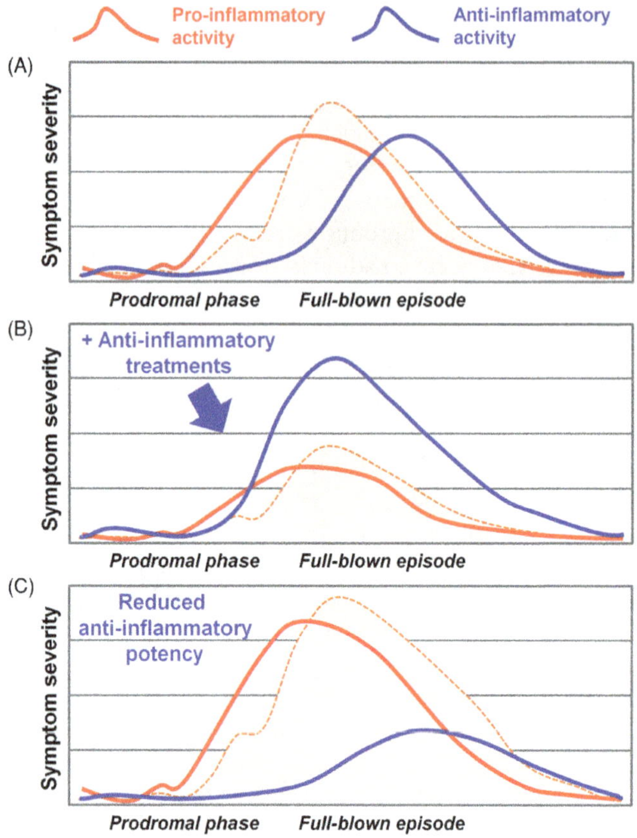

Figure 21.2 Inflammatory responses and disease progression in schizophrenia. The figure provides a hypothetical model illustrating potential relationships between temporal changes in inflammatory responses and disease progression in schizophrenia. (A) Increased pro-inflammatory activity (represented by solid red lines) may be particularly prominent in the early stage of schizophrenic disease, including the (initial) prodromal phase and onset of full-blown psychotic episodes. The subsequent enhancement in anti-inflammatory activity (represented by solid blue lines) may provide a compensatory response to the initial pro-inflammatory stimulus and may contribute to the resolution of psychotic episodes and abnormally enhanced pro-inflammatory activity. The enhancement of anti-inflammatory activity may partly be driven by endogenous response mechanisms, and partly by the anti-inflammatory effects of antipsychotic drug treatment (not shown). (B) Pharmacologically induced enhancement of anti-inflammatory activity by administration of primary anti-inflammatory agents during the early phase of schizophrenic disease may attenuate gradual increases in pro-inflammatory activity and progression into full-blown psychotic disease. (C) Reduced potency to mount anti-inflammatory responses (during the early phase of schizophrenic disease) may facilitate the gradual elevation of pro-inflammatory activity and may increase symptom severity and duration.

to resemble an exaggeration of gray matter reduction occurring as a result of normal adult development (Wood *et al.*, 2008), and it is matter of current debate whether or not this process may involve (transient) neurodegenerative processes (Archer, 2010). A recent study by de la Fuente-Sandoval *et al.* (2011) shows increased brain glutamate levels in subjects with ultra-high risk for schizophrenia, and first-episode patients. This has been taken as circumstantial evidence to support the possibility of (transient) processes of neurodegeneration in the early stages of schizophrenia (Lahti and Reid, 2011), primarily because excess synaptic glutamate levels are highly neurotoxic (Lau and Tymianski, 2010). In the present context it is highly interesting to point out that activated microglia release substantial levels of glutamate (Barger, Goodwin, Porter, and Beggs, 2007), and such microglia-mediated toxicity may readily contribute to neuronal damage in the event of neuroinflammation (Block, Zecca, and Hong, 2007).

Microglia overactivation also leads to elevated production of quinolinic acid (QUIN) and 3-hydroxykynurenine (3-OHKY), both of which have potent neurotoxic properties too (Wonodi and Schwarcz, 2010). In a recent study, Condray *et al.* (2011) showed that drug-naïve first-episode schizophrenic patients displayed enhanced 3-OHKY levels, and that the levels of 3-OHKY predicted clinical improvement following anti-psychotic drug treatment in as much as the lowest concentrations of 3-OHKY were associated with the greatest improvement in symptoms. Taken together, the excess in glutamate and 3-OHKY release during the early (prodromal) stages of schizophrenic disease would fit with the hypothetical model emphasizing a critical role of enhanced neuroinflammatory processes in the progressive development of overt schizophrenic disease (Figure 21.2).

Conclusions

An appreciable number of studies support the hypothesis of activated peripheral and central inflammatory responses in schizophrenia. There is also accumulating evidence to suggest that activated inflammatory responses can contribute to disease-relevant affective, emotional, social, and cognitive dysfunctions. Against this background, anti-inflammatory therapies in schizophrenia appear to be a promising approach to improve psychopathological symptoms, and the extension of anti-inflammatory therapies to the early stages of schizophrenia seems feasible.

The available neuroimmunological and clinical data leave many questions unanswered, especially with regards to the precise cellular and molecular mechanisms underlying the beneficial therapeutic effects of anti-inflammatory drugs against schizophrenic symptoms. However, these data readily provide testable hypotheses, given the fact that the cellular and molecular effects of most currently available anti-inflammatory drugs are relatively well described. Animal models of schizophrenia, particularly those which recapitulate inflammatory components of the disorder (Meyer and Feldon, 2010), may further help to identify the relevant neuroimmunological mechanisms pertinent to the beneficial clinical effects of anti-inflammatory therapies in schizophrenia. Given the limited efficacy of currently available APDs to ameliorate especially the negative and cognitive symptoms, the further exploration of inflammatory mechanisms and anti-inflammatory strategies may open fruitful avenues for a better treatment of symptoms undermining affective, emotional, social and cognitive functions relevant for schizophrenic disease.

References

Abi-Dargham, A., Laruelle, M., Aghajanian, G.K., Charney, D., and Krystal, J. (1997). The role of serotonin in the pathophysiology and treatment of schizophrenia. *The Journal of Neuropsychiatry and Clinical Neurosciences*, 9, 1–17.

Akhondzadeh, S., Tabatabaee, M., Amini, H., Ahmadi Abhari, S.A., Abbasi, S.H., and Behnam, B. (2007). Celecoxib as adjunctive therapy in schizophrenia: a double-blind, randomized and placebo-controlled trial. *Schizophrenia Research*, 90, 179–185.

Anisman, H., Kokkinidis, L., and Merali, Z. (2002). Further evidence for the depressive effects of cytokines: anhedonia and neurochemical changes. *Brain, Behavior, and Immunity*, 16, 544–556.

Archer, T. (2010). Neurodegeneration in schizophrenia. *Expert Review of Neurotherapeutics*, 10, 1131–1141.

Barger, S.W., Goodwin, M.E., Porter, M.M., and Beggs, M.L. (2007). Glutamate release from activated microglia requires the oxidative burst and lipid peroxidation. *Journal of Neurochemistry*, 101, 1205–1213.

Bauer, S., Kerr, B.J., and Patterson, P.H. (2007). The neuropoietic cytokine family in development, plasticity, disease and injury. *Nature Reviews Neuroscience*, 8, 221–232.

Bernstein, H.G., Steiner, J., and Bogerts, B. (2009). Glial cells in schizophrenia: pathophysiological significance and possible consequences for therapy. *Expert Review of Neurotherapeutics*, 9, 1059–1071.

Block, M.L., Zecca, L., and Hong, J.S. (2007). Microglia-mediated neurotoxicity: uncovering the molecular mechanisms. *Nature Reviews Neuroscience*, 8, 57–69.

Brydon, L., Harrison, N.A., Walker, C., Steptoe, A., and Critchley, H.D. (2008). Peripheral inflammation is associated with altered substantia nigra activity and psychomotor slowing in humans. *Biological Psychiatry*, 63, 1022–1029.

Chess, A.C., Simoni, M.K., Alling, T.E., and Bucci, D.J. (2007). Elevations of endogenous kynurenic acid produce spatial working memory deficits. *Schizophrenia Bulletin*, 33, 797–804.

Condray, R., Dougherty, G.G. Jr., Keshavan, M.S., Reddy, R.D., Haas, G.L., Montrose, D.M., et al. (2011). 3-Hydroxykynurenine and clinical symptoms in first-episode neuroleptic-naive patients with schizophrenia. *International Journal of Neuropsychopharmacology*, 14, 756–767.

Dantzer, R., O'Connor, J.C., Freund, G.G., Johnson, R.W., and Kelley, K.W. (2008). From inflammation to sickness and depression: when the immune system subjugates the brain. *Nature Reviews Neuroscience*, 9, 46–56.

de la Fuente-Sandoval, C., León-Ortiz, P., Favila, R., Stephano, S., Mamo, D., Ramírez-Bermúdez, J., et al. (2011). Higher levels of glutamate in the associative-striatum of subjects with prodromal symptoms of schizophrenia and patients with first-episode psychosis. *Neuropsychopharmacology*, 36, 1781–1791.

Doorduin, J., de Vries, E.F., Willemsen, A.T., de Groot, J.C., Dierckx, R.A., and Klein, H.C. (2009). Neuroinflammation in schizophrenia-related psychosis: a PET study. *Journal of Nuclear Medicine*, 50, 1801–1807.

Drexhage, R.C., Hoogenboezem, T.A., Cohen, D., Versnel, M.A., Nolen, W.A., van Beveren, N.J., et al. (2011). An activated set point of T-cell and monocyte inflammatory networks in recent-onset schizophrenia patients involves both pro- and anti-inflammatory forces. *International Journal of Neuropsychopharmacology*, 14, 746–755.

Drexhage, R.C., Knijff, E.M., Padmos, R.C., Heul-Nieuwenhuijzen, L., Beumer, W., Versnel, M.A., et al. (2010). The mononuclear phagocyte system and its cytokine inflammatory networks in schizophrenia and bipolar disorder. *Expert Review of Neurotherapeutics*, 10, 59–76.

Drzyzga, L., Obuchowicz, E., Marcinowska, A., and Herman, Z.S. (2006). Cytokines in schizophrenia and the effects of antipsychotic drugs. *Brain, Behavior, and Immunity*, 20, 532–545.

Dunn, A.J. (2006). Effects of cytokines and infections on brain neurochemistry. *Clinical Neuroscience Research*, 6, 52–68.

Fatemi, S.H., and Folsom, T.D. (2009). The neurodevelopmental hypothesis of schizophrenia, revisited. *Schizophrenia Bulletin*, 35, 528–548.

García-Bueno, B., Caso, J.R., and Leza, J.C. (2008). Stress as a neuroinflammatory condition in brain: damaging and protective mechanisms. *Neuroscience and Biobehavioral Reviews*, 32, 1136–1151.

Holden, J.M., Meyers-Manor, J.E., Overmier, J.B., Gahtan, E., Sweeney, W., and Miller, H. (2008). Lipopolysaccharide-induced immune activation impairs attention but has little effect on short-term working memory. *Behavioural Brain Research*, 194, 138–145.

Howes, O.D., and Kapur, S. (2009). The dopamine hypothesis of schizophrenia: version III – the final common pathway. *Schizophrenia Bulletin*, 35, 549–562.

Javitt, D.C. (2007). Glutamate and schizophrenia: phencyclidine, N-methyl-D-aspartate receptors, and dopamine-glutamate interactions. *International Review of Neurobiology*, 78, 69–108.

Kim, Y.K., Myint, A.M., Lee, B.H., Han, C.S., Lee, H.J., Kim, D.J., et al. (2004). Th1, Th2 and Th3 cytokine alteration in schizophrenia. *Progress in Neuro-Psychopharmacology and Biological Psychiatry*, 28, 1129–1134.

Laan, W., Grobbee, D.E., Selten, J.P., Heijnen, C.J., Kahn, R.S., and Burger, H. (2010). Adjuvant aspirin therapy reduces symptoms of schizophrenia spectrum disorders: results from a randomized, double-blind, placebo-controlled trial. *The Journal of Clinical Psychiatry*, 71, 520–527.

Lahti, A.C., and Reid, M.A. (2011). Is there evidence for neurotoxicity in the prodromal and early stages of schizophrenia? *Neuropsychopharmacology*, 36, 1779–1780.

Lau, A., and Tymianski, M. (2010). Glutamate receptors, neurotoxicity and neurodegeneration. *Pflügers Archiv: European Journal of Physiology*, 460, 525–542.

Levkovitz, Y., Mendlovich, S., Riwkes, S., Braw, Y., Levkovitch-Verbin, H., Gal, G., et al. (2010). A double-blind, randomized study of minocycline for the treatment of negative and cognitive symptoms in early-phase schizophrenia. *The Journal of Clinical Psychiatry*, 71, 138–149.

Martin, L.F., and Freedman, R. (2007). Schizophrenia and the alpha7 nicotinic acetylcholine receptor. *International Review of Neurobiology*, 78, 225–246.

McAfoose, J., and Baune, B.T. (2009). Evidence for a cytokine model of cognitive function. *Neuroscience and Biobehavioral Reviews*, 33, 355–366.

Meyer, J.M., and Stahl, S.M. (2009). The metabolic syndrome and schizophrenia. *Acta Psychiatrica Scandinavica*, 119, 4–14.

Meyer, U. (2011). Anti-inflammatory signaling in schizophrenia. *Brain, Behavior, and Immunity*, 25, 1507–1518.

Meyer, U., and Feldon, J. (2010). Epidemiology-driven neurodevelopmental animal models of schizophrenia. *Progress in Neurobiology*, 90, 285–326.

Meyer, U., Schwarz, M.J., and Müller, N. (2011). Inflammatory processes in schizophrenia: a promising neuroimmunological target for the treatment of negative/cognitive symptoms and beyond. *Pharmacology and Therapeutics*, 132, 96–110.

Miyaoka, T., Yasukawa, R., Yasuda, H., Hayashida, M., Inagaki, T., and Horiguchi, J. (2008). Minocycline as adjunctive therapy for schizophrenia: an open-label study. *Clinical Neuropharmacology*, 31, 287–292.

Monji, A., Kato, T., and Kanba, S. (2009). Cytokines and schizophrenia: Microglia hypothesis of schizophrenia. *Psychiatry and Clinical Neurosciences*, 63, 257–265.

Müller, N., Dobmeier, P, Empl, M., Riedel, M., Schwarz, M., and Ackenheil, M. (1997). Soluble IL-6 receptors in the serum and cerebrospinal fluid of paranoid schizophrenic patients. *European Psychiatry*, 12, 294–299.

Müller, N., Krause, D., Dehning, S., Musil, R., Schennach-Wolff, R., Obermeier, M., et al. (2010). Celecoxib treatment in an early stage of schizophrenia: results of a randomized, double-blind, placebo-controlled trial of celecoxib augmentation of amisulpride treatment. *Schizophrenia Research*, 121, 118–124.

Müller, N., Riedel, M., Scheppach, C., Brandstätter, B., Sokullu, S., Krampe, K., et al. (2002). Beneficial antipsychotic effects of celecoxib add-on therapy compared to risperidone alone in schizophrenia. *The American Journal of Psychiatry*, 159, 1029–1034.

Müller, N., Riedel, M., Schwarz, M.J., and Engel, R.R. (2005). Clinical effects of COX-2 inhibitors on cognition in schizophrenia. *European Archives of Psychiatry and Clinical Neuroscience*, 255, 149–151.

Müller, N., and Schwarz, M.J. (2010). Immune system and schizophrenia. *Current Immunology Reviews*, 6, 213–220.

Phillips, L.J., McGorry, P.D., Garner, B., Thompson, K.N., Pantelis, C., Wood, S.J., et al. (2006). Stress, the hippocampus and the hypothalamic-pituitary-adrenal axis: implications for the development of psychotic disorders. *Australian and New Zealand Journal of Psychiatry*, 40, 725–741.

Ransohoff, R.M., and Perry, V.H. (2009). Microglial physiology: unique stimuli, specialized responses. *Annual Review of Immunology*, 27, 119–145.

Rapaport, M.H., Delrahim, K.K., Bresee, C.J., Maddux, R.E., Ahmadpour, O., and Dolnak, D. (2005). Celecoxib augmentation of continuously ill patients with schizophrenia. *Biological Psychiatry*, 57, 1594–1596.

Rothermundt, M., Ahn, J.N., and Jörgens, S. (2009). S100B in schizophrenia: an update. *General Physiology and Biophysics*, 28, F76–81.

Schnieder, T.P., and Dwork, A.J. (2011). Searching for neuropathology: gliosis in schizophrenia. *Biological Psychiatry*, 69, 134–139.

Serhan, C.N., and Savill, J. (2005). Resolution of inflammation: the beginning programs the end. *Nature Immunology*, 6, 1191–1197.

Tandon, R., Keshavan, M.S., and Nasrallah, H.A. (2008). Schizophrenia, "just the facts": what we know in 2008. 2. Epidemiology and etiology. *Schizophrenia Research*, 102, 1–18.

Tandon, R., Nasrallah, H.A., and Keshavan, M.S. (2009). Schizophrenia, "just the facts" 4. Clinical features and conceptualization. *Schizophrenia Research*, 110, 1–23.

van Os, J., and Kapur, S. (2009). Schizophrenia. *Lancet*, 374, 635–645.

Weinberger, D.R. (1987). Implications of normal brain development for the pathogenesis of schizophrenia. *Archives of General Psychiatry*, 44, 660–669.

Wonodi, I., and Schwarcz, R. (2010). Cortical kynurenine pathway metabolism: a novel target for cognitive enhancement in schizophrenia. *Schizophrenia Bulletin*, 36, 211–218.

Wood, S.J., Pantelis, C., Velakoulis, D., Yücel, M., Fornito, A., and McGorry, P.D. (2008). Progressive changes in the development toward schizophrenia: studies in subjects at increased symptomatic risk. *Schizophrenia Bulletin*, 34, 322–329.

Yamamoto, K., and Hornykiewicz, O. (2004). Proposal for a noradrenaline hypothesis of schizophrenia. *Progress in Neuro-Psychopharmacology and Biological Psychiatry*, 28, 913–922.

22

Neuroimmune Mechanisms in Autism

Veronica M. Miller,[1,2] Rachael Racine,[3] and Steven S. Zalcman[4]

[1] *Wadsworth Center, New York State Department of Health, Empire State Plaza, Albany, NY, USA*

[2] *School of Public Health, University at Albany, State University of New York, Albany, NY, USA*

[3] *Department of Immunobiology, Yale University of Medicine, The Anlyan Center for Medical Research & Education, New Haven, CT, USA*

[4] *Department of Psychiatry, The University of Medicine and Dentistry of New Jersey, New Jersey Medical School, Newark, NJ, USA*

Introduction

Autism is a neurodevelopmental disorder associated with abnormalities in three behavioral domains: 1) social interaction; 2) language, communication and imaginative play; and 3) range of interests and activities (DSM IV, 2000). Symptoms of autism usually arise before 2 years of age and the diagnosis is usually made by 4 years of age. The first cases of autism were diagnosed in the 1930s, although it is unknown whether the disorder existed before then. In the 1970s, epidemiological studies conducted in the US, UK and Japan estimated the prevalence of autism at ~0.05%. Since then, more recent studies in the UK, US and South Korea estimate that autism affects ~1–2% of children under the age of 8 years (Baron-Cohen *et al.*, 2009; Hoshino *et al.*, 1982; Kim *et al.*, 2011; Treffert, 1970; Wing and Gould, 1979). This alarming 20-fold increase in the prevalence of autism since the 1970s has led to a surge in studies aimed at determining the mechanisms underscoring the pathophysiology of the disorder.

It should be noted that part of the increasing prevalence of autism could be attributed to changes in the diagnostic criteria for the disorder. A study by King and colleagues on the prevalence of autism in California (King and Bearman, 2009) observed *diagnostic substitution*, a situation where people who previously have been labeled with something else are diagnosed as autistic. This meant that children who had a diagnosis of mental retardation were more likely to be diagnosed with autism, and this likely accounted for ~25% of the increased prevalence of autism in California. Another study by Hertz-Picciotto and colleagues (2009) into the factors which precipitated the 600% increase in autism prevalence in California (1990 to 2006) suggested that earlier diagnosis of autism accounted for ~24% of the rate increase (Hertz-Picciotto and Delwiche, 2009). Therefore, changes in the timing and type of diagnostic

The Wiley-Blackwell Handbook of Psychoneuroimmunology, First Edition. Edited by Alexander W. Kusnecov and Hymie Anisman.

criteria used to define autism could account for 50% of the increased prevalence of autism; however this leaves ~50% of the increase in prevalence unaccounted for.

Genetic factors are involved in autism and may play a role in the pathophysiology of the disease. For example, the risk of developing autism is higher in siblings of children with autism, than found in the general population (Jorde *et al.*, 1991). However, autism is not fully penetrant in monozygotic twins, affecting between 60 and 91%, which suggests that genetic factors are not necessarily causative of autism (Muhle,Trentacoste, and Rapin, 2004). In fact, it is more likely, as Landrigan suggested (2010), that a complex interaction between environmental and genetic factors underscores the increasing prevalence of autism (Landrigan, 2010). Moreover, it is even more likely that abnormal immune responses to environmental pathogens and stressors play a role in the increasing prevalence of autism.

Abnormal immune responses and increased susceptibility to fungal and bacterial infections are reported in both autistic children and their parents (Ashwood, Wills, and Van de Water, 2006; Wei *et al.*, 2011). The latter finding has led to speculation that dysfunctional immune responses may not only be a symptom, but also a potential trigger of autism. In this chapter, we discuss the evidence from human and animal modeling studies that abnormal maternal immune responses during pregnancy contribute to the etiology disorder. We also discuss how an array of insults to the immune system may give rise to the spectrum of symptoms in autism and whether medications which remediate immune responses in children or mothers of children with autism can reduce behavioral abnormalities. Before we delve too deeply into the neuroimmune mechanisms associated with autism, firstly we will introduce the key cellular components which mediate immune responses in the central and peripheral nervous system, and how they are altered in autism.

Mediators of Central and Peripheral Immune Responses

On a gross level, the brain is protected from perturbances in the local environment via protective structures such as the skull and cerebrospinal fluid, not to mention the blood–brain-barrier (BBB) which serves as a semi-permeable barrier to prevent toxins or pathogens from entering the brain. On a cellular basis there are three kinds of cell, or glia, which mediate the majority of neuroimmune responses: there are microglia, the "small" cells, are also known as the brain's macrophages, which can scavenge debris from dead and dying cells as well as mounting responses based on superoxide, cytokines, and growth factors to immune challenges; there are oligodendrocytes, or the "many" armed myelin-synthesizing cells, which are essential to promote axonal function, both in terms of speed of conducting impulses and also connecting cortical regions; and, finally, there are the astrocytes, the "star-shaped" cells, responsible for maintaining the integrity of the BBB via their end-feet which form a core composite of the vessel's outer wall. Astrocytes also recycle, store, and synthesize growth factors and metabolites necessary for neuronal survival. All three neuroglia are involved in regulating the growth of the brain from gestation until the early postnatal period, and also in maintaining the integrity of the brain structure and function from early adulthood until old-age.

In the peripheral nervous system, immune responses can be divided on a simplistic level into those which are innate and those that are adaptive. Innate immune responses are immediate and non-specific reactions to infectious agents or allergens. Adaptive responses are slower and involve immunological memory, or pre-exposure to the pathogen, but are also more specific. These two types of responses are mediated by a variety of cells, including those of a type made in the bone marrow (B-cells) or the thymus (T-cells). Depending on the immune trigger, different types of cells are activated and may try to phagocytose invading pathogens, or release a wide array of immune-related signaling molecules (cytokines), growth factors, superoxide radicals, or antibodies. Interestingly, there is good evidence for abnormal central and peripheral immune responses in autistic individuals, which raises the question we will discuss in later sections, whether immune changes are a cause or consequence of the disorder.

Core Neuropathological Changes in Autism

Autism is a neurobehavioral disorder, which naturally suggests there should be neurological correlates to the disorder. Neuropathological and neuroimaging studies suggest both gross morphological and cell based differences between autistic and non-autistic individuals. For example there are differences in brain volume in autistic individuals compared with age-matched controls. In addition, there are white matter alterations in autism, displaced neurons, changes in the density and branching or arborisation of neurons, particularly in the cerebellum. There is also good evidence that the layers of cortical neurons are not placed in discrete columns in autistic brains as perfectly as they are in control cases, and that there are fewer than normal numbers of neurons in the amygdala, which is the almond-shaped structure that mediates emotion in the brain (Figure 22.1) (Polsek *et al.*, 2011). It is likely that changes in neuronal density in these key regions, which regulate movement and attentive behavior (the cerebellum and frontal cortex) or emotions (the amygdala) contribute to the behavioral symptoms of autism. However the causes of these neuropathological changes remain unknown.

Is Inflammation Central to Autism?

It is possible that dysfunctional neuroimmune processes may be involved in abnormal brain development in autistic children. For example, white matter is comprised chiefly of glial cells

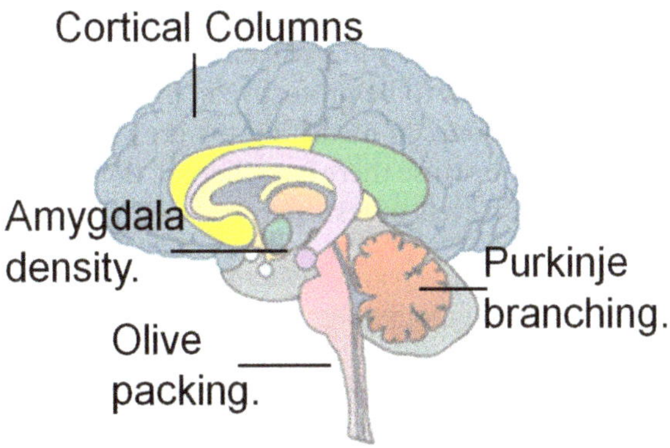

Figure 22.1 Some of the brain regions implicated in the pathophysiology of autism. Abnormal packing density or branching of neurons is reported in the cerebellum (Purkinje cells), brainstem (olivary neurons), frontal cortex (neuron column structure) and amygdala. These neurological changes may underscore some autistic-like behaviors.

Table 22.1 Autoimmune and Allergic Disorders with an Increased Prevalence in Parents of Children with Autism

Immune disease	*Family member*	*Reference*
Auto-immune:		
Psoriasis	Mother or father	Atladottir *et al.*, 2009; Comi *et al.*, 1999; Croen *et al.*, 2005; Keil *et al.*, 2010
Type-1 diabetes	Mother or father	Atladottir *et al.*, 2009; Comi *et al.*,1999; Croen *et al.*, 2005; Keil *et al.*, 2010
Systemic lupus erythematosus	Mother	Comi *et al.*,1999; Keil *et al.*, 2010
Rheumatoid arthritis	Mother	Atladottir *et al.*, 2009; Comi *et al.*,1999
Celiac disease	Mother	Atladottir *et al.*, 2009
Asthma	Mother	Croen *et al.*, 2005; Keil *et al.*, 2010
Rheumatic fever	Mother or father	Keil *et al.*, 2010
Allergies:		
Allergic rhinitis	Mother	Croen *et al.*, 2005
Atopic eczema	Mother	Croen *et al.*, 2005

a complex interaction between sex, immune dysfunction in parents, and additional stressors during the gestational and postnatal period. In the following sections we will discuss the types of stressors that may trigger additional aberrant immune responses in mothers of autistic individuals, in addition to during the postnatal period.

The term, "stress," refers to one of the most common concepts in neurobiology. For example, stress can be defined in terms of activation of the classical hypothalamic–pituitary–adrenal axis (HPA), a physiological or endocrine response, or the more molecular-driven descriptions of intracellular stress-activated proteins. For this review, we are defining immune stressors, as factors, such as infections, environmental toxicants and genetic changes which are likely associated with immune changes in mothers of children with autism. The reason we are taking a broad approach to describe stressors associated with autism, is because even though the initial stress-related event may be a virus, or exposure to an environmental contaminant, the types of immune responses associated with these stressors converge on several common mechanisms, which may precipitate the autistic phenotype.

Maternal Immune Activation (MIA) and Autism

The developing fetus is a chimera comprised of both maternal and paternal genes. Thus, the fetus expresses paternal antigens that would normally be recognized as foreign and subsequently eliminated by the maternal immune system. During pregnancy, the mother's immune system must maintain a unique balance to prevent fetal rejection, yet still provide adequate defenses against microbial pathogens. Multiple mechanisms exist to support the fetus's development. Specifically, the pregnancy-induced expansion of regulatory T-cells, or T_{reg}s, in mothers, is crucial for maintaining fetal tolerance by suppressing the production of pro-inflammatory cytokines. These changes in the maternal immune system contribute to the enhanced risk of infection and/or immune disorders in pregnant females, thereby increasing the risk of the fetus developing autism.

One Danish study found that mothers who were hospitalized for a bacterial infection in the second trimester of pregnancy or for a viral infection during the first trimester had children who were at a greater risk of developing autism (Atladottir *et al.*, 2010a, 2010b). Early prenatal viral infections, in particular, showed a greater autism hazard ratio, 2.98 for example, as compared with 1.42 for bacterial infections. It is hypothesized that maternal infection results in alterations in the development of the fetal neural network development, which contribute to the development of autistic-related behaviors. Support for this hypothesis can be found in a variety of animal studies which have attempted to model maternal immune infection, described in the following sections.

A note on the use of laboratory animals to model autism

While results obtained from clinical and epidemiological studies have revealed important immune disorders potentially associated with autism, animal models are an essential tool to allow researchers to directly assess the interplay between sex, immune responses, neuropathology, and behavior. Rodent behaviors, such as social interactions, repetitive movements, and the ability to communicate food preference to a cage mate, can be extrapolated to more sophisticated human behaviors. For example, a well-used animal model of social changes related to autism is the three-chamber test. This test involves two larger chambers connected by a passageway. One chamber contains a novel mouse in a cage, and a second chamber contains an empty cage. Mice that exhibit normal social behaviors will prefer to spend more time in the chamber with the novel mouse, than in the chamber with the empty cage; whereas mice which have social deficits will spend equal time in the chamber with the empty cage as they will in the chamber with the novel mice (Bolivar, Walters, and Phoenix, 2007). Moreover, the time spent sniffing the novel mouse can give more sophisticated analysis of social deficits in mice. It is important to note that neuro-behaviorists do not consider the aforementioned behaviors as being identical to those found in humans, rather they are reproducible, recognizable phenotypes which echo simple behaviors that may reflect changes associated with autism. By extension, neurological, neuroimmune and neuropathological changes found in animal models of autism also carry the caveat that their relevance to the human condition must be extrapolated with caution (Figure 22.2).

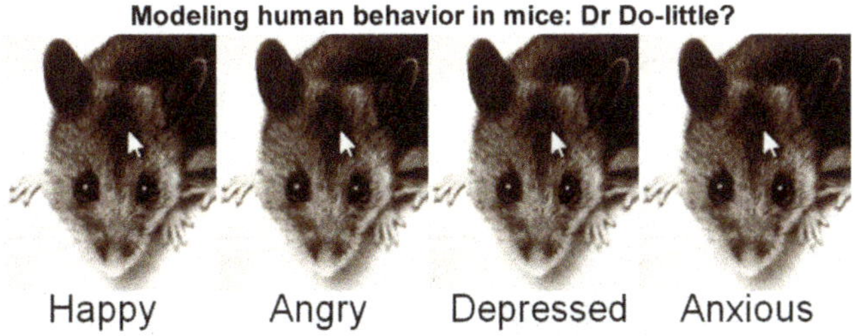

Figure 22.2 Mouse behaviors are not identical to human ones. However, they do display reproducible social, movement and emotionally related behaviors which can be quantified. Adapted from Zalcman (2011).

Immune and behavioral changes associated with Maternal Immune Activation (MIA)

Infection with bacterial pathogens is associated with MIA. Lipopolysaccharides (LPS) are large molecules found on the outer membrane of Gram-negative bacterial pathogens, and mediate the toxic effects associated with infection by these pathogens. In rodents, administration of LPS results in a robust production of pro-inflammatory cytokines, which include: TNF-α, IL-1, IL-6, IL-8, and IL-12. In rodents, LPS injection during the early post-conception zygote period is associated with abnormal implantation of the embryo and subsequent developmental abnormalities. Moreover, LPS administration to pregnant females causes sex-specific changes in the progeny, which have the capacity to persist in male offspring after they have been infected early post-conception (Williams, Teeling, Perry, and Fleming, 2011). The effects of LPS infection in rodents, associated with sex-specific abnormal development of offspring, suggest a similar phenomenon may occur in pregnant mothers. These studies also illustrate that a single maternal immune challenge can lead to immune abnormalities which persist into adulthood of the offspring. Moreover, we cannot implicate infection in the pathogenesis of autism, without highlighting the potential contribution of epigenetic changes during the pre- and postnatal period associated with the infection. For example, LPS stimulation is associated with epigenetic changes, which includes the phosphorylation of serine 10 on histone 3 (H3S10) on a number of immune-related genes (Medzhitov and Horng, 2009). This type of epigenetic change may contribute to the persistence of abnormal immune changes in offspring of infected mothers, and by extension the abnormal immune and potentially behavioral responses found in children with autism.

To mimic viral infection, laboratory animals can be challenged with viral pathogens or treated with synthetic analogs of viruses. Polyinosinic:polycytidylic acid (Poly I:C) is an immunostimulatant that is structurally similar to double-stranded RNA, which is produced by certain viruses, and is also recognized by Toll-like receptor 3 (TLR-3). Similar to viral infections, poly I:C is a strong inducer of type I interferon (α and β) responses. Moreover, IL-6, IL-12, and TNF-α are also generated following stimulation with poly I:C in both murine and human cell cultures. A study by Smith *et al.* (2007) found that a single injection of poly I:C to pregnant mice produced sex-specific exploratory and social behavior in male offspring. A second series of experiments by the same group found that a similar infection in IL-6-deficient mice resulted in no behavioral deficits in offspring. Therefore, the authors concluded that IL-6 triggers behavioral changes in offspring after prenatal maternal viral exposure. However, it should be noted that even though poly I:C-induced changes in IL-6 may underscore behavioral abnormalities in offspring, poly I:C infection is actually more commonly utilized to mimic the robust type-I IFN responses elicited associated with viral infection. The IFN cytokine family are implicated in the pathogenesis of autoimmune diseases. Therefore we suggest that studies are warranted to investigate the potential contribution of IFN-α and β in to the progression of autism.

If immune responses are toxic then is *dose* the poison?

To better understand the relationship between maternal viral infection and neuropsychiatric disorders, such as autism, Zalcman and colleagues performed an illuminating series of experiments. Pregnant females were challenged with a variety of doses of the influenza virus during the second trimester (Zalcman, 2011). At higher infectious doses of the virus, 300 plaque-forming units (PFU), the male offspring showed significant movement abnormalities, including increased locomotion and stereotypic behaviors, compared with male offspring of sham-infected mothers. These behaviors were not related to changes in sensorimotor coordination. Moreover, there was no difference in the performance on the rotorod test, which consists of a rotating rod, on which the mice are obliged to use motor activity, in a coordinated and balanced fashion, in order for them to stay on. At the same dose, female offspring did not exhibit any stereotypic changes, however they did display impaired locomotor function.

More intriguingly, at a lower infectious dose, 75 PFU, male offspring did not display any behavioral changes, but the female offspring exhibited increased anxiety like behavior (Zalcman, 2011). It should be noted that the behavioral changes caused by viral infection were not due to the direct infection of the fetal brain, as influenza viral RNA was not detected in these tissues. Collectively, these intriguing studies on the interplay between the dose of a viral infection and sex-specific behaviors raise the question as to whether the dose of an infection during behavior will contribute to a range of diverse behavioral abnormalities, which occasionally may manifest as autism-like changes.

MIA induced neurological changes in animal models

A vital question that needs to be better addressed in the MIA field is, what is the specific mechanism underlying behavioral changes after infection? To date, studies using MIA model systems, whether viral or bacterial mimics, have yet to hit on a common mechanism to explain why infection alters behavior. One possibility is that infection directly alters the structure of the brain. Support for this hypothesis comes from animal model studies that demonstrate changes in the volume of the cerebellum of offspring from mothers infected with a sublethal challenge dose of the influenza virus. These findings mirror results obtained from imaging studies of patients with autism. Furthermore, viral infection also causes alterations in the expression of certain genes required for myelin synthesis, such as myelin basic protein and myelin associated glycoprotein (Fatemi *et al.*, 2009). Other groups have reported that poly I:C treatment is associated with cerebellar abnormalities and changes in Purkinje cell density similar to those found in autistic individuals (Shi *et al.*, 2009).

Alternatively, microbial infection may induce behavioral changes via a different mechanism. For example, LPS induced changes in social and locomotor behavior (Lin, Lin, and Wang, 2011), are thought to be due to changes in the function of dopaminergic and serotonergic neurons in prefrontal cortical regions. However, we do not yet know if this mechanism is specific to LPS infection models only, because alterations in dopamine or serotonin neuron densities have yet to be characterized in the offspring of virally infected mice. Correspondingly, white matter changes have also not been determined in offspring from bacterially-infected mothers. This is an important point, because unless we complete side-by-side studies comparing the behavioral and pathological effects of maternal immune stressors, we will be unable to determine if there are common mechanisms underscoring behavioral and neurological changes in offspring. The identification of common mechanisms may give hope for the generation of common treatments or preventative strategies in the future. Although we have yet to identify the specific mechanisms underscoring abnormal behavior of offspring in MIA models there is some evidence that cytokines are involved.

How Cytokines Could Affect Brain Development and Function in Autism

Our defense responses against infection are typically associated with robust production of pro-inflammatory cytokines. Recent studies have provided evidence that cytokines are not only important for inflammatory responses but that they also function as growth factors and are crucial for normal brain development. For example, IL-6 is critical for the division and maintenance of oligodendrocyte precursors (Deng *et al.*, 2011) while TNF-α is important for the development and maintenance of synaptic connections (Lee *et al.*, 2010). Thus, alterations in cytokine levels associated with MIA, during critical periods when fetal neural networks are developing may be associated with autism.

In fact, not only is it possible that cytokines may alter the development of the brain, these cellular mediators may also contribute to behavioral changes in adult autistic individuals by directly and tonically modulating neurochemical transmission. Neurochemical deficits such as altered circulating serotonin levels, perhaps associated with reduced activity of tryptophan hydroxylase, the enzyme catalyzing the rate-limiting step in serotonin synthesis, or reduced efficacy of the serotonin reuptake transporter (SERT), are reported in people with autism (Polsek *et al.*, 2011). As previously mentioned, increased levels of cytokines such as IL-1β, are reported in sera of individuals with autism compared with controls. Interestingly, IL-1β can regulate SERT activity, and IL-1β, TNF-α and IFN-γ can all modulate serotonin levels in the hypothalamus, hippocampus and cortex (Zhao and Schwartz, 1998). Moreover, alterations in the glutamate decarboxylase (GAD), a key enzyme for the synthesis of gamma amino butyric acid (GABA; one of the most important inhibitory neurotransmitters in the brain), in tandem with reductions in GABA receptor activity, are reported in brain tissues from individuals with autism (Polsek *et al.*, 2011).

Interestingly, a physiological study using brainstem tissue slices from rats found that IL-1β not only directly inhibits the firing of serotonergic neurons, but also increased GABA-ergic inhibitory processes (Brambilla, Franciosi, Opp, and Imeri, 2007). In addition, other studies suggest a role for IL-1β in altering GABA-ergic activity in individuals with epilepsy. This is important because currently it is estimated that approximately 30% of individuals with autism also have epileptic seizures during their lifetime (Polsek *et al.*, 2011; Vezzani, Balosso, and Ravizza, 2008). Moreover, IL-6 can induce sleep, and TNF-α can induce anorexia, and both sleep disruption and altered eating habits are found in individuals with autism (Suzuki *et al.*, 2011; Tracey *et al.*, 1988). Therefore we suggest it is very likely that alterations in the levels of cytokines including, but not limited to, IL-1β could perturb normal release and regulation of neurotransmitters such as serotonin and GABA and thus contribute to the autism phenotype in some individuals. And changes in the GABA inhibitory neurotransmitter may underscore seizure activity in autism.

Maternal Autoantibody Responses and Autism

Antibodies are critical for host defense against microbial challenge. However, antibodies that are formed against self-antigens (known as "autoantibodies") are involved in both the onset and maintenance of certain autoimmune diseases including systemic lupus erthyrematosus, rheumatoid arthritis, and multiple sclerosis, all of which affect females more so than males.

One theory regarding the pathophysiology of autism is that maternally-derived autoantibodies may alter the course of the development of the fetal brain. Maternal IgG can traverse the placenta, and this is an important process in helping to build fetal immune responses, with the greatest transfer rates occurring between 20 and 32 weeks gestation. The severity of autoimmune diseases is known to subside during pregnancy. This would suggest that the improved disease symptoms would most likely correlate with decreased production of autoantibodies, thereby reducing transmission rates to the fetus. However, due to the longer half-life of serum IgG, approximately 21 days, the sustained presence of these autoantibodies can mediate its pathogenic effects during crucial developmental milestones, particularly during the first trimester. As we have discussed previously in this chapter, timing is likely the critical component that dictates the risk for developing autism.

An alternative hypothesis is that autoantibodies are of fetal origin, but we doubt this possibility despite the fact that immunoglobulin synthesis begins as early as 10 weeks post-conception. Firstly, the overall antibody levels in fetal tissues are significantly reduced compared to those detected in adults. Secondly, IgM is the predominant subclass generated, and neonates are largely unable to produced class-switched antibodies, which are responsible for the pathogenesis caused by autoimmune conditions. Thirdly, the development of brain regions associated with autism, such as olives (or olivary bodies), or cerebellar Purkinje cells, occurs prior to the ability of the fetus to synthesize its own immunoglobulins. In later stages of gestation, the reduced antibody levels are likely not sufficient to alter the structures that develop during this time period (i.e., cortical mini-columns). Regardless of whether the autoantibodies are of maternal or fetal origin, the mechanism by which autoantibodies contribute to the pathophysiology of autism remains unresolved.

Autoantibodies in animal models of autism

Some support for the autoantibody hypothesis of autism can be found in animal model systems. For example, studies in non-human primates have revealed that exposure to sera containing autoantibodies derived from mothers of children with autism induces anti-social and stereopathy behavioral changes (Ashwood, Wills, and Van de Water, 2006), although the specific autoantibodies which underpin these behavioral changes remain to be found.

Other evidence to support a role for autoantibodies in autism comes from the mouse modeling field. Currently, the best behavioral model of autism is the inbred BTBR mouse strain, which displays reduced social behavior, increased stereopathies such as self grooming, and increased levels of cytokines, mast cells, and brain-reactive antibodies (Heo *et al.*, 2011). Moreover, the BTBR mouse strain is raised on an autoimmune genetic background and has high levels of autoantibodies, suggesting that autoimmune responses may contribute to its abnormal anti-social behavioral phenotype (Heo *et al.*, 2011).

Mechanisms of autoantibody-mediated autism

If autoantibodies are involved in autism this may be because: a) they bind to brain-specific antigens; b) they inadvertently mimic an infectious antigen and trigger an immune response; or c) they provoke a non-specific reaction in developing brain tissues associated with abnormal brain development. Autoantibodies directed against certain CNS proteins have been detected in both the sera of autistic individuals and their mothers, which include: myelin basic protein, glial fibrillary acid proteins, neuron axon fillaments, nerve growth factor, and endothelial cells (Ashwood, Wills, and Van de Water, 2006). Thus, they may specifically interfer with the normal function of these proteins during development.

Alternatively they may mimic pathogens. Toll-like receptors in the brain are responsible for mediating some innate immune responses, and recognize pathogens via specific motifs known as pathogen associated molecular patterns (PAMPs). There are many forms of Toll-like receptors, and although originally they were only thought to be expressed on extracranial immune cells, now they are known to be expressed on a variety of cells, including epithelial, endothelial, cancerous, neuronal, and glial cells. Moreover, they may play an important role during brain development (Crack and Bray, 2007). For instance, it is possible that autoantibody initiated activation of Toll-like receptors could contribute to aberrant development of the brain, either a) via initiating unusual apoptosis in neurons, or b) via altered apoptosis of glia cells such as astrocytes which are involved in axonal patterning, which would change neuronal connectivity in the developing brain.

One problem with the autoantibody theory of autism is that certain autoantibodies to proteins are found in the general population in healthy individuals. Moreover, mothers with autoimmune diseases such as type-I diabetes have autoantibodies against pancreatic islet cells, associated with the disease severity (Orban *et al.*, 2009). This means that if autoantibodies can transfer to the developing fetus and interfere with the development of organs such as the brain, then autoantibodies against pancreatic islet cells should also transfer, yielding a diabetic phenotype in tandem with an autistic one in offspring from mothers with type-1 diabetes. This is not the case.

The aforementioned examples raise two important questions, which need to be addressed. Firstly, we need to know what the normal function of autoantibodies is, and to identify the autism-specific autoantibodies in mothers at risk of having children with autism. Secondly, we need to determine whether autoantibodies which are associated with autism are present prior to pregnancy in mothers at risk of having children with autism, or if they are developed in response to an immune challenge during pregnancy.

Environmental Contaminants as a Perinatal Immune Challenge in Autism

Infectious agents are not the only factors which can alter maternal, fetal and neonatal immune responses. Environmental contaminants are known to have similar effects. Moreover, it was suggested that the increasing rate of autism may be directly attributable to increased likelihood of exposure to environmental contaminants (Herbert, 2010). It would be difficult to describe all of the environmental contaminants reportedly associated with autism in one section, therefore, we will introduce only a few of the contaminants which have been associated with autism including polycyclic aromatic hydrocarbons (PAHs), metals such as cadmium and mercury, valproic acid, and thalidomide.

The term PAHs describes a range of persistent environmental contaminants including polychlorinated biphenyls (PCBs), and polybrominated diphenyl ethers (PBDEs), or flame retardants, as they are more commonly termed. PAHs are particularly toxic to the developing fetus, because they are lipophilic and are easily transferred to fetal and infant brains via the placenta and breast milk. Epidemiological studies suggest a link between higher maternal sera and cord blood PDBE and PCB levels and abnormal behaviors associated with autism. In addition, exposure to inorganic contaminants, such as the heavy metals, mercury, cadmium, arsenic and lead, is linked with developmental abnormalities in children, as well as reduced sociability and exploratory movement in rodents (Dietert and Dietert, 2008). Furthermore, exposures to thalidomide (originally used to treat morning sickness and found to be a mutagen), valproic acid (an anti-elliptic drug found to induce developmental abnormalities in children of mothers who used it), and consumption of monosodium glutamate, are also associated with a greater risk of autism and autistic-like behavioral changes in animal model systems (McGinnis, Miller, and Audhya, 2010).

It is striking that such a range of diverse environmental toxicants, from endocrine disrupters to heavy metals, to food additives, to drugs which modify immune responses, are all associated with autism. This raises the question whether there is a common immune disturbance associated with exposure to all the aforementioned contaminants, or if the divergent toxicants are associated with the range and severity of symptoms associated with autism (Hertz-Picciotto *et al.*, 2008)

Immune changes associated with autism-related toxicants

The thymus is critical for T-lymphocyte development, thus perturbances in thymus function will affect T-lymphocyte function. Higher maternal serum levels of PCBs are associated with reduced thymus size in neonates (Hertz-Picciotto *et al.*, 2008). Disrupted $T_H1{:}T_H2$ balance is also found *in vitro* after exposure to PCBs, suggesting they may augment autism risk via dysregulation of T-cell homeostasis. Animal studies suggest that PCB exposures also alter cerebellar tissue development in a sex-specific fashion possibly associated with changes in IL-6 (Miller *et al.*, 2010). It is unlikely that PCB-induced developmental changes are antibody-related because a Slovakian study on 384 mother–infant pairs found no association between maternal and early postnatal PCB concentrations, and infant serum IgG, IgA, IgM or IgE levels (Jusko *et al.*, 2011). Cytokines are also implicated in the pathogenic changes associated with other contaminants. For example, organic mercury is associated with changes in T-lymphocyte populations, in tandem with alterations in cytokines such as IFN-γ (Dietert and Dietert, 2008). Thalidomide also alters levels of IFN-γ and TNF-α in humans and animals, suggesting that alterations in cytokines and T-lymphocytes associated with toxicant exposures may provide a common mechanism underscoring increased risk of autism in children living in areas high in these environmental contaminants, or to mothers with higher contaminant levels.

However, it should be noted that as with animal models of infection, toxicological studies rarely are set up to identify common mechanisms associated with divergent compounds. In addition, behavioral changes associated with toxicant exposures are rarely conducted pari passu with neuropathological examinations, and vice versa. Thus, it is unclear whether there is a unique or common pathway associated with toxicant exposures. In addition, it is very unlikely that all toxicants associated with autism share a common neuroimmune mechanism. In fact, with regards to Valproic acid, one study suggests that pre-treatment of mothers with IFN-γ can remediate birth defects in offspring (Hrubec *et al.*, 2006). This raises the intriguing possibility that infection prior to pregnancy could actually mitigate the effects of some autism-related toxicants on the developing fetus.

Autistic Regression and Postnatal Exposure to Stressors

Autism is distinguished from other developmental disorders by alterations in three behavioral domains: sociability, language, and range of interests and activities. However, not all patients with autism present with identical symptoms, since some patients will manifest greater deficits in one domain over the other. In addition, not all individuals with autism develop the condition at the same time point. It is thought there may be two forms of autism, the early-onset form, which children are born with, and a regressive form, which develops after birth. Some children with autism develop normally until ~18 months of age, but thereafter they lose vocabulary, interest in social play, eye contact with parents, and/or have reduced vocalization. Currently it is estimated that 20–30% of autistic individuals undergo what is termed "autistic regression" (McGinnis, Miller, and Audhya, 2010).

The pathophysiology of regressive autism likely differs from that of early-onset autism, because the onset of symptoms suggests there is "normal" development of the brain up to the postnatal period. Therefore it is likely that exposure to environmental contaminants or pathogens during the postnatal period may be involved with the pathophysiology of regressive autism. However, after birth, certain brain regions should be protected from environmental pathogens via protective structures such as the blood–brain-barrier (BBB). In addition, certain environmental contaminants such as monosodium glutamate, paraquat, organic mercury and cadmium only poorly traverse the blood brain barrier (BBB), which raises the question as to how they enter and interfere with development of the postnatal brain.

One hypothesis to explain the vulnerability of the postnatal brain to stressors, including infiltrating IgG, autoantibodies, or cytokines, is that certain areas act as portals for toxicants or pathogens into the developing brain because they: a) lack a BBB, such as the area postrema or pineal gland; b) they are adjacent to cerebrospinal fluid and exposure to contaminants within CSF, for example the circumventricular organs (CVO); or c) they lack protective myelin, such as the vagal sensory C fibers within the brainstem (McGinnis, Miller, and Audhya, 2010). Support for the toxicant portal theory stems from the fact that many symptoms found in regressive autism, such as speech replaced by a whisper, gastro-intestinal disturbances, and reduced heart rate regulation, could be associated with reduced brainstem vagal activity or CVO function (McGinnis, Miller, and Audhya, 2010). Unfortunately much of the research using animal models of autism fails to distinguish between regressive and early onset forms of autism, thus mechanistic understanding as to how the timing of insults may precipitate divergent behaviors associated with autism is limited at this time.

With Insults, Timing is Everything

The fact that patients with autism present with symptoms of an early-onset or regressive nature suggests that cytokine and/or antibody changes at different time points during fetal brain development contributes different autism phenotypes. Studies on thalidomide use have revealed that mothers who used thalidomide while the brainstem was developing in the first trimester are more likely to have had children with autism, (Dietert and Dietert, 2008; McGinnis, Miller, and Audhya, 2010). It is also likely that at later stages in gestation when the brain is more fully formed, perturbances in the maternal environment would likely have less destructive effects (Figure 22.3). Few if any previously published studies on maternal infection or

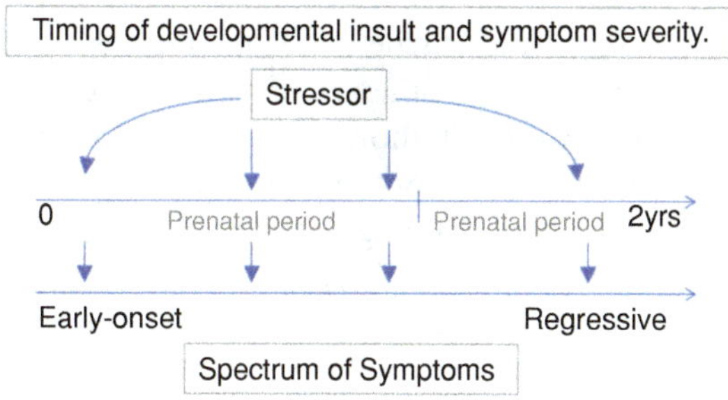

Figure 22.3 The spectrum and severity of symptoms associated with autism may be underpinned by the timing and type of developmental insult.

toxicant exposures were designed to compare the divergent effects of the time of the insult on behavioral changes in offspring. Moreover, in the real world, coexposures to infectious agents and toxicants is extremely likely, but animal modeling studies rarely model the effects of such coexposures. Thus, while animal model systems and cell-based assays are incredibly useful to help us understand behavioral pathological and cell-based changes associated with autism, by failing to generate more complete and "real-life" type models we may be left with an incomplete understanding of the true etiology of autism.

Vaccinations and Autism

It is very important that we address the role of vaccinations in autism, given the current belief that vaccinations play a role in the autism "epidemic." Currently, according to Landrigan (2000), "there is no credible evidence that vaccines cause autism" (Landrigan, 2010).

The controversy surrounding the potential role for adverse immune responses to vaccines in autism was initiated in 1988. A study, originally published in *The Lancet*, suggested a new form of autism, titled *autism–enterocolitus syndrome*, associated with the measles, mumps, and rubella vaccine. In 2010 after a lengthy investigation process *The Lancet* retracted the paper.

In the interim, 20 years since the retracted study was published, there was a slump in the uptake of MMR vaccines in the UK from 98% to 76%. There also followed a string of investigations as to whether MMR vaccines, or thimerosol, a mercury-containing preservative in vaccines, may contribute to neurological abnormalities in children. Thimerosol is toxic at high doses to animals, and mercury is known to be a mutagen, however, published studies have found no association between the MMR vaccine or thimerosol and autism. Recently, given the association between immune challenge during pregnancy and ASDs, there has also been worry regarding whether flu vaccine during pregnancy is beneficial. However, studies have found that flu vaccination during pregnancy is associated with a reduced risk of ASD in offspring.

Are Immune Changes a Symptom Rather Than Trigger of Autism-Related Neuropathology?

To play devil's advocate, we should address the possibility that immune changes associated with autism neuropathology could be a symptom rather than cause of the disorder. In this scenario, neuronal changes would cause neuroinflammatory and immune changes in autistic individuals. So far, due to a scarcity of tissues, the question as to whether the severity of autism depends on the severity and range of neuroinflammatory changes remains unresolved. Thus, unlike in other disorders, we can't show a connection between increasing symptom severity and increasing neuroinflammation. Some researchers suggest that autism-related neuroinflammatory changes be part of an ongoing pathophysiology or in response to neuronal stress (Herbert, 2010). Moreover, it is noteworthy that some of the pathology associated with autism could suggest that dysfunctional neural control of immune responses is involved with the disorder.

Immune responses are regulated, in part, by autonomic parasympathetic and sympathetic nerve fibers, and neurotransmitters originating from the brainstem. In fact the maturation of immune responses is dependent on autonomic innervations of the thymus, spleen, and lymph nodes. In children with autism, pathological studies have revealed increased density of Paneth cell granules. The activity of Paneth cells is regulated by autonomic vagal parasympathetic fibers. Paneth cells line the intestine and release granules which are important for regulating the bacterial flora and fauna in the gut, and maintaining digestive processes. Impaired Paneth cell function may underscore the increased and unusual *Clostridia* colonies found in children with autism. In addition, there are reports of abnormal heart rate and gastrointestinal problems in children with autism (Figure 22.4). Thus, aberrant signaling of autonomic nerve fibers regulated by the brainstem, associated with abnormal development of the brainstem, could contribute to "top-down" immune dysfunction, in the absence of infections or infectious agents in people with autism.

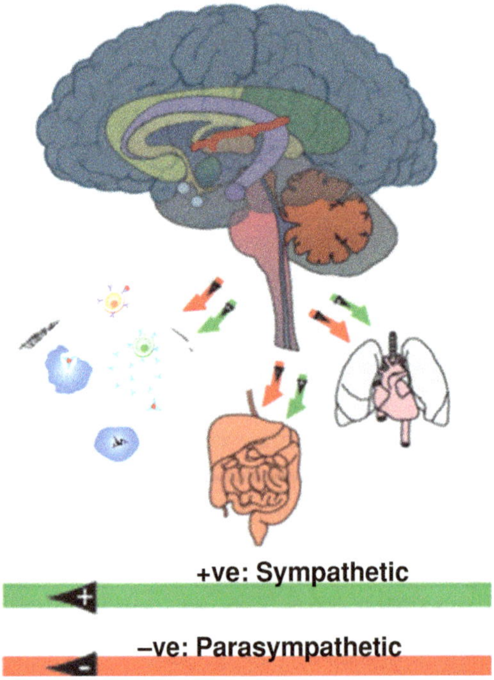

Figure 22.4 Top-down neural regulation of sympathetic and parasympathetic nerve fibers which regulate gastrointestinal, cardiovascular (eg., heart rate) and immune responses.

Neuroinflammation to excise ectopic neurons

Neuroinflammation in autism could also be a response to abnormal neuronal development. Ectopic neurons are cells localized to inappropriate regions. Their function is unknown, but they are usually bordered by activated glial cells, and are found in white matter, brainstem and cerebellar tissues of individuals with autism (Polsek *et al.*, 2011). Ectopic neurons are associated with gliosis, which suggest a localized immune response to these neurons, perhaps in an attempt to remove or eradicate them as the brain recognizes that they are out of place. The ectopic neurons may be the most obvious manifestation of a trigger of a brain-specific autoimmune apoptotic response. But in other brain regions disrupted neuronal growth associated with neurons of an unusual size or packing density may trigger the activation of the brain's immune system, which recognizes these abnormal phenomena. This may then precipitate a persistent pruning machine, which does not necessarily kill off neurons but attempts to cut them back during development. This pruning or cutting back may be normal or abnormal, i.e. just enough to put neurons back to where they should be to normalize the development of an otherwise abnormal brain, or it may be excessive, killing off neurons and leading to neuronal depletion in the amygdala, for example.

Why is Autism More Common in Some Families?

It is notable that while autism is not fully a hereditary disorder, it appears to be more common in some families than others. Epidemiological studies have found an association between a number of immune-related genes, including IL-6, ubiquitin, HLA-DRB1*04, complement C4B (Ashwood, Wills, and Van de Water, 2006), and autism. It is also notable that parents with autoimmune diseases are more likely to have children with autism, as discussed previously. This raises the intriguing possibility that autism is a hereditary disorder, and part of a broader family of autoimmune diseases that may be precipitated by different triggers and present with different symptoms. However, it could be argued that the increased likelihood of siblings developing autism is a consequence of them being exposed to similar environmental contaminants and pathogens. Moreover, it is likely that parents of autistic children are more vigilant about symptoms of autism in other family members, which could contribute to the increased diagnosis of autism in families.

Notwithstanding the role for increased vigilance among siblings, there are other aspects of autism which suggest that hereditary factors play a strong, if latent role. For example, facial asymmetry is associated with developmental insults. Studies have found that children with autism have greater facial asymmetry than children without autism. Indeed, photographs of children as young as 10 months are proposed as useful tools for the early diagnosis of autism. Moreover, studies of parents with autism reveal that mothers of children with autism, who were not diagnosed with autism themselves, have greater facial asymmetry than mothers of developmentally normal children. In addition, facial asymmetry is not found in siblings or fathers of children with autism (Hammond *et al.*, 2008). This, in tandem with the increased prevalence of autoimmune diseases in mothers of children with autism, and the fact that some of the candidate genes for autism directly regulate immune responses, strongly suggests an interaction between genes and the immune system which leads to the autism phenotype in later generations. In addition, sexually divergent maturation processes of the immune system

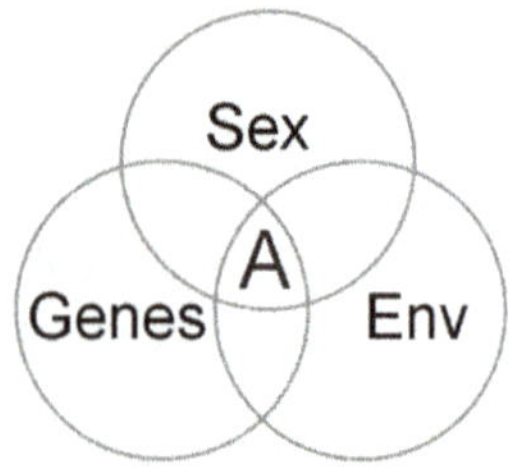

Figure 22.5 Autism is likely associated with a complex interplay between genetic, environmental and sex-specific factors.

may render the male fetus more sensitive to neuroimmune and developmental perturbances than the female fetus (Figure 22.5).

If We Manipulate Immune Responses Can We Manage Autism Better?

Vancomycin is an antibiotic which works by preventing cell wall synthesis by Gram-positive bacteria, and has been proposed as a treatment for autism. One small clinical study of 10 children with regressive autism found that 8 of them reported improvements in symptoms with vancomycin treatment (Sandler *et al.*, 2000). These improvements were not lasting, and the study has yet to be followed up with a large-scale clinical trial. However, its results suggest that the manipulation of immune responses in children with regressive autism may help improve behaviors. Vancomycin may improve gastrointestinal function, leading to improved sleep, nutrition, and reduced pain associated with digestive discomfort, all of which could improve behavior. In addition, if cytokine alterations in autism play a tonic role in altering neurochemical responses, it is plausible, albeit unproven, that modulating cytokine levels by reducing gastrointestinal infections may result in improved behaviors associated with neurochemical deficits in some children with autism.

With regard to maternal immune stress, some studies in rodents suggest that immune modulation may reduce behavioral abnormalities after maternal immune activation. For example, in order to reduce behavioral changes associated with viral exposure, one group used an inhibitor of NF- κB (an important intracellular messenger for transducing immune responses) in pregnant mice which had been injected with Poly I:C. The inhibitor molecule used was pyrrolidine dithiocarbamate, and it protected against behavioral changes in offspring of dams which had been exposed to Poly I:C injection (Song *et al.*, 2011). This experiment illustrates that interventions to remediate abnormal immune responses during pregnancy may be important, and help prevent the development of autism in the future.

In addition it should be noted that not all maternal infections are bad, and to a certain extent some may be necessary in order for offspring to develop better immune responses. For example, immune priming of female mice with *Babesia microti* (a protozoan parasite that infects the blood) results in the mice gaining more weight during pregnancy and spending more time nursing offspring. More importantly, immune responses in offspring subsequently exposed to *Babesia microti* infection as adults is better, with more rapid clearing of the infection and interestingly, reduced testosterone release in response to social stress (Curno *et al.*, 2011).

This study illustrates why the transfer of IgG from mother to fetus during development is important to help build fetal immune responses. Thus, maternal infections, at the right time, may actually be useful to offspring in the future. In the future it will be important for us to better understand the role of previous infections, in tandem with infections during pregnancy, in protecting against and producing developmental neuropsychiatric disorders.

Inflammation in Autism: The Beginning of the End

Aberrant immune responses in parents are associated with increased likelihood of offspring developing autism. In addition children with autism have aberrant immune responses. This raises the inevitable chicken-or-egg question which dogs so many neurological disorders associated with inflammation: Is inflammation a cause or consequence of the disorder? Furthermore, with regard to autism, it is possible that inflammation is not only a cause or consequence, but also a key part of the disorder and its persistence. In order to better address whether neuroinflammation is a cause or consequence of autism we suggest that the following research questions need to be addressed in the future.

1 What are the common neuroimmune mechanisms shared by autism-related maternal stressors, inclusive of infectious agents and environmental contaminants associated with abnormal behaviors in offspring?
2 More extensive translational studies are needed to determine if remediation of cytokine, immunoglobulin and/or autoantibody synthesis results in remediation of autistic behaviors in animals.
3 Is there a particular profile of autoantibodies or cytokines during pregnancy which can predict risk of autism in offspring, as this will help with early diagnosis.

We have yet to achieve agreement as to whether there is a true increase in the prevalence of autism, or whether it reflects changing diagnostic criteria. However, we are aware that boys are four times more likely to develop autism than girls, that abnormal immune responses are common in autism, and that parents with autoimmune diseases such as type-1 diabetes, or who have had a virus infection during pregnancy, are more likely to have children with autism. The fact that there are such strong sex differences in the development and function of neuroimmune responses, and sex-specific behaviors in animal models of autism, associated with viral or toxicant exposure, strongly suggests sex-specific immune factors are involved in autism. We need greater emphasis on delineating the neurobiology of the spectrum of autism disorders, and better translation of this to animal models to encourage a specific focus on the comparative effects of maternal stressors of different doses at different times on behavior in offspring. By delineating specific neuroimmune mechanisms associated with specific symptoms we will also be able to improve treatment of the disorder.

Acknowledgements

This review was funded in part by a grant from the Autism Research Institute award, a gift by Bo and Sandy McGinnis to Dr Veronica Miller, and a New Jersey Governor's Council on Autism award to Dr Stephen Zalcman.

References

Abdallah, M.W., Larsen, N., Grove, J., Norgaard-Pedersen, B., Thorsen, P., Mortensen, E.L., et al. (2011). Amniotic fluid inflammatory cytokines: potential markers of immunologic dysfunction in autism spectrum disorders. *World Journal of Biological Psychiatry*, December 19, 2011, epub ahead of print.

Ashwood, P., Krakowiak, P., Hertz-Picciotto, I., Hansen, R., Pessah, I., and Van de Water, J. (2011). Elevated plasma cytokines in autism spectrum disorders provide evidence of immune dysfunction and are associated with impaired behavioral outcome. *Brain, Behavior, and Immunity*, 25, 40–45.

Ashwood, P., Wills, S., and Van de Water, J. (2006). The immune response in autism: a new frontier for autism research. *Journal of LeukocyteBiology*, 80, 1–15.

Atladottir, H.O., Pedersen, M.G., Thorsen, P., Mortensen, P.B., Deleuran, B., Eaton, W.W., et al. (2009). Association of family history of autoimmune diseases and autism spectrum disorders. *Pediatrics*, 124, 687–694.

Atladottir, H.O., Thorsen, P., Ostergaard, L., Schendel, D.E., Lemcke, S., Abdallah, M., et al. (2010a). Maternal infection requiring hospitalization during pregnancy and autism spectrum disorders. *Journal of Autism and Developmental Disorders*, 40, 1423–1430.

Atladottir, H.O., Thorsen, P., Schendel, D.E., Ostergaard, L., Lemcke, S., and Parner, E.T. (2010b). Association of hospitalization for infection in childhood with diagnosis of autism spectrum disorders: a Danish cohort study. *Archives of Pediatrics and Adolescent Medicine*, 164, 470–477.

Barbeau, E.B., Mendrek, A., and Mottron, L. (2009). Are autistic traits autistic?. *British Journal of Psychology*, 100, 23–28.

Baron-Cohen, S., Lombardo, M.V., Auyeung, B., Ashwin, E., Chakrabarti, B., and Knickmeyer, R. (2011). Why are autism spectrum conditions more prevalent in males?. *Public Library of Science Biology*, 9:e1001081.

Baron-Cohen, S., Scott, F.J., Allison, C., Williams, J., Bolton, P., Matthews, F.E., et al. (2009). Prevalence of autism-spectrum conditions: UK school-based population study. *British Journal of Psychiatry*, 194, 500–509.

Bolivar, V.J., Walters, S.R., and Phoenix, J.L. (2007). Assessing autism-like behavior in mice: variations in social interactions among inbred strains. *Behavioural Brain Research*, 176, 21–26.

Brambilla, D., Franciosi, S., Opp, M.R., and Imeri, L. (2007). Interleukin-1 inhibits firing of serotonergic neurons in the dorsal raphe nucleus and enhances GABAergic inhibitory post-synaptic potentials. *European Journal of Neuroscience*, 26, 1862–1869.

Comi, A.M., Zimmerman, A.W., Frye, V.H., Law, P.A., and Peeden, J.N. (1999). Familial clustering of autoimmune disorders and evaluation of medical risk factors in autism. *Journal of Child Neurology*, 14, 388–394.

Crack, P.J., and Bray, P.J. (2007). Toll-like receptors in the brain and their potential roles in neuropathology. *Immunology and Cell Biology*, 85, 476–480.

Croen, L.A., Grether, J.K., Yoshida, C.K., Odouli, R., and Van de Water, J. (2005). Maternal autoimmune diseases, asthma and allergies, and childhood autism spectrum disorders: a case-control study. *Archives of Pediatrics and Adolescent Medicine*, 159, 151–157.

Curno, O., Reader, T., McElligott, A.G., Behnke, J.M., and Barnard, C.J. (2011). Infection before pregnancy affects immunity and response to social challenge in the next generation. *Philosophical Transactions of the Royal Society B: Biological Sciences*, 366, 3364–3374.

Deng, M.Y., Lam, S., Meyer, U., Feldon, J., Li, Q., Wei, R., et al. (2011). Frontal-subcortical protein expression following prenatal exposure to maternal inflammation. *Public Library of Science One*, 6:e16638.

Dietert, R.R., and Dietert, J.M. (2008). Potential for early-life immune insult including developmental immunotoxicity in autism and autism spectrum disorders: focus on critical windows of immune vulnerability. *Journal of Toxicology and Environmental Health B, Critical Reviews*, 11, 660–680.

DSM IV (2000). *Diagnostic and Statistical Manual of Mental Disorders: DSM-IV/TR.*, 4th ed. Washington, D.C.: American Psychiatric Association.

Fairweather, D., Frisancho-Kiss, S., and Rose, N.R. (2008). Sex differences in autoimmune disease from a pathological perspective. *American Journal of Pathology*, 173, 600–609.

Fatemi, S.H., Folsom, T.D., Reutiman, T.J., Abu-Odeh, D., Mori, S., Huang, H., et al. (2009). Abnormal expression of myelination genes and alterations in white matter fractional anisotropy following prenatal viral influenza infection at E16 in mice. *Schizophrenia Research*, 112, 46–53.

Hammond, P., Forster-Gibson, C., Chudley, A.E., Allanson, J.E., Hutton, T.J., Farrell, S.A., et al. (2008). Face-brain asymmetry in autism spectrum disorders. *Molecular Psychiatry*, 13, 614–623.

Heo, Y., Zhang, Y., Gao, D., Miller, V.M., and Lawrence, D.A. (2011). Aberrant immune responses in a mouse with behavioral disorders. *Public Library of Science One*, 6:e20912.

Herbert, M.R. (2010). Contributions of the environment and environmentally vulnerable physiology to autism spectrum disorders. *Current Opinion in Neurology*, 23, 103–110.

Hertz-Picciotto, I. and Delwiche, L. (2009). The rise in autism and the role of age at diagnosis. *Epidemiology*, 20, 84–90.

Hertz-Picciotto, I., Park, H.Y., Dostal, M., Kocan, A., Trnovec, T., and Sram, R. (2008). Prenatal exposures to persistent and non-persistent organic compounds and effects on immune system development. *Basic and Clinical Pharmacology and Toxicology*, 102, 146–154.

Hoshino, Y., Kumashiro, H., Yashima, Y., Tachibana, R., and Watanabe, M. (1982). The epidemiological study of autism in Fukushima-ken. *Folia Psychiatrica et Neurologica Japonica*, 36, 115–124.

Hrubec, T.C., Yan, M., Ye, K., Salafia, C.M., and Holladay, S.D. (2006). Valproic acid-induced fetal malformations are reduced by maternal immune stimulation with granulocyte-macrophage colony-stimulating factor or interferon-gamma. *Anatomical Record A, Discovories in Molecular, Cellular, and Evolutionary Biology*, 288, 1303–1309.

Jorde, L.B., Hasstedt, S.J., Ritvo, E.R., Mason-Brothers, A., Freeman, B.J., Pingree, C., et al. (1991). Complex segregation analysis of autism. *American Journal of Human Genetics*, 49, 932–938.

Jusko, T.A., De Roos, A.J., Schwartz, S.M., Lawrence, B.P., Palkovicova, L., Nemessanyi, T., et al. (2011). Maternal and early postnatal polychlorinated biphenyl exposure in relation to total serum immunoglobulin concentrations in 6-month-old infants. *Journal of Immunotoxicology*, 8, 95–100.

Jyonouchi, H., Geng, L., Cushing-Ruby, A., and Quraishi, H. (2008). Impact of innate immunity in a subset of children with autism spectrum disorders: a case control study. *Journal of Neuroinflammation*, 5, 52.

Keil, A., Daniels, J.L., Forssen, U., Hultman, C., Cnattingius, S., Soderberg, K.C., et al. (2010). Parental autoimmune diseases associated with autism spectrum disorders in offspring. *Epidemiology*, 21, 805–808.

Kim, Y.S., Leventhal, B.L., Koh, Y.J., Fombonne, E., Laska, E., Lim, E.C., et al. (2011). Prevalence of autism spectrum disorders in a total population sample. *American Journal of Psychiatry*, 168, 904–912.

King, M., and Bearman, P. (2009). Diagnostic change and the increased prevalence of autism. *International Journal of Epidemiology*, 38, 1224–1234.

Landrigan, P.J. (2010). What causes autism? Exploring the environmental contribution. *Current Opinion in Pediatrics*, 22, 219–225.

Lee, R.H., Mills, E.A., Schwartz, N., Bell, M.R., Deeg, K.E., Ruthazer, E.S., et al. (2010). Neurodevelopmental effects of chronic exposure to elevated levels of pro-inflammatory cytokines in a developing visual system. *Neural Development*, 5, 2.

Lin, Y.L., Lin, S.Y., and Wang, S. (2011). Prenatal lipopolysaccharide exposure increases anxiety-like behaviors and enhances stress-induced corticosterone responses in adult rats. *Brain, Behavior, and Immunity*, 26, 459–468.

Lutchmaya, S., Baron-Cohen, S., and Ragatt, P. (2002). Foetal testosterone and eye contact in 12 month old infants. *Infant Behavior and Development*, 25, 327–335.

McGinnis, W., Miller, V.M., and Audhya, T. (2010), Neurotoxic brainstem impairment as proposed threshold event in autistic regression. In A. Chauhan, V. Chauhan, and T. Brown, (eds.) *Autism: Oxidative Stress, Inflammation and Immune Abnormalities* (pp. 153–176).Boca Raton, FL: CRC Press.

Medzhitov, R. and Horng, T. (2009). Transcriptional control of the inflammatory response. *Nature Reviews. Immunology*, 9, 692–703.

Miller, V.M., Kahnke, T., Neu, N., Sanchez-Morrissey, S.R., Brosch, K., Kelsey, K., et al. (2010). Developmental PCB exposure induces hypothyroxinemia and sex-specific effects on cerebellum glial protein levels in rats. *International Journal of Developmental Neuroscience*, 28, 553–560.

Molloy, C.A., Morrow, A.L., Meinzen-Derr, J., Schleifer, K., Dienger, K., Manning-Courtney, P., et al. (2006). Elevated cytokine levels in children with autism spectrum disorder. *Journal of Neuroimmunology*, 172, 198–205.

Muhle, R., Trentacoste, S.V., and Rapin, I. (2004). The genetics of autism. *Pediatrics*, 113, e472–e486.

Orban, T., Sosenko, J.M., Cuthbertson, D., Krischer, J.P., Skyler, J.S., Jackson, R., et al. (2009). Pancreatic islet autoantibodies as predictors of type 1 diabetes in the Diabetes Prevention Trial-Type 1. *Diabetes Care*, 32, 2269–2274.

Polsek, D., Jagatic, T., Cepanec, M., Hof, P.R., and Simic, G. (2011). Recent developments in neuropathology of autism spectrum disorders. *Translational Neuroscience*, 2, 256–264.

Sandler, R.H., Finegold, S.M., Bolte, E.R., Buchanan, C.P., Maxwell, A.P., Vaisanen, M.L., et al. (2000). Short-term benefit from oral vancomycin treatment of regressive-onset autism. *Journal of Child Neurology*, 15, 429–435.

Santos-Galindo, M., Acaz-Fonseca, E., Bellini, M.J., and Garcia-Segura, L.M. (2011). Sex differences in the inflammatory response of primary astrocytes to lipopolysaccharide. *Biology of Sex Differences*, 2, 7.

Schwarz, J.M., Sholar, P.W., and Bilbo, S.D. (2011). Sex differences in microglial colonization of the developing rat brain. *Journal of Neurochemistry*, 120, 948–963.

Shi, L., Smith, S.E., Malkova, N., Tse, D., Su, Y., and Patterson, P.H. (2009). Activation of the maternal immune system alters cerebellar development in the offspring. *Brain, Behavior, and Immunity*, 23, 116–123.

Smith, S.E., Li, J., Garbett, K., Mirnics, K., and Patterson, P.H. (2007). Maternal immune activation alters fetal brain development through interleukin-6. *Journal of Neuroscience*, 27, 10695–10702.

Song, X., Li, W., Yang, Y., Zhao, J., Jiang, C., Li, W., et al. (2011). The nuclear factor-kappaB inhibitor pyrrolidine dithiocarbamate reduces polyinosinic-polycytidilic acid-induced immune response in pregnant rats and the behavioral defects of their adult offspring. *Behavioral and Brain Functions*, 7, 50.

Suzuki, K., Matsuzaki, H., Iwata, K., Kameno, Y., Shimmura, C., Kawai, S., et al. (2011). Plasma cytokine profiles in subjects with high-functioning autism spectrum disorders. *Public Library of Science One*, 6:e20470.

Tracey, K.J., Wei, H., Manogue, K.R., Fong, Y., Hesse, D.G., Nguyen, H.T., et al. (1988). Cachectin/tumor necrosis factor induces cachexia, anemia, and inflammation. *Journal of Experimental Medicine*, 167, 1211–1227.

Treffert, D.A. (1970). Epidemiology of infantile autism. *Archives of General Psychiatry*, 22, 431–438.

Vargas, D.L., Nascimbene, C., Krishnan, C., Zimmerman, A.W., and Pardo, C.A. (2005). Neuroglial activation and neuroinflammation in the brain of patients with autism. *Annals of Neurology*, 57, 67–81.

Vezzani, A., Balosso, S., and Ravizza, T. (2008). The role of cytokines in the pathophysiology of epilepsy. *Brain, Behavior, and Immunity*, 22, 797–803.

Wei, H., Zou, H., Sheikh, A.M., Malik, M., Dobkin, C., Brown, W.T., et al. (2011). IL-6 is increased in the cerebellum of autistic brain and alters neural cell adhesion, migration and synaptic formation. *Journal of Neuroinflammation*, 8, 52.

Williams, C.L., Teeling, J.L., Perry, V.H., and Fleming, T.P. (2011). Mouse maternal systemic inflammation at the zygote stage causes blunted cytokine responsiveness in lipopolysaccharide-challenged adult offspring. *BioMed Central Biology*, 9, 49.

Wing, L. and Gould, J. (1979). Severe impairments of social interaction and associated abnormalities in children: epidemiology and classification. *Journal of Autism and Developmental Disorders*, 9, 11–29.

Zalcman, S. (2011). Sex differences in behavioral disturbances associated with maternal infection and periadolescent cytokine challenge. Fifth Annual Meeting of the Organization for the Study of Sex Differences, Oklahoma.

Zhao, B. and Schwartz, J.P. (1998). Involvement of cytokines in normal CNS development and neurological diseases: recent progress and perspectives. *Journal of Neuroscience Research*, 52, 7–16.

23

Depression, Inflammation and Tryptophan Metabolism

Robert H. McCusker,[4] Annemieke Kavelaars,[*,1,2,3,4,5] Cobi J. Heijnen,[*,5] Robert Dantzer,[*,4] and Keith W. Kelley[4]

[1] *Integrated Immunology and Behavior Program,*
[2] *Neuroscience Program,*
[3] *Department of Animal Sciences,*
[4] *Department of Pathology University of Illinois at Urbana-Champaign Urbana, Illinois, USA*
[5] *Laboratory of Neuroimmunology and Developmental Origins of Disease, University Medical Center Utrecht, Utrecht*

Overview

From both a clinical and preclinical perspective, it has become widely accepted that inflammatory stimuli can initiate or accentuate symptoms of depression. In both human and animal models, symptoms of depression appear after pro-inflammatory cytokines are produced within the body or administered exogenously, suggesting that immune activation can precipitate depression. On the flipside of the coin, several symptoms of depression are frequently associated with elevated levels of systemic inflammatory markers.

With the development of drugs that alleviate depression, particularly those that putatively act via inhibition of serotonin reuptake in the brain, a link between tryptophan metabolism and depression became evident leading to the *Monoamine/5-HT Theory of Depression*. Nevertheless, a direct connection between changes in monoaminergic neurotransmission and depression has never been definitively proven. Other research efforts based on this theory have led to an alternative hypothesis. In this scenario, shifting tryptophan metabolism from serotonin synthesis to the generation of neuroactive metabolites, such as quinolinic acid and kynurenic acid, by the kynurenine pathway is now considered to play an important a role in the pathogenesis of inflammation-dependent depression. The balance between serotonergic and kynurenine pathways is controlled by expression of three rate-limiting enzymes within a class of dioxygenases that convert tryptophan to kynurenine: indolamine 2,3 dioxygenase (IDO1), IDO2 and tryptophan 2,3 dioxygenase (TDO2). Expression of these enzymes is tightly regulated by the innate

* Current address for Annemieke Kavelaars, Cobi Heijnen and Robert Dantzer: MD Anderson Cancer Center, Division of Internal Medicine, Department of Symptom Research, Houston, TX 77030.

The Wiley-Blackwell Handbook of Psychoneuroimmunology, First Edition. Edited by Alexander W. Kusnecov and Hymie Anisman.

immune system. A now-defined linear sequence of inflammation → cytokines → IDO/TDO → kynurenine → behavioral changes provides a newly developing link between inflammation, tryptophan metabolism and depression. This sequence is the basis for the *Kynurenine Theory of Depression*.

Impact

Major clinical depression is a major cause of disability (Moussavi *et al.*, 2007). Clinical depression affects over 120 million people worldwide, with a lifetime prevalence ranging from 10 to 15%. Depression-related absenteeism and presenteeism (non-productive work time) represent an estimated $36 billion per year loss in the USA alone. More important than this work-related loss is the 20-fold greater chance of suicide among patients with clinical depression compared to the general population (Lepine and Briley, 2011; Maes, Leonard, Myint, Kubera, and Verkerk, 2011) and the high psychosocial burden of depression to the patient, relatives and society as a whole. In addition to the increased chance of suicide, depression has additional health burdens. For example, the chance of mortality 5 years after a myocardial infarction is greater in depressed patients than in non-depressed patients. Depressed patients, particularly men, are prone to engage in risky behaviors, such as smoking and overconsumption of alcohol, and patients may fail to adhere to their medication schedules. Since clinical depression is predicted to overcome infectious diseases as the major health burden worldwide by 2030, there is considerable need to discover additional means to cure or treat major depression.

A Balance

The body is in a state of constant flux, with compensation maintained by homeostatic mechanisms. These regulatory systems maintain a balance (Figure 23.1) in an attempt to sustain body functions within a narrow range or homeostasis. Any failure to maintain this balance results in

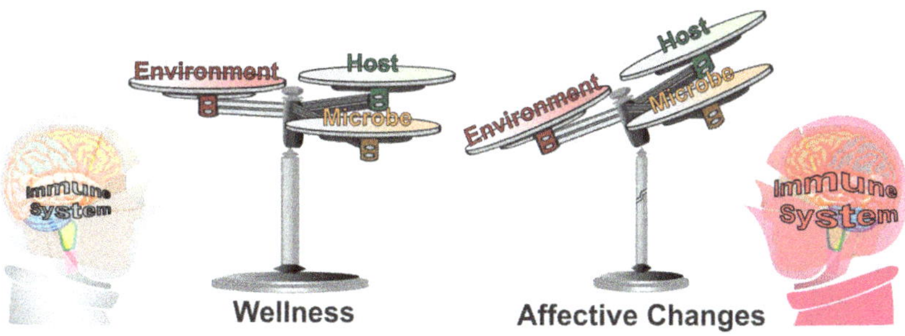

Figure 23.1 Host defense: a balancing act. The immune system, and in particular the innate immune system, represents the first line of defense in the body. Stimuli from the environment, genetic predisposition of the host and the constant microbial attack on the body produce a tempered state of activation. This baseline immune response is critical for a sense of wellness, optimal learning and memory and positive affect. Changes in the level of stimuli activate the immune system, resulting in acute immune responses that are accompanied by behavioral changes termed sickness behavior. Several affective disorders are associated with a prolonged imbalance of the immune response to these stimuli.

physical and behavioral changes. From a global perspective, homeostatic mechanisms function to balance input from external stimuli (e.g., environmental signals such as noise and temperature), to protect the body from infectious agents, and to maintain optimal physiological function on a background of host differences (e.g. genetic susceptibility/resistance).

The ability of the body to protect itself against these changing inputs is dependent on a number of support mechanisms. The classic five sensory systems of sight, sound, taste, touch, and smell inform humans and animals about their environment. Animals respond by avoiding danger, searching for food, and finding shelter. Part of the body's homeostatic response is mediated by the immune system. Even before cytokines were discovered, it was proposed that the immune system is a sensory organ that informs the brain that infectious microorganisms have invaded the body proper (Blalock, 1984). Activation of the immune system is clearly important in defense against infectious agents, but the innate immune system also is activated by environmental stress, and the degree of immune activation is controlled by host susceptibility/resistance.

It was once believed that the brain was immune-privileged, making it blind to many of the detrimental signals that peripheral tissues are exposed to on a daily basis. It is now widely accepted that the brain is not only affected by the immune system, but in many ways the brain attempts to mirror immune changes that occur at the periphery as a mechanism to transmit appropriate counterregulatory signals. Most important for this review is the discovery that the immune system communicates with the brain by both neuronal (fast) and humoral (slower) systems, leading to important changes in behavior (Dantzer, O'Connor, Freund, Johnson, and Kelley, 2008).

Inflammation and Depression

Major depressive disorders encompass a number of symptoms (Table 23.1). A depressed patient is identified by self-reported experiences or by a score on a questionnaire (such as the Montgomery–Asberg Depression Rating Scale (MADRS), which is an adjunct to the Hamilton Rating Scale for Depression (HAMD); both commonly used among researchers, especially to quantify therapeutic efficacy). These scales were designed to identify the presence of symptoms, with the goal of improving and standardizing the detection of depression.

Table 23.1 Clinical Signs of Depression

memory deficits, difficulty concentrating
lack of energy: fatigue
feelings of helplessness or hopelessness
feelings of worthlessness or guilt; self-loathing
sleep pattern changes: insomnia or hypersomnia
escapist behavior; recklessness, compulsive behavior
changes in mood; irritable, short-tempered, over-aggressive
lack of interest in daily or pleasurable activities; anhedonia
changes in appetite or weight; over or under eating; weight gain or weight loss
unexplained aches and pains; headaches, muscle pain, stomach pain
suicidal thoughts/attempts
For diagnosis, $\geq$ 5 symptoms, including ↓ mood or interest over 2 weeks

However, many of the symptoms of depression are ambiguous in nature (e.g., over- or under-eating; insomnia or hypersomnia) or associated with other conditions (e.g., memory deficits and Alzheimer's). To make this even more complicated, depression is associated with a number of factors such as endocrine changes that occur with postpartum depression, mental abuse as with prior emotional abuse, medications such as beta-blockers for high blood pressure that can increase the risk of depression, current personal problems such a social isolation or rejection, or inflammation, as when associated with infections or stress. In many cases, the etiology of a patient's depression remains unclear. In striking contrast, depression associated with inflammation has now been clearly recognized as a distinct cause–effect phenomenon.

A systemic inflammatory component associated with depression is evident by the increased concentrations of pro-inflammatory cytokines such as IL-6 and TNF-α, and acute-phase proteins such as haptoglobin and C-reactive protein, that have been reported in the circulation of depressed patients. Also, several conditions or diseases with a chronic inflammatory component such as aging, obesity, atherosclerosis, rheumatoid arthritis, and congestive heart failure are associated with an increased prevalence of depressive disorders (Evans *et al.*, 2005). These findings do not confirm cause–effect relationships, especially in cross-sectional clinical studies, but they do support the idea that more research needs to examine the potential role between systemic inflammation and depression. After all, where there is smoke, there is often fire, and fire just happens to be the root Latin meaning of "inflammare."

A cause–effect relationship between inflammation and depression is supported by several clinical examples. There is a significantly elevated incidence of depressive symptoms reported by patients undergoing cancer immunotherapy and cytokine treatment for hepatitis C infection (Capuron and Dantzer, 2003; Capuron *et al.*, 2002). With these examples involving activation of the immune system in humans, depressive symptoms develop on a background of neurovegetative symptoms (Figure 23.2, top) that are commonly referred to as inflammation-induced sickness behavior (Dantzer *et al.*, 2008). Symptoms of sickness either overlap with or precede symptoms of depression (Figure 23.2, middle). In contrast, a recent study presented data supporting dissociation between depression and overt sickness (Reichenberg *et al.*, 2001). When challenged with low-dose endotoxemia, *Salmonella abortus equi* endotoxin, patients lacked physical symptoms of sickness despite elevated circulating pro-inflammatory cytokine levels. Patients treated with endotoxin reported increased anxiety and depressed mood. This latter finding provided evidence that depression in humans does not fully overlap with sickness but confirmed that depression is associated with elevated peripheral cytokines. Data such as these suggest that elevated cytokine production may result in sickness behaviors, whereas some level of immune activation results in the more subtle expression of symptoms associated with depression (Figure 23.2, middle). It is obvious that not all patients with an underlying chronic inflammatory component are depressed, and those that become depressed do not remain depressed. A low level of cytokine expression may not be sufficient to cause depression by itself, as for aged patients or patients with obesity, atherosclerosis, rheumatoid arthritis, and congestive heart failure. However, cytokines may well be a predisposing factor involved in the development of clinical symptoms associated with a physiological stressor (Figure 23.2, bottom), thus providing a physiological basis for host-environment interactions.

Preclinical animal models frequently employ an inflammatory stimulus, such as an intraperitoneal injection of lipopolysaccharide (LPS), to initiate an acute cytokine response that ultimately leads to both sickness and depression-like behaviors. An acute inflammatory response is associated with transient sickness that is accompanied by a neuroinflammatory response as

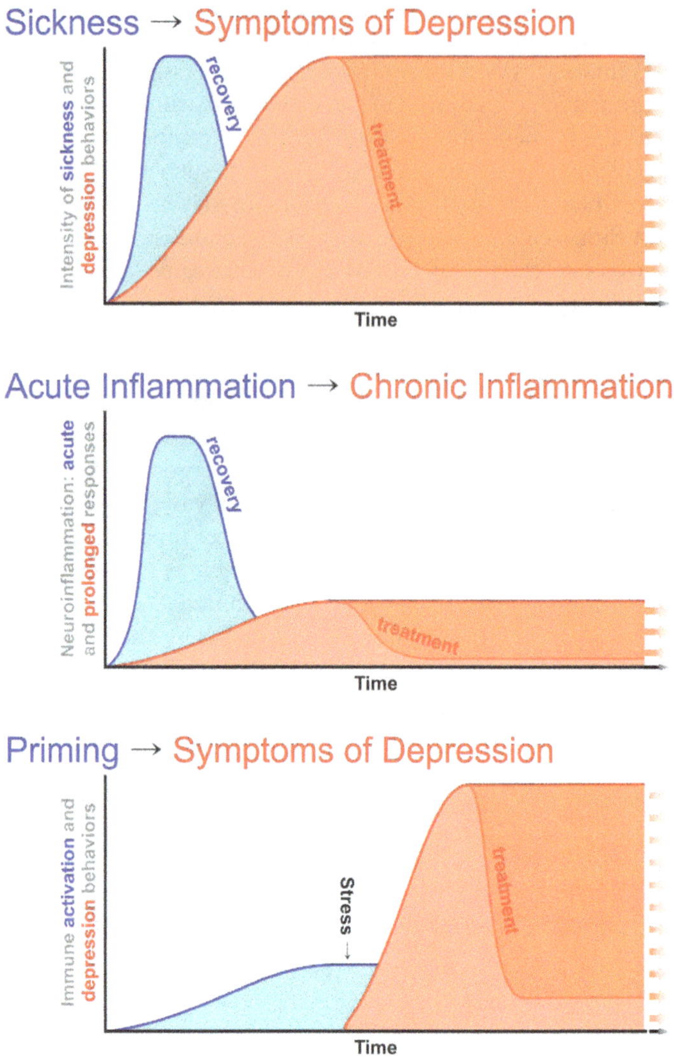

Figure 23.2 Associations between behavior and neuroinflammation. The acute sickness response (top panel, blue) is typically manifested by a reduction in food consumption, fever, decreased activity, social isolation, achiness, and sleep changes. These symptoms reflect a robust, but acute, systemic inflammatory response (middle panel, blue). This change in peripheral inflammatory status is conveyed to the brain, where a mirror image of the systemic inflammatory response is elicited, leading to elevated cytokine synthesis in the brain. Depressive symptoms (top panel, orange) are usually manifested as irritability, feelings of hopelessness and helplessness, inability to concentrate, overwhelming sadness, alterations in sleep, loss of interest in life's activities, and self-loathing. These affective changes typically disappear when the acute bout of inflammation resolves. If the acute inflammatory response inappropriately continues and develops into chronic, low-grade systemic or central inflammation (middle panel, orange); symptoms of depression can be sustained and lead to full-blown clinical depression. Many anti-depressants possess anti-inflammatory activity, a property that correlates with clinical efficacy. With patients undergoing remission, a previous inflammatory response (bottom panel, blue) may sensitize the immune system, leading to an earlier, heightened, and often sustained immune response, a property that is known as priming. Acute stress, which has been shown to elicit an acute inflammatory response, may subsequently elicit symptoms of depression (bottom panel, orange).

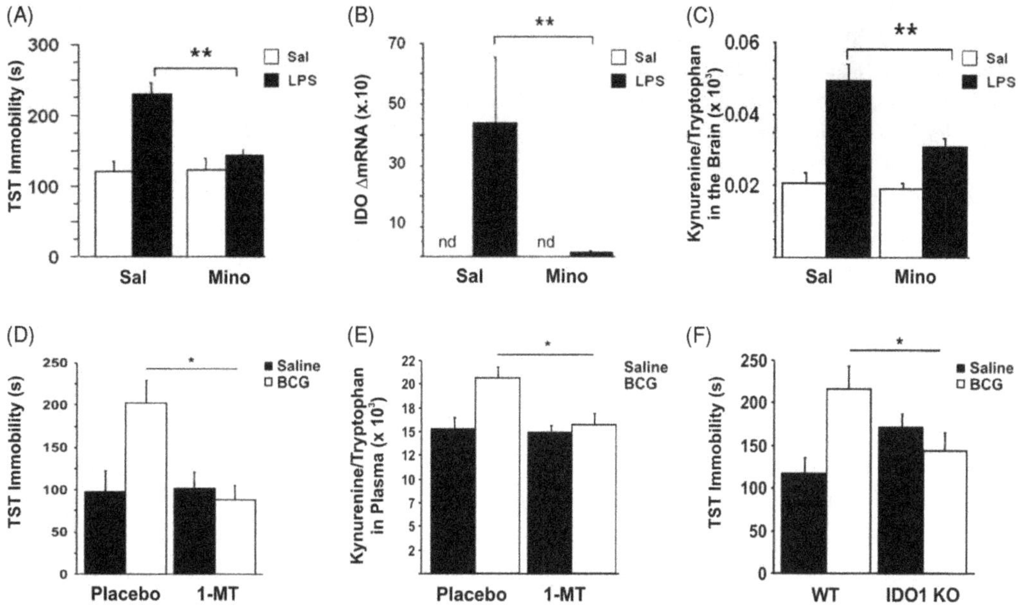

Figure 23.3 Depression-like behaviors of mice are dependent on an active immune response and IDO1 enzymatic activity. In mouse models, depression-like behavior is frequently assessed as duration of immobility during the tail suspension test (TST). An i.p. injection of LPS induces acute activation of the immune system that causes an increase in immobility when measured 24 hours after the injection. Minocycline (Mino), which attenuates microglial activation and subsequent cytokine release (data not shown), attenuates this behavioral response (A). Minocycline also blocks the ability of LPS to induce IDO1 expression in the brain (B) and reduces the kynurenine/tryptophan ratio in the brain (C). An i.p. injection of the live bacteria, BCG, induces prolonged activation of the immune system and causes an increase in immobility during the TST up to a few weeks following exposure to the bacteria. This increase in immobility is absent with mice pre-treated with 1-methyltryptophan (1-MT), an inhibitor of IDO activity (D). Treatment with 1-MT normalizes the plasma kynurenine/tryptophan ratio (E). Mice lacking IDO1 (IDO1 KO) do not have an increase in time of immobility in the TST following injection of BCG (F). These data establish that IDO1 expression and activity are required for inflammation-induced depression-like behavior of mice. Data in A, B and C (O'Connor *et al.*, 2009c) and D, E and F (O'Connor *et al.*, 2009b) were adapted from published manuscripts.

determined by elevated cytokine production by cells within the brain. This central inflammatory response is associated with depression-like behaviors. An example is shown in Figure 23.3. Treatment with LPS causes depression-like behavior of mice, assessed as an increase in time of immobility during the tail suspension test (TST) and sickness behavior. In this example, minocycline attenuated the sickness response (data not shown), assessed by a loss of body weight, food consumption, and general locomotor activity (O'Connor, Lawson, Andre, Moreau *et al.*, 2009).

Minocycline, which blocks microglial activation, attenuates the cytokine response (not shown) and importantly blocks LPS-induced depression-like behaviors, shown by an elevated time of immobility during TST (Figure 23.3A). This inflammation-induced depression-like behavior is paralleled by expression of IDO1 in the brain (Figure 23.3B) and an increase in the kynurenine/tryptophan ratio within the brain (Figure 23.3C). However, it is possible to distinguish depression-like behaviors from sickness of mice. Neurotrophins, insulin-like growth factor-I and its metabolite (consisting of only the first three amino acids of insulin-like growth factor-I, GPE), diminish central inflammation and LPS-induced depression-like behaviors of mice, independent of changes in sickness behavior (Park, Dantzer, Kelley, and McCusker, 2011; Park, Lawson, Dantzer, Kelley, and McCusker, 2011).

In addition to an acute inflammatory response, systemic infections can be used to initiate a sustained inflammatory response. In such animal models, the acute immune response elicits sickness behaviors, but as the infection is cleared, sickness behaviors diminish and continuing low-grade neuroinflammation leads to depression-like behaviors (Moreau *et al.*, 2005). Importantly, the induction of depression-like behaviors by Bacille Calmette–Guerin (BCG) is cytokine-dependent (O'Connor *et al.*, 2009a) and absent in mice lacking IDO1 (O'Connor *et al.*, 2009b). An example of data from this model was published in O'Connor *et al.*, 2009b. Immobility in the TST is elevated 7 d after inoculation with BCG (Figure 23.3D). In this mouse model, administration of a D and L isoform mix of 1-methyltryptophan (1-MT) that inhibits both IDO1 and IDO2 enzymatic activity (Metz *et al.*, 2007) alleviated depression-like behavior of mice (Figure 23.3D). Treatment with 1-MT did not attenuate BCG-induced IDO1 expression in the brain (Figure 23.3E) and lungs (not shown) or cytokine expression, but normalized the kynurenine:tryptophan ratio in the circulation (Figure 23.3F). These examples, using LPS and BCG as inflammatory stimuli to induce an inflammatory response, as well as similar studies, support a key role for neuroinflammation in the induction of depression-like behavior and the importance of kynurenine production from tryptophan as a downstream but requisite event involved in inflammation-induced depression-like behaviors.

Two major theories of depression arose from early studies in this field. The *Macrophage Theory of Depression* was proposed in 1991and it implicated elevated pro-inflammatory cytokines as a causative factor for depression (Smith, 1991). The *Monoamine/serotonin (5-HT) Theory of Depression* was proposed in 1967 and implicated an alteration in tryptophan and other monoamine activities in the etiology of depression (Coppen, 1967). With the discovery that several pro-inflammatory cytokines induce the expression of IDO1, the two theories were united (Maes *et al.*, 2011). The *New Kynurenine Theory of Depression* ties activation of the immune system to a shift in tryptophan metabolism. Activation of TDO2 by stress (via glucocorticoids that are often elevated in depressed patients) and activation of IDO1 by an inflammatory response (via cytokines that are elevated in depressed patients) reduce the availability of tryptophan while producing kynurenine for conversion to neuroactive metabolites (Figure 23.4). The delivery of kynurenine to the brain or generation of kynurenine within the brain is proposed as a causative factor for development of inflammation-dependent depression.

Tryptophan Metabolism

Tryptophan may be one of the original multitaskers. It cannot be synthesized by the body, which is why it is defined as an essential amino acid. Every good nutritionist could easily provide a list of foods with high levels of this essential amino acid. Adequate intake of these foods is necessary to maintain health and growth, largely because of tryptophan's role in protein synthesis (Figure 23.5A). Biochemists could wax poetic about the exchange of carbons and nitrogens upon complete metabolism of tryptophan to 2-acetyl-CoA for the production of ATP upon entry into the Krebs cycle (Figure 23.5E). These biochemists would then join nutritionists to further describe metabolism by extending the nutritional value of tryptophan

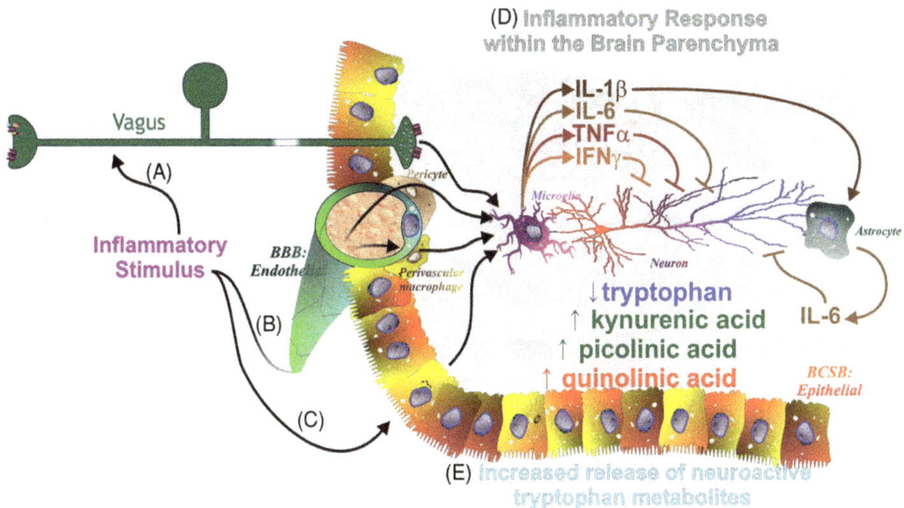

Figure 23.4 Immune system-to-brain dialogue can culminate in cytokine synthesis in the brain and an increase in kynurenine metabolites derived from tryptophan. The brain receives input by several venues in its quest to monitor the immune status. (A) Afferent neuronal signals can be induced by i.p. injection of inflammatory agents, such as those that occur via vagal input into the lower brain stem (nucleus tractus solitaries). Neural circuits convey these stimuli to the hypothalamus and amygdala where they can induce the synthesis of cytokines within the brain. Although all cells in the brain are capable of synthesizing cytokines, microglia and resident macrophages display a strong and early response to neuronal and humoral systemic inflammatory stimuli. (B) Humoral inflammatory input can directly deliver infectious agents to the brain. However, most often blood-borne inflammatory signals, including peripheral immune cells, arrive at the brain in the form of toxins and cytokines from the periphery. These signals either initiate a response from endothelial cells, that form the blood–brain barrier (BBB), or directly within the brain parenchyma, after transport across the BBB. In either case, perivascular macrophages, microglia or astrocytes propagate the inflammatory response within the CNS. (C) Although rare, inflammatory responses can be initiated by direct interaction of cytokines with epithelial cells of the blood cerebrospinal barrier (BCSB). (D) Under any of these conditions, a cytokine cascade (including IL-1β, TNF-α, IL-6 and nitric oxide (NO) is initiated within the brain parenchyma that forms a mirror image of the peripheral inflammatory status. (E) This loop is a feedforward response that results in a shift in tryptophan metabolism within the brain, resulting in the generation of neuroactive metabolites.

as a precursor for the endogenous generation of the vitamin, nicotinamide (NAD, Figure 23.5D) and then describe the role of NAD as an electron donor. All of these processes occur intracellularly without the requisite extracellular release of intermediates, and, indeed, most cells of the body utilize tryptophan for these purposes, although in varying proportions. Under normal conditions, approximately 80% of tryptophan within the brain is converted to nicotinamide, emphasizing the importance of this diversity in contrast to the laic perception that tryptophan is just necessary for protein synthesis.

Tryptophan is also converted into several neuroactive compounds that may be released from cells, not the least of which is serotonin, a critical neurotransmitter (Figure 23.5B). The release of products derived from tryptophan into the extracellular space provides for cell-to-cell communication and subsequent regulatory mechanisms that are largely independent of its use for protein synthesis, energy or the generation of NAD. Quinolinic acid, picolinic

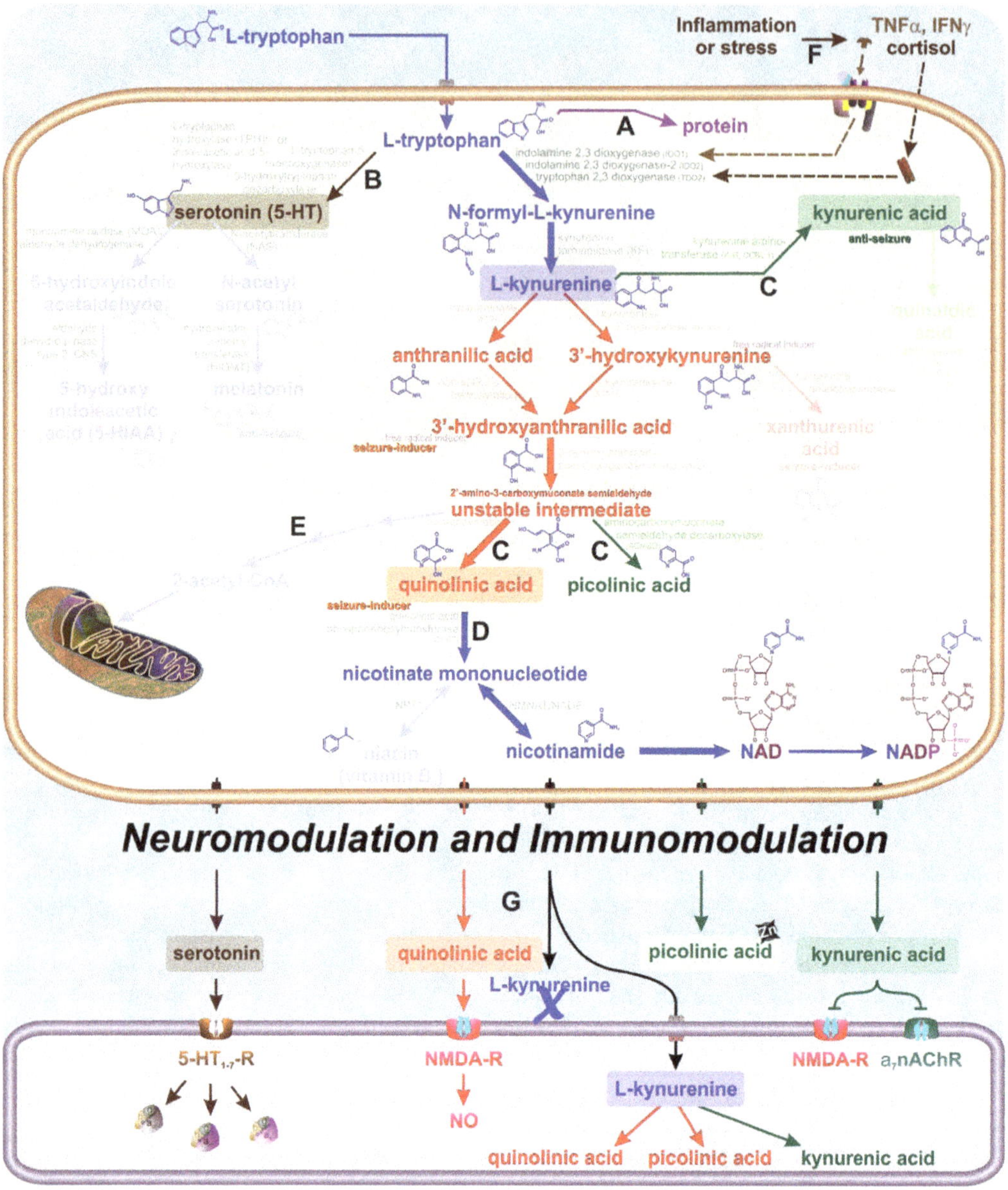

Figure 23.5 Tryptophan metabolism. A truly versatile molecule, tryptophan serves as an: (A) essential amino acid for protein synthesis, (B) a precursor for the neurotransmitter, serotonin, (C) a source of neuromodulators, such as kynurenic acid and quinolinic acid, (D) a building block for an electron transporter, NAD, and the vitamin niacin, and (E) as a source of energy upon complete catabolism. These numerous routes of tryptophan metabolism have immense behavioral consequences through shifts in the amounts of the various intermediary products, some of which can have opposing effects on neuronal function. (F) Inflammation or stress markedly alters this balance via induction of dioxygenase expression within various tissues, including the brain. (G) Inflammation increases intracellular metabolism of tryptophan towards the production of kynurenine, which is inactive on neurons. However, this change is accompanied by the subsequent production and release of downstream neuro-active compounds; including *quinolinic acid*, *kynurenic acid* and picolinic acid. The proportion of the various active metabolites is dependent on the cell type where kynurenine is generated and further metabolized.

acid, and kynurenic acid are three of the metabolic products of considerable interest into the study of behavior because each has distinct neuronal activity. Kynurenic acid (Hilmas *et al.*, 2001; Perkins and Stone, 1982) and picolinic acid (Kalisch, Jhamandas, Boegman, and Beninger, 1994) are neuroprotective and antagonize the neurotoxic n-methyl-D-aspartate receptor (NMDA-R) dependent action of quinolinic acid (Stone and Perkins, 1981). Quinolinic acid excites neurons by directly interacting with the NMDA-R with agonist activity, and it also increases glutamate release and depresses glutamate uptake by astrocytes. All of these quinolinic acid-induced processes accentuate NMDA-R activation. In contrast, kynurenic acid is a strong antagonist of the NDMA-R and this inhibitory activity is responsible for its neuroprotective properties (Perkins and Stone, 1982). In addition, kynurenic acid inhibits the α7 nicotinic receptor (α7 nAChR) activity with a lower IC50 than for the NMDA-R (Hilmas *et al.*, 2001). Via its interaction with the α7 nAChR, kynurenic acid also depresses glutamate release thus amplifying its antagonism of NMDA-R activity (Nemeth, Toldi, and Vecsei, 2005). The mechanism for neuroprotection by picolinic acid is independent of the NMDA-R and may involve its ability to bind zinc which accentuates NMDA-R activation (Jhamandas, Boegman, Beninger, Miranda, and Lipic, 2000).

It might be of interest to note here that during the generation of NAD from tryptophan, quinolinic acid is a requisite intermediate (Figure 23.5D). Thus, under normal conditions, quinolinic acid is a major metabolite of tryptophan within the brain but it is not neurotoxic because of its intracellular location (Beagles, Morrison, and Heyes, 1998). Quinolinic acid must be released from cells to activate the NMDA-R or to increase the extracellular level of glutamate for activation of the NMDA-R. Similarly, kynurenic acid generation within cells does not affect neuronal activity. Instead, kynurenic acid must be exported to the interstitial fluid to be active by binding to the extracellular region of membrane receptors. Also of particular interest is the fact that extracellular kynurenine is inactive and must be taken up into cells for conversion to active compounds (Figure 23.5G). When using tryptophan as a starting substrate, the generation of kynurenine competes with the production of serotonin. Similarly, quinolinic acid and kynurenic acid compete with each other for kynurenine as a common precursor. Three dioxygenases are present in most tissues including the brain, and the generation of kynurenine from tryptophan is proportional to their combined activity: IDO1, IDO2 and TDO2 activity are rate-limiting along the kynurenine pathway.

Tryptophan Metabolism and Disease

Changes in tryptophan metabolism within the brain have been implicated in several neurodegenerative and psychiatric conditions (Table 23.2). IDO1 activity is increased in patients with idiopathic epilepsy (Liimatainen *et al.*, 2011). An increase in IDO1 activity, with resultant quinolinic acid release from microglia, at the expense of kynurenic acid production, is a likely direct inducer of seizure activity(Schwarcz, Speciale, and French, 1987; Schwarcz, Speciale, Okuno, French, and Kohler, 1986). Diminished levels of kynurenic acid have been reported in the frontal cortex, putamen and substantia nigra pars compacta of Parkinson's patients (Ogawa *et al.*, 1992). Together with elevated levels of 3-hydroxykynurenine, suggesting a potential for elevated levels of the neurotoxic quinolinic acid; the loss of the neuroprotective kynurenic acid may well contribute to oxidative damage to dopaminergic neurons.

In patients with Huntington's disease, quinolinic acid levels vary considerably from elevated in early stage disease to unchanged in later stage disease within the cortex and striatum

Table 23.2 Changes in Brain Tryptophan Metabolites Associated with Clinical Outcomes

Condition	*Quinolinic acid*	*Ratio*	*Kynurenic acid*	*Neurodegeneration*
Seizures	↑	>	↓	+
Parkinson's	probable↑	>	↓	+
Huntington's	↑–	>	↓	+
Multiple sclerosis	speculated↑	>	?	+
Alzheimer's	↑↑	>	↑	+
Schizophrenia		<	↑	
Cognitive deficits	↑	or	↑	+ or –
Depression, non-inflammatory	—	=	—	
Depression, inflammatory	↑	=	↑↑	
Site of synthesis:	*microglia or periphery*		*astrocytes, neurons, blood–brain barrier or periphery*	

Alteration in tryptophan metabolism is common to several neurodegenerative and psychiatric disorders. Several seizure-inducing and neurotoxic metabolites are released within the brain following an increased rate of metabolism of tryptophan down the kynurenine pathway, most notable quinolinic acid. Neuronal loss is highly associated with the neurotoxic index: quinolinic > kynurenic acid ratio. Reversal of this ratio with higher kynurenic acid appears to be associated with a greater incidence of schizophrenia and non-neurodegenerative cognitive deficits. In contrast, an increase in levels of both quinolinic and kynurenic acid within the brain may be a hallmark of inflammation-induced non-neurodegenerative depression.

(Guidetti, Luthi-Carter, Augood, and Schwarcz, 2004). In contrast, kynurenic acid is low in the striatum of Huntington's patients (Beal, Matson, Swartz, Gamache, and Bird, 1990; Jauch *et al.*, 1995). These findings suggest that an elevated quinolinic acid to kynurenic acid ratio enhances Huntington-mediated neurotoxicity. Although proposed as a mediator of seizures and neurodegeneration associated with multiple sclerosis (MS) (Anderson and Rodriguez, 2011), direct evidence for changes in brain quinolinic or kynurenic acid levels in MS patients is lacking. Microglia and astrocyte levels of IDO1 are elevated in the brains of Alzheimer's patients, as is immunoreactive quinolinic acid (Guillemin, Brew, Noonan, Takikawa, and Cullen, 2005a), which may contribute to neurodegeneration. An increase in IDO1 activity is probably also responsible for increased kynurenic acid in the caudate nucleus and putamen of postmortem brains of patients with Alzheimer's (Baran, Jellinger, and Deecke, 1999) which, although elevated, may not be adequate to prevent the neuronal damage associated with highly elevated quinolinic acid. All of these conditions are associated with an increase in the neurotoxic index within the brain (calculated various ways but usually as the ratio of either quinolinic acid or kynurenine to kynurenic acid or tryptophan). These conditions are primarily driven by marked microglial activation, and all lead to neuronal death.

In contrast, elevated levels of the neuroprotective kynurenic acid within the brain are associated with psychosis and schizophrenia (Anderson, 2011). Kynurenic acid in the brain of schizophrenic patients is likely derived from an increased expression of TDO2 within astrocytes, as found in the frontal cortex (Miller *et al.*, 2004). Unlike most of the other conditions that are listed in Table 23.2, cognitive impairment found in schizophrenia is believed to be a result of neuronal dysfunction rather than neurodegeneration (Wonodi and Schwarcz, 2010). Although there are a considerable number of reports showing that memory and learning are affected by quinolinic acid, these deficits are largely attributed to neurodegeneration rather than a strict alteration in cognitive processes. In contrast, elevated kynurenic acid levels may cause cognitive dysfunction and, indeed, a reduction in kynurenic acid generation may be a useful target for cognitive improvement (Pocivavsek *et al.*, 2011). The extreme cognitive deficits that are found in Alzheimer's may not only be attributed to neurodegeneration, but may be accentuated by the elevation in kynurenic acid (Baran *et al.*, 1999).

Collectively, these clinical data strongly support a causative role for the release of specific tryptophan metabolites in the etiology of neurodegenerative (↑ quinolinic acid ± ↓ kynurenic acid) as well as psychiatric and cognitive (↑ kynurenic acid) diseases. Neurodegeneration is strongly associated with an elevated quinolinic acid to kynurenic acid ratio and subsequent alterations in cognition and behavior. In contrast, an elevated kynurenic acid to quinolinic acid ratio is associated with neuronal dysfunction and cognitive impairment, independent of neurodegeneration. The possible association between brain levels of quinolinic acid and kynurenic acid with depressive disorders remains less clear.

Depressive disorders are not necessarily associated with neurodegeneration or even changes in cognition, although cognitive changes frequently occur. Depressive disorders are viewed as a state of dysfunctional neuron circuits. Unfortunately, there is a complete lack of information regarding quinolinic acid or kynurenic acid levels within the brain parenchyma of depressed patients without co-morbid somatic disorders. This represents a major information void in knowledge regarding tryptophan metabolism and depression. In depressed patients without an inflammatory disease, neither quinolinic or kynurenic acid levels were changed in the CSF compared to controls (Heyes *et al.*, 1992). There was lower kynurenic acid in the plasma of depressed patients without a change in circulating kynurenine. This later finding provided evidence that in patients without inflammatory disease the circulating neurotoxic index is higher in depressed patients compared to controls (Myint *et al.*, 2007). Since kynurenine itself is inactive, this finding assumes that kynurenine is converted to an active metabolite such as quinolinic acid before entering or upon entering the nervous system.

The findings above contrast with those using subjects in an inflammation-dependent model of depression. In patients with hepatitis C, following 12 weeks of treatment with IFN-α (Raison *et al.*, 2010), a ~79% increase in kynurenic acid, a ~65% increase in kynurenine, and a ~59% increase in quinolinic acid levels in the CSF were observed as compared to placebo-treated patients. IFN-α also caused a significant increase in scores for depression (MADRS; Montgomery-Asberg depression Rating Scale). This increase in kynurenic acid with a similar increase in kynurenine and quinolinic acid presents a unique scenario for depression compared to the other conditions in Table 23.2. Thus, IFN-α induced depression presents without an increase in the brain (CSF) neurotoxic index. This finding suggests that the increase in the neuroprotective kynurenic acid offsets a possible NMDA-R-dependent neurodegeneration that has been associated with elevated levels of quinolinic acid, which in turn leads to the interesting question as to whether an increase in kynurenic acid within the CNS may be involved in non-neurodegenerative depression. Intrastriatal administration of kynurenic acid to rodents reduces extracellular dopamine in the striatum (Wu, Rassoulpour, and Schwarcz, 2007). A reduction of brain dopamine following administration of IFN-α to monkeys is involved in the induction of depression-like behavior (Felger *et al.*, 2007). These data suggest that elevated kynurenic acid within the brain is likely to be involved in IFN-α-induced depression.

The source of kynurenine metabolites within the brain is of major interest especially relative to inflammation-dependent depression. The finding of Raison and colleagues (Raison *et al.*, 2010) that circulating quinolinic acid and kynurenine levels in humans correlate significantly with quinolinic acid and kynurenine levels in the CSF suggests that these metabolites within the brain arise from the circulation. Like tryptophan, kynurenine is transported by the large amino acid transporter (L-system) and is readily taken up by the rat brain from the circulation (Fukui, Schwarcz, Rapoport, Takada, and Smith, 1991). In contrast, quinolinic acid, 3-hydroxykynurenine and kynurenic acid have limited access to the brain (Fukui *et al.*, 1991). Thus, the source of the elevated levels of kynurenine, quinolinic acid and kynurenic acid in the CSF of IFN-treated patients is unclear. They probably result from elevated generation in situ based on the increased production of all metabolites by several cell types when challenged with cytokines.

Tryptophan Metabolism in the Brain

The brain is normally protected from peripheral kynurenine or quinolinic acid by their metabolism at the blood–brain barrier with subsequent release of non-toxic metabolites. Within the brain parenchyma, there is a balance between the production of neuroprotective metabolites by pericytes, astrocytes, oligodendrocytes and neurons and the production of neurotoxic products by microglia and macrophages. An inflammatory response stimulates all of the cell types to increase metabolism of kynurenine metabolites via their respective pathways and the net effect on behavior depends on how the balance of tryptophan metabolites is shifted within the brain.

All three dioxygenases are present in the brain, with a combination of IDO1, IDO2 and TDO2 activity controlling conversion of tryptophan to kynurenine. IDO1 is found in most cell types within the brain (Guillemin *et al.*, 2000, 2001, 2005b, 2007; Owe-Young *et al.*, 2008). The cellular localization of IDO2 within the brain has not been characterized, although it may reside in resident dendritic cells, based on its high expression by bone marrow-derived dendritic cells (Simones and Shepherd, 2011). TDO2 is expressed almost exclusively by neurons in the normal mouse hippocampus (Ohira *et al.*, 2010), although levels are detectible in astrocytes of schizophrenic patients (Miller *et al.*, 2004). With a commitment of 80% of tryptophan to NAD generation, it is obvious that these enzymes are at adequate levels to compete with tryptophan hydroxylase, and thus the production of serotonin, for tryptophan utilization. It should also be obvious that IDO1, IDO2 and TDO2 activity must be tightly controlled to avoid under-availability of tryptophan for protein and neurotransmitter synthesis.

Most cell types are capable of metabolizing tryptophan, so it is critical to evaluate the role of each cell type in the production of active tryptophan derivatives (Figure 23.6). Tryptophan is delivered to the brain via the circulation, and the first cells that are encountered are those associated with blood vessels. When placed in culture under basal conditions, endothelial cells produce kynurenic acid when provided with tryptophan, 3-hydroxyanthranilic acid or quinolinic acid as a substrate (Figure 23.6A). When these endothelial cells are provided with 3-hydroxyanthranilic acid they also produce kynurenine (Owe-Young *et al.*, 2008). This secretory profile remains after challenge with pro-inflammatory cytokines to mimic an inflammatory response. Thus, even under inflammatory conditions induced by interferon (IFN)-γ or tumor necrosis factor (TNF)-α, endothelial cells do not produce neurotoxic tryptophan metabolites. More importantly endothelial cells metabolize the potentially harmful quinolinic acid and

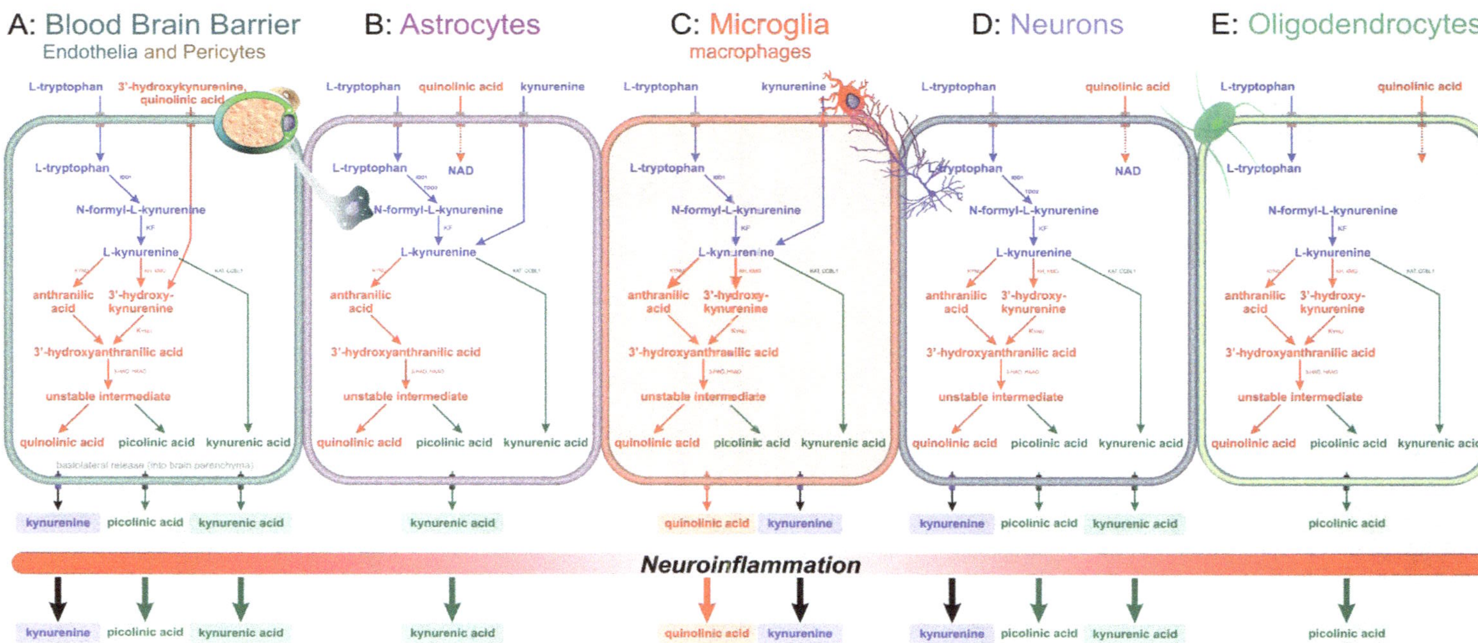

Figure 23.6 Metabolism of tryptophan within the brain depends on location. Changes in tryptophan metabolism result in a different pattern of metabolites that depend on the cellular site of metabolism. Microglia and macrophages are responsible in large part for the generation of the neurotoxic metabolite, quinolinic acid, within the brain using tryptophan or kynurenine as a substrate. Astrocytes, neurons, oligodendrocytes, endothelial cells, and pericytes produce a combination of neuroprotective tryptophan metabolites. These cells also inactivate quinolinic acid and 3-hydroxykynurenine by either conversion to NAD or to non-neurotoxic compounds, which constitutes an additional neuroprotective mechanism. All of the cells types respond to an inflammatory stimulus by increasing the production of tryptophan metabolites with relatively little change in the profile of released products. This balanced increase in tryptophan metabolites may be a hallmark of inflammation-dependent depression.

3-hydroxyanthranilic acid metabolites to either the neuroprotective kynurenic acid or the inactive metabolite kynurenine.

Pericytes (Figure 23.6A) produce primarily picolinic acid and kynurenine under identical conditions, but secrete elevated amounts of kynurenic acid and kynurenine when challenged simultaneously with both IFN-γand TNF-α. Thus, cells of the blood–brain barrier produce neuroprotective (kynurenic acid and picolinic acids) or neutral (kynurenine) metabolites, or they convert the neurotoxic quinolinic acid and its precursor, 3-hydroxyanthranilic acid, to neuroprotective metabolites. This activity buffers the brain from peripheral insults, and, indeed, the conversion of neurotoxic quinolinic acid and 3-hydroxyanthranilic acid to non-toxic or protective metabolites is increased following cytokine challenges. These data indicate that inflammatory responses stimulate cells of the blood–brain barrier to protect the brain.

Second-in-line within the CSN with access to circulating substrates are astrocytes (Figure 23.6B). It has been widely accepted that the major tryptophan metabolite produced by astrocytes is kynurenic acid. Astrocytes lack kynurenine 3′-hydroxylase (Guillemin *et al.*, 2001), thus limiting kynurenine conversion to quinolinic acid through 3-hydroxykynurenine. Under basal conditions human fetal astrocytes release primarily kynurenic acid and after challenge with IFN-γ release higher levels of kynurenic acid along with kynurenine (Guillemin *et al.*, 2001). It was suggested that this profile of metabolite release is neuroprotective, analogous to endothelial cells and pericytes, even under conditions associated with inflammation. This protective role was further supported by the uptake and metabolism of quinolinic acid by astrocytes to remove the neurotoxin from extracellular fluids (Guillemin *et al.*, 2001, 2005b). However, this protective environment is altered by the presence of microglia or macrophages. In the same study, macrophages were exposed to kynurenine at concentrations produced by astrocytes. Under these conditions, macrophages converted kynurenine to quinolinic acid and the rate of conversion was augmented by IFN-γ. Unlike astrocytes, microglia (Figure 23.6C) release quinolinic acid and this release is augmented by IFN-γ (Guillemin *et al.*, 2005a).

Microglia also release kynurenine. Upon stimulation with IFN-γ or LPS, microglia increase kynurenine production, which is an event that corresponds with the induction of IDO1 expression by microglia (Wang, Lawson, Kelley, and Dantzer, 2010). Thus, microglia, which are considered the primary immune cells of the brain, produce primarily the neurotoxic tryptophan metabolite quinolinic acid or the inactive kynurenine.

Oligodendrocytes (Figure 23.6D) are the only cell within the brain that do not express IDO1 or TDO2 (IDO2 expression unknown) and thus are unable to metabolize tryptophan to kynurenine. Oligodendrocytes, like astrocytes, do metabolize quinolinic acid, with the exception that picolinic acid is released instead of kynurenic acid, and this occurs in both the presence or absence of IFN-γ (Lim, Smythe, Stocker, Brew, and Guillemin, 2007). Thus, as would be expected, oligodendrocytes have a net neuroprotective role within the brain via the removal of quinolinic acid.

Neurons (Figure 23.6E), the workhorse of the brain and center of behavior, also have a unique role in the kynurenine pathway. Like astrocytes and oligodendrocytes, neurons take up quinolinic acid (Guillemin *et al.*, 2005b), even converting low levels of this neurotoxic chemical into NAD (Braidy, Grant, Adams, Brew, and Guillemin, 2009). Primary cultures of human neurons release the neuroprotective picolinic acid but not the neurotoxic quinolinic acid (Guillemin *et al.*, 2007). Stimulation of serotonergic neurons with IFN-γ has been shown to increase IDO1 expression (Roy, Takikawa, Kranz, Brown, and Thomas, 2005) without causing neuronal death (Hochstrasser, Ullrich, Sperner-Unterweger, and Humpel, 2011), suggesting that even under inflammatory conditions neurons to not release quinolinic acid at high enough concentrations to cause cell death (Guillemin *et al.*, 2005b).

In summary, each cell type within the brain has a unique role in the metabolism of tryptophan and its metabolites. An inflammatory stimulus does not appear to change the intracellular processing pattern within any type of cell, but accelerates the rate of metabolism through the kynurenine pathway. The effect of inflammation on neuronal function and behavior depends on the degree to which microglial neurotoxic products are released relative to the degree by which neuroprotective products are produced by all the other cell types. This general and balanced increase in tryptophan, or conversion to neurotoxic and neuroprotective metabolites, supports the increase in levels of central quinolinic acid, kynurenic acid, and kynurenine that have been reported in IFN-γ-challenged patients and the resulting increase in symptoms of depression (Raison *et al.*, 2010).

Dioxygenase Expression in the Brain

It is clear that a systemic inflammatory response results in an increase in circulating cytokines and alteration in circulating tryptophan metabolites. Human models of entodoxemia (Reichenberg *et al.*, 2001), IFN-γ therapy for hepatitis C (Raison *et al.*, 2010) and numerous animal models such as injection of LPS or BCG (O'Connor *et al.*, 2009c; Park *et al.*, 2011) support this statement. The inflammatory response initiated in the periphery is mirrored within the brain by increased central cytokine expression and a shift in the metabolism of tryptophan. Ensuing depression-like behaviors are a central event mediated by changes in neuronal function that is regulated by several tryptophan metabolites. The logical questions are: What is the effect of neuroinflammation on expression of the rate-limiting enzymes for the kynurenine pathway? and are these changes relevant to development of depression?

It has been widely accepted that induction of IDO1 within microglia is responsible for quinolinic acid generation and ensuing neurodegeneration. Several studies support this hypothesis and have shown that IDO1 is present in microglia and/or resident macrophages under inflammatory conditions such as Alzheimer's and experimental encephalomyelitis (Guillemin *et al.*, 2005a; Kwidzinski *et al.*, 2003, 2005). It should be noted that support for this hypothesis does not come from models of depression *per se*, but instead derives from models of inflammation-dependent neurodegeneration. Whether IDO1 is elevated in microglia of patients with depression but without co-morbid somatic diseases is not known. Preclinical animal models however support this hypothesis. Injection of LPS, via the intraperitoneal route, into mice induces depression-like behavior (Corona *et al.*, 2010; Henry *et al.*, 2008; Henry, Huang, Wynne, and Godbout, 2009). Microglia isolated from these mice have elevated IDO1 expression compared to controls, and this expression is associated with an elevated kynurenine:tryptophan ratio in the brain. Whether IDO1, IDO2 or TDO2 are also induced in other cell types or if brain extracellular fluid quinolinic acid or kynurenic acid are elevated in this model has yet to be defined. This model may only appropriately model human depression associated with an acute immune response such as the recent study of patients undergoing low-dose endotoxemia (Reichenberg *et al.*, 2001).

Chronic inflammation or neuroinflammation may have a different profile of dioxygenase expression. IDO1 is expressed primarily in the vascular endothelium of malaria-infected tissue (Hansen, Driussi, Turner, Takikawa, and Hunt, 2000), suggesting that chronic inflammation induces the production of kynurenic acid, kynurenine, and picolinic acid, but not quinolinic acid within the brain. Similarly, IDO1 is induced in mouse astrocytes following treatment with IFN-γ (Kwidzinski *et al.*, 2003). These treated cells would be induced to produce kynurenic acid and to increase conversion of extracellular quinolinic acid to kynurenic acid (Guillemin *et al.*, 2001; Guillemin *et al.*, 2005b). *In vitro*, IDO1 is induced specifically in neurons following treatment of dorsal raphe nucleus slice cultures with LPS, IFN-γ, TNF-α, or ß-amyloid$_{1\text{-}42}$. IDO1 was not induced within astrocytes or microglia, despite activation of glia by the inflammatory stimuli (Hochstrasser *et al.*, 2011). In this same study, IFN-γ did not induce neuronal death or microglial activation. These results lead to the possibility that inflammation-induced depression in humans (Raison *et al.*, 2010) is not a result of direct microglial activation or central quinolinic acid synthesis, and that elevated kynurenic acid in the brain of IFN-γ-treated patients derives from neurons, or astrocytes, via the induction of IDO1 within neurons of the mouse hippocampus by IFN-γ (Roy *et al.*, 2005).

Levels of TDO2 protein are elevated in brains of patients with major depression (Miller, Llenos, Dulay, and Weis, 2006). The elevation in TDO2 protein occurred in astrocytes which produce primarily kynurenic acid from tryptophan. In an animal trial of inflammation-induced depression, we recently reported that an intraperitoneal injection of LPS induced depression-like behavior as well as elevated steady-state mRNA expression of TDO2, IDO2 and IDO1 in the prefrontal cortex of mice (Park *et al.*, 2011b). Whether the increase in TDO2 occurred within neurons or astrocytes was not determined but, in either case, this would result primarily in kynurenic acid rather than quinolinic acid production. This study also established for the first time that elevation of all three dioxygenases is induced in an animal model of inflammation-induced depression. Thus, elevated TDO2 in the brain in major depression would protect neurons from the quinolinic acid produced by microglia.

Summary

Systemic inflammation results in elevated peripheral cytokine expression that is associated with an increase in the prevalence of depression. The systemic inflammatory response increases circulating quinolinic acid and kynurenine levels. Current dogma places considerable emphasis on these findings and suggests that elevated parenchymal quinolinic acid, acting via its neurotoxic pathway, may be responsible for depression. However, this neurotoxic tryptophan metabolite has limited if any access to the parenchyma of the brain from the circulation, and most cases of depression are not associated with neurotoxicity. An inflammatory response induces IDO1 in all cell types of the brain, including microglia, neurons and astrocytes, as well as TDO2 in the brain, with the net production of both neuroprotective, kynurenic acid, and neurotoxic, quinolinic acid, tryptophan metabolites within the parenchyma. Thus, inflammation results in an increase in parenchymal tryptophan metabolites produced by resident cells, possibly without a change in the neurotoxic index. This balanced increase in tryptophan metabolites may be a hallmark of inflammation-independent depression in the general population.

Conclusion and Future Direction

The long standing *Macrophage* and *5-HT Theories* of depression have provided valuable insight into the etiology of depression. In particular, pharmaceuticals have been developed largely with these hypotheses in mind, including the development of serotonin, dopamine, and norepinephrine reuptake inhibitors and the testing of anti-inflammatory agents. However, the newer *Kynurenine Theory* of depression has been gaining support based on independent evidence and the fact that it combines the two original theories into a specific plausible causative pathway. Recent data show that several classic antidepressants (fluoxetine, imipramine – SSRIs, and citalopram, amitriptyline – TCAs) directly alter the kynurenine pathway of rat astroglial cultures (Kocki *et al.*, 2011). These data suggest that existing antidepressant drugs, many of which have anti-inflammatory activity, may also act in part by regulating the kynurenine pathway and provide a clue to the future validation and acceptance of the *Kynurenine Theory.* Since inflammation-associated depression is a distinct clinical entity, characterized as a non-neurodegenerative mood disorder with alterations in tryptophan metabolism, developing pharmaceuticals that directly target the kynurenine pathway within the brain may provide a promising route for development of novel potent antidepressants.

Acknowledgements

This work is supported by National Institutes of Health grants RO1 MH083767 to RHM, RO1 AG029573 to KWK, RO1 NS073939 to AK, RD and KWK and RO1 NS074999 to AK.

References

Anderson, G. (2011). Neuronal–immune interactions in mediating stress effects in the etiology and course of schizophrenia: role of the amygdala in developmental co-ordination. *Medical Hypotheses*, 76(1), 54–60.

Anderson, G., and Rodriguez, M. (2011). Multiple sclerosis, seizures, and antiepileptics: role of IL-18, IDO, and melatonin. *European Journal of Neurology*, 18(5), 680–685.

Baran, H., Jellinger, K., and Deecke, L. (1999). Kynurenine metabolism in Alzheimer's disease. *Journal of Neural Transmission*, 106(2), 165–181.

Beagles, K. E., Morrison, P. F., and Heyes, M. P. (1998). Quinolinic acid in vivo synthesis rates, extracellular concentrations, and intercompartmental distributions in normal and immune-activated brain as determined by multiple-isotope microdialysis. *Journal of Neurochemistry*, 70(1), 281–291.

Beal, M. F., Matson, W. R., Swartz, K. J., Gamache, P. H., and Bird, E. D. (1990). Kynurenine pathway measurements in Huntington's disease striatum: evidence for reduced formation of kynurenic acid. *Journal of Neurochemistry*, 55(4), 1327–1339.

Blalock, J. E. (1984). The immune system as a sensory organ. *Journal of Immunology*, 132(3), 1067–1070.

Braidy, N., Grant, R., Adams, S., Brew, B. J., and Guillemin, G. J. (2009). Mechanism for quinolinic acid cytotoxicity in human astrocytes and neurons. *Neurotoxicity Research*, 16(1), 77–86.

Capuron, L., and Dantzer, R. (2003). Cytokines and depression: the need for a new paradigm. *Brain, Behavior, and Immunity*, 17 Suppl 1, S119–124.

Capuron, L., Gumnick, J. F., Musselman, D. L., Lawson, D. H., Reemsnyder, A., Nemeroff, C. B., and Miller, A. H. (2002). Neurobehavioral effects of interferon-alpha in cancer patients: phenomenology and paroxetine responsiveness of symptom dimensions. *Neuropsychopharmacology*, 26(5), 643–652.

Coppen, A. (1967). The biochemistry of affective disorders. *British Journal of Psychiatry*, 113(504), 1237–1264.

Corona, A. W., Huang, Y., O'Connor, J. C., Dantzer, R., Kelley, K. W., Popovich, P. G., and Godbout, J. P. (2010). Fractalkine receptor (CX3CR1) deficiency sensitizes mice to the behavioral changes induced by lipopolysaccharide. *Journal of Neuroinflammation*, 7, 93.

Dantzer, R., O'Connor, J. C., Freund, G. G., Johnson, R. W., and Kelley, K. W. (2008). From inflammation to sickness and depression: when the immune system subjugates the brain. *Nature Reviews Neuroscience*, 9(1), 46–56.

Evans, D. L., Charney, D. S., Lewis, L., Golden, R. N., Gorman, J. M., Krishnan, K. R., . . . Valvo, W. J. (2005). Mood disorders in the medically ill: scientific review and recommendations. *Biological Psychiatry*, 58(3), 175–189.

Felger, J. C., Alagbe, O., Hu, F., Mook, D., Freeman, A. A., Sanchez, M. M., . . . Miller, A. H. (2007). Effects of interferon-alpha on rhesus monkeys: a nonhuman primate model of cytokine-induced depression. *Biological Psychiatry*, 62(11), 1324–1333.

Fukui, S., Schwarcz, R., Rapoport, S. I., Takada, Y., and Smith, Q. R. (1991). Blood–brain barrier transport of kynurenines: implications for brain synthesis and metabolism. *Journal of Neurochemistry*, 56(6), 2007–2017.

Guidetti, P., Luthi-Carter, R. E., Augood, S. J., and Schwarcz, R. (2004). Neostriatal and cortical quinolinate levels are increased in early grade Huntington's disease. *Neurobiology of Disease*, 17(3), 455–461.

Guillemin, G. J., Brew, B. J., Noonan, C. E., Takikawa, O., and Cullen, K. M. (2005a). Indoleamine 2,3 dioxygenase and quinolinic acid immunoreactivity in Alzheimer's disease hippocampus. *Neuropathology and Applied Neurobiology*, 31(4), 395–404.

Guillemin, G. J., Cullen, K. M., Lim, C. K., Smythe, G. A., Garner, B., Kapoor, V., . . . Brew, B. J. (2007). Characterization of the kynurenine pathway in human neurons. *Journal of Neuroscience*, 27(47), 12884–12892.

Guillemin, G. J., Kerr, S. J., Smythe, G. A., Smith, D. G., Kapoor, V., Armati, P. J., . . . Brew, B. J. (2001). Kynurenine pathway metabolism in human astrocytes: a paradox for neuronal protection. *Journal of Neurochemistry*, 78(4), 842–853.

Guillemin, G. J., Smith, D. G., Kerr, S. J., Smythe, G. A., Kapoor, V., Armati, P. J., and Brew, B. J. (2000). Characterisation of kynurenine pathway metabolism in human astrocytes and implications in neuropathogenesis. *Redox Report*, 5(2–3), 108–111.

Guillemin, G. J., Smythe, G., Takikawa, O., and Brew, B. J. (2005b). Expression of indoleamine 2,3-dioxygenase and production of quinolinic acid by human microglia, astrocytes, and neurons. *Glia*, 49(1), 15–23.

Hansen, A. M., Driussi, C., Turner, V., Takikawa, O., and Hunt, N. H. (2000). Tissue distribution of indoleamine 2,3-dioxygenase in normal and malaria-infected tissue. *Redox Report*, 5(2–3), 112–115.

Henry, C. J., Huang, Y., Wynne, A., Hanke, M., Himler, J., Bailey, M. T., . . . Godbout, J. P. (2008). Minocycline attenuates lipopolysaccharide (LPS)-induced neuroinflammation, sickness behavior, and anhedonia. *Journal of Neuroinflammation*, 5, 15.

Henry, C. J., Huang, Y., Wynne, A. M., and Godbout, J. P. (2009). Peripheral lipopolysaccharide (LPS) challenge promotes microglial hyperactivity in aged mice that is associated with exaggerated induction of both pro-inflammatory IL-1beta and anti-inflammatory IL-10 cytokines. *Brain, Behavior, and Immunity*, 23(3), 309–317.

Heyes, M. P., Saito, K., Crowley, J. S., Davis, L. E., Demitrack, M. A., Der, M., . . . et al. (1992). Quinolinic acid and kynurenine pathway metabolism in inflammatory and non-inflammatory neurological disease. *Brain*, 115 (Pt 5), 1249–1273.

Hilmas, C., Pereira, E. F., Alkondon, M., Rassoulpour, A., Schwarcz, R., and Albuquerque, E. X. (2001). The brain metabolite kynurenic acid inhibits alpha7 nicotinic receptor activity and increases non-alpha7 nicotinic receptor expression: physiopathological implications. *Journal of Neuroscience*, 21(19), 7463–7473.

Hochstrasser, T., Ullrich, C., Sperner-Unterweger, B., and Humpel, C. (2011). Inflammatory stimuli reduce survival of serotonergic neurons and induce neuronal expression of indoleamine 2,3-dioxygenase in rat dorsal raphe nucleus organotypic brain slices. *Neuroscience*, 184, 128–138.

Jauch, D., Urbanska, E. M., Guidetti, P., Bird, E. D., Vonsattel, J. P., Whetsell, W. O., Jr., and Schwarcz, R. (1995). Dysfunction of brain kynurenic acid metabolism in Huntington's disease: focus on kynurenine aminotransferases. *Journal of Neurological Science*, 130(1), 39–47.

Jhamandas, K. H., Boegman, R. J., Beninger, R. J., Miranda, A. F., and Lipic, K. A. (2000). Excitotoxicity of quinolinic acid: modulation by endogenous antagonists. *Neurotoxicity Research*, 2(2–3), 139–155.

Kalisch, B. E., Jhamandas, K., Boegman, R. J., and Beninger, R. J. (1994). Picolinic acid protects against quinolinic acid-induced depletion of NADPH diaphorase containing neurons in the rat striatum. *Brain Research*, 668(1–2), 1–8.

Kocki, T., Wnuk, S., Kloc, R., Kocki, J., Owe-Larsson, B., and Urbanska, E. M. (2011). New insight into the antidepressants action: modulation of kynurenine pathway by increasing the kynurenic acid/3-hydroxykynurenine ratio. *Journal of Neural Transmission*, 119(2), 235–243.

Kwidzinski, E., Bunse, J., Aktas, O., Richter, D., Mutlu, L., Zipp, F., . . . Bechmann, I. (2005). Indolamine 2,3-dioxygenase is expressed in the CNS and down-regulates autoimmune inflammation. *FASEB Journal*, 19(10), 1347–1349.

Kwidzinski, E., Bunse, J., Kovac, A. D., Ullrich, O., Zipp, F., Nitsch, R., and Bechmann, I. (2003). IDO (indolamine 2,3-dioxygenase) expression and function in the CNS. *Adv Exp Med Biol*, 527, 113–118.

Lepine, J. P., and Briley, M. (2011). The increasing burden of depression. *Neuropsychiatric Disease and Treatment*, 7(Suppl 1), 3–7.

Liimatainen, S., Lehtimaki, K., Raitala, A., Peltola, M., Oja, S. S., Peltola, J., and Hurme, M. A. (2011). Increased indoleamine 2,3-dioxygenase (IDO) activity in idiopathic generalized epilepsy. *Epilepsy Research*, 94, 206–212

Lim, C. K., Smythe, G. A., Stocker, R., Brew, B. J., and Guillemin, G. J. (2007). Characterization of the kynurenine pathway in human oligodendrocytes. *International Congress Series*, 1304, 213–217.

Maes, M., Leonard, B. E., Myint, A. M., Kubera, M., and Verkerk, R. (2011). The new '5-HT' hypothesis of depression: cell-mediated immune activation induces indoleamine 2,3-dioxygenase, which leads to lower plasma tryptophan and an increased synthesis of detrimental tryptophan catabolites (TRYCATs), both of which contribute to the onset of depression. *Progress in Neuropsychopharmacology and Biological Psychiatry*, 35(3), 702–721.

Metz, R., Duhadaway, J. B., Kamasani, U., Laury-Kleintop, L., Muller, A. J., and Prendergast, G. C. (2007). Novel tryptophan catabolic enzyme IDO2 is the preferred biochemical target of the antitumor indoleamine 2,3-dioxygenase inhibitory compound D-1-methyl-tryptophan. *Cancer Research*, 67(15), 7082–7087.

Miller, C. L., Llenos, I. C., Dulay, J. R., Barillo, M. M., Yolken, R. H., and Weis, S. (2004). Expression of the kynurenine pathway enzyme tryptophan 2,3–dioxygenase is increased in the frontal cortex of individuals with schizophrenia. *Neurobiology of Disease*, 15(3), 618–629.

Miller, C. L., Llenos, I. C., Dulay, J. R., and Weis, S. (2006). Upregulation of the initiating step of the kynurenine pathway in postmortem anterior cingulate cortex from individuals with schizophrenia and bipolar disorder. *Brain Research*, 1073–1074, 25–37.

Moreau, M., Lestage, J., Verrier, D., Mormede, C., Kelley, K. W., Dantzer, R., and Castanon, N. (2005). Bacille Calmette–Guerin inoculation induces chronic activation of peripheral and brain indoleamine 2,3-dioxygenase in mice. *Journal of Infectious Diseases*, 192(3), 537–544.

Myint, A. M., Kim, Y. K., Verkerk, R., Scharpe, S., Steinbusch, H., and Leonard, B. (2007). Kynurenine pathway in major depression: evidence of impaired neuroprotection. *Journal of Affective Disorders*, 98(1–2), 143–151.

Nemeth, H., Toldi, J., and Vecsei, L. (2005). Role of kynurenines in the central and peripheral nervous systems. *Current Neurovascular Research*, 2(3), 249–260.

O'Connor, J. C., Andre, C., Wang, Y., Lawson, M. A., Szegedi, S. S., Lestage, J., . . . Dantzer, R. (2009). Interferon-gamma and tumor necrosis factor-alpha mediate the upregulation of indoleamine 2,3-dioxygenase and the induction of depressive-like behavior in mice in response to bacillus Calmette–Guerin. *Journal of Neuroscience*, 29(13), 4200–4209.

O'Connor, J. C., Lawson, M. A., Andre, C., Briley, E. M., Szegedi, S. S., Lestage, J., . . . Kelley, K. W. (2009). Induction of IDO by bacille Calmette–Guerin is responsible for development of murine depressive-like behavior. *Journal of Immunology*, 182(5), 3202–3212.

O'Connor, J. C., Lawson, M. A., Andre, C., Moreau, M., Lestage, J., Castanon, N.,...Dantzer, R. (2009). Lipopolysaccharide-induced depressive-like behavior is mediated by indoleamine 2,3-dioxygenase activation in mice. *Molecular Psychiatry*, 14(5), 511–522.

Ogawa, T., Matson, W. R., Beal, M. F., Myers, R. H., Bird, E. D., Milbury, P., and Saso, S. (1992). Kynurenine pathway abnormalities in Parkinson's disease. *Neurology*, 42(9), 1702–1706.

Ohira, K., Hagihara, H., Toyama, K., Takao, K., Kanai, M., Funakoshi, H.,...Miyakawa, T. (2010). Expression of tryptophan 2,3-dioxygenase in mature granule cells of the adult mouse dentate gyrus. *Molecular Brain*, 3(1), 26.

Owe-Young, R., Webster, N. L., Mukhtar, M., Pomerantz, R. J., Smythe, G., Walker, D.,...Brew, B. J. (2008). Kynurenine pathway metabolism in human blood–brain-barrier cells: implications for immune tolerance and neurotoxicity. *Journal of Neurochemistry*, 105(4), 1346–1357.

Park, S. E., Dantzer, R., Kelley, K. W., and McCusker, R. H. (2011). Central administration of insulin-like growth factor-I decreases depressive-like behavior and brain cytokine expression in mice. *Journal of Neuroinflammation*, 8, 12.

Park, S. E., Lawson, M. A., Dantzer, R., Kelley, K. W., and McCusker, R.H. (2011). Insulin-like growth factor-I peptides act centrally to decrease depression-like behavior of mice treated intraperitoneally with lipopolysaccharide. *Journal of Neuroinflammation*, 8 179.

Perkins, M. N., and Stone, T. W. (1982). An iontophoretic investigation of the actions of convulsant kynurenines and their interaction with the endogenous excitant quinolinic acid. *Brain Research*, 247(1), 184–187.

Pocivavsek, A., Wu, H. Q., Potter, M. C., Elmer, G. I., Pellicciari, R., and Schwarcz, R. (2011). Fluctuations in endogenous kynurenic Acid control hippocampal glutamate and memory. *Neuropsychopharmacology*, 36(11), 2357–2367.

Raison, C. L., Dantzer, R., Kelley, K. W., Lawson, M. A., Woolwine, B. J., Vogt, G.,...Miller, A. H. (2010). CSF concentrations of brain tryptophan and kynurenines during immune stimulation with IFN-alpha: relationship to CNS immune responses and depression. *Molecular Psychiatry*, 15(4), 393–403.

Reichenberg, A., Yirmiya, R., Schuld, A., Kraus, T., Haack, M., Morag, A., and Pollmacher, T. (2001). Cytokine-associated emotional and cognitive disturbances in humans. *Archives of General Psychiatry*, 58(5), 445–452.

Roy, E. J., Takikawa, O., Kranz, D. M., Brown, A. R., and Thomas, D. L. (2005). Neuronal localization of indoleamine 2,3-dioxygenase in mice. *Neuroscience Letters*, 387(2), 95–99.

Schwarcz, R., Speciale, C., and French, E. D. (1987). Hippocampal kynurenines as etiological factors in seizure disorders. *Polish Journal of Pharmacology and Pharmacy*, 39(5), 485–494.

Schwarcz, R., Speciale, C., Okuno, E., French, E. D., and Kohler, C. (1986). Quinolinic acid: a pathogen in seizure disorders? *Advances in Experimental Medicine and Biology*, 203, 697–707.

Simones, T., and Shepherd, D. M. (2011). Consequences of AhR activation in steady-state dendritic cells. *Toxicological Sciences*, 119(2), 293–307.

Smith, R. S. (1991). The macrophage theory of depression. *Medical Hypotheses*, 35(4), 298–306.

Stone, T. W., and Perkins, M. N. (1981). Quinolinic acid: a potent endogenous excitant at amino acid receptors in CNS. *European Journal of Pharmacology*, 72(4), 411–412.

Wang, Y., Lawson, M. A., Kelley, K. W., and Dantzer, R. (2010). Primary murine microglia are resistant to nitric oxide inhibition of indoleamine 2,3-dioxygenase. *Brain, Behavior, and Immunity*, 24(8), 1249–1253.

Wonodi, I., and Schwarcz, R. (2010). Cortical kynurenine pathway metabolism: a novel target for cognitive enhancement in Schizophrenia. *Schizophrenia Bulletin*, 36(2), 211–218.

Wu, H. Q., Rassoulpour, A., and Schwarcz, R. (2007). Kynurenic acid leads, dopamine follows: a new case of volume transmission in the brain? *Journal of Neural Transmission*, 114(1), 33–41.

24

An Inflammatory Perspective of Stress and Human Depressive Disorder

Marie-Claude Audet, Shlomit Jacobson-Pick, Robyn J. McQuaid, and Hymie Anisman

Department of Neuroscience, Carleton University, Ottawa, Ontario, Canada

Monoamines, such as serotonin and norepinephrine, have historically been implicated as mediators of major depressive disorder. Although several lines of evidence have supported this perspective, there has been increasing attention devoted to the analysis of other processes that might contribute to this illness. To a significant extent this has come about because of the moderate success achieved in resolving depressive symptoms using pharmacological treatments that target monoamines. Specifically, the available antidepressants appear to have a positive effect in only 50–60% of patients, symptom amelioration is often incomplete, and relapse rates exceed 50% over a 5-year period (Moncrieff and Kirsch, 2005). Furthermore, simply increasing serotonin or norepinephrine availability does not immediately attenuate symptoms of the disorder, as the therapeutic effects of antidepressants are usually observed only after 2–3 weeks of treatment. To be sure, the effectiveness of antidepressant medication can be improved through strategies that involve multiple targets (Millan, 2006), but this in itself speaks to the limited contribution of monoamines in the promotion of major depression.

Several alternative propositions have been offered regarding the neurochemical processes supporting depressive illness. These have included the potential involvement of corticotropin-releasing hormone (CRH), arginine vasopressin (AVP), glucocorticoids, and gamma-aminobutyric acid (GABA), as well as brain-derived neurotrophic factor (BDNF) and nerve growth factor (NGF) functioning (reviewed in Anisman, Merali, and Hayley, 2008). In addition, there have been numerous reports implicating activation of the inflammatory immune system in the pathogenesis of depressive disorders. Among other things, elevated concentrations of peripheral and of mitogen-stimulated pro-inflammatory cytokines were reported in depressed patients (Maes, 1995). Likewise, depressive symptoms were described in patients suffering from chronic illnesses or acute pathological conditions associated with elevated peripheral inflammation (Cremeans-Smith *et al.*, 2009; Musselman *et al.*, 2001). Treatments that influence immune functioning in humans, such as vaccines (e.g., for typhoid) or immunotherapy using the pro-inflammatory cytokine interferon (IFN)-α in patients suffering from chronic hepatitis C or certain types of cancers (e.g., malignant melanoma), were also reported to promote the development and exacerbation of depressive symptoms (Capuron and Miller, 2004; Harrison *et al.*, 2009).

The Wiley-Blackwell Handbook of Psychoneuroimmunology, First Edition. Edited by Alexander W. Kusnecov and Hymie Anisman.

As impressive as the data have been linking cytokine functioning to depressive illness, the processes by which this comes about remain to be fully established. For instance, it is uncertain whether a single cytokine is of particular relevance in regard to the provocation of depression, or whether symptoms (or clusters of symptoms) evolve owing to multiple cytokine actions. Moreover, it is unsure to what extent depressive symptoms elicited by peripheral inflammatory activation (e.g., through cytokine immunotherapy) reflect a genuine depressive disorder or are actually a reflection of a more general syndrome that includes behavioral manifestations reminiscent of depression (e.g., neurovegetative features such as fatigue, malaise). Finally, the relative contributions of peripheral and central inflammation in the etiology of depressive symptoms remain to be determined.

To further complicate the issue, associations between inflammation and depression may be related to or moderated by the effects of stressors on peripheral and central processes, including cytokine functioning. Indeed, stressful events elicit several neurochemical changes congruent with those associated with inflammatory challenges, including elevated cytokine variations in blood and brain. Thus, it is possible that depression evolves as a result of the interactive biological changes elicited by stressors and inflammation (Anisman, Merali, and Hayley, 2008).

The current chapter will discuss the contributions of inflammatory activation, particularly that of pro-inflammatory cytokines, in depressive illness and the specific role of stressors may have in this regard. In so doing, we will necessarily consider the various approaches used to link cytokine functioning and depressive illness. As well, beyond assessing the influence of peripheral cytokine variations in the provocation of depression, we will consider the cytokine changes that occur in specific areas of the brain that might also contribute to the illness (including central cytokine variations secondary to an inflammatory challenge). Of course, changes that occur in the brain cannot be assessed in human depressed populations (other than in postmortem tissue of individuals that died by suicide relative to non-suicidal controls) and thus, most of the studies on brain cytokine changes in relation to depression and/or stressors will be based on animal models of the pathology.

Elevated Inflammation in Individuals with Depressive Disorders

The suggestion that pro-inflammatory cytokines might be related to depressive illness was supported by several reports indicating that elevated circulating levels of interleukin (IL)-6 and tumor necrosis factor (TNF)-α were evident in patients with major depression, especially melancholic depression (Maes, 1995). In contrast, relations between IL-1β elevations and depressive illness were less consistently demonstrated (Dowlati *et al.*, 2010; Liu, Ho, and Mak, 2011), possibly because of the difficulty in detecting the very low levels of circulating IL-1β in humans. Based on a meta-analysis, Liu, Ho, and Mak (2011) established that circulating levels of IL-6, TNF-α, and soluble IL-2 receptor were significantly higher in depressed patients than in healthy controls, whereas those for IL-1β, IFN-γ, IL-2, IL-8, and and the antiinflammatory cytokines IL-4 and IL-10 did not differ. Unfortunately, in their analysis severity of depressive symptoms was not taken into account, a factor that was shown to be fundamental for the cytokine differences to be evident (Maes, 1995). Indeed, positive associations between depression and blood elevations of IL-6 and the endogenous antagonist IL-1ra were more pronounced among clinically depressed patients (i.e., clinical populations diagnosed with major depression) than among community-based individuals presenting with depressive symptoms, possibly reflecting stronger cytokine–depression associations in more severely depressed individuals (Howren, Lamkin, and Suls, 2009).

Consistent with a role for pro-inflammatory cytokines in major depression, resolution of depressive episodes after antidepressant treatment was associated with the normalization of circulating cytokine elevations (Maes, 2011). A meta-analysis indicated that treatment with selective serotonin reuptake inhibitors (SSRIs) was associated with a reduction of IL-6 and IL-1β and to a lesser extent, TNF-α levels normalized after treatment as well (Hannestad, dellaGioia, and Bloch, 2011a). Interestingly, depressed patients resistant to SSRI treatment produced more IL-6 and TNF-α compared to currently euthymic patients that had formerly been SSRI-resistant or to normal controls, suggesting that suppression of these specific cytokines might be necessary for clinical recovery (O'Brien *et al.*, 2007). Similarly, elevated levels of IL-6 and TNF-α that were present prior to antidepressant medication normalized only among those patients who displayed a positive response to the treatment (Lanquillon *et al.*, 2000; Yoshimura *et al.*, 2009).

Although these studies revealed a connection between depressive illness and pro-inflammatory cytokine elevations, even though not necessarily a causal one, several reports indicated that despite showing clinical improvement circulating cytokine levels were unchanged in depressed patients treated with antidepressant medication. For example, administration of bupropion (a norepinephrine–dopamine reuptake inhibitor) in the treatment of SSRI-resistant depressed patients diminished depressive symptoms, but without changes of peripheral TNF-α levels (Eller *et al.*, 2009). Likewise, higher basal production of IL-1β in dysthymic patients was not normalized by SSRI treatment, even though depressive symptoms were attenuated (Anisman *et al.*, 1999). In the meta-analysis described earlier (Hannestad, DellaGioia, and Bloch, 2011a), it was established that although the severity of depressive symptoms was attenuated by 50–60%, antidepressants in general (without differentiation by class of medication) did not influence TNF-α levels and had exceptionally small effects on IL-6. In fact, it was only when stratified subgroup analyses were performed based on the class of antidepressant administered that more significant effects on peripheral cytokines emerged. As mentioned earlier, when SSRIs were specifically considered in this meta-analysis, treatment was associated with a modest reduction of IL-6 levels, and possibly of TNF-α. In addition, few studies in this meta-analysis included IL-1β, likely owing to measurement problems; however, of the six studies that did assess IL-1β changes, five were performed with depressed patients treated with SSRIs, thus precluding comparisons between particular drug classes in modifying IL-1β levels (Hannestad, DellaGioia, and Bloch, 2011a).

Considering that individuals with major depression frequently display elevated levels of IL-6 and TNF-α (and less often IL-1β) and that these cytokine elevations are not systematically attenuated by antidepressants, despite their clinical efficacy, the fundamental question that needs to be addressed concerns the specific contribution of circulating pro-inflammatory cytokines in mediating depressive symptoms. That is, are these cytokines peripheral markers or trait characteristics of depressive illness, are they indicative of those individuals who are at risk for depression, or are they informative of an ongoing biological dysfunction that signifies which individuals will be most prone to relapse following successful therapy? Ultimately, it will also be necessary to assess the effects of more protracted antidepressant treatments on cytokine variations (especially as many investigators have concluded that depressive illness may be a lifelong disorder), as well as whether the cytokine response to antidepressant treatments predicts illness recurrence, particularly in the presence of contextual factors (e.g., distressing events) that have been linked to depression.

Most studies that assessed the link between circulating cytokines and depression, as well as the effects of antidepressants in moderating this relationship, have considered depression from a broad perspective (i.e., overall depression levels), rather than one that focused on specific symptoms. Likewise, although participants in some studies were classified as being major depressive or melancholic, among major depressive patients it was usually unclear in most studies whether they presented with typical or atypical symptoms. Typical and atypical depression can be distinguished from one another on the basis of neurovegetative features that are present (reduced appetite, weight, and sleep being evident in typical depression, whereas increased appetite/eating, weight and sleep characterizes atypical depression). As cytokines may influence these neurovegetative characteristics, it might be especially important to distinguish subtypes of depression from one another. The fact that this was rarely done might have contributed to the inconsistencies regarding cytokine variations reported in depressed patients and, to some extent, to the incompatibilities between clinical efficacy of antidepressants and cytokine normalization.

It has been suggested that particular biological markers (e.g., neuroendocrine, neurochemical) could distinguish between subtypes of depressive syndromes (Gibb *et al.*, 2009). For instance, among individuals with typical features of major depression, hypothalamic-pituitary-adrenal (HPA) axis and sympathetic nervous system activity may be stimulated, whereas in individuals with atypical depression, activity of the HPA axis and sympathetic nervous system might be attenuated (Gold and Chrousos, 2002). In relation to peripheral cytokine activation, it was reported that dysthymic patients (which comprises low grade depression of two years or more), but not those with major depression, displayed higher mitogen-stimulated production of IL-1β than healthy controls and that this was related to the duration of illness (Anisman *et al.*, 1999). Unlike IL-1β, levels of IL-6 and BDNF were comparably elevated in major depressive and dysthymic patients (Yoshimura *et al.*, 2010). This might suggest that IL-1β is associated with specific features of depression, whereas IL-6 and BDNF might represent more general biomarkers of depressive illnesses. Whether links exist between other cytokines and specific features of the illness remains to be determined.

Although suicidality may be associated with several psychological disturbances, and in the case of depression is not uniformly related to illness severity, suicide attempts in depressed patients have also been associated with cytokine variations, in some instances being greater than in individuals with major depression but without history of suicidal ideation. Plasma concentrations of IL-6 and TNF-α were higher and IL-2 levels were lower in suicide attempters, compared to either depressed individuals that did not attempt suicide or to healthy controls (Janelidze *et al.*, 2011). Likewise, elevated IL-6 levels were found in the cerebrospinal fluid of suicidal patients; interestingly, the extent of cytokine elevations was related to depression severity and was also found to be higher in patients that made efforts of violent suicide (Lindqvist *et al.*, 2009). However, it was also reported that mitogen-provoked production of IL-6 was greater in non-suicidal depressed patients compared to those with major depression that were suicidal and healthy controls (Kim *et al.*, 2008). The source for these different outcomes is not certain, but could be related to differences of the cytokine measures (i.e., circulating levels versus mitogen-stimulated production of cytokines) or to characteristics of the patients (presence or absence of aggressive or violent tendencies).

As informative as plasma cytokine levels might be, ultimately depressive behaviors are more likely to involve brain cytokine functioning or effects secondary to the altered brain cytokine changes, including variations of neurotransmitters, peptides, or growth factors. Moreover, it is uncertain what the plasma cytokine variations might actually reflect in relation to depression, although indices of inflammation might represent biomarkers of depressive illness, as suggested earlier. For obvious reasons, there have been very few studies concerning brain cytokine variations associated with depressive illness. Nevertheless, it was reported that mRNA expression of IL-4 (in women) and IL-13 (in men) was elevated in postmortem orbitofrontal cortex of individuals that died by suicide relative to those that died suddenly of causes unrelated to suicide, whereas no differences were evident with respect to IL-1β, TNF-α, or IL-6 (Tonelli *et al.*, 2008). More recently, it was reported that among teenaged individuals that died by suicide, mRNA and protein expression levels of IL-1β, IL-6, and TNF-α were increased in Brodmann area 10 (corresponding to frontopolar cortex) relative to normal controls (Pandey *et al.*, 2011). However, in these reports, not all individuals that died by suicide had been diagnosed with major depression. Although suicidal thoughts or ideations may be a symptom of major depression, actual suicide attempts are not necessarily reflective of depressive illness. Acting out in suicidal individuals might also be indicative of additional factors, such as impulsivity and extreme or violent behaviors, which themselves can contribute to neurochemical variations. In addition, the act of suicide itself could potentially elicit biological changes. Thus, inflammatory variations in individuals who have attempted suicide or have died by suicide, whether they were depressed or not, might also result from characteristic traits (impulsivity) or from emotional or physical impacts of acting out, or even with respect to how death occurred, rather than being uniquely associated with depression (see Anisman, 2009).

In sum, although elevated peripheral inflammation has consistently been associated with depression in both clinical populations and community-based individuals, it seems that a definite picture of cytokine variations in depressive disorders has yet to emerge and it remains uncertain how peripheral cytokine changes are translated into depressive states. It has been suggested that cytokines, along with growth factors, hormones, metabolic and neurotransmitters, might serve as biomarkers or endophenotypes for depression (Gibb *et al.*, 2009). In this regard, it will be useful to identify how specific cytokine markers might align with particular symptoms of depression. Moreover, beyond peripheral variations of cytokines, an important issue that will need to be considered is the implication of central inflammatory changes in the etiology of major depression.

In recent years, there has been an increased push for individualized treatment of depressed patients, coupled with a growing acknowledgement that there has been limited success in defining the genetic and biological complements that are associated with this illness. This has led, among other things, to the view that analyses of major depressive disorder might not be well served by considering it as a syndrome or a phenotype, particularly as depressive symptoms may vary widely across depressed individuals, as do the efficacy of pharmacological treatment strategies. As an alternative, it was suggested that the research approach should instead be one that focuses on the endophenotypes that make up the disorder (i.e., focusing on specific symptoms of the illness in relation to specific neurochemical processes and potential genetic polymorphisms) (e.g., Hasler et al., 2004). Endophenotypic analyses likely represents a highly effective and valid approach, but it has also been suggested that this could turn out to be exceptionally difficult, particularly as the constellation of symptoms and neurochemical characteristics associated with depressive illness might involve complex neurochemical (and receptor) interactions across multiple brain regions. Thus, even assuming a best case scenario, a huge number of participants would be needed, involving multiple centers following identical protocols, and considering not only symptoms of illness, but other experiential factors (e.g., early-life neglect or abuse) that might feed into the evolution of depressive illness. This said, the inclusion of immune system markers in such an effort would be highly advantageous.

Co-morbidities Between Depression and Inflammatory Conditions

Support for a role for peripheral inflammation in depression has also come from the high prevalence of depressive episodes in patients suffering from chronic inflammatory illnesses as well as in individuals recovering from acute inflammatory insults associated with surgery or stroke. Indeed, elevated circulating levels of pro-inflammatory cytokines associated with chronic physical illnesses have been related to depressive symptoms, raising the possibility that cytokine elevations might be a common factor for these pathologies (Anisman, Merali, and Hayley, 2008). Higher plasma concentrations of TNF-α were reported in non-medicated hepatitis C patients compared to non-infected individuals, and these TNF-α elevations were associated with severity of depressive symptoms (Loftis *et al.*, 2008). Elevated TNF-α levels in patients with Parkinson's disease were also correlated with greater cognitive problems and more severe depression (Menza *et al.*, 2010). Likewise, depressed cancer patients displayed higher plasma concentrations of IL-6 relative to cancer patients that were not depressed, or depressed patients who were cancer-free (Musselman *et al.*, 2001). Even if depressive episodes in these chronically ill patients arose from nonspecific factors, such as general malaise or emotional distress, it is also possible that persistent activation of inflammatory processes might contribute to the co-morbid depression, although emotional distress associated with ongoing physical illnesses could contribute to inflammation as well as to the clinical conditions (Anisman, Merali, and Hayley, 2008; Gibb *et al.*, 2009).

As in the case of chronic inflammatory illnesses, depression has frequently been observed after acute inflammation resulting from peripheral or central insults, including surgery and stroke. Elevated IL-6 levels measured early following total knee replacement surgeries were reported to predict higher prevalence of subsequent depressive symptoms (Cremeans-Smith *et al.*, 2009). Likewise, following a central damage in the form of stroke, serum IL-18 levels, but not that of IL-6 and TNF-α, were higher in patients that later developed depression (Yang *et al.*, 2010). In addition, risk of depression following stroke was elevated among individuals who carried alleles associated with reduced anti-inflammatory cytokine function (IL-4 and IL-10), whereas no such association was found with respect to pro-inflammatory cytokines (Kim *et al.*, 2011). It is interesting that cytokine changes related to poststroke depression (e.g., IL-18) appeared to differ from the cytokine variations ordinarily observed in patients with major depression unrelated to stroke (IL-6, TNF-α), suggesting that these forms of depression might actually involve different processes.

The occurrence of depression following stroke has been suggested to predict a poor prognosis for functional recovery and future global functioning (Bilge *et al.*, 2008). Moreover, early depressive symptoms after stroke were associated with the maintenance of poststroke depression as well as with increased mortality over the ensuing 1–2 years (Kouwenhoven *et al.*, 2011). As elevated peripheral inflammation following stroke has been related to later development of depression, it is possible that specific cytokines could mediate functional recuperation and constitute a clinical marker of later functional recovery, later incidence of stroke, persistence of depression, and mortality. In fact, plasma concentrations of IL-6 collected within 24 hours after acute ischemic stroke predicted mortality at 12 months (although in this study depressive symptoms were not evaluated) (Shenhar-Tsarfaty *et al.*, 2010). It has, indeed, been suggested that the identification of the cytokine sequelae of ischemic stroke might be instrumental in the development of novel targets to treat stroke or limit the downstream consequences that typically are associated with stroke (Thompson and Hakim, 2005).

Influence of Immune Challenges on Human Depressive and Cognitive Behaviors

Associations between circulating levels of pro-inflammatory cytokines and depressive disorders have provided valuable information concerning the implications of peripheral inflammation in relation to depressive illness. It should be considered, however, that these associations are correlational, thus precluding causal conclusions regarding the cytokine–depression relationship. Causal links between peripheral inflammation and depressive states have, however, been supported by reports showing that triggering an inflammatory response using immunogenic agents, such as vaccines (e.g., typhoid) or bacterial endotoxins (e.g., lipopolysaccharide: LPS), elicited depressive-like mood changes concomitant with pro-inflammatory cytokines changes. For example, plasma IL-6 elevations induced by typhoid vaccination were accompanied by depressed mood as well as fatigue, confusion and impaired concentration (Harrison *et al.*, 2009). Interestingly, the relationship between cytokine and depressed mood was related to increased activity within the subgenual anterior cingulate cortex (a brain region implicated in depression), and to reduced functional connectivity of this region to the amygdala, medial prefrontal cortex and nucleus accumbens (Harrison *et al.*, 2009). Increased plasma TNF-α, IL-6, and IL-1ra levels elicited by a low dose of the endotoxin *Salmonella abortus equi* (which did not affect physical symptoms of sickness, blood pressure or heart rate) were also positively correlated with anxiety and depression as well as with memory impairments (Reichenberg *et al.*, 2001). Moreover, mild depressive-like symptoms (e.g., lassitude, social anhedonia), paralleling IL-6 and TNF-α elevations induced by the endotoxin LPS, were limited in individuals that had initially been treated with the SSRI citalopram (Hannestad *et al.*, 2011b). However, peripheral cytokine effects elicited by LPS were not changed in citalopram-treated individuals, suggesting that elevated pro-inflammatory markers, although being associated with depressive-like manifestations, might not be direct modulators of neuroaffective states, or at least not the only ones that acted in this capacity (Hannestad *et al.*, 2011b).

Depressive Episodes elicited by IFN-α immunotherapy in Hepatitis C and Cancer Patients

In addition to reports of depressive mood and cognitive impairments elicited by vaccine or endotoxin challenges, causal involvement of pro-inflammatory cytokines in the pathogenesis of depression has largely been supported by studies on the neuropsychiatric effects elicited by IFN-α immunotherapy among chronic hepatitis C or cancer patients. Surprisingly, although this issue has been extensively examined, there might still be some question as to whether IFN-α promotes the emergence of a general state of malaise, leading to a diffuse syndrome where depression is a cogent feature, or is actually a genuine depressive disorder like that associated with stressors.

Despite its therapeutic effects, cytokine-based therapy with IFN-α has been associated with neuropsychiatric complications in about 50% of treated patients, sometimes severe enough to necessitate discontinuation of medication (Capuron and Miller, 2004). Within 6–8 hours following the initial IFN-α treatment and lasting for about 2 weeks, patients may experience side-effects in the form of an acute flu-like syndrome, characterized by non-specific neurovegetative symptoms such as fever, chills, fatigue, malaise, sleep disturbances, myalgia, nausea, reduced appetite/anorexia, and psychomotor slowing/lethargy (Capuron and Miller, 2004). Some of these features are reminiscent of the sickness behaviors elicited by pro-inflammatory cytokines or endotoxins in rodent models. Later in the course of IFN-α therapy, within about 3 months after the start of treatment, patients may experience depressed mood and cognitive dysfunction (Capuron and Miller, 2004).

The mechanisms by which IFN-α exerts its side-effects are not entirely clear, but it has been suggested that it could stimulate the synthesis and secretion of other pro-inflammatory cytokines that are important for the clearance of the hepatitis C virus, but that also act to elicit the neurovegetative symptoms. One explanation for the effects of IFN-α therapy that has received considerable traction is that this cytokine causes the activation of indoleamine 2,3-dioxygenase (IDO), an enzyme responsible for tryptophan degradation, thus accelerating tryptophan depletion (and limiting its availability), resulting in diminished serotonin synthesis, and culminating in depressive illness (Dantzer *et al.*, 2011; Maes *et al.*, 2011). An alternative perspective in this regard is that the increased rate of tryptophan catabolism caused by IDO activation may lead to elevated production of kynurenic acid, 3-hydroxy kynurenine, and quinolinic acid, which may activate oxidative pathways, elicit mitochondrial dysfunctions, and engender neurotoxic effects that culminate in neurodegeneration, hence leading to anxiety and depression (Dantzer *et al.*, 2011; Maes *et al.*, 2011). While not dismissing a role for these processes in depressive illness, it is also possible that IFN-α has effects on brain processes beyond those involving serotonin and neurotoxic changes subsequent to IDO activation. Indeed, development of depressive symptoms during IFN-α therapy in hepatitis C patients has been associated with decreased serum levels of BDNF (Kenis *et al.*, 2011). As well, in patients that developed depression following IFN-α therapy, serum levels of soluble IL-2 receptor and of IL-1ra prior to treatment were associated with subsequent lower BDNF levels (Kenis *et al.*, 2011). Thus, as attractive as an IDO-based hypothesis might be, it is premature to dismiss a role for other inflammatory factors, particularly as depressive symptoms might be a consequence of multiple variables.

Consistent with a role of IFN-α in the pathophysiology of depression, prophylactic antidepressant treatment was found to prevent the emergence of depressive symptoms in cytokine-treated cancer or hepatitis C patients. The antidepressants tended to limit the depressed mood and cognitive impairments elicited by IFN-α, but hardly affected the early neurovegetative features (Capuron and Miller, 2004). Moreover, based on a meta-analysis it was concluded that preventive administration of antidepressants among patients that had received IFN-α was most effective in reducing depressive symptoms in those patients that exhibited depressive features prior to cytokine therapy (Galvao-de Almeida *et al.*, 2010). Considering that multiple pathways might be affected during IFN-α immunotherapy (e.g., serotonin, neurotoxicity, BDNF), it is possible that the limited clinical efficacy of prophylactic antidepressant treatment in some cytokine-treated patients (or for some neurovegetative symptoms) result from the use of pharmacological treatment strategies that uniquely (or primarily) target monoamines, rather than a multi-targeted approach

The fact that depressive features elicited by IFN-α could be attenuated by antidepressants, even if it does not occur in all patients or for all symptoms, is nevertheless consistent with a view that inflammatory factors are associated with depression. However, this does not mean that IFN-α therapy engenders a syndrome that is, essentially, the same as idiopathic major depression nor does it mean that the depressive symptoms comprised in these two conditions involve identical processes. It has been suggested that flu-like neurovegetative symptoms and later depression associated with IFN-α therapy could be linked to the same initial cytokine activation or, alternatively, that depressed mood could actually be a consequence of the flu-like syndrome experienced at the start of treatment (Charlton, 2000). In fact, it was shown that early onset of neurovegetative symptoms during IFN-α therapy predicted greater depressive–cognitive problems later in treatment (Wichers *et al.*, 2005). However, the symptoms elicited by IFN-α treatment and those experienced during idiopathic major depression in otherwise healthy individuals could be distinguished from one another. Specifically, even if depressive symptoms in the two conditions substantially overlapped, psychomotor retardation and weight loss were more pronounced among IFN-α-treated patients, whereas feelings of guilt, suicidal thoughts, and agitation were more characteristic of idiopathic major depression (Capuron *et al.*, 2009).

Although IFN-α promotes depressive symptoms in some patients, behavioral symptoms elicited by the cytokine might also reflect toxicity rather than changes that underlie idiopathic depression. It is possible that cognitive and depressive symptoms reported over the course of cytokine therapy might be a sign of non-specific cognitive impairments or a mental cloudiness similar to that of postchemotherapy cognitive impairment (PCCI; also known as "chemo brain" or "chemo fog") often reported in breast, ovarian or prostate cancer patients during chemotherapy (Argyriou *et al.*, 2011). This syndrome has been linked to oxidative stress and DNA damage, altered neuroendocrine levels, reduction of BDNF levels and cell proliferation in hippocampus (in rats), as well as deregulation of cytokine release (Kannarkat, Lasher, and Schiff, 2007). It has been suggested that one mechanism by which chemotherapy might affect cognitive processes involves altered TNF-α functioning (Aluise *et al.*, 2011). It will be recalled that elevated plasma TNF-α levels in chronic hepatitis C and Parkinson's patients were correlated with severity of depression and cognitive dysfunction (Loftis *et al.*, 2008; Menza *et al.*, 2010). It is thus possible that brain toxicity stemming from IFN-α, possibly through actions on TNF-α, could trigger a diffuse state of emotional and cognitive impairment that might not necessarily correspond to idiopathic major depression. Whether this applies to other cytokines remains to be determined. Nevertheless, as suggested earlier, at this point it is premature to dismiss the possibility that certain cytokines might be associated with malaise or lethargy, whereas others might be more aligned with mood changes.

Impacts of Stressors on Peripheral Inflammation and Depression

As indicated earlier, the relationships between elevated inflammation and depression may be moderated by stressors, or alternatively, inflammatory processes might give rise to stressor-like neurochemical changes (e.g., monoamine variations) that come to elicit depressive symptoms. In fact, stressful events provoke several neurochemical changes that have been associated with the pathophysiology of depression, including peripheral cytokine variations. This said, it is not unusual for depressed individuals to adopt unhealthy lifestyles, including poor diet, smoking, neglect of self appearance, and social isolation that may aggravate emotional distress and accentuate depressive state, and these poor lifestyle factors could also influence immune functioning (Irwin, 1999). Thus, immune changes could be secondary to depression or stressful experiences as opposed to playing a causal role in the emergence (or recurrence) of this disorder.

Psychosocial stressors in humans have been associated with elevated levels of circulating pro-inflammatory cytokines, especially IL-6 (Carroll *et al.*, 2011). It has also been reported that the link between IL-6 and depression may be moderated by the presence of social isolation that often accompanies depressed mood (Hafner *et al.*, 2011).Whether elevated inflammatory markers in depressed individuals are actually due to the individuals' mood, other neurochemical disturbances (e.g., monoamine variations), stressor experiences or unhealthy lifestyle, or a combination of these factors is uncertain. Nevertheless, it has been suggested that stressors may interact with pro-inflammatory markers through their synergistic action, ultimately promoting depressive behaviors (Anisman, Merali, and Hayley, 2008). As will be seen in the ensuing section, the impact of a variety of immune challenges on brain neurotransmitters, hormones, as well as on peripheral and central cytokine expression, may be influenced by the stressor backdrop upon which these treatments are administered.

Not surprisingly, it has been suggested that stressful life-events or emotional distress that often accompanies hepatitis C or cancer interact with IFN-α therapy to elicit the depressive symptoms reported in treated patients (Anisman, Merali, and Hayley, 2008). The presence of depressive features prior to the start of IFN-α therapy (Galvão-de Almeida *et al.*, 2010) as well as elevated HPA activation after the initial IFN-α treatment (Capuron *et al.*, 2003) were associated with the development of depression later in treatment. Likewise, the inflammatory cascade in response to the initial IFN-α injection (in this case manifested by p38 mitogen-activated protein kinase – MAPK) was strongly correlated with the presence of depressive symptoms prior to the cytokine therapy and with the cortisol response to the first IFN-α injection (Felger *et al.*, 2011). Moreover, the cytokine-induced p38 MAPK response was predictive of the severity of depressive symptoms evident during the first few weeks of treatment (Felger *et al.*, 2011), suggesting that increased sensitivity of p38 MAPK signaling might be a vulnerability marker for the depression elicited by IFN-α. It is also possible that this inflammatory pathway might have been sensitized through stressor experiences (or a previous depressive episode), resulting an exaggerated response to IFN-α, ultimately contributing to a pattern of depressive behaviors (Felger *et al.*, 2011).

Beyond the immediate effects elicited, certain cytokines (e.g., IL-1β, TNF-α) can enhance the response to stressors applied weeks later, and conversely, stressors may augment the effects of subsequent cytokine treatments (Anisman, Merali, and Hayley, 2003). Whether a similar sensitization effect occurs with respect to IFN-α has not been established. However, it is conceivable that the depressive effects of this cytokine may be related to the sensitization of neurochemical processes associated with previously encountered stressful experiences or distress experienced during the illness (Anisman, Merali, and Hayley, 2008; Felder *et al.*, 2011).

Although it would be efficient to consider the effects of immune challenges independently of other variables, it seems likely that the effects elicited by the immune treatments are largely influenced by contextual factors (e.g., whether the immune challenge was applied on a stressor backdrop). As well, the impact of immune challenges may vary with other stressor-related processes, including stressor appraisal and coping, although these aspects of the stress response are not readily assessed. Furthermore, given the potential sensitization (and synergy) of neurochemical responses elicited by stressful experiences, it seems appropriate to consider that the effects of IFN-α on depressive behaviors might not only be determined by ongoing stressor, but also by stressors experienced earlier in life.

Animal Models of Cytokine-induced Depressive Behaviors

It has not been possible to evaluate thoroughly all aspects of inflammatory activation in relation to depressive disorders in human populations, especially the cytokine variations that occur in the brain. Animal models have thus provided useful information concerning the associations between inflammation and depressive disorders and on the moderating influence of stressors on these relationships, although it is the case that animal models cannot fully capture all aspects of depression (e.g., feelings of guilt, worthlessness, suicidal ideation).

Several animal studies have been conducted in an effort to describe the behavioral syndrome associated with inflammatory activation and to define the factors responsible for the behavioral and biological effects of cytokines. One of the most common effects observed in response to pro-inflammatory cytokine (e.g., IL-1β and TNF-α) or bacterial endotoxin (e.g., LPS) administration comprises short-lived behavioral variations referred to as sickness behaviors. These behaviors include neurovegetative symptoms such as fever, anorexia, decreased activity and lethargy, ptosis, piloerection, and curled body posture, which as a group are reminiscent of the flu-like syndrome experienced during the first weeks of IFN-α therapy. As sickness symptoms are attenuated by antidepressant treatments (Yirmiya *et al.*, 2000), this behavior has at times been used as a proxy for the symptoms of depression in humans.

In addition to inducing sickness behaviors, it was shown that IL-1β reliably promotes monoamine variations within stress-related brain regions (Anisman, Merali, and Hayley, 2008) and that blockade of IL-1β functioning limits behavioral, monoamine, and inflammatory changes associated with stressor or inflammatory challenges (Johnson *et al.*, 2004). Yet, as indicated earlier, there is still some question as to whether this cytokine is, in fact, the most closely aligned with human depressive illness (Liu, Ho, and Mak, 2011). Curiously, the cytokines that have been found to be elevated in depressed individuals (i.e., IL-6, TNF-α) do not seem to be the most effective in eliciting sickness behaviors in rodent models of the disorder. Along the same line, although IFN-α therapy in hepatitis C or cancer patients has been associated with incidence of depression, its effects on depressive-like behaviors in rodent models have been much less consistent (Kosel *et al.*, 2011). The reasons for this are not entirely clear, but at least in the case of IFN-α, it seems that in many of the studies that examined cytokine effects in mice, the human isoform of the compound was used even though it has limited effects in this rodent species. Additional factors that might have contributed to the limited effects of IFN-α in rodents are related to the doses used, routes of administration, and times of behavioral measurements that were often not optimal to make parallels to the human condition. As well, in humans, immunotherapy is usually administered over many months, but most animal studies with IFN-α have used relatively acute treatment, likely accounting for the modest cytokine effects that have been observed.

It will be recalled that in humans treated with IFN-α, a period of neurovegetative symptoms emerges in the first weeks of treatment initiation, after which the mood and cognitive changes become apparent. It is thus surprising that in rodent models most of the behaviors associated with endotoxin or pro-inflammatory cytokine administration, including IFN-α, have typically been restricted to sickness behaviors. Far fewer studies, it seems, have focused on cytokine elicitation of core symptoms of major depression (e.g., anhedonia and cognitive-like dysfunctions), again limiting the conclusions that can be drawn relevant to the depressive actions stemming from cytokine treatments.

To deal with the bind concerning the value of assessing sickness symptoms to model depression, it has been suggested that pro-inflammatory cytokines might primarily be influencing atypical features of depression (e.g., increased lethargy, increased sleep). One would hope that this would, in fact, be a valid analogy, but these cytokines also resulted in reduced eating, which is a feature of typical depression. One could legitimately argue that these behavioral outcomes (e.g., lethargy and anorexia) are indeed a reflection of sickness, but in itself, sickness might not be at all informative of a depressive-like state (unless, of course, animals became depressed as a result of feeling sick). To be sure, there have been reports that antidepressant treatments may attenuate the sickness behaviors elicited by inflammatory agents (Yirmiya *et al.*, 2000), providing support for the validity of the sickness model of depression. However, one also needs to determine whether the antidepressants act directly on mood state or whether the drugs are actually altering the immune response elicited, thereby reducing the sickness. In this regard, it was reported that SSRI treatment reduced the fatigue elicited by LPS in humans, but did not normalize plasma cytokine elevations induced by the endotoxin (Hannestad *et al.*, 2011b), thus challenging the notion that peripheral cytokines are involved in depressive-like behaviors elicited by LPS.

As already indicated there have been few reports in rodents that assessed the effects of inflammatory activation on core features of depression, such as anhedonia. Nevertheless, it was demonstrated that both pro-inflammatory cytokines and LPS elicited anhedonic actions in relatively sophisticated behavioral paradigms. For instance, these treatments disrupted responding for rewarding brain stimulation, as well as responding on a progressive ratio schedule of reinforcement (or other reinforcement schedules) that allowed for dissociation of sickness effects from anhedonia elicited by the treatments (Merali *et al.*, 2003). Furthermore, it was reported that antidepressants attenuated the performance disturbances elicited by an inflammatory challenge in these paradigms (Merali *et al.*, 2003). To date, not unexpectedly, there has been limited information available concerning the effect of IFN-α on progressive ratio performance or responding for rewarding brain stimulation using appropriate treatment doses. At this point, additional measures of depressive and cognitive functions in animal models are needed to better dissociate neurovegetative symptoms (sickness behaviors) from depressive and cognitive disturbances associated with inflammatory activation.

In addition to the impact of cytokines on sickness and depressive-like symptoms, rodent models have also served in the analysis of stressor effects on peripheral and central inflammatory processes as well as in moderating the relation between cytokines and depression. Naturalistic psychosocial stressors such as social defeat, which have been widely used in rodent models of depression and anxiety, were found to elicit peripheral and central variations of pro-inflammatory cytokines, and it seemed that IL-6 was particularly affected in this regard (Audet *et al.*, 2011; Gibb *et al.*, 2011). It was also reported that sickness behaviors as well as plasma and brain cytokine variations elicited by LPS were markedly enhanced if the endotoxin had been administered on the backdrop of a social stressor (Gibb *et al.*, 2011). Such a finding was also observed with respect to IFN-α, although as indicated earlier, the cytokine has limited effects on behaviors in rodent models (Anisman *et al.*, 2007). In addition, variations of cytokine mRNA expression triggered by a social stressor or by LPS were moderated by whether mice had previously experienced a chronic social stressor (Audet *et al.*, 2011). It is interesting that in these studies IL-6 was particularly affected by the combined actions of the social stressor and the LPS treatment, irrespective of whether the stressor and inflammatory challenges were applied in close temporal congruity (reflecting a potential synergistic action or were spaced further apart (sensitization) (Audet *et al.*, 2011; Gibb *et al.*, 2011). Since IL-6 appears to be particularly affected in major depression (Liu, Ho, and Mak, 2011) and sensitive to stressors in humans (Carroll *et al.*, 2011), it seems essential that animal-based studies continue to focus on the role of this cytokine in the pathogenesis of depressive behaviors as well as on its interactions with stressors and other pro-inflammatory markers. Yet, it could be argued that the IL-6 changes are too sensitive to stressors and hence might not be effective in differentiating those treatments that effectively elicit depressive symptoms and those that do not.

In relation to cytokine-induced depression, it ought to be considered that reciprocal relations may exist between peripheral and central cytokine variations and that stressors might moderate these relations, ultimately resulting in depressive disorders. It has been shown in rodent models that peripheral LPS or cytokine challenges (e.g., IFN-α treatment) may elicit variations of circulating cytokines as well as concomitant or subsequent changes of various neurotransmitters (e.g., norepinephrine and serotonin), peptides (e.g., CRH) or inflammatory cytokines (e.g., IL-6) in stress-related brain regions linked to depression, such as the PFC and hippocampus (Audet *et al.*, 2011; Gibb *et al.*, 2011). As described earlier, stressors may also influence both plasma cytokine levels and cytokine mRNA expression in these same areas of the mouse brain (Audet *et al.*, 2011; Gibb *et al.*, 2011). It is possible that these peripheral cytokine variations might contribute to the central cytokine elevations, although the central effects do not always parallel those seen peripherally (Gibb *et al.*, 2011). Thus, although peripheral cytokines might not directly promote depressive symptoms, they might represent a biomarker for this illness, particularly as this affective state might itself be a profound stressor that elicits peripheral and central inflammatory immune activation. A schematic representation of the link between stressor and inflammatory actions is presented in Figure 24.1.

In line with the latter proposition, brain inflammatory insults have been reported to elicit peripheral cytokine changes, thus suggesting that central insults may act like stressors, thereby triggering peripheral cytokine variations. Indeed, acute stroke in humans was accompanied by increased cytokine levels in plasma (Shenhar-Tsarfaty *et al.*, 2010; Yang *et al.*, 2010), just as ischemic stroke in rat models resulted in elevated peripheral inflammation. Although peripheral cytokine changes have not been correlated with depressive symptoms that often accompanied stroke (not because such correlations do not exist, but because depression outcomes were not thoroughly investigated in these studies), these data support the possibility that peripheral cytokine changes in relation to major depression might be a consequence of central variations elicited by stressors or from depression itself (acting as a stressor), and thus might be limited to being a biomarker of the illness.

One final issue warrants consideration in relation to the inflammation–stress synergies that could be associated with depressive features. Specifically, it has been suggested that the timing of HPA axis (e.g., triggered by stressor experience or condition) and inflammatory activation might be of considerable importance for the provocation of depressive behaviors and of biological changes implicated in depression. Specifically, it is possible that pre-existing stressful states might be necessary to prime the system for subsequent inflammatory challenges to be effective in eliciting depressive symptoms. It has been reported that exposure to glucocorticoids (e.g., corticosterone) prior to an inflammatory challenge with LPS (e.g., 2 hours or 24 hours before)

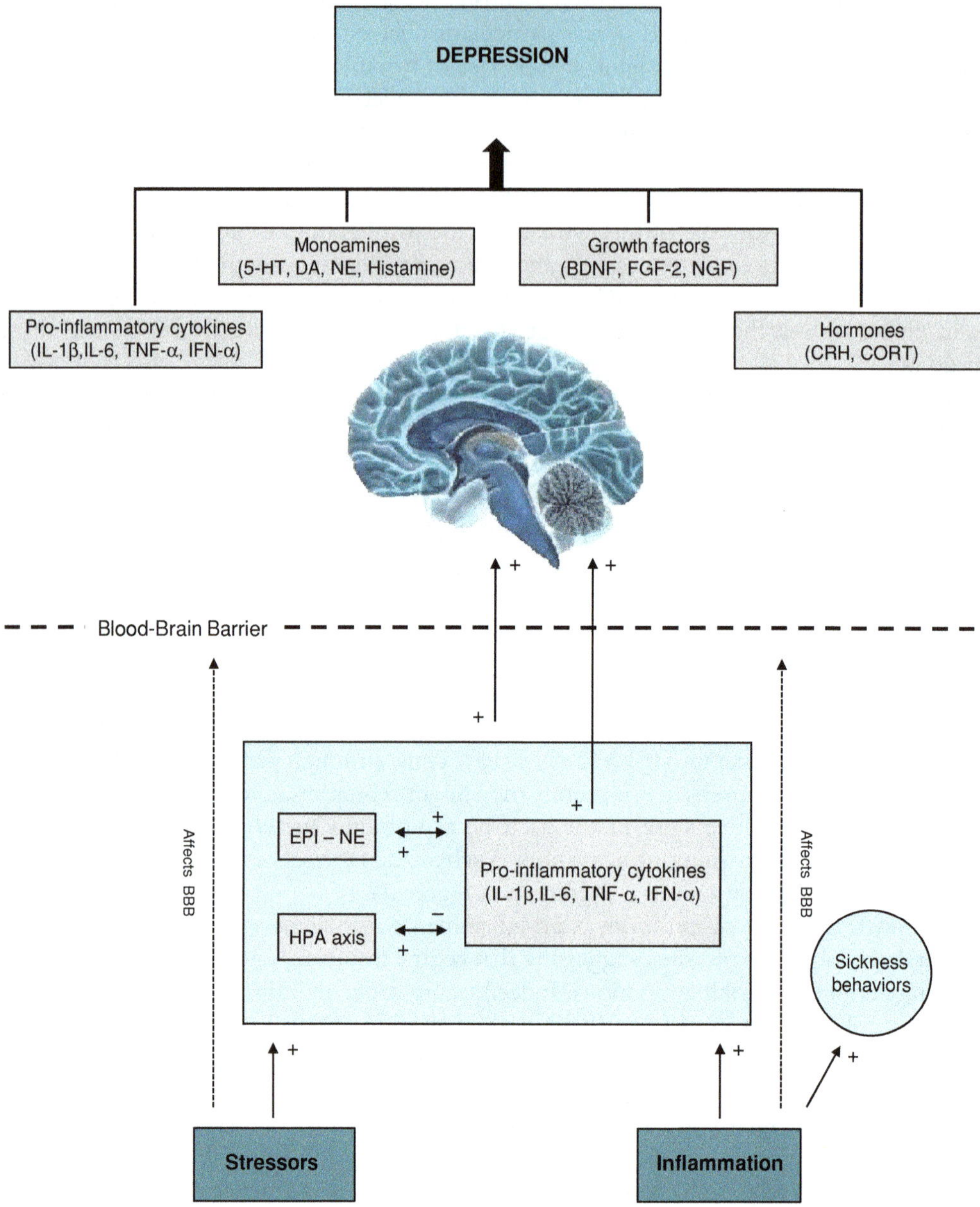

Figure 24.1 Schematic representation of the effects of stressors and inflammation on the peripheral and central nervous systems in relation to depression. It is suggested that stressors promote both hypothalamic-pituitary-adrenal (HPA) axis activity, culminating in cortisol secretion, and autonomic functioning, characterized by epinephrine (EPI) and norepinephrine (NE) release. The EPI and NE release promotes pro-inflammatory cytokine secretion from immune cells, whereas at physiological levels

enhanced liver and hippocampal variations of IL-1β, IL-6, and TNF-α levels. However, when glucocorticoids were administered after the LPS challenge, cytokine elevations in liver and hippocampus were not apparent (Frank *et al.*, 2010). Essentially, these data support the possibility that stress-activated systems might be required for subsequent inflammation to exert optimal effects and for depression to emerge, whereas the opposite sequence (inflammation preceding the stressor) might be less likely to engender these outcomes.

Conclusion

After more than two decades of research regarding the implications of inflammatory processes for depression, the mechanisms supporting these associations are only now being defined. Although it seems clear that circulating markers of inflammation are elevated in individuals with major depression and that peripheral inflammatory challenges (e.g., IFN-α treatment) result in depression in a substantial number of patients, the occurrence of illness appear to be governed by several further variables and risk factors.

There have been several issues that might have limited forward movement in defining the relationship between the inflammatory system and depressive disorders. This has included a failure to distinguish between depressive illnesses based on specific symptoms or even illness subtypes that might involve different mechanisms. Moreover, it is not necessarily the case that all cytokines (or their downstream sequelae) are involved in the same aspects or symptoms of depression. As well, studies examining the effects of immune challenges on depression in humans often did not consider the stressor context upon which these immune/cytokine challenges were overlaid, even though there is ample evidence suggesting that cytokines and stressors act synergistically in the promotion of depression. Finally, to a degree, the behavioral analyses in animal studies have not kept pace with the sophisticated approaches used in the analyses of the biological changes associated with inflammatory challenges. This said, many of these issues are being recognized, and it can reasonably be expected that it won't be long before a coherent picture emerges concerning the conditions under which inflammatory immune activation gives rise to behavioral and cognitive psychopathology.

Figure 24.1 (*continued*) the corticosterone release limits immune activation, and at high levels may promote suppression of immune functioning. Inflammation likewise causes release of pro-inflammatory cytokines from activated immune cells. The cytokine release, in turn, activates HPA functioning and autonomic activity (EPI and NE) and independently elicits sickness behaviors. Although cytokines do not readily pass through blood-brain barrier (BBB) mechanisms, access can be gained at some sites, and the possibility exists that inflammatory factors induced by both stressors and inflammation can increase brain permeability. As well, psychological stressors and physical insults (concussive injury, head trauma) can directly elicit release of pro-inflammatory cytokines from brain glial cells, and concurrently promote variations in brain monoamines, growth factors (e.g., brain-derived neurotrophic factor: BDNF, basic fibroblast growth factor: FGF-2, nerve growth factor: NGF), corticotropin-releasing hormone (CRH) and other peptides. The effects of inflammatory challenges on the brain changes are thus more pronounced when administered on a backdrop of strong stressors, which might promote greater mood changes. Likewise, stressor experiences may result in the sensitization of neurochemical processes, so that the responses to later inflammatory challenges favor the evolution of depressed mood or anxiety disorders.

References

Aluise, C.D., Miriyala, S., Noel, T., Sultana, R., Jungsuwadee, P., Taylor, T.J., et al. (2011). 2-mercaptoethane sulfonate prevents doxorubicin-induced plasma protein oxidation and TNF-α release: implications for the reactive oxygen species-mediated mechanisms of chemobrain. *Free Radical Biology and Medicine*, 50, 1630–1638.

Anisman, H. (2009). Cascading effects of stressors and inflammatory immune activation: implications for major depressive disorder. *Journal of Psychiatry and Neuroscience*, 34, 4–20.

Anisman, H., Merali, Z., and Hayley, S. (2003). Sensitization associated with stressors and cytokine treatments. *Brain, Behavior, and Immunity*, 17, 86–93.

Anisman, H., Merali, Z., and Hayley, S. (2008). Neurotransmitter, peptide and cytokine processes in relation to depressive disorder: comorbidity between depression and neurodegenerative disorders. *Progress in Neurobiology*, 85, 1–74.

Anisman, H., Poulter, M.O., Gandhi, R., Merali, Z., and Hayley, S. (2007). Interferon-alpha effects are exaggerated when administered on a psychosocial stressor backdrop: cytokine, corticosterone, and monoamine variations. *Journal of Neuroimmunology*, 186, 45–53.

Anisman, H., Ravindran, A.V., Griffiths, J., and Merali, Z. (1999). Interleukin-1 beta production in dysthymia before and after pharmacotherapy. *Biological Psychiatry*, 46, 1649–1655.

Argyriou, A.A., Assimakopoulos, K., Iconomou, G., Giannakopoulou, F., and Kalofonos, H.P. (2011). Either called "chemobrain" or "chemofog," the long-term chemotherapy-induced cognitive decline in cancer survivors is real. *Journal of Pain and Symptom Management*, 41, 126–139.

Audet, M.C., Jacobson-Pick, S., Wann, B.P., and Anisman, H. (2011). Social defeat promotes specific cytokine variations within the prefrontal cortex upon subsequent aggressive or endotoxin challenges. *Brain, Behavior, and Immunity*, 25, 1197–1205.

Bilge, C., Koçer, E., Koçer, A., and Turc Boru, U. (2008). Depression and functional outcomes after stroke: the effects of antidepressant therapy on functional recovery. *European Journal of Physical and Rehabilitation Medicine*, 44, 13–18.

Capuron, L., Fornwalt, F.B., Knight, B.T., Harvey, P.D., Ninan, P.T., and Miller, A.H. (2009). Does cytokine-induced depression differ from idiopathic major depression in medically healthy individuals? *Journal of Affective Disorders*, 119, 181–185.

Capuron, L., and Miller, A.H. (2004). Cytokines and psychopathology: lessons from interferon-alpha. *Biological Psychiatry*, 56, 819–824.

Capuron, L., Raison, C.L., Musselman, D.L., Lawson, D.H., Nemeroff, C.B., and Miller, A.H. (2003). Association of exaggerated HPA axis response to the initial injection of interferon-alpha with development of depression during interferon-alpha therapy. *American Journal of Psychiatry*, 160, 1342–1345.

Carroll, J.E., Low, C.A., Prather, A.A., Cohen, S., Fury, J.M., Ross, D.C., et al. (2011). Negative affective responses to a speech task predict changes in interleukin (IL)-6. *Brain, Behavior, and Immunity*, 25, 232–238.

Charlton, B.G. (2000). The malaise theory of depression: major depressive disorder is sickness behavior and antidepressants are analgesic. *Medical Hypotheses*, 54, 126–130.

Cremeans-Smith, J.K., Soehlen, S., Greene, K., Alexander, T., and Delahanty, D.L. (2009). In-hospital levels of C-reactive protein and IL-6 predict post-operative depressive symptoms among patients undergoing total knee replacement surgery. *Brain, Behavior, and Immunity*, 23, 1096–1103.

Dantzer, R., O'Connor, J.C., Lawson, M.A., and Kelley, K.W. (2011). Inflammation-associated depression: from serotonin to kynurenine. *Psychoneuroendocrinology*, 36, 426–436.

Dowlati, Y., Herrmann, N., Swardfager, W., Liu, H., Sham, L., Reim, E.K., et al. (2010). A meta-analysis of cytokines in major depression. *Biological Psychiatry*, 67, 446–457.

Eller, T., Vasar, V., Shlik, J., and Maron, E. (2009). Effects of bupropion augmentation on pro-inflammatory cytokines in escitalopram-resistant patients with major depressive disorder. *Journal of Psychopharmacology*, 23, 854–858.

Felger, J.C., Alagbe, O., Pace, T.W., Woolwine, B.J., Hu, F., Raison, C.L., et al. (2011). Early activation of p38 mitogen activated protein kinase is associated with interferon-alpha-induced depression and fatigue. *Brain, Behavior, and Immunity*, 25, 1094–1098.

Frank, M.G., Miguel, Z.D., Watkins, L.R., and Maier, S.F. (2010). Prior exposure to glucocorticoids sensitizes the neuroinflammatory and peripheral inflammatory responses to E. Coli lipopolysaccharide. *Brain, Behavior, and Immunity*, 24, 19–30.

Galvão-de Almeida, A., Guindalini, C., Batista-Neves, S., de Oliveira, I.R., Miranda-Scippa, A., and Quarantini, L.C. (2010). Can anti-depressants prevent interferon-alpha-induced depression? A review of the literature. *General Hospital Psychiatry*, 32, 401–405.

Gibb, J., Audet, M.C., Hayley, S., and Anisman, H. (2009). Neurochemical and behavioral responses to inflammatory immune stressors. *Frontiers in Bioscience (Scholar Edition)*, 1, 275–295.

Gibb, J., Hayley, S., Poulter, M.O., and Anisman, H. (2011). Effects of stressors and immune activating agents on peripheral and central cytokines in mouse strains that differ in stress responsivity. *Brain, Behavior, and Immunity*, 25, 468–482.

Gold, P.W., and Chrousos, G.P. (2002). Organization of the stress system and its dysregulation in melancholic and atypical depression: high vs low CRH/NE states. *Molecular Psychiatry*, 7, 254–275.

Häfner, S., Emeny, R.T., Lacruz, M.E., Baumert, J., Herder, C., Koenig, W., et al. (2011). Association between social isolation and inflammatory markers in depressed and non-depressed individuals: results from the MONICA/KORA study. *Brain, Behavior, and Immunity*, 25, 1701–1707.

Hannestad, J., DellaGioia, N., and Bloch, M. (2011a). The effect of antidepressant medication treatment on serum levels of inflammatory cytokines: a meta-analysis. *Neuropsychopharmacology*, 36, 2452–2459.

Hannestad, J., DellaGioia, N., Ortiz, N., Pittman, B., and Bhagwagar, Z. (2011b). Citalopram reduces endotoxin-induced fatigue. *Brain, Behavior, and Immunity*, 25, 256–259.

Harrison, N.A., Brydon, L., Walker, C., Gray, M.A., Steptoe, A., and Critchley, H.D. (2009). Inflammation causes mood changes through alterations in subgenual cingulated activity and mesolimbic connectivity. *Biological Psychiatry*, 66, 407–414.

Hasler, G., Drevets, W.C., Manji, H.K., and Charney, D.S. (2004). Discovering endophenotypes for major depression. *Neuropsychopharmacology*, 29, 1765–1781.

Howren, M.B., Lamkin, D.M., and Suls, J. (2009). Associations of depression with C-reactive protein, IL-1, and IL-6: a meta-analysis. *Psychosomatic Medicine*, 71, 171–186.

Irwin, M. (1999). Immune correlates of depression. *Advances in Experimental Medicine and Biology*, 461, 1–24.

Janelidze, S., Mattei, D., Westrin, Å., Träskman-Bendz, L., and Brundin, L. (2011). Cytokine levels in the blood may distinguish suicide attempters from depressed patients. *Brain, Behavior, and Immunity*, 25, 335–339.

Johnson, J.D., O'Connor, K.A., Watkins, L.R., and Maier, S.F. (2004). The role of IL-1b in stress-induced sensitization of proinflammatory cytokine and corticosterone response. *Neuroscience*, 127, 569–577.

Kannarkat, G., Lasher, E.E., and Schiff, D. (2007). Neurological complications of chemotherapy agents. *Current Opinion in Neurology*, 20, 719–725.

Kenis, G., Prickaerts, J., Van Os, J., Koek, G.H., Robaeys, G., Steinbusch, H.W., et al. (2011). Depressive symptoms following interferon-α therapy: mediated by immune-induced reductions in brain-derived neurotrophic factor? *International Journal of Neuropsychopharmacology*, 14, 247–253.

Kim, Y.K., Lee, S.W., Kim,S.H., Shim, S.H., Han, S.W., Choi, S.H., et al. (2008). Differences in cytokines between non-suicidal patients and suicidal patients in major depression. *Progress in Neuropsychopharmacology and Biological Psychiatry*, 32, 356–361.

Kim, J.M., Stewart, R., Kim, S.W., Shin, I.S., Kim, J.T., Park, M.S., et al. (2011). Associations of cytokine gene polymorphisms with post-stroke depression. *World Journal of Biological Psychiatry*, 13, 579–587.

Kosel, M., Bilkei-Gorzo, A., Zawatzky, R., Zimmer, A., and Schlaepfer, T.E. (2011). Pegylated human interferon alpha 2a does not induce depression-associated changes in mice. *Psychiatry Research*, 185, 243–247.

Kouwenhoven, S.E., Kirkevold, M., Engedal, K., and Kim, H.S. (2011). Depression in acute stroke: prevalence, dominant symptoms and associated factors. A systemic literature review. *Disability and Rehabilitation*, 33, 539–556.

Lanquillon, S., Krieg, J.C., Bening-Abu-Shach, U., and Vedder, H. (2000). Cytokine production and treatment response in major depressive disorder. *Neuropsychopharmacology*, 22, 370–379.

Lindqvist, D., Janelidze, S., Hagell, P., Erhardt, S., Samuelsson, M., Minthon, L., et al. (2009). Interleukin-6 is elevated in the cerebrospinal fluid of suicide attempters and related to symptom severity. *Biological Psychiatry*, 66, 287–292.

Liu, Y., Ho, R.C., and Mak, A. (2011). Interleukin (IL)-6, tumour necrosis factor alpha (TNF-α) and soluble interleukin-2 receptors (sIL-2R) are elevated in patients with major depressive disorder: a meta-analysis and meta-regression. *Journal of Affective Disorders*, 139, 230–239.

Loftis, J.M., Huckans, M., Ruimy, S., Hinrichs, D.J., and Hauser, P. (2008). Depressive symptoms in patients with chronic hepatitis C are correlated with elevated plasma levels of interleukin-1beta and tumor necrosis factor-alpha. *Neuroscience Letters*, 430, 264–268.

Maes, M. (1995). Evidence for an immune response in major depression: a review and hypothesis. *Progress in Neuropsychopharmacology and Biological Psychiatry*, 19, 11–38.

Maes, M. (2011). Depression is an inflammatory disease, but cell-mediated immune activation is the key component of depression. *Progress in Neuropsychopharmacology and Biological Psychiatry*, 35, 664–675.

Maes, M., Leonard, B.E., Myint, A.M., Kubera, M., and Verkerk, R. (2011). The new "5-HT" hypothesis of depression: cell-mediated immune activation induces indoleamine 2,3-dioxygenase, which leads to lower plasma tryptophan and an increased synthesis of detrimental tryptophan catabolites (TRYCATs), both of which contribute to the onset of depression. *Progress in Neuropsychopharmacology and Biological Psychiatry*, 35, 702–721.

Menza, M., Dobkin, R.D., Marin, H., Mark, M.H., Gara, M., Bienfait, K., et al. (2010). The role of inflammatory cytokines in cognition and other non-motor symptoms of Parkinson's disease. *Psychosomatics*, 51, 474–479.

Merali, Z., Brennan, K., Brau, P., and Anisman, H. (2003). Dissociating anorexia and anhedonia elicited by interleukin-1beta: antidepressant and gender effects on responding for "free chow" and "earned" sucrose intake. *Psychopharmacology (Berlin)*, 165, 413–418.

Millan, M.J. (2006). Multi-target strategies for the improved treatment of depressive states: conceptual foundations and neuronal substrates, drug discovery and therapeutic application. *Pharmacology and Therapeutics*, 110, 135–370.

Moncrieff, J., and Kirsch, I. (2005). Efficacy of anti-depressants in adults. *British Medical Journal*, 331, 155–157.

Musselman, D.L., Miller, A.H., Porter, M.R., Manatunga, A., Gao, F., Penna, S., et al. (2001). Higher than normal plasma interleukin-6 concentrations in cancer patients with depression: preliminary findings. *American Journal of Psychiatry*, 158, 1252–1257.

O'Brien, S.M., Scully, P., Fitzgerald, P., Scott, L.V., and Dinan, T.G. (2007). Plasma cytokine profiles in depressed patients who fail to respond to selective serotonin reuptake inhibitor therapy. *Journal of Psychiatric Research*, 41, 326–331.

Pandey, G.N., Rizavi, H.S., Ren, X., Fareed, J., Hoppensteadt, D.A., Roberts, R.C., et al. (2011). Proinflammatory cytokines in the prefrontal cortex of teenage suicide victims. *Journal of Psychiatry Research*, 46, 57–63.

Reichenberg, A., Yirmiya, R., Schuld, A., Kraus, T., Haack, M., Morag, A., et al. (2001). Cytokine-associated emotional and cognitive disturbances in humans. *Archives of General Psychiatry*, 58, 445–452.

Shenhar-Tsarfaty, S., Ben Assayag, E., Bova, I., Shopin, L., Fried, M., Berliner, S., et al. (2010). Interleukin-6 as an early predictor for one-year survival following an ischaemic stroke/transient ischaemic attack. *International Journal of Stroke*, 5, 16–20.

Thompson, C.S., and Hakim, A.M. (2005). Cortical spreading depression modifies components of the inflammatory cascade. *Molecular Neurobiology*, 32, 51–57.

Tonelli, L.H., Stiller, J., Rujescu, D., Giegling, I., Schneider, B., Maurer, K., et al. (2008). Elevated cytokine expression in the orbitofrontal cortex of victims of suicide. *Acta Psychiatrica Scandinavica*, 117, 198–206.

Wichers, M.C., Koek, G.H., Robaeys, G., Praamstra, A.J., and Maes, M. (2005). Early increase in vegetative symptoms predicts IFN-alpha-induced cognitive-depressive changes. *Psychological Medicine*, 35, 433–441.

Yang, L., Zhang, Z., Sun, D., Xu, Z., Zhang, X., and Li, L. (2010). The serum interleukin-18 is a potential marker for development of post-stroke depression. *Neurological Research*, 32, 340–346.

Yirmiya, R., Pollak, Y., Morag, M., Reichenberg, A., Barak, O., Avitsur, R., et al. (2000). Illness, cytokines, and depression. *Annals of the New York Academy of Sciences*, 917, 478–487.

Yoshimura, R., Hori, H., Ikenouchi-Sugita, A., Umene-Nakano, W., Ueda, N., and Nakamura, J. (2009). Higher plasma interleukin-6 (IL-6) level is associated with SSRI- or SNRI-refractory depression. *Progress in Neuropsychopharmacology and Biological Psychiatry*, 33, 722–726.

Yoshimura, R., Umene-Nakano, W., Hoshuyama, T., Ikenouchi-Sugita, A., Hori, H., Katsuki, A., et al. (2010). Plasma levels of brain-derived neurotrophic factor and interleukin-6 in patients with dysthymic disorder: comparison with age- and sex-matched major depressed patients and healthy controls. *Human Psychopharmacology*, 25, 566–569.

25

Interaction Between Immune and Energy-Balance Signals in the Regulation of Feeding and Metabolism

Alfonso Abizaid,[1] Giamal Luheshi,[2] and Barbara C. Woodside[3]

[1]*Department of Neuroscience, Carleton University, Ottawa, Ontario, Canada*
[2]*Douglas Hospital Research Centre, Department of Psychiatry, McGill University, Montreal, Quebec, Canada*
[3]*Centre for Studies in Behavioral Neurobiology, Concordia University, Montreal, Quebec, Canada*

Introduction

The rapid increase in obesity rates worldwide together with the well-established relation between obesity and a number of health risks, including type-2 diabetes and cardiovascular disease, has provided a strong impetus for the study of the neural and neurochemical systems that control energy balance. With these studies came the understanding that organs, such as white adipose tissue and gut, that had not previously been recognized as endocrine organs actually secrete hormones and immune mediators that act in the brain to affect food intake, energy expenditure, and other aspects of metabolism. This has led to new conceptualizations of the control of energy balance. In this review, we describe current advances in research linking immunity with the central control of energy balance, and interactions between hormones commonly associated with the regulation of energy balance, such as ghrelin and leptin, and immune mediators.

Central Regulation of Energy Balance

It is now well established that the mediobasal hypothalamus and in particular, hypothalamic nuclei surrounding the third ventricle including the arcuate nucleus (ARC), the paraventricular nucleus (PVN), the ventromedial hypothalamic nucleus (VMH), dorsomedial hypothalamic

The Wiley-Blackwell Handbook of Psychoneuroimmunology, First Edition. Edited by Alexander W. Kusnecov and Hymie Anisman.

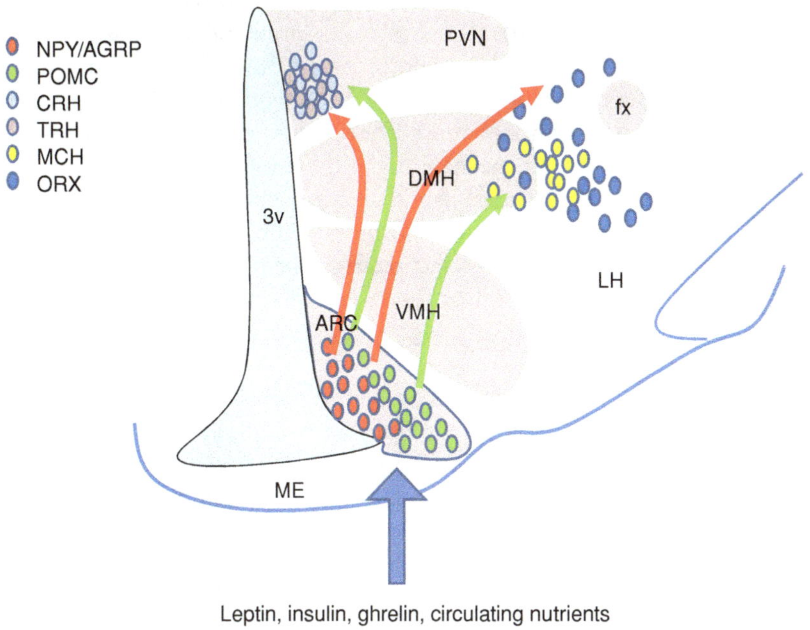

Figure 25.1 Hypothalamic nuclei implicated in the control of energy balance. Peripheral signals, including hormones and circulating nutrients, alter the activity of neurons in the arcuate nucleus (ARC) of the hypothalamus. Orexigenic hormones like ghrelin will increase the secretion of anabolic peptides such as neuropeptide Y (NPY) and agouti-related peptide (AGRP), whereas leptin and insulin will increase the activity of catabolic peptides such as αMSH. These first-order neurons stimulate other hypothalamic regions to ultimately modulate a number of regulatory processes that include changes in arousal and feeding behavior, metabolic rate, and cognitive processes associated with hunger. *Abbreviations:* Paraventricular nucleus (PVN), Dorsomedial nucleus of the hypothalamus (DMH), Ventromedial Nucleus of the hypothalamus (VMH), Lateral hypothalamus (LH), fornix (fx), Median eminence (ME), third ventricle (3v).

nucleus (DMH), and the lateral hypothalamus (LH) play a primary role in the regulation of energy homeostasis (Abizaid and Horvath, 2008).The ARC contains two sets of neuronal populations that produce several peptides with opposing effects on energy balance (Abizaid and Horvath, 2008). One set of cells produces the peptide ER (POMC), a precursor for a number of biologically active peptides including α-melanocyte stimulating hormone (α-MSH). This hormone binds to melanocortin receptors 3 (MC3) and 4 (MC4) located in the PVN, DMH and LH as well as in forebrain regions. Activation of these receptors produces a pronounced decrease *of* food intake and an increase of energy expenditure (see Figure 25.1).

Other neurons in the ARC co-express and release neuropeptide Y (NPY) and the agouti-related protein (AGRP). In contrast to α-MSH, these are potent orexigenic peptides. Interestingly, AGRP is an endogenous antagonist at MC3 and MC4 receptors. The existence of two sets of neurons that produce natural agonists or antagonists for MC3 and MC4 receptors, and the sensitivity of both neuronal populations to fluctuations in hormone and nutritional signals, have led to the proposition that energy balance is maintained by this "melanocortin system" (Abizaid and Horvath, 2008).

Both POMC and NPY/AGRP cells within the ARC are considered by some to be first order sensory cells since they constitute a significant target of multiple hormonal signals. Prominent amongst these signals are three hormones: leptin, insulin, and ghrelin, each of which originates from a peripheral organ: white adipose tissue (WAT), the pancreas and the stomach, respectively. These hormones most likely access ARC neurons through multiple pathways, including active transport mechanisms in the choroid plexus, and direct access to the CNS at areas such as the medial basal hypothalamus where the blood–brain barrier is less effective. It has also been suggested that these hormones influence the ARC indirectly through their ability to affect activity in neurons projecting from the nucleus of the solitary tract to the hypothalamus, neurons that are themselves the targets of satiating gastrointestinal cues that signal through the afferent portion of the vagus nerve (see Abizaid and Horvath, 2008, for review).

The discovery of the hormone leptin was a watershed in the unraveling of the brain mechanisms regulating short- and long-term energy availability. Leptin is the protein product of the *Ob* gene that is expressed mainly in WAT, and circulating levels of this hormone are positively correlated with adiposity. When administered either peripherally or directly into the brain, leptin decreases food intake and promotes energy expenditure (Abizaid and Horvath, 2008). POMC neurons within the ARC are activated by, and secrete α-MSH in response to leptin, while NPY/AGRP neurons reduce their peptidergic output in response to these same signals. Mice that do not produce leptin or that bear genes coding for mutant forms of the leptin receptor become obese (reviewed in Abizaid and Horvath, 2008).

The contribution of insulin to glucose metabolism has been known for close to 100 years, but for much of that time insulin was regarded as having effects only in the periphery. More recently, insulin receptors were identified in the brain, and it has been demonstrated that central elimination of insulin receptors results in a phenotype that includes increased food intake and obesity (Bruning *et al.*, 2000). Although the evidence that acute central insulin administration decreases food intake is mixed (Jessen *et al.*, 2010), acute administration of insulin into the ARC increases sympathetic outflow and hence energy expenditure (Porte *et al.*, 2002). Activation of the insulin receptor stimulates multiple downstream events and there is considerable crosstalk between leptin and insulin signaling cascades (Porte *et al.*, 2002).

During the past ten years another hormone, ghrelin, has emerged as a key regulator of energy balance. Ghrelin is secreted primarily by the P/D1 cells lining the stomach and, in contrast to leptin, this hormone increases appetite and decreases energy expenditure, promoting the accumulation of adipose tissue (reviewed in Kirchner *et al.*, 2010). Ghrelin levels show circadian variations that have predictable peaks prior to the natural feeding time of animals, and that can be entrained to environmental food availability (Kirchner *et al.*, 2010). Thus, in humans and most other mammals, ghrelin levels peak in anticipation of a scheduled meal (Kirchner *et al.*, 2010). As with leptin receptors, ghrelin receptors are found in multiple brain areas, including the hypothalamus. In contrast, to leptin, however, and in keeping with its orexigenic function, ghrelin stimulates the secretion of NPY and AGRP while decreasing POMC expression and the release of α-MSH (Kirchner *et al.*, 2010).

It is clear that the maintenance of energy balance is a tightly regulated complex process that involves multiple peripheral satiety signals and several central mediators, all acting in concert to maintain homeostasis. It is not surprising, therefore, that disruption of the normal functioning of these pathways either in the periphery or the brain can lead to serious consequences, some of which result in chronic metabolic disorders. Recent findings also suggest that a dysregulated immune system could contribute to the disease states linked with metabolic disorders, such

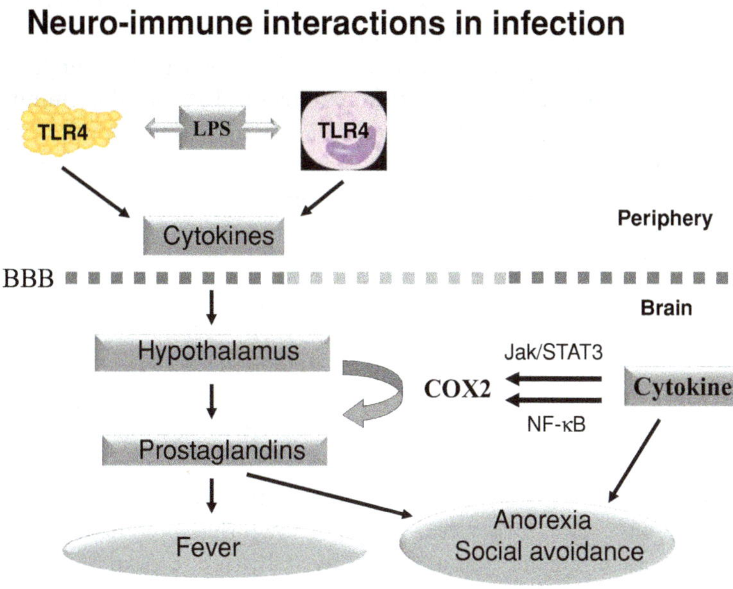

Figure 25.2 Pathways through which acute systemic inflammation induces hypothalamically regulated sickness behaviors. LPS and other bacterial pathogens activate TLR4 receptors in various tissues including white adipose tissue, resulting in cytokine production and release. The peripheral inflammatory signal then induces cytokine production within the brain, leading to the activation of the Jak/STAT and NF-κB signaling pathways in the hypothalamus, resulting in prostaglandin-mediated fever as well as anorexia. *Abbreviations:* Lipopolysaccharide (LPS), Toll-like receptor 4 (TLR4), blood–brain barrier (BBB), janus kinase/signal transducers and activators of transcription protein 3 (Jak/STAT3), nuclear factor kappa-light chain enhancer of activated B cells (NF-κB), cyclooxygenase 2 (COX2).

as obesity (Hotamisligil, 2006). As a result, a great deal of attention has been focused on how inflammation can influence the mechanisms regulating energy balance and the role of the inflammatory cytokines in this process.

Inflammation or infection results in the rapid peripheral release of a family of cytokines from macrophages and monocytes as well as from white adipose tissue (see Figure 25.2). Some cytokines such as interleukin (IL)-1β, IL-6 and tumor necrosis factor (TNF)-α are pro-inflammatory, whereas others, for example IL-10 and the endogenous antagonist to the IL-1 receptor, IL-1 receptor antagonist (ra), are anti-inflammatory (Luheshi and Rothwell, 1996, Rothwell *et al.*, 1996). Associated with these alterations is a pattern of behavioral and physiological changes which are referred to as sickness behavior. These include fever and general malaise as well as a decrease in both appetite and interest in the external environment (Dantzer *et al.*, 1998). Administration of lipopolysaccharide (LPS), a cell wall product of Gram-negative bacteria, has been used extensively to model these effects of acute inflammation in animals. LPS activates Toll-like receptors 2 and 4 to induce both the sickness symptoms and changes in circulating cytokines characteristic of acute inflammation. Using this model it has also been demonstrated that the increase of circulating cytokines is mirrored by alterations in levels of cytokines within the brain. Systemic inflammation results in the induction of IL-1β, TNF-α and other pro-and anti-inflammatory cytokines throughout the brain and it is the action of these cytokines that induce signaling cascades that lead to the behavioral responses to inflammation, such as fever and other sickness behaviors (Dantzer *et al.*, 1998).

The induction of the central cytokine response by LPS is mediated through multiple pathways including: activation of vagal afferents; a direct effect of LPS or other immune mediators on the endothelial cells lining the blood–brain barrier (BBB); active transport of peripheral cytokines across the BBB, or direct entry of circulating cytokines through areas of the CNS devoid of BBB protection such as the circumventricular organs (Rothwell *et al.*, 1996).

Cytokines and Energy Regulation

The last two decades have seen rapid growth in research linking inflammatory signals with changes in energy balance. This research has shown that the actions of pro-inflammatory cytokines are linked to anorexia as well as to obesity and its associated disorders, and some have argued that dysregulation of cytokine signaling pathways are a necessary step in the development of the obese state. Other evidence has shown that alterations in metabolic state or specific nutrients can modulate immune responses. In this section we briefly review the evidence for each of these effects.

Inflammatory cytokines and negative energy balance

A precipitous decline of food intake is perhaps one of the most dramatic behavioral effects of acute inflammation. The anorectic effect of LPS treatment has been attributed to the actions of IL-1ß in the brain because central administration of IL-1ß is sufficient to induce a decrease in food intake and in food-motivated behavior, and central administration of IL-1ra blocks this effect (Kent *et al.*, 1996). Recent evidence suggests that IL-1β-induced anorexia may be mediated through the melanocortin system. Specifically, IL-1ß receptors are found in a number of hypothalamic nuclei known to control energy balance and have been localized on subsets of pro-opiomelanocortin (POMC) and AGRP neurons in the arcuate nucleus. In addition, administration of IL-1ß increases α-MSH release from hypothalamic explants (Scarlett *et al.*, 2007), whilst reducing AGRP release (Scarlett *et al.*, 2008) and the anorectic effects of IL-1ß are eliminated by treatment with an α-MSH antagonist (Lawrence and Rothwell, 2001).

It should be noted that IL-1ß is not the only cytokine to target POMC neurons. Ciliary neurotrophic factor (CNTF) and Leukemia inhibitory factor (LIF) target and stimulate POMC neurons, and produce anorectic effects that are mediated by the activation of the gp130 receptor family (Janoschek *et al.*, 2006, Grossberg *et al.*, 2010b). Unlike other anorectic agents, the effects of CNTF on POMC expression and on body weight are long lasting, which has made CNTF an attractive alternative to leptin as a potential therapeutic compound for the treatment for obesity (Janoschek *et al.*, 2006, Grossberg *et al.*, 2010b).

Chronic conditions such as cancer, AIDS, tuberculosis, and hormone deficiency are frequently associated with another metabolic syndrome: cachexia. Unlike anorexia, cachexia involves not only a prolonged loss in appetite but also fatigue, weakness and muscle loss (Grossberg, Scarlett, and Marks, 2010a). A defining characteristic of this syndrome is that muscle loss persists even when caloric intake is restored. Patients suffering from cachexia typically show high levels of circulating pro-inflammatory cytokines including TNF-α, IL-1β, and IL-6 (see Carson and Baltgalvis, 2010, for review), and experimental models of cancer-induced cachexia have shown increased hypothalamic expression of IL-1β, and TNF-α (Lira *et al.*, 2011). Cachexia, like the anorectic response to IL-1β, has been linked to increased activation of the melanocortin system and specifically to prolonged activation of the MC4 receptor, which appears to be of primary importance in modulating energy expenditure (Grossberg, Scarlett, and Marks, 2010a) (see Figure 25.2).

Inflammatory cytokines in obesity

Perhaps the strongest impetus for proposing a link between obesity and the immune system came from the recognition that white adipose tissue (WAT) is not merely a passive energy store, but is actually an endocrine organ and both an important source, and target, of cytokines. White fat is a complex tissue comprised of macrophages, fibroblasts, and adipocytes (Murphy and Bloom, 2006). In contrast to TNF-α, IL-10 and IL-1ra are secreted primarily from macrophages and fibroblasts (Fain, 2006), the primary source of IL-6 is adipocytes, although it is also secreted by macrophages (Fain *et al.*, 2004). Increases of both pro- and anti-inflammatory cytokines have been reported in obese humans (Trayhurn and Beattie, 2001). Circulating IL-6, for example, has consistently been found to correlate with body mass index and with waist circumference (Fenkci *et al.*, 2006) with this relationship being most apparent at greater levels of obesity. Higher levels of circulating IL-6 have also been found in genetically obese mice (Harkins *et al.*, 2004) and in sedentary, but not exercised, obese Zucker rats (Xiang, Naik, and Hester, 2005). The situation with respect to TNF-α is more controversial: although some studies revealed elevated levels of this cytokine in circulation (e.g. Malavazos *et al.*, 2007), others have found no differences between obese and lean subjects (e.g., Bruun *et al.*, 2003). Only a few studies investigated levels of circulating anti-inflammatory cytokines such as IL-10 and IL-1ra in obesity (e.g., Somm *et al.*, 2006), but most of these suggested that levels of anti-inflammatory cytokines also increase.

Cachexia and prolonged obesity are frequently associated with insulin resistance (Grossberg, Scarlett, and Marks, 2010a) and, as described earlier, both of these states are associated with a chronic increase in basal cytokine secretion. The association between insulin sensitivity and pro-inflammatory cytokines, specifically IL-6 and TNF-α has been demonstrated in both rodents and humans (Kern *et al.*, 2001, Klover *et al.*, 2003). Indeed, the presence of higher titers of IL-6 may even predict the development of type-2 diabetes (Pradhan *et al.*, 2001). In addition, *in vivo* and *in vitro* studies in mice have demonstrated that IL-6 can induce insulin resistance in hepatocytes (Senn *et al.*, 2002), and that IL-6 depletion enhances liver insulin sensitivity (Klover *et al.*, 2003). It is likely that diverse mechanisms mediate the association between increased circulating levels of cytokines and insulin resistance, including the stimulation of mediators, such as inducible nitric oxide, that reduce insulin sensitivity, and a number of signaling pathways that interact with those downstream of insulin receptor activation (see Wellen and Hotamisligil, 2005, for review).

Other evidence in support of a causal role for inflammatory pathways in the development of metabolic disorders comes from the finding that obesity-induced insulin resistance is attenuated in mice lacking the TLR4 receptor (Shi *et al.*, 2006). Further, Toll-like receptor activation is not the only pathway through which immune responses are induced: recently, considerable attention has been paid to the role of another class of receptors, NOD-like receptors (NLRs), in the development of obesity (Stienstra *et al.*, 2011). Activation of NLRs, as with TLRs, is linked to cytokine production and is implicated in the innate immune response. Moreover, like TLRs, NLRs are expressed in white adipose tissue. Some NLRs, notably Nlrp3, not only recognize external pathogens but also pathogens that are produced endogenously as a result of tissue damage, and these have been implicated in autoimmune disease. Activation of Nlrp3 results in the formation of a protein complex that is referred to as the "inflammasone" by inducing activation of caspase 1, a process that depends on the interaction of both molecules with apoptosis-associated speck-like protein. In turn, activation of caspase 1 facilitates the production of IL-1β and IL-18. Recent evidence suggests that targeted deletion of the genes associated with these proteins resulted in protection from high-fat diet (HFD)-induced obesity (see Stienstra *et al.*, 2011). One might expect, given the relationship between circulating and central cytokines, that the chronic low-level inflammatory state that accompanies obesity would result in cytokine induction within the brain, and this is indeed the case. De Souza *et al.* (2005) showed that 16 weeks of high-fat diet feeding resulted in increased expression of a number of pro-inflammatory cytokines, such as IL-1β and TNF-α within the hypothalamus. It appears, however, that at least in rodent models, systemic inflammation is not a necessary precursor to hypothalamic inflammation, because as little as 3 days of exposure to a cafeteria diet comprising palatable foodstuffs such as bread, chocolate and cookies is sufficient to induce an upregulation of IL-1β and TNF-α (Hansen *et al.*, 1998).

Free fatty acids, and in particular saturated fatty acids, activate Toll-like receptor 4 to induce inflammatory cytokine production both in peripheral macrophages (Shi *et al.*, 2006) and in the hypothalamus (Milanski *et al.*, 2009). Further, Posey *et al.* (2009) showed that intracerebroventricular administration of a saturated fatty acid was sufficent to induce hypothalamic inflammation. The same interactions between cytokine and insulin signaling pathways are likely to occur in the brain as they do in the periphery, providing a mechanism through which central proinflammatory cytokines can induce central insulin and perhaps leptin resistance and thereby facilitate the development/and or maintenance of obesity. Indeed, Posey *et al.* (2009) have demonstrated that the same fatty acid infusion that induced proinflammatory cytokines in the hypothalamus also produced hypothalamic insulin insensitivity. Other evidence linking central proinflammatory pathways to energy balance come from a study showing that mice deficient in MyD88, an adaptor molecule required for TLR4 receptor signaling, only within the brain, do not show HFD-induced weight gain (Bruning, 2009).

Although saturated fats appear to exacerbate inflammatory pathways, long-chain polyunsaturated fatty acids tend to decrease cytokine production (Browning, 2003), perhaps by suppressing endoplasmic stress, and modulate the behavioral changes typically induced by IL-1β (Song, Manku, and Horrobin, 2008). Interestingly, these types of fats also protect against the development of metabolic syndome (Poudyal *et al.*, 2011).

The studies described to this point have linked inflammation to the development of the obese and/or insulin resistant state. However, there is also evidence that obesity or high blood glucose can trigger inflammation in some tissues. Several studies have associated the increased endoplasmic stress placed on cells by obesity, as well as the increased reactive oxidative species production induced by increased glucose metabolism, to activation of inflammatory pathways (reviewed in Wellen and Hotamisligil, 2005). Together, these data indicate the presence of positive feedback in the obesity/immune system relationship such that activating inflammatory pathways may promote insulin resistance and/or obesity; the high blood glucose levels and the resulting endoplasmic stress provide a further inflammatory stimulus.

Chronic low levels of inflammatory cytokines may be key in mediating some of the associations between obesity and illnesses, such as type-2 diabetes and cardiovascular disease; however, the implications of this state for responses to acute immune challenges is not clear. There is some evidence showing that obese individuals are more susceptible to opportune infections, such as those seen postoperatively (Falagas and Kompoti, 2006), and increased susceptibility to experimentally induced infection has been seen in genetically obese rats (Plotkin *et al.*, 1996) and diet-induced obese mice (Smith *et al.*, 2007).

Studies of acute immune responses in animal models of obesity resulting from targeted deletions of the *ob* gene or mutations in the leptin receptor have produced varying results, with some studies finding no effects and others indicating either increases or decreases in responses, perhaps because of varying effects of lifelong elimination or diminution of leptin signaling. In diet-induced obese rats, however, LPS injection produces a fever of a higher magnitude and a longer duration than in lean controls without affecting basal body temperature (Pohl, Woodside, and Luheshi, 2009). The exacerbated fever response is accompanied by increases of circulating levels of IL-6, TNF-α and the anti-inflammatory cytokine IL-1ra, as well as leptin, at varying time-points during the fever response. The increase of circulating IL-6 concentrations correlated with the acute rise in body temperature in both obese rats and their lean counterparts, a finding consistent with previous data showing that circulating IL-6 is the primary mediatory of the fever response. The prolonged fever of obese rats, however, was more closely associated with circulating leptin concentrations, which started to deviate from basal levels at 8 hours. The changes of circulating cytokines were associated with changes in the hypothalamic expression of both pro-inflammatory cytokines (IL-6 and IL-1β) and markers of activation of the fever pathway e.g. COX2 and suppressor of cytokine signaling 3 (SOCS3) (Pohl, Woodside, and Luheshi, 2009)

In the same studies these authors showed that the changes in peripheral and central cytokine responses to acute inflammation were associated with qualitative changes of white adipose tissue. *In vitro*, LPS stimulated more IL-6 release/gm from the WAT extracted from obese than from lean rats, suggesting that a qualitative difference in the ability of this tissue to secrete cytokines might contribute to the greater acute immune response in obese rats. Further, retroperitoneal fat pads from obese rats showed higher TLR4 mRNA expression than those of their lean counterparts, suggesting that increased sensitivity may indeed be a factor in the altered fever response. Notably, the changes in the acute immune response observed in this study were seen in young rats with moderate levels of obesity (15%) increases in weight and were not associated with increases of basal cytokines, suggesting that qualitative changes in adipose tissue depots may precede the chronic inflammatory state associated with greater and more prolonged obese states (Pohl, Woodside, and Luheshi, 2009).

Interactions of Hormone and Cytokine Signaling

The close association between pathways mediating the immune response, and those modulating energy balance is indicated by the fact that circulating levels of both leptin and ghrelin are altered following an acute immune challenge. For leptin, there now exists a great deal of evidence supporting its role in immunity, where it has been demonstrated to act in a cytokine-like fashion in concert with other mediators from the cytokine family (reviewed in La Cava and Matarese, 2004). For example, exogenous leptin has been shown to upregulate LPS-induced phagocytosis and pro-inflammatory cytokine expression ex vivo in mouse macrophages and in human circulating monocytes (Loffreda *et al.*, 1998; Santos-Alvarez, Goberna, and Sanchez-Margalet, 1999). Additionally, leptin-deficient *(ob/ob)* mice and the obese *(fa/fa)* Zucker rats exhibit attenuated levels of serum TNF-α and IL-6 in response to LPS administration. A subsequent study demonstrated that the reduction of TNF-α secretion causes resistance to endotoxin toxicity in fasted, leptin receptor deficient *(db/db)*, obese mice, thus reinforcing the importance of pro-inflammatory cytokines in mediating some actions of leptin (Madiehe, Mitchell, and Harris, 2003). Other studies in rats revealed that peripheral or central injection of leptin induced the production of hypothalamic IL-1β, and that the effects of leptin on appetite are absent in the presence of IL-1ra and in IL-1 type-I receptor knockout mice. In the same study, an appetite-suppressing dose of leptin induced a marked increase in core body temperature (fever), which was IL-1β-driven and prostaglandin-dependent (Luheshi *et al.*, 1999). In other studies (Sachot, Poole, and Luheshi, 2004) the role of endogenous leptin in mediating the inflammatory responses (fever and anorexia) induced by a systemic injection of LPS was tested. By utilizing a neutralizing antiserum raised specifically against endogenous rat leptin, it was demonstrated that this hormone is involved in propagating the inflammatory signal from the periphery to the brain by a process that involves the induction of hypothalamic IL-1β as well as COX-2. These findings, in particular, coupled with those of others showing that leptin levels increase following a systemic pathogenic stimulus (Mastronardi *et al.*, 2001) strongly suggested that endogenous leptin may be acting as a circulating neuroimmune signal of systemic inflammatory responses in the same mode as do pro-inflammatory cytokines such as IL-1β and, in particular, IL-6. In more recent studies, the role of leptin in acute responses to immunogen stimulation was functionally linked to its energy-regulating effects. This was done in studies where inducing a decrease in endogenous leptin levels by fasting, a manipulation that decreased both basal body temperature and LPS-induced fever, were reversed by leptin replacement (Inoue and Luheshi, 2010).

Similar to their opposing effects on energy balance, ghrelin and leptin appear to play opposite roles in modulation of immune pathways. In contrast to the pro-inflammatory effects of leptin, ghrelin has been shown in a wide variety of studies to have anti-inflammatory effect, which has led some authors to argue that ghrelin might have therapeutic value in inflammatory disease states (Baatar, Patel, and Taub, 2011). Ghrelin administration either before or after the challenge has been shown to suppress the induction of inflammatory cytokines in a wide variety of both *in vivo* and *in vitro* models (see review in Baatar, Patel, and Taub, 2011). Indeed, monocytes not only express the growth hormone secretagogue receptor, but it also appeared that ghrelin reduced cytokine secretion in a dose–response fashion (Dixit *et al.*, 2004, reviewed in Baatar, Patel, and Taub, 2011). Moreover, ghrelin was able to suppress leptin-induced increases in pro-inflammatory cytokine release from human T cells. In the same set of studies these authors also demonstrated that LPS-treated mice treated with ghrelin and LPS showed reduced levels of circulating cytokines IL-1β, IL-6 and TNF-α, as well as gene expression for these cytokines in liver and spleen, and also attenuated anorexia compared to mice treated with LPS alone. More recently, the ability of ghrelin to have anti-inflammatory effects in other systems including lung and kidney has been reported (Chen *et al.*, 2008; Wang *et al.* 2009).

White adipose tissue is also a target of ghrelin, where it acts to facilitate the storage of fats through upregulation of enzymes, such as lipoprotein lipase. Whether ghrelin can also modulate inflammatory pathways within this tissue remains to be determined. It has been demonstrated that the potent neuroprotective effect of ghrelin in animal models of stroke and Parkinson's disease is mediated through the downregulation of the inflammatory responses that accompany damage induced by increases in oxidative stress in these models (Andrews, 2011). These data are particularly interesting given the suggestion that inflammatory markers in obese organisms are associated with increased intracellular metabolic stress and induction of reactive oxygen species (ROS) (see Wellen and Hotamisligil, 2005) and might indicate a pathway through which ghrelin could modulate the induction of inflammation both in peripheral tissues and the central nervous system.

Intracellular Signaling Pathways Linking Leptin, Ghrelin and Immune Signals to Energy Balance

The studies reviewed provide clear evidence for a role for inflammatory signals in the control of energy balance and interactions between the primary circulating signals of energy balance and immune mediators. Here we describe some of the signaling mechanisms through which these effects are mediated, with particular emphasis on central pathways.

Several cytokines, including IL-6, CNTF and LIF, as well as leptin, have receptors that are members of the gp 130 cytokine-receptor family that are coupled to the JAK/STAT signaling pathway. Activation of these receptors results in phosphorylation of JAK, with the result that STAT3 molecules are phosphorylated, dimerized, and translocated to the nucleus, where they act as transcription factors. This common signaling pathway represents an obvious point of interaction among cytokines, and the fact that targeted mutations of the STAT3 gene cause a morbid obesity syndrome that is more pronounced than that of leptin or leptin-receptor mutant mice supports the notion that other signals that also phosphorylate STAT3 proteins may regulate energy balance (Gao *et al.*, 2004). One of the transcripts stimulated by DNA-bound pSTAT3 is the suppressor of cytokine signaling 3 (SOCS3) protein, an intracellular signal that prevents further phosphorylation of JAK and STAT proteins and thus has a negative feedback effect on the signaling pathway. Induction of SOCS3 within a particular neuron through prolonged activation of the JAK/STAT pathway would be expected to reduce signaling through other receptors coupled to the same signaling pathway, thus providing a means through which overactivation of one receptor-type could downregulate the response to activation of another. This might potentially provide a mechanism for the induction of leptin resistance by other cytokines targeting this signaling pathway. SOCS3 has also been shown to interfere with insulin receptor substrate 1 and 2 function, perhaps by targeting these proteins for degradation, and thus could potentially be a mechanism through which prolonged exposure to pro-inflammatory cytokines such as IL-6 might induce insulin resistance (Wellen and Hotamisligil, 2005).

Overexpression of SOCS 3 also suppresses the ability of leptin and other cytokines to modulate the activity of another signaling pathway: the AMP kinase pathway. AMPK is a protein kinase complex that works as a fuel sensor in the cell, and, when phosphorylated, can increase intracellular energy levels through the stimulation of fatty acid and glucose oxidation. Changes in AMPK activity are regulated in a tissue-dependent manner. Within the hypothalamus, decreasing metabolic fuel availability or increasing ghrelin signaling results in increased AMPK activity, whereas refeeding following a fast, leptin, or insulin decreased hypothalamic AMPK activity. AMPK activity appears to be upstream of the melanocortin system, as drugs that promote AMPK activity not only increase food intake and promote the expression of orexigenic peptides like NPY and AGRP, but also attenuate the anorectic effects of leptin. In contrast, drugs that block the phosphorylation of AMPK prevent ghrelin from increasing hypothalamic expression of NPY/AGRP, and ghrelin-induced food intake. Interestingly, IL-6 and CNTF stimulate the activity of AMPK in peripheral tissues like muscle. In the brain, however, both IL-6 and CNTF treatment reduce food intake and this is mediated through a decrease of AMPK activity (Steinberg *et al.*, 2009). These effects are reminiscent of the central and peripheral effects of leptin described earlier, and given the convergence in signaling pathways, IL-6- and CNTF-mediated effects on AMPK and overall energy balance may also be related to activation of JAK/STAT/SOCS3 signaling cascades.

Not all cytokines signal through the JAK/STAT pathway. A major downstream signal of IL-1 receptor activation is NF-κB. NF-κB is a transcription factor that resides in the cytoplasm, and upon stimulation is translocated to the nucleus, a process that requires phosphorylated IKKβ. Jang *et al.* (2010) showed that LPS treatment induced NF-κB activation within POMC neurons of the arcuate nucleus, presumably through activation of IL-1 receptors on POMC neurons. Inhibiting NF-κB eliminated both the ability of LPS to induce POMC transcription and LPS-induced anorexia. The fact that inhibiting NF-κB activity also eliminated the anorectic effects of leptin suggests that NF-κB maybe acting directly downstream of leptin signaling, and that there is commonality between signaling pathways for the anorectic effects of both leptin and cytokines (Jang *et al.*, 2010).

Zhang *et al.* (2008) demonstrated that hypothalamic NF-κB activation is increased in animals exposed to a high-fat diet, and that this increase is mediated by endoplasmic reticular (ER)

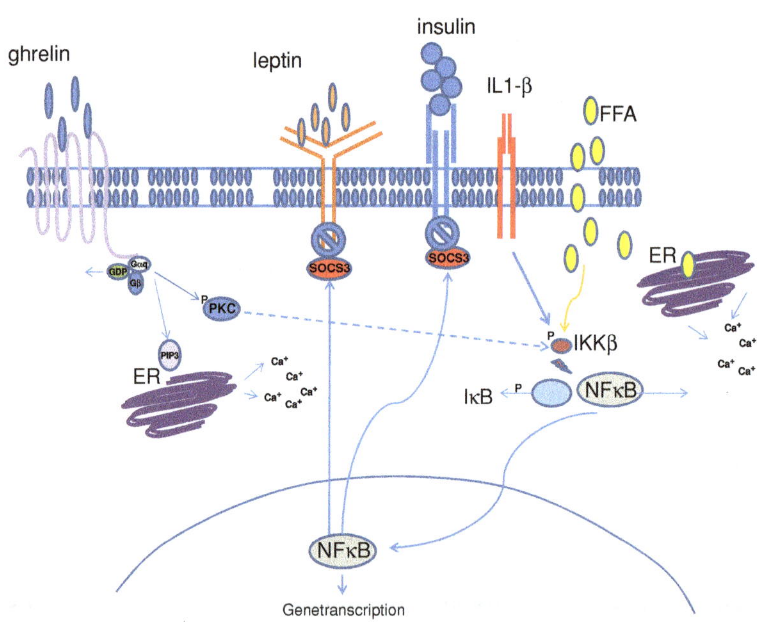

Figure 25.3 Potential mechanisms by which continuous induction of ER stress, Toll-like receptor activation, and/or ghrelin receptor activation could result in NF-κB activation, SOCS3-mediated leptin resistance, and ultimately obesity. In this model, free fatty acids (FFA) derived from overconsumption of high-fat diets produce intracellular responses associated with inflammation, including the release of intracellular calcium, stimulation of the NF-κB pathway, and ultimately metabolic stress induced by the inability of hypothalamic cells to sense feedback from adipocytes that are critical for body weight regulation, as are leptin, and insulin.

stress. Further, they administered an inducer of ER stress into the 3rd ventricle and found increased levels of NF-κB activation, suggesting a feedforward relationship between these two factors. In contrast to the role of NF-κB in mediating the anorectic response of an acute immune challenge via its effects on POMC transcription, Zhang *et al.* showed that deletion of the gene encoding IKKβ protein selectively in AGRP neurons prevents obesity induced by a high-fat diet. Transgenic mice with overactive IKKβ, and thus with increased translocation of NF-κB into the nucleus of AGRP neurons, are vulnerable to diet-induced obesity and overexpress SOCS3 (Zhang *et al.*, 2008). These data suggest that when the cells that regulate energy balance in the hypothalamus are exposed to excessive amounts free fatty acids, there is an activation of immune responses that mimic inflammatory processes. These then culminate in intracellular cell signals that attenuate leptin signaling, and thus, promote an obese phenotype (see Figure 25.3).

Remaining Questions

In spite of the progress made to this point, the current understanding of the links between metabolic and immune systems is at a relatively early stage. It is clear that immune mediators interact with metabolic pathways in multiple tissues. Similarly there is considerable evidence that energy status affects immune function, and that peripheral signals of energy balance, such as leptin and ghrelin, have important roles in this modulation. There is also ample evidence that inflammatory cytokines can target those areas of the brain and signaling pathways that have been implicated in the central control of energy balance. However, although it is clear that metabolic disorders are associated with dysregulation of immune function, whether this dysregulation has a role to play in the etiology of metabolic disorders is uncertain. Thus, while there is clear evidence for a role of immune signals in the induction of insulin resistance in peripheral tissues it is uncertain whether this occurs independently of some upstream metabolic stressor.

One of the complications in unraveling these pathways is the crosstalk amongst them, the fact that different cell types may provide different opportunities for interactions between intracellular signals and that acute versus chronic activation of these pathways can produce very different functional outcomes. How hypothalamic cells integrate these incoming signals as well as those coming from nutrients is only partially understood, yet this interaction may be critical for our understanding of how our body regulates energy balance and may hold the answers that will lead to treatments for metabolic disorders such as obesity, hypertension or cachexia.

References

Abizaid, A., and Horvath, T.L. (2008). Brain circuits regulating energy homeostasis. *Regulatory Peptides*, 149, 3–10.

Andrews, Z.B. (2011). The extra-hypothalamic actions of ghrelin on neuronal function. *Trends in Neurosciences*, 34, 31–40.

Baatar, D., Patel, K., and Taub, D.D. (2011). The effects of ghrelin on inflammation and the immune system. *Molecular and Cellular Endocrinology*, 340, 44–58.

Browning, L.M. (2003). n-3 Polyunsaturated fatty acids, inflammation and obesity-related disease. *Proceedings of the Nutrition Society*, 62, 447–453.

Bruning, J.C., Gautam, D., Burks, D.J., Gillette, J., Schubert, M., Orban, P.C., et al. (2000). Role of brain insulin receptor in control of body weight and reproduction. *Science*, 289, 2122–2125.

Bruun, J.M., Verdich, C., Toubro, S., Astrup, A., and Richelsen, B. (2003). Association between measures of insulin sensitivity and circulating levels of interleukin-8, interleukin-6 and tumor necrosis factor-alpha. *Effect of weight loss in obese men. European Journal of Endocrinology*, 148, 535–542.

Carson, J.A., and Baltgalvis, K.A. (2010). Interleukin 6 as a key regulator of muscle mass during cachexia. *Exercise and Sport Sciences Reviews*, 38, 168–176.

Chen, J, Liu, X, Shu, Q, Li, S, and Luo, F. (2008). Ghrelin attenuates lipopolysaccharide-induced acute lung injury through NO pathway. *Medical Science Monitor*, 14(7), 141–146.

Dantzer, R., Bluthe, R.M., Gheusi, G., Cremona, S., Laye, S., Parnet, P., et al. (1998). Molecular basis of sickness behavior. *Annals of the New York Academy of Sciences*, 856, 132–138.

De Souza, C.T., Araujo, E.P., Bordin, S., Ashimine, R., Zollner, R.L., Boschero, A.C., et al. (2005). Consumption of a fat-rich diet activates a proinflammatory response and induces insulin resistance in the hypothalamus. *Endocrinology*, 146, 4192–4199.

Dixit, V.D., Schaffer, E.M., Pyle, R.S., Collins, G.D., et al. (2004). Ghrelin inhibits leptin- and activation-induced proinflammatory cytokine expression by human monocytes and T cells. *Journal of Clinical Investigation*, 114(1), 57–66.

Fain, J.N. (2006). Release of interleukins and other inflammatory cytokines by human adipose tissue is enhanced in obesity and primarily due to the nonfat cells. *Vitamins and Hormones*, 74, 443–477.

Fain, J.N., Madan, A.K., Hiler, M.L., Cheema, P., and Bahouth, S.W. (2004). Comparison of the release of adipokines by adipose tissue, adipose tissue matrix, and adipocytes from visceral and subcutaneous abdominal adipose tissues of obese humans. *Endocrinology*, 145, 2273–2282.

Falagas, M.E., and Kompoti, M. (2006). Obesity and infection. *Lancet Infectious Diseases*, 6, 438–446.

Fenkci, S., Rota, S., Sabir, N., Sermez, Y., Guclu, A., and Akdag, B. (2006). Relationship of serum interleukin-6 and tumor necrosis factor alpha levels with abdominal fat distribution evaluated by ultrasonography in overweight or obese postmenopausal women. *Journal of Investigative Medicine*, 54, 455–460.

Gao, Q., Wolfgang, M.J., Neschen, S., Morino, K., Horvath, T.L., Shulman, G.I., et al. (2004). Disruption of neural signal transducer and activator of transcription 3 causes obesity, diabetes, infertility, and thermal dysregulation. *Proceedings of the National Academy of Sciences of the United States of America*, 101, 4661–4666.

Grossberg, A.J., Scarlett, J.M., and Marks, D.L. (2010a). Hypothalamic mechanisms in cachexia. *Physiology and Behavior*, 100, 478–489.

Grossberg, A.J., Scarlett, J.M., Zhu, X., Bowe, D.D., Batra, A.K., Braun, T.P., et al. (2010b). Arcuate nucleus proopiomelanocortin neurons mediate the acute anorectic actions of leukemia inhibitory factor via gp130. *Endocrinology*, 151, 606–616.

Hansen, M.K., Taishi, P., Chen, Z., and Krueger, J.M. (1998). Cafeteria feeding induces interleukin-1beta mRNA expression in rat liver and brain. *American Journal of Physiology*, 274, R1734–1739.

Harkins, J.M., Moustaid-Moussa, N., Chung, Y.J., Penner, K.M., Pestka, J.J., North, C.M., et al. (2004). Expression of interleukin-6 is greater in preadipocytes than in adipocytes of 3T3-L1 cells and C57BL/6J and ob/ob mice. *Journal of Nutrition*, 134, 2673–2677.

Hotamisligil, G.S. (2006). Inflammation and metabolic disorders. *Nature*, 444, 860–867.

Inoue, W., and Luheshi, G.N. (2010). Acute starvation alters lipopolysaccharide-induced fever in leptin-dependent and -independent mechanisms in rats. *American Journal of Physiology. Regulatory, Integrative, and Comparative Physiology*, 299, R1709–1719.

Jang, P.G., Namkoong, C., Kang, G.M., Hur, M.W., Kim, S.W., Kim, G.H., et al. (2010). NF-kappaB activation in hypothalamic pro-opiomelanocortin neurons is essential in illness- and leptin-induced anorexia. *Journal of Bioligcal Chemistry*, 285, 9706–9715.

Janoschek, R., Plum, L., Koch, L., Munzberg, H., Diano, S., Shanabrough, M., et al. (2006). gp130 signaling in proopiomelanocortin neurons mediates the acute anorectic response to centrally applied ciliary neurotrophic factor. *Proceedings of the National Academy of Sciences of the United States of America*, 103, 10707–10712.

Jessen, L., Clegg, D.J., and Bouman, S.D. (2010). Evaluation of the lack of anorectic effect of intracerebroventricular insulin in rats. *American Journal of Physiology. Regulatory, Integrative, and Comparative Physiology*, 298, R43–50.

Kent, S., Bret-Dibat, J.L., Kelley, K.W., and Dantzer, R. (1996). Mechanisms of sickness-induced decreases in food-motivated behavior. *Neuroscience and Biobehavioral Reviews*, 20, 171–175.

Kern, P.A., Ranganathan, S., Li, C., Wood, L., and Ranganathan, G. (2001). Adipose tissue tumor necrosis factor and interleukin-6 expression in human obesity and insulin resistance. *American Journal of Physiology. Endocrinology, and Metabolism*, 280, E745–7451.

Kirchner, H., Tong, J., Tschop, M.H., and Pfluger, P.T. (2010). Ghrelin and PYY in the regulation of energy balance and metabolism: lessons from mouse mutants. *American Journal of Physiology. Endocrinology, and Metabolism*, 298, E909–919.

Klover, P.J., Zimmers, T.A., Koniaris, L.G., and Mooney, R.A. (2003). Chronic exposure to interleukin-6 causes hepatic insulin resistance in mice. *Diabetes*, 52, 2784–2789.

La Cava, A., and Matarese, G. (2004). The weight of leptin in immunity. *Nature Reviews. Immunology*, 4, 371–379.

Lawrence, C.B., and Rothwell, N.J. (2001). Anorexic but not pyrogenic actions of interleukin-1 are modulated by central melanocortin-3/4 receptors in the rat. *Journal of Neuroendocrinology*, 13, 490–495.

Lira, F.S., Yamashita, A.S., Rosa, J.C., Tavares, F.L., Caperuto, E., Carnevali, L.C., Jr, et al. (2011). Hypothalamic inflammation is reversed by endurance training in anorectic-cachectic rats. *Nutrition and Metabolism (London)*, 8, 60.

Loffreda, S., Yang, S.Q., Lin, H.Z., Karp, C.L., Brengman, M.L., Wang, D.J., et al. (1998). Leptin regulates proinflammatory immune responses. *FASEB Journal*, 12, 57–65.

Luheshi, G.N., Gardner, J.D., Rushforth, D.A., Loudon, A.S., and Rothwell, N.J. (1999). Leptin actions on food intake and body temperature are mediated by IL-1. *Proceedings of the National Academy of Sciences of the United States of America*, 96, 7047–7052.

Luheshi, G., and Rothwell, N. (1996). Cytokines and fever. *International Archives of Allergy and Immunology*, 109, 301–307.

Madiehe, A.M., Mitchell, T.D., and Harris, R.B. (2003). Hyperleptinemia and reduced TNF-alpha secretion cause resistance of db/db mice to endotoxin. *American Journal of Physiology. Regulatory, Integrative, and Comparative Physiology*, 284, R763–770.

Malavazos, A.E., Corsi, M.M., Ermetici, F., Coman, C., Sardanelli, F., Rossi, A., et al. (2007). Proinflammatory cytokines and cardiac abnormalities in uncomplicated obesity: relationship with abdominal fat deposition. *Nutrition, Metabolism, and Cardiovascular Diseases*, 17, 294–302.

Mastronardi, C.A., Yu, W.H., Srivastava, V.K., Dees, W.L., and McCann, S.M. (2001). Lipopolysaccharide-induced leptin release is neurally controlled. *Proceedings of the National Academy of Sciences of the United States of America*, 98, 14720–14725.

Milanski, M., Degasperi, G., Coope, A., Morari, J., Denis, R., Cintra, D.E., et al. (2009). Saturated fatty acids produce an inflammatory response predominantly through the activation of TLR4 signaling in hypothalamus: implications for the pathogenesis of obesity. *Journal of Neuroscience*, 29, 359–370.

Murphy, K.G., and Bloom, S.R. (2006). Are all fats created equal? *Nature Medicine*, 12, 32–33.

Plotkin, B.J., Paulson, D., Chelich, A., Jurak, D., Cole, J., Kasimos, J., et al. (1996). Immune responsiveness in a rat model for type II diabetes (Zucker rat, fa/fa): susceptibility to Candida albicans infection and leucocyte function. *Journal of Medical Microbiology*, 44, 277–283.

Pohl, J., Woodside, B., and Luheshi, G.N. (2009). Changes in hypothalamically mediated acute-phase inflammatory responses to lipopolysaccharide in diet-induced obese rats. *Endocrinology*, 150, 4901–4910.

Porte, D., Jr, Baskin, D.G., and Schwartz, M.W. (2002). Leptin and insulin action in the central nervous system. *Nutrition Reviews*, 60, S20–29; discussion S68–84, 85–87.

Posey, K.A., Clegg, D.J., Printz, R.L., Byun, J., Morton, G.J., Vivekanandan-Giri, A., et al. (2009). Hypothalamic proinflammatory lipid accumulation, inflammation, and insulin resistance in rats fed a high-fat diet. *American Journal of Physiology. Endocrinology, and Metabolism*, 296, E1003-1012.

Poudyal, H., Panchal, S.K., Diwan, V., and Brown, L. (2011). Omega-3 fatty acids and metabolic syndrome: Effects and emerging mechanisms of action. *Progress in Lipid Research*, 50, 372–387.

Pradhan, A.D., Manson, J.E., Rifai, N., Buring, J.E., and Ridker, P.M. (2001). C-reactive protein, interleukin 6, and risk of developing type 2 diabetes mellitus. *Journal of the American Medical Association*, 286, 327–334.

Rothwell, N.J., Luheshi, G., and Toulmond, S. (1996). Cytokines and their receptors in the central nervous system: physiology, pharmacology, and pathology. *Pharmacology and Therapeutics*, 69, 85–95.

Sachot, C., Poole, S., and Luheshi, G.N. (2004). Circulating leptin mediates lipopolysaccharide-induced anorexia and fever in rats. *Journal of Physiology*, 561, 263–272.

Santos-Alvarez, J., Goberna, R., and Sanchez-Margalet, V. (1999). Human leptin stimulates proliferation and activation of human circulating monocytes. *Cellular Immunology*, 194, 6–11.

Scarlett, J.M., Jobst, E.E., Enriori, P.J., Bowe, D.D., Batra, A.K., Grant, W.F., et al. (2007). Regulation of central melanocortin signaling by interleukin-1 beta. *Endocrinology*, 148, 4217–4225.

Scarlett, J.M., Zhu, X., Enriori, P.J., Bowe, D.D., Batra, A.K., Levasseur, P.R., et al. (2008). Regulation of agouti-related protein messenger ribonucleic acid transcription and peptide secretion by acute and chronic inflammation. *Endocrinology*, 149, 4837–4845.

Senn, J.J., Klover, P.J., Nowak, I.A., and Mooney, R.A. (2002). Interleukin-6 induces cellular insulin resistance in hepatocytes. *Diabetes*, 51, 3391–3399.

Shi, H., Kokoeva, M.V., Inouye, K., Tzameli, I., Yin, H., and Flier, J.S. (2006). TLR4 links innate immunity and fatty acid-induced insulin resistance. *Journal of Clinical Investigation*, 116, 3015–3025.

Smith, A.G., Sheridan, P.A., Harp, J.B., and Beck, M.A. (2007). Diet-induced obese mice have increased mortality and altered immune responses when infected with influenza virus. *Journal of Nutrition*, 137, 1236–1243.

Somm, E., Cettour-Rose, P., Asensio, C., Charollais, A., Klein, M., Theander-Carrillo, C., et al. (2006). Interleukin-1 receptor antagonist is upregulated during diet-induced obesity and regulates insulin sensitivity in rodents. *Diabetologia*, 49, 387–393.

Song, C., Manku, M.S., and Horrobin, D.F. (2008). Long-chain polyunsaturated fatty acids modulate interleukin-1beta-induced changes in behavior, monoaminergic neurotransmitters, and brain inflammation in rats. *Journal of Nutrition*, 138, 954–963.

Steinberg, G.R., Watt, M.J., Ernst, M., Birnbaum, M.J. et al. (2009). Ciliary neurotrophic factor stimulates muscle glucose uptake by a PI3-kinase-dependent pathway that is impaired with obesity. *Diabetes*, 58(4), 829–839.

Stienstra, R., van Diepen, J.A., Tack, C.J., Zaki, M.H., van de Veerdonk, F.L., Perera, D., et al. (2011). Inflammasome is a central player in the induction of obesity and insulin resistance. *Proceedings of the National Academy of Sciences of the United States of America*, 108, 15324–15329.

Trayhurn, P., and Beattie, J.H. (2001). Physiological role of adipose tissue: white adipose tissue as an endocrine and secretory organ. *Proceedings of the Nutrition Society*, 60, 329–339.

Wang, W., Bansal, S., Falk, S., Ljubanovic, D., and Schrier, R. (2009). Ghrelin protects mice against endotoxemia-induced acute kidney injury. *American Journal of Physiology. Renal Physiology*, 297(4), F1032–7.

Wellen, K.E., and Hotamisligil, G.S. (2005). Inflammation, stress, and diabetes. *Journal of Clinical Investigation*, 115, 1111–1119.

Xiang, L., Naik, J., and Hester, R.L. (2005). Exercise-induced increase in skeletal muscle vasodilatory responses in obese Zucker rats. *American Journal of Physiology. Regulatory, Integrative, and Comparative Physiology*, 288, R987–991.

Zhang, X., Zhang, G., Zhang, H., Karin, M., Bai, H., and Cai, D. (2008). Hypothalamic IKKbeta/NF-kappaB and ER stress link overnutrition to energy imbalance and obesity. *Cell*, 135, 61–73.

26

Psychoneuroimmunological Processes in Coronary Artery Disease and Heart Failure

Willem J. Kop and Paula M.C. Mommersteeg

Department of Medical Psychology and Neuropsychology, Center of Research on Psychology in Somatic diseases (CoRPS), Tilburg University, the Netherlands

Morbidity and mortality related to cardiovascular diseases are major clinical and public health problems. Coronary artery disease (CAD) and heart failure (HF) are the primary diseases of the heart. The immune system plays a critical role in the underlying pathophysiological processes of atherosclerosis in CAD and myocardial hypertrophy in HF. Inflammation reflects the immune response to ongoing disease processes and inflammation also adversely affects disease progression (Hansson, 2005; Libby and Theroux, 2005; Ross, 1999). In addition to the biological aspects of CAD and HF, it is also known that chronic and acute psychological factors increase the risk of CAD (Dimsdale, 2008; Suls and Bunde, 2005) and HF (Rutledge *et al.*, 2006). Because of the interplay between psychological and immunological processes in cardiovascular disease, the knowledge base of the psychoneuroimmunological (PNI) processes in CAD (Kop and Cohen, 2007; Kop, 1994) and HF (Kop, Synowski, and Gottlieb, 2011) has increased substantially over the past decade. The general conceptual model outlining the interactions between psychological factors, immune system responses, and cardiovascular disease processes is outlined in Figure 26.1.

This chapter reviews the interactions between psychological and immunological factors in the pathophysiology of CAD and HF. A distinction will be made between gradual CAD progression versus acute clinical manifestations of CAD such as myocardial infarction and sudden cardiac death (i.e., acute coronary syndromes). This distinction is important because it partly explains the different time-trajectories of various psychological risk factors for CAD and HF. The psychological risk factors associated with increased cardiovascular risk can be categorized into chronic (e.g., personality traits such as hostility), episodic (e.g., depression), and acute factors (triggers such as outbursts of anger) (Kop, 1999). This categorization of psychological factors is also relevant to HF (Rutledge *et al.*, 2006; Kop, Synowski, and Gottlieb, 2011). In the following sections an overview will be provided of: (1) clinical manifestations of CAD and HF; (2) atherosclerotic and hypertrophic disease processes; (3) immunological processes in atherosclerosis and myocardial hypertrophy; and (4) psychoneuroimmunological pathways of CAD and HF.

The Wiley-Blackwell Handbook of Psychoneuroimmunology, First Edition. Edited by Alexander W. Kusnecov and Hymie Anisman.

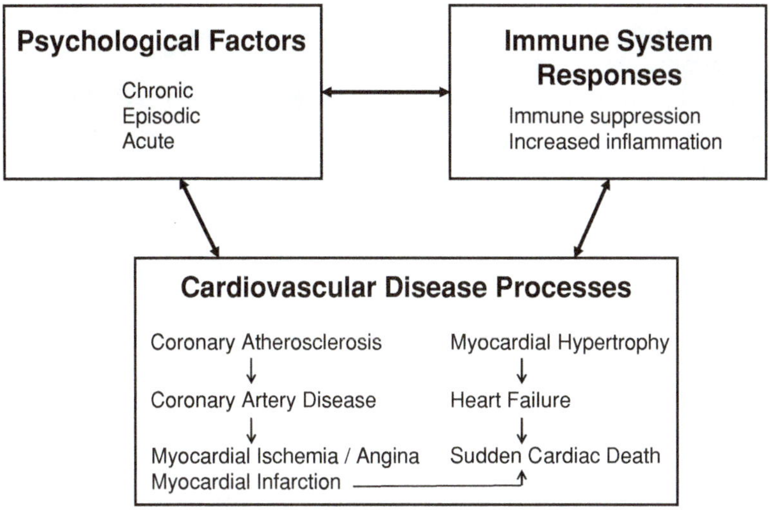

Figure 26.1 Interrelation of psychological factors and immune system responses as related to disease processes in coronary artery disease (CAD) and heart failure (HF). Early disease processes are often asymptomatic (non-obstructive coronary atherosclerosis and myocardial hypertrophy), but at later stages result in clinical conditions (in CAD: myocardial ischemia and related angina complaints or myocardial infarction; or symptomatic HF). These clinical conditions increase the risk of life-threatening arrhythmias and sudden cardiac death.

Clinical Manifestations of Coronary Artery Disease and Heart Failure

Coronary artery disease is part of the comprehensive category of cardiovascular diseases that also includes heart failure, stroke, hypertension, and congenital heart diseases among many others. Coronary artery disease involves gradual atherosclerotic plaque formation and subsequent narrowing of the coronary arteries (i.e., reduced coronary supply) which can result in myocardial ischemia (i.e., impaired blood perfusion of the heart muscle; see below for additional details). Heart diseases resulting from CAD are therefore often referred to as coronary heart disease or ischemic heart disease; terms that will not be used in the remainder of this chapter. In addition to CAD and its clinical manifestations, we also address the pathophysiological issues involved in heart failure (HF) because HF is a common consequence of myocardial infarction, and the prevalence of HF has increased substantially as a consequence of improved survival post myocardial infarction and the increased life expectancy at the population level.

The typical symptomatic manifestation of stable CAD is angina pectoris (chest pain). Angina pectoris results from ischemia (impaired blood perfusion) to the myocardium (heart muscle). Myocardial ischemia is caused by an imbalance between coronary supply (related to narrowed coronary arteries) and cardiac demand (related to factors that increase the workload of the heart muscle, such as increased heart rate and blood pressure induced by physical exertion). In stable CAD, myocardial ischemia is commonly transient and resolves when patients discontinue activities that result in increased cardiac demand (e.g., discontinue exercising) or take medications that increase coronary supply (e.g., nitroglycerine). Chest pain with physical exertion is therefore one of the typical clinical characteristics of stable CAD, as it often reflects myocardial ischemia. While chest pain is the typical manifestation of myocardial ischemia, multiple other symptoms can be considered as "angina equivalents," among which are shortness of breath, pain in other locations, and (exertion-related) fatigue.

In the majority of patients CAD remains asymptomatic and undetected until the development of a (life threatening) acute coronary syndrome (Krantz, Kop, Santiago, and Gottdiener, 1996). One reason for this phenomenon of asymptomatic CAD is that advanced atherosclerotic lesions (damaged areas) do generally not impair coronary blood flow (<75% luminal narrowing) (Ambrose *et al.*, 1988). In other words, acute coronary syndromes are often the first clinical manifestations of CAD and occur in vulnerable individuals with advanced lesions that suddenly rupture. These underlying lesions are themselves not yet obstructive enough to result in decreased coronary supply and inducible myocardial ischemia, and these lesions are therefore rarely accompanied by chest pain or other anginal symptoms.

Acute coronary syndromes include unstable angina pectoris (angina with minimal exertion or even at rest), myocardial infarction (MI) and sudden cardiac death. These acute coronary syndromes may develop if myocardial ischemia is severe and persists for more than 10 minutes (Naghavi *et al.*, 2003; Alonzo, Simon, and Feinleib, 1975). Myocardial ischemia increases the risk of cardiac electrical instability and hence life threatening arrhythmias and sudden cardiac death (Verrier, 1987).

Myocardial infarction can lead to transient or sustained poor cardiac pump function as a consequence of damage to the heart muscle, which can result in heart failure (HF). HF is a clinical syndrome of impaired cardiac function during the ejection and/or filling phase of the cardiac cycle. HF in the context of CAD is referred to ischemic HF, which accounts for approximately half of HF patients. Other etiologies of HF include alcohol overuse and hypertension, among others. HF can reflect poor cardiac pump function (low ejection fraction) or poor filling of the ventricle but with preserved ejection fraction (sometimes called "diastolic HF") and is accompanied by neurohormonal dysregulation, effort intolerance, and fluid retention. Primary symptoms of HF include fatigue and dyspnea on exertion. Approximately 5 million people in the United States have HF, and HF is associated with a 5-year mortality rate of 50%.

Thus, the risk of acute coronary syndromes and heart failure is determined by vulnerability factors in three areas: the atherosclerotic plaque, blood particles related to clot formation, and myocardial tissue (relevant to arrhythmias and heart failure) (Naghavi *et al.*, 2003). The relationship between CAD severity and acute coronary syndromes is non-linear. The rate of atherosclerotic disease progression, plaque instability, and other vulnerability factors are influenced by the immune system. Heart failure is an increasingly important area, both clinically and also in research on the interface between PNI and cardiovascular behavioral medicine (Kop *et al.*, 2011). Myocardial hypertrophy is the primary underlying disease process of HF and also involves immune-system related processes. In this chapter, we will use the severity of coronary disease to elucidate the immunological and psychosocial factors contributing to CAD progression and its clinical manifestations as acute coronary syndromes.

Atherosclerotic and Hypertrophic Disease Processes

The initial stages of coronary atherosclerosis (fatty streaks) are associated with functional alterations of the endothelium (the lining cells of the vessel wall). Endothelial damage is promoted by several factors including inflammatory processes, hypercholesterolemia, hypertension and chemical irritants (e.g., smoke and pollutants). These early lesions in the vascular wall provide a site in which lipids, macrophages and T-lymphocytes accumulate (Ross, 1999; Hansson, 2005). Fatty streaks are not associated with cardiac symptoms and may either disappear or develop into atheromata (i.e., atherosclerotic lesions) (Hansson, 2005). The next phase in early atherosclerosis is that growth factors, secreted by platelets, endothelial cells, and macrophages result in smooth muscle cell growth and migration. Endothelial dysfunction and smooth muscle cell proliferation may result in lesions of more inward layers of the coronary vascular wall.

Intermediate stages of atherosclerotic lesions involve atheromata with vessel damage of the endothelium, fibrin deposits in the intima, and/or lipid-laden phagocytes (i.e., foam cells). In addition, these lesions also include immune cells such as T-cells, macrophages, and mast cells. Because these cells are activated they produce inflammatory cytokines. The arterial luminal narrowing is generally minimal at this stage because of compensatory vessel dilatation (remodeling) and an inward growth of the lesion. These lesions are covered by a fibrous layer of smooth muscle cells and collagen. This layer is thin and can easily rupture, causing severe vascular lesions and blood clot formation.

The advanced stage of CAD is characterized by damage to all three layers of the vessel wall: endothelium, intima and the elastic lamina. Ruptured lesions can (temporarily) obstruct the lumen (i.e., the open "tube" part of a blood vessel). In addition, collagen is exposed to the blood when these lesions rupture, which is highly thrombogenic. Subsequent platelet adhesion and aggregation as well as coagulation and fibrinolytic processes are involved in the formation and stabilization of the thrombus (blood clot). These blood clots can cause a permanent complete blockage of the coronary artery, in turn causing damage to the heart tissue that is dependent on the affected vessel (i.e., myocardial infarction).

Acute coronary syndromes commonly occur as a result of plaque rupture or endothelial erosion often combined with occlusive thrombus formation. As mentioned, these conditions generally develop in the setting of relatively stable but non-obstructive atherosclerotic plaques (< 75% narrowing of the coronary artery diameter) (Ambrose *et al.*, 1988). Advanced coronary lesions lead three times as often to a total coronary artery occlusion compared with less severe lesions (Ambrose *et al.*, 1988). However, the relationship between atherosclerotic disease severity and risk of acute coronary syndromes is complex and atherosclerotic disease progresses in periodic spurts of growth (Yokoya *et al.*, 1999). Nonetheless, physical disruption of the atherosclerotic plaque accounts for virtually all acute coronary syndromes (Libby and Theroux, 2005).

In addition to atherosclerotic disease processes relevant to CAD, hypertrophy of the cardiac muscle often co-occurs with ischemic CAD. Myocardial hypertrophy can lead to stiffening of the heart muscle, poor cardiac pump function and subsequently HF. Myocardial hypertrophy and atherosclerosis are distinct disease processes, although there are several common immunological processes involved (see below). Hypertrophy can also develop in the absence of CAD resulting from hypertension or in the setting of various cardiovascular diseases.

In summary, atherosclerosis progresses from minor endothelial injury (fatty streaks) via intimal damage (atheromata) to plaques that involve all layers of the vessel wall. The nature and speed of the processes causing progression from moderate to severe lesions are mediated by immunological factors and are associated with major clinical consequences, including unstable anginal complaints and acute coronary syndromes. Initially, platelet adhesion and aggregation, arterial engulfment of lipids, macrophages and T-cells, as well as smooth muscle cell proliferation play a crucial role. At later CAD stages, thrombosis and impaired fibrinolysis contribute to the development of severe coronary lesions. Prolonged coronary disease often results in gradual vessel narrowing, which may be accompanied by anginal complaints. The disruption of relatively small atherosclerotic plaques plays a crucial role in the pathogenesis of acute myocardial infarction. Myocardial infarction can lead to sustained reduced pump function of the heart and HF. Myocardial hypertrophy can also lead to impaired cardiac pump function in the absence of coronary atherosclerosis and CAD. Immune system processes play an important role at early and late stages of CAD and HF and will be discussed in the next section.

Immunological Processes in Atherosclerosis and Myocardial Hypertrophy

The "response to injury" model of cardiovascular disease builds on the observation that vascular wall and subclinical myocardial tissue damage are an essential aspects of the disease process (Ross, 1999). Research on the inflammatory component of atherosclerosis can be found in reports from the 19th century by pioneers such as von Rokitansky and Virchow. Clinical observations further support immune system involvement in cardiovascular diseases. Several clinical examples highlight the importance of immunological processes in CAD and HF. Rheumatic arthritis and HIV are associated with adverse cardiovascular consequences (Wolfe *et al.*, 1994). Patients undergoing splenectomy have an increased risk of myocardial infarction (Robinette and Fraumeni, Jr., 1977). Another example is that influenza vaccinations among post-MI patients have beneficial cardiovascular effects (Gurfinkel, de la Fuente, Mendiz, and Mautner, 2002). Monoclonal antibody and DNA studies technology have shown that immunological and growth-mediating factors affect endothelial cells and smooth muscle cells at various stages of CAD and abnormal collagen metabolism in HF.

Longitudinal epidemiological investigations further support the immunological processes in CAD. Non-specific markers of systemic inflammation, such as C-reactive protein (CRP), are associated with an increased risk for cardiovascular events (Danesh *et al.*, 2004). CRP is a nonspecific marker of systemic inflammation, which activates coronary endothelium and accumulates in plaques. CRP levels tend to be stable over time (e.g., the within-person correlation coefficient of CRP over 12 years = 0.59; Danesh *et al.*, 2004) and may therefore reflect sustained low-grade inflammation related to subclinical atherosclerosis. Other predictors of CAD are pro-inflammatory cytokines, particularly interleukin 6 (IL-6), and tumor necrosis factor α (TNF-α) (Danesh, Collins, and Peto, 1997; Cesari *et al.*, 2003).

All stages of CAD involve immune system-related processes. Early stages of atherosclerosis are characterized by immunological effector molecules involved in lesion progression. Primary processes involve arterial lipid deposition and engulfment of T-lymphocytes in the atherosclerotic wall as well as the proliferation and migration of smooth muscle cells. The initial inflammatory response to arterial injury is adaptive. However, if the inflammatory reaction does not remove the damaging agent and inflammation persists, then this protective response can turn pathogenic. The subsequent "walling off" of the damaged area may perpetuate an inflammation-impaired response to injury cascade similar to other chronic inflammatory diseases (Ross, 1999). A vicious circle may then develop characterized by inflammation, lipid modification and oxidation, arterial damage, and further inflammation (Ross, 1999; White, 1997).

Once atherosclerotic plaques have developed, the onset of acute coronary syndromes is promoted by inflammation-related plaque activation and thrombus formation. Cardiac myocytes produce cytokines in response to ischemia. Inflammatory processes at this stage of atherosclerosis also interact with thrombogenic and fibrinolytic factors, resulting in plaque instability and higher risk of coronary thrombosis.

The primary immune system markers involved in CAD and HF involve macrophages (specialized monocytes), lymphocytes (T-cells, B-cells, natural killer (NK) cells), cytokines (messenger molecules), acute-phase reactants (acute inflammation markers, e.g., CRP and clotting factors such as fibrinogen and factor VII) and cell adhesion molecules (extracellular attractors binding cells of the immune system). In addition, microorganisms (e.g. bacteria, viruses) purportedly contribute to CAD and HF. Macrophageous foam cells in the vascular wall originate from circulating monocytes. The differentiation of these circulating monocytes into macrophages that occurs in the vascular wall is essential to atherosclerosis because it results in upregulation of scavenger receptors and Toll-like receptors on the outside of these cells. These receptors result in activation of the innate immune response, leading to enhanced lipid uptake, oxidation and metabolism by macrophages. As a consequence, the lipid-ridden macrophageous foam cells release cytokines and induce growth factors, which further attracts inflammatory cells. Lymphocytes can be passively deposited or actively engulfed in the arterial wall via the cellular adhesion molecules. B-lymphocytes and NK cells do not seem to substantially contribute to atherosclerosis whereas T-lymphocytes play a critical role, particularly when they become activated (Hansson, 2005). T-cells in atherosclerotic plaques are primarily T_H1 ($CD4^+$) cells involved in the defense against intra-cellular pathogens (anti-inflammatory), and to a lesser extent T_H2 ($CD8^+$) cells (pro-inflammatory). T-cell activation leads to cytokine release, which explains why elevated circulating levels of the cytokine IL-6 can be detected in the peripheral circulation of patients at risk of clinical CAD. Pro-inflammatory cytokines (particularly IL-1 and TNF-α) stimulate cellular adhesion molecules which contribute to the binding of monocytes, T-lymphocytes and platelets to the vascular endothelium. In addition to cytokines, chemokines, stem/muscle progenitor cell homing, and chemotaxis play a role in ischemic cardiac tissue (Bosch *et al.*, 2003). Activated macrophages and T-cells produce cytokines and metalloproteases (MMPs: protein and/or peptide dissolving enzymes) resulting in local extracellular matrix disruption and hence rupture of advanced atherosclerotic plaques and subsequent acute coronary syndromes.

Based on these observations, several studies have examined the role of anti-inflammatory interventions in CAD and HF. A systematic literature review indicated that TNF-α antagonists appear to reduce the risk of cardiac events in patients with rheumatic arthritis (Westlake *et al.*, 2011). However, subsequent clinical trials in HF patients using TNF-α antagonists have been negative, and the use of these agents is now contraindicated in patients with rheumatic arthritis with co-morbid moderate to severe HF (Cacciapaglia *et al.*, 2011).

Microorganisms have received special scientific attention in the etiology of CAD. Elevated levels of antibodies to various pathogens are found in patients with CAD. These "seroepidemiological" studies indicate that chronic infections can contribute to CAD. Research on pathogens in CAD was initiated in the 1950s showing that avian herpes virus (Marek) can induce atherosclerosis in chickens (Paterson and Cottral, 1950). Later evidence confirmed that gingivitis (inflammation of the gums) in humans is related to an increased risk of cardiovascular events (Beck *et al.*, 1996). Pathogens associated with increased risk include *Helicobacter pylori*, *Chlamydia pneumoniae* and cytomegalovirus (CMV) (Danesh *et al.*, 1997). It appears that *C. pneumonia* and CMV are associated with a two-fold risk of acute coronary syndrome (ACS), but that risks associated with *H. pylori* may reflect low socioeconomic status and other common factors (Danesh *et al.*, 1997). A wide range of other pathogens have been identified as CAD risk factors and some investigations have focused on the total number of infections (pathogen burden) (Zhu *et al.*, 2001). The effects of microorganisms do not necessarily require a productive (active) infection. Pathogens can have direct effects and indirect effects on the pathophysiology of cardiovascular diseases (Danesh *et al.*, 1997; Libby, Egan, and Skarlatos, 1997). The "innocent bystander" is probably the most plausible explanation of the microorganisms–CAD association. It has, for example, been challenging to culture microorganisms from atherosclerotic tissue. Furthermore, common causal factors (e.g., age, low socioeconomic status, access to health care, adverse environmental exposures and pollution, and possibly chronic psychological distress) may explain the observed associations (Wald, Law, Morris, and Bagnall, 1997). Finally, intervention trials using antibiotics targeting *C. pneumoniae* have not been successful in reducing recurrent cardiac events (Cercek *et al.*, 2003; Grayston *et al.*, 2005). It is possible that microorganisms trigger the onset of atherosclerotic disease without persisting in the infected tissue, but this hypothesis remains to be confirmed (Libby *et al.*, 1997). Fever is also known to increase the vascular wall-stress which may lead to plaque rupture and ACS in vulnerable patients with advanced CAD (Libby *et al.*, 1997).

Regarding HF, multiple studies show that CRP and pro-inflammatory cytokines (primarily IL6 and TNF-α) predict mortality among HF patients (for reviews see Kapadia, 1999; Pasic, Levy, and Sullivan, 2003). Pro-inflammatory cytokines are activated following myocardial injury as well as hemodynamic overload. Immune system-related factors involved in left ventricular or atrial remodeling include hypertrophy, apoptosis, and altered gene expression in cardiac myocytes (Kapadia, 1999). Poor cardiac pump function in HF results from myocardial muscle stiffness caused by fibrosis (de Souza, 2002), which is influenced by inflammatory processes (Funder, 1995). Inflammation also plays a major role in a syndrome of wasting in end-stage HF (i.e., cardiac cachexia). Pharmacological trials aimed at antagonizing cytokine activity (e.g., the anti-TNF-α agents etanercept and infliximab) have thus far been unsuccessful in improving HF outcomes (Anker and Coats, 2002; Cacciapaglia *et al.*, 2011). The myocardium itself also produces pro-inflammatory cytokines in response to HF. In addition to a response to tissue damage, activation of the sympathetic nervous system plays a role in HF-related cytokine elevation as well (Parthenakis *et al.*, 2003). Thus, evidence indicates a bidirectional association between the immune system and HF.

In summary, inflammatory processes contribute to CAD and HF, but further research is needed to determine whether inflammation is a primary precipitant of CAD and/or HF, or whether inflammation reflects a secondary response to the ongoing atherosclerotic or hypertrophic disease processes. Parallel to these immune-system-related processes directly related to atherosclerosis and hypertrophy, the immunological correlates of CAD and HF can also reflect correlates of risk factors such as hypertension, diabetes, renal dysfunction, dyslipidemia, obesity, and smoking.

Psychological Risk Factors for Coronary Artery Disease and Heart Failure

An extensive literature addresses the role of psychological factors in the progression of CAD (Kop, 1999; Suls and Bunde, 2005) and heart failure (Rutledge *et al.*, 2006; Kop *et al.*, 2011). The underlying disease severity influences the nature and magnitude of the associations between psychological factors with clinical disease outcomes. Psychological risk factors for cardiovascular disease can be classified into three categories, based on their duration and temporal proximity to the onset of clinical syndromes: 1) chronic psychological and social factors, such as negative personality traits (e.g., hostility) and low socioeconomic status; 2) episodic factors with a duration of several months up to 2 years, among which are depression and exhaustion; and 3) acute triggers, including acute mental distress and outbursts of anger (Kop, 1999).

It is also known that the exposure duration of psychological distress influences the nature of its immunological correlates (Segerstrom and Miller, 2004). Furthermore, epidemiological studies indicate that the association of psychological factors with future cardiovascular events and mortality is partly attributable to immunological processes, particularly inflammation (Whooley *et al.*, 2008; Kop *et al.*, 2010). In the following sections, we will selectively review evidence for the adverse cardiovascular risks associated with each of these three categories of psychological factors. Per category, we will describe the potential immunological mediators involved as possible pathophysiological mechanisms.

The primary pathways by which the central nervous system (CNS) affects the immune system are the hypothalamic–pituitary–adrenal (HPA) axis and the autonomic nervous system. Corticotropin-releasing hormone (CRH) responses characterize acute and chronic psychological distress-induced HPA activation. CRH release results in a wide range of immune system responses, particularly those related to inflammation. The autonomic nervous system also plays an important role in the acute-phase reaction via the parasympathetically mediated "cholinergic anti-inflammatory pathway" (Tracey, 2002). As is shown in Figure 26.2, chronic psychological risk factors may promote the onset of initial stages of atherosclerosis by sympathetic nervous system-mediated pathophysiological consequences (e.g., lipid deposition and inflammatory processes) and/or as a result of their association with known cardiovascular risk factors (e.g., hypertension, smoking, lipids, and obesity). At advanced disease stages, acute psychological risk factors may trigger cardiac ischemia or malignant arrhythmias leading to acute coronary syndromes.

Chronic psychological risk factors

Relationship with cardiac disease Chronic psychological factors include personality traits such as hostility and the Type A behavior pattern, neuroticism, Type D personality, and trait anxiety. These personality traits have genetic underpinnings and are also influenced by an individual's environment during early development and possibly throughout the lifespan. In addition to personality traits, chronic factors relevant to cardiovascular disease also involve socioeconomic factors associated with psychological distress, including poverty, low socioeconomic status, racism, and lack of resources.

Chronic psychological risk factors may promote the onset of initial stages of atherosclerosis by various biobehavioral pathways starting in young adulthood, including sympathetic nervous system-mediated processes (e.g., lipid deposition and inflammation), adverse health behaviors (e.g., smoking, poor dietary habits, reduced physical activity) and/or their association with known CAD risk factors (e.g., hypertension, smoking, lipids, and obesity). At advanced disease stages, these chronic psychological factors may increase the effects of acute psychological risk factors thereby triggering acute coronary syndromes.

Hostility and the Type A behavior pattern have been extensively investigated as cardiovascular risk factors. This line of research was started by Friedman and Rosenman in the late 1950s

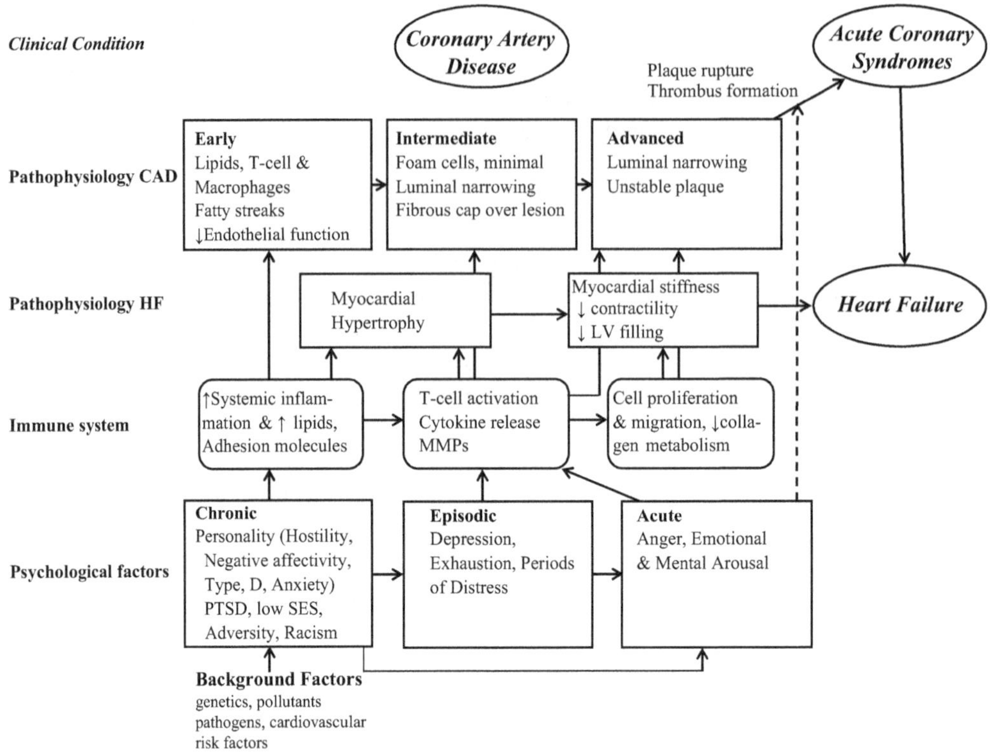

Figure 26.2 Conceptual model of the relationships between cardiovascular disease progression (atherosclerosis and hypertrophy), immune system-related disease processes and psychological risk factors. A distinction is made between chronic, episodic, and acute psychological risk factors for CAD and HF. Chronic psychological factors increase the risk of early atherosclerosis, especially in the setting of genetic vulnerability, adverse health behaviors, and other environmental risk factors. Chronic psychological factors are also related to an increased risk of developing episodic factors and more frequent occurrence of and exaggerated responses to acute psychological factors. Episodic psychological factors have immune system correlates that are involved in the progression of severe coronary disease to acute coronary syndromes. Acute psychological factors result in a partial immune system activation that may cause plaque instability and increased blood clotting tendencies. In vulnerable patients, these cardiac effects may result in plaque instability and rupture with subsequent myocardial infarction. (Modified from Kop and Cohen, 2001.)

(e.g., (Rosenman *et al.*, 1975)). Later studies have indicated that hostility is probably the toxic component of Type A behavior. Hostility is a trait characterized by cynical mistrust, aggressive responding, and an overall antagonistic attitude (Barefoot, Dahlstrom, and Williams, 1983). Hostility/Type A behavior is associated with more severe CAD and also with an increased risk of incident (i.e., first) myocardial infarction during follow-up (Barefoot, Dahlstrom, and Williams, 1983). The association between hostility and myocardial infarction is stronger in younger (< 55 years of age) than older men. In contrast, evidence for the predictive value of hostility/Type A behavior for *recurrent* coronary events is less consistent.

In addition to hostility, other psychological traits such as trait anxiety as well as sociological factors – particularly low socioeconomic status – may act as additional sources of persistent exposure to psychological distress. A general underlying trait factor that predisposes individuals to chronic distress may explain some of the overlap in the predictive value of these traits. The "distressed" or Type D personality refers to a chronic form of distress characterized by an individual's inclination to experience negative emotions (negative affectivity) combined with the inhibition of self-expression in social interaction (social inhibition) (Denollet, Schiffer, and Spek, 2010). Several studies have shown that Type D personality reflects a general propensity to psychological distress that adversely affects cardiovascular outcomes, although some studies have not found such associations, particularly in HF patients (for review see Denollet *et al.*, 2010). More research is needed to establish the content as well as divergent validity of the Type D construct versus more established constructs such as neuroticism. A general psychosocial (trait)vulnerability factor seems nonetheless plausible (Denollet *et al.*, 2010).

Post-traumatic stress disorder can be viewed as an "acquired" chronic risk factor and is predictive of increased healthcare use, adverse cardiovascular risk factors, and increased cardiovascular morbidity and mortality (Boscarino, 2008). Rumination about the adverse event may be the key factor in the risk of PTSD for adverse cardiac outcomes. Repeated intrusions and ruminations can lead to continuously elevated central and autonomic nervous system activity, thereby promoting atherosclerosis and cardiac hypertrophy (Brosschot, Gerin, and Thayer, 2006).

Little is known about chronic psychological risk factors in HF, particularly constructs related to anger and hostility. Studies on Type D personality have been largely negative for HF, in contrast to the positive findings with other cardiovascular outcomes (Denollet *et al.*, 2010). Low socioeconomic status is associated with poor HF prognosis (Philbin, Dec, Jenkins, and DiSalvo, 2001), which may have important implications for PNI research in HF, and socioeconomic status may be an important contributor to chronic psychological factors in HF.

Immunological correlates Atherosclerosis may initially be promoted by low-grade inflammation as a consequence of the immunosuppressive effects of chronic persistent psychological distress (Kop and Cohen, 2007). Hostility is associated with elevated plasma IL-6 in otherwise healthy individuals and with the percentage of monocytes in patients with acute coronary syndromes. Chronic factors, particularly low socioeconomic status and relative deprivation may result in increased exposure to a wide range of pathogens. In addition to these cross-sectional correlations, hostility is also related to higher immune responses during laboratory challenge tasks, including elevated levels of NK cells and more NK cell cytotoxicity (for details and references see Kop and Cohen, 2007).

No studies to date have examined the interaction between hostility and immune parameters in HF patients. One study has demonstrated elevated TNF-α as well as sTNFR1 and sTNFR2 (soluble receptors of TNF-α) levels in HF with the Type D personality (Denollet *et al.*, 2003). These soluble receptors can be understood as a "slow release reservoir," reflecting local activation of TNF-α rather than acting as independent immune system molecules. The PNI component of chronic psychological and social risk factors in HF remains largely unexplored.

Summary Chronic psychological traits are associated with persistent alterations in immunological parameters. In addition to the sustained biobehavioral correlates, chronic psychological factors may also increase the likelihood of developing proximate psychological risk factors such as episodes of exhaustion and frequent occurrences of acute psychological distress, which have immune system correlates relevant to cardiovascular disease (see below). For example, hostility is associated with elevated immune responses to acute challenging conditions over and above an elevated low-grade inflammatory state during rest. Chronic psychological factors other than hostility (e.g., trait anxiety, neuroticism, Type D personality, and PTSD) and socioeconomic factors may affect CAD and HF because of their association with persistent and or intermittent experiences of psychological distress. Exaggerated reactivity has not been consistently found in these chronic conditions (other than hostility) and other response patterns may be relevant, including delayed recovery. Cardiovascular risk factors (e.g., dyslipidemia and hypertension), and adverse health behaviors (smoking and poor dietary habits) are disproportionately elevated in individuals with chronic psychological risk factors. The immunological processes associated with these cardiovascular risk factors and health behaviors may further enhance the association between chronic psychological factors and cardiovascular disease risk (Winkleby, Jatulis, Frank, and Fortmann, 1992; Mommersteeg and Pouwer, 2012).

Episodic psychological risk factors

Relationship with cardiac disease Episodic psychological risk factors are transient and recurring, with durations ranging from several weeks to 2 years. In this section we will first summarize research on depressive episodes, followed by investigations on episodes of vital exhaustion and psychological distress.

Depression is predictive of first and recurrent myocardial infarction and sudden cardiac death (for review see for example Nicholson, Kuper, and Hemingway, 2006). Prevalence estimates of depressive mood disorder range from 15% to 40% in patients with CAD (Kop, 1999) and depression is even more prevalent in clinical HF (Kop *et al.*, 2011). The need for a coordinated detection and treatment plan for depression has been outlined by the American Heart Association (Lichtman *et al.*, 2008). Although multiple practical and theoretical concerns remain, this statement emphasizes the importance of depression in CAD and HF.

The onset of depressive episodes in cardiac patients can be precipitated by: 1) biological and physiological changes that are a consequence of cardiovascular disease (e.g., atherosclerosis-related inflammation) which can affect the CNS; 2) psychological reactions to disease-related symptoms, functional limitations and/or having a life-threatening disease; and 3) environmental challenges that are unrelated to cardiac disease *per se* (e.g., economic factors, living alone/social isolation, alcohol overuse). Common genetic predisposing factors for cardiovascular disease and depression may also contribute to the high prevalence in CAD and HF (McCaffery *et al.*, 2006).

The risk for incident and recurrent cardiovascular events associated with depression is approximately two-fold (Nicholson *et al.*, 2006). The predictive value of depression decreases when the follow-up period exceeds 2 years (Nicholson *et al.*, 2006). It has therefore been hypothesized that the duration of depression and other episodic risk factors may not be long enough to initiate and sustain an atherosclerotic process. Rather than gradual disease progression, plaque activation may be primarily involved in the adverse risk associated with depression and other episodic psychological risk factors (Kop, 1999).

The clinical presentation of depression in cardiac patients is often very different from those observed in psychiatric patients. Fatigue or lack of energy, and irritability occur more frequently in cardiac patients than typical symptoms of depression, such as sad or depressed mood states or feelings of guilt and low self-esteem (for reviews see Kop, 1999).

As in CAD, depression is also the best-documented psychological factor associated with clinical HF progression, with a greater than two-fold risk of mortality, hospitalizations and functional decline (Rutledge *et al.*, 2006; Kop *et al.*, 2011). Functional status plays a primary role in HF-related depression, with the most severe depression occurring at the time of acute HF exacerbations and functional decline (Koenig, 1998).

Fatigue is among the most common premonitory symptoms of acute coronary syndromes and one of the core symptoms of CAD and HF. The state of extreme fatigue that precedes acute cardiac events is referred to as "vital exhaustion." The term "vital" is used in this construct to emphasize the far-reaching consequences of this condition on daily life functioning, and will be omitted in the remainder of this chapter. Exhaustion consists of a combination of lack of energy, increased irritability, and feelings of demoralization. Exhaustion is of predictive value for cardiovascular events disease (Kop, 1999). There is substantial overlap in the constructs of exhaustion and depression, but there seem to be important differences in biological concomitants (Kop, 1999). Exhaustion purportedly reflects the end-stage of prolonged uncontrollable psychological distress, which is not necessarily an etiological condition for depression. The importance of exhaustion is further supported by the recent scientific developments indicating that "somatic depressive symptoms" (fatigability, sleep problems, appetite changes, and psychomotor alterations) are associated with better predictive value of post-myocardial infarction mortality and hospitalization than "cognitive-affective depressive symptoms" (depressed mood, lack of interest/anhedonia, negative feelings about self, concentration problems and suicidal ideation) (Smolderen *et al.*, 2009). In relatively rare cases, exhaustion may reflect severe underlying cardiac pathology, particularly if this state is of recent onset and occurs immediately post exertion.

Psychological distress may be the common factor involved in both depression and exhaustion as cardiovascular risk factors (Gold, Goodwin, and Chrousos, 1988). Various domains of psychological distress have been identified (e.g., job strain, loss of employment, marital distress, prolonged distress following natural disasters, and care giving of a chronically ill family member). A large international study (INTERHEART) used a case-control design of 11,119 patients hospitalized for myocardial infarction versus 13,648 age- and sex-matched controls. Participants were enrolled from continents across the world. Higher levels of perceived stress, depression and low locus of control were associated with myocardial infarction (p-values all <0.0001). General distress (at work and/or home) was associated with an increased risk of myocardial infarction (odds ratio (OR) = 1.45, 95%CI = 1.30–1.61 for several periods of distress and OR = 2.17, 95%CI = 1.84–2.55 for permanent distress). A dose–response relationship was found for psychological distress but not for depression.

A (transient) homeostatic imbalance may be characteristic of episodic risk factors. The most common finding is that depression, especially melancholia, is associated with increased activation of the corticotropin releasing hormone (CRH) system and hence elevated cortisol levels. In addition to neuroendocrine correlates, episodic risk factors are related to sympathetic overactivity and decreased parasympathetic activity, hemostatic cardiovascular risk factors including impaired fibrinolysis, increased platelet adhesion and aggregation, and increased blood clotting tendencies (von Kanel, Mills, Fainman, and Dimsdale, 2001). Studies have found elevated hemodynamic responsiveness among individuals with episodic risk factors (Kibler and Ma, 2004), although this has not been consistently documented in CAD patients (Kop, 1999). These findings may in part reflect what has been described as increased allostatic load (physiological burden) in individuals with episodic risk factors (depression, exhaustion and periods of prolonged psychological distress) (Seeman *et al.*, 1997).

Immunological correlates The immunological correlates of depression are relatively well established (Kop and Cohen, 2007). Depression is associated with elevated cytokine levels, increased numbers of neutrophils and monocytes, decreased lymphocytes, elevated CRP levels, and reduced "functional" immune measures (e.g., lower NK cell activity and a decreased proliferative lymphocytic response to mitogens) (Ladwig *et al.*, 2003; Segerstrom and Miller, 2004). Patients with clinical depression also have increased antibody levels of herpes viruses, including cytomegalovirus (CMV) (Miller, Freedland, Duntley, and Carney, 2005) which is associated with reduced T-helper cells and other markers of immunosuppression, which in turn could be accompanied by increased innate immune system activity. These associations are, at least partially affected by adverse health behaviors such as overweight (Douglas, Taylor, and O'Malley, 2004). It is likely that multiple pathways are involved in the immune system correlates of depression because inflammation markers are not consistently interrelated among depressed individuals. The immune system correlates of depression are quite similar to those observed in exhaustion and periods of psychological distress (Segerstrom and Miller, 2004) and may link episodic risk factors to clinical manifestations of CAD and HF.

The condition referred to as "sickness behavior" provides an explanation for the association between symptoms of depression and fatigue with inflammation markers (Dantzer and Kelley, 1989; Goodkin and Appels, 1997). Sickness behavior includes reduced social and sexual behaviors, increased pain sensitivity, reduced activity levels, depressed mood, cognitive alterations, and decreased food and liquid intake. This behavioral phenotype can be provoked by administration of cytokines and pathogens. It is likely that sickness behavior has adaptive functions because it results in reduced energy expenditure. Infection can result in non-specific sickness behavior responses via cytokines, resulting in symptoms such as fatigue, fever, apathy, general malaise, and irritability. Fatigue and malaise are common side effects of cytokine administration (e.g. IL-1) (Dantzer and Kelley, 1989). In addition to the effects of the CNS on the immune system, via neurohormonal and/or autonomic pathways, the immune system (e.g., IL-1 and TNF-α) can activate the HPA axis, which in turn has been associated with depression (Sapolsky *et al.*, 1987; Dantzer and Kelley, 1989). Thus, animal studies on sickness behavior and clinical observations in humans support a bidirectional relationship between immune system parameters and depressive symptoms.

Summary The relationship between episodic psychological factors and immune system parameters is bidirectional, such that CNS correlates of depression, fatigue, and prolonged psychological distress result in immune system changes, and vice versa. Immunosuppression of the specific adaptive immune system is well-documented in depression and may also play a role in other episodic risk factors. Some of the immunological correlates of episodic risk factors (e.g., increased levels of leukocytes, cytokines, and antibodies to viruses) are also associated with elevated risk for acute coronary syndromes and HF. In patients at risk of myocardial infarction, these low-grade inflammation processes may destabilize atherosclerotic plaques, thus increasing the risk of plaque rupture and subsequent acute coronary syndromes. It is hypothesized that plaque activation, rather than gradual CAD progression, plays a key role in the adverse risk associated with *episodic* psychological risk factors. Prospective clinical and epidemiological studies may clarify the time-trajectory of immunological and psychological factors in patients at risk for acute coronary syndromes and HF exacerbations.

Acute psychological risk factors

Relationship with cardiac disease Approximately one in five acute coronary syndromes are "triggered" by physical or psychological factors. Cardiac events that are triggered by acute psychological factors are commonly referred to as "mental stress-induced events." Outbursts of anger are associated with a two-fold risk of myocardial infarction, as documented in a case-crossover study of 1623 patients interviewed about their activities and psychological state prior to their event (Mittleman *et al.*, 1995). Myocardial infarctions that are triggered by acute physical or emotional stressors are not necessarily associated with more severe underlying CAD and also not with a worse 1-year prognosis (Brodov *et al.*, 2008). HF is in general a chronic condition, with intermittent exacerbations (i.e., decompensation, pump-failure, and arrhythmias). The immediate precipitants of HF exacerbations are not well documented, and it is possible that health behaviors such as dietary control and medication adherence are more pertinent factors contributing to HF exacerbations and acute coronary syndromes.

The pathophysiological mechanisms associated with acute psychological factors, such as anger, involve CNS-mediated autonomic, neuroendocrine and homeostatic responses. The autonomic nervous system response is characterized by a shift toward increased activity of the sympathetic nervous system and decreased parasympathetic (vagal) activity. The neurohormonal response includes increased release of catecholamines into the circulation. Homeostatic responses include decreases in plasma volume, increased platelet activity, and higher blood clotting tendency (Krantz *et al.*, 1996). Physiologically, stress-induced elevations in blood pressure, heart rate, and cardiac contractility result in increased cardiac demand. In patients with CAD these increases in cardiac demand may be accompanied by decreased coronary blood supply to the heart muscle, hence leading to myocardial ischemia (Krantz *et al.*, 1996). The pattern of the actual biological and physiological acute response to psychological and mental challenges is determined by multiple factors, task characteristics, and the type of perturbation and presence of cardiovascular risk factors and/or co-morbidities. The mechanisms accounting for cardiac arrhythmias induced by mental arousal have been reviewed elsewhere (Verrier, 1987) and do not involve a primary immune system component.

Immunological correlates The effects of acute mental arousal on the immune system are complex (Ader, Cohen, and Felten, 1995). In general, acute psychological distress results in increased $CD8^+$ T-cells, decreased $CD4^+$ T-cells, increased B-cells, elevated pro-inflammatory cytokine levels (IL-1β and IL-2), suggesting at least a partial activation of the immune system (Dantzer and Kelley, 1989). Acute phase proteins (CRP and fibrinogen) (Kop *et al.*, 2004) and adhesion molecules (Mills and Dimsdale, 1996) increase in response to acute psychological distress. The acute stress response also may involve increased T-cell expression of chemokines (CXCR2, CXCR3, and CCR5) (Bosch *et al.*, 2003). This complex immune response can vary substantially across individuals and challenge tasks and partly depend on stress-induced reductions in plasma volume (Marsland *et al.*, 1997). Although it is theoretically plausible that acute psychological factors increase plaque vulnerability via immune system-related processes, this has not been demonstrated by experimental studies. The evidence to date mostly focuses on the physiological and subsequent ischemic and arrhythmic responses to acute mental stress in vulnerable patients.

Summary Acute psychological factors induce activation of the immune system, particularly increased levels of $CD8^+$ T-cells, pro-inflammatory cytokines, acute-phase proteins and circulating adhesion molecules. These immune system reactions may lead to activation and subsequent rupture of vulnerable atherosclerotic plaques and thus result in myocardial infarction (Libby *et al.*, 1997). In addition, these acute immune system responses may interfere with normal endothelial function and cause local vasoconstriction. Immune activation also interacts with the blood-clotting process, thereby further increasing the risk of myocardial infarction.

Concluding Remarks

Figure 26.2 presents a simplified diagram that distinguishes between: 1) the atherosclerotic and hypertrophic disease stages in CAD and HF; 2) physiological and immunological correlates; and 3) psychological factors involved In CAD and HF. Psychological risk factors are involved in the early progression of CAD and cardiac hypertrophy by processes of gradual disease progression. At later stages of the disease, psychological factors play a potentially critical role in the transition from advanced atherosclerotic lesions to acute coronary syndromes.

This model also provides a conceptual framework for the "clustering" of psychological risk factors for CAD and HF (Suls and Bunde, 2005). The clustering of psychological risk factors is important from a longitudinal perspective, particular when considered in parallel to the underlying cardiovascular disease processes. Chronic psychological factors may not only promote early atherosclerotic and hypertrophic disease processes, but also increase the likelihood of developing episodic and acute risk factors. For example, chronic psychological risk factors for coronary syndromes are associated with elevated responsiveness to acute challenges (Kop and Cohen, 2007).

Pharmacological interventions that directly target sytemic inflammation have been largely ineffective in reducing CAD or HF progression. Corticosteroid interventions have been ineffective in preventing re-narrowing of coronary vessels after successful revascularization (Stone *et al.*, 1989; Pepine *et al.*, 1990), and corticosteroid administration upon admission for myocardial infarction results in adverse clinical outcomes (Roberts, De Mello, and Sobel, 1976). Azithromyzin (an antibiotic) trials have also been largely unsuccessful in reducing cardiac events among CAD patients. Only local immunosuppressive agents supplied with intracoronary stents have shown some benefits as these agents reduce intimal hyperplasia by inhibiting growth factors (for review see Fattori and Piva, 2003). Some pharmacological agents that target risk factors that do not directly involve the immune system (e.g., lipid-lowering statins and aspirin) may have beneficial cardiovascular effects that are nonetheless mediated via immunological (anti-inflammatory) processes (Ikonomidis *et al.*, 1999; Ridker *et al.*, 2005). In HF, most anti-inflammation pharmacological trials have been unsuccessful (Anker and Coats, 2002; Cacciapaglia *et al.*, 2011). None of the pharmacological intervention trials targeting inflammation in cardiovascular disease patients have included psychological or behavioral factors as potential effect modifiers, which may be an interesting area of future research.

Behavioral and psychological interventions can result in positive outcomes in CAD and HF patients, although the magnitude of the effect is generally small, difficult to reproduce in independent studies, and dependent on characteristics of the therapists as well as the patients (for review see Linden, Stossel, and Maurice, 1996). These interventions include: relaxation, stress management, Type A behavior/hostility intervention, and social support. Several negative studies have also been reported (see Linden *et al.*, 1996). Nonetheless, it seems that the incidence of adverse cardiac events is twice as high in patients who do not receive psychosocial interventions. The mechanisms underlying these positive effects remain insufficiently understood.

This selective review provides a few domains of future research on biobehavioral pathways in the onset and progression of CAD and HF. More information is needed in the following areas:

1 Fundamental animal and human research to determine whether inflammation is a primary precipitant of CAD and/or HF, or whether inflammation reflects a secondary response to the ongoing atherosclerotic or hypertrophic disease processes
2 Research on the role of specific CNS, HPA axis and autonomic correlates of psychological risk factors such as depression and exhaustion, by longitudinally examining these conditions in relation to pro-inflammatory cytokines and CAD and HF progression
3 Studies examining chronic psychological risk factors such as personality factors, PTSD, long-term consequences of early-life adversities, and socioeconomic factors in relation to inflammatory markers in the onset and progression of CAD and heart failure
4 Investigations on acute psychological factors and other triggers as related to the immune system-related processes of plaque instability in patients with vulnerability for acute coronary syndromes.

These investigations may help develop and improve behavioral and pharmacological interventions for CAD and HF. It is not known to what extent the beneficial effects of psychological and behavioral interventions can be explained by their immune system-related consequences. These psychoneuroimmunological pathways may be of particular importance in chronic cardiac conditions such as coronary artery disease and heart failure in which the burden of disease is high and multiple immunological, neurohormonal, and psychosocial processes are interrelated in the prediction of adverse outcomes (Pasic *et al.*, 2003; Kop *et al.*, 2011).

References

Ader, R., Cohen, N., and Felten, D. (1995). Psychoneuroimmunology: interactions between the nervous system and the immune system. *Lancet*, 345, 99–103.

Alonzo, A.A., Simon, A.B., and Feinleib, M. (1975). Prodromata of myocardial infarction and sudden death. *Circulation*, 52, 1056–1062.

Ambrose, J.A., Tannenbaum, M.A., Alexopoulos, D., Hjemdahl-Monsen, C.E., Leavy, J., Weiss, M., et al. (1988). Angiographic progression of coronary artery disease and the development of myocardial infarction. *Journal of the American College of Cardiology*, 12, 56–62.

Anker, S.D., and Coats, A.J. (2002). How to RECOVER from RENAISSANCE? The significance of the results of RECOVER, RENAISSANCE, RENEWAL and ATTACH. *International Journal of Cardiology*, 86, 123–130.

Barefoot, J.C., Dahlstrom, W.G., and Williams, R.B. (1983). Hostility, CHD incidence, and total mortality: a 25-year follow-up study of 255 physicians. *Psychosomatic Medicine*, 45, 59–63.

Beck, J., Garcia, R., Heiss, G., Vokonas, P.S., and Offenbacher, S. (1996). Periodontal disease and cardiovascular disease. *Journal of Periodontology*, 67, 1123–1137.

Boscarino, J.A. (2008). A prospective study of PTSD and early-age heart disease mortality among Vietnam veterans: implications for surveillance and prevention. *Psychosomatic Medicine*, 70, 668–676.

Bosch, J.A., Berntson, G.G., Cacioppo, J.T., Dhabhar, F.S., and Marucha, P.T. (2003). Acute stress evokes selective mobilization of T cells that differ in chemokine receptor expression: a potential pathway linking immunologic reactivity to cardiovascular disease. *Brain, Behavior, and Immunity*, 17, 251–259.

Brodov, Y., Sandach, A., Boyko, V., Matetzky, S., Guetta, V., Mandelzweig, L., et al. (2008). Acute myocardial infarction preceded by potential triggering activities: angiographic and clinical characteristics. *International Journal of Cardiology*, 130, 180–184.

Brosschot, J.F., Gerin, W., and Thayer, J.F. (2006). The perseverative cognition hypothesis: a review of worry, prolonged stress-related physiological activation, and health. *Journal of Psychosomatic Research*, 60, 113–124.

Cacciapaglia, F., Navarini, L., Menna, P., Salvatorelli, E., Minotti, G., and Afeltra, A. (2011). Cardiovascular safety of anti-TNF-alpha therapies: facts and unsettled issues. *Autoimmunity Reviews*, 10, 631–635.

Cercek, B., Shah, P.K., Noc, M., Zahger, D., Zeymer, U., Matetzky, S., et al. (2003). Effect of short-term treatment with azithromycin on recurrent ischaemic events in patients with acute coronary syndrome in the Azithromycin in Acute Coronary Syndrome (AZACS) trial: a randomised controlled trial. *Lancet*, 361, 809–813.

Cesari, M., Penninx, B.W., Newman, A.B., Kritchevsky, S.B., Nicklas, B.J., Sutton-Tyrrell, K., et al. (2003). Inflammatory markers and onset of cardiovascular events: results from the Health ABC study. *Circulation*, 108, 2317–2322.

Danesh, J., Collins, R., and Peto, R. (1997). Chronic infections and coronary heart disease: is there a link? *Lancet*, 350, 430–436.

Danesh, J., Wheeler, J.G., Hirschfield, G.M., Eda, S., Eiriksdottir, G., Rumley, A., et al. (2004). C-reactive protein and other circulating markers of inflammation in the prediction of coronary heart disease. *New England Journal of Medicine*, 350, 1387–1397.

Dantzer, R., and Kelley, K.W. (1989). Stress and immunity: an integrated view of relationships between the brain and the immune system. *Life Sciences*, 44, 1995–2008.

de Souza, R.R. (2002). Aging of myocardial collagen. *Biogerontology*, 3, 325–335.

Denollet, J., Conraads, V.M., Brutsaert, D.L., De Clerck, L.S., Stevens, W.J., and Vrints, C.J. (2003). Cytokines and immune activation in systolic heart failure: the role of Type D personality. *Brain, Behavior, and Immunity*, 17, 304–309.

Denollet, J., Schiffer, A.A., and Spek, V. (2010). A general propensity to psychological distress affects cardiovascular outcomes: evidence from research on the type D (distressed) personality profile. *Circulation: Cardiovascular Quality and Outcomes*, 3, 546–557.

Dimsdale, J.E. (2008). Psychological stress and cardiovascular disease. *Journal of the American College of Cardiology*, 51, 1237–1246.

Douglas, K.M., Taylor, A.J., and OMalley, P.G. (2004). Relationship between depression and C-reactive protein in a screening population. *Psychosomatic Medicine*, 66, 679–683.

Fattori, R., and Piva, T. (2003). Drug-eluting stents in vascular intervention. *Lancet*, 361, 247–249.

Funder, J.W. (1995). Steroids, hypertension and cardiac fibrosis. *Blood Pressure. Supplement*, 2, 39–42.

Gold, P.W., Goodwin, F.K., and Chrousos, G.P. (1988). Clinical and biochemical manifestations of depression. Relation to the neurobiology of stress (1). *New England Journal of Medicine*, 319, 348–353.

Goodkin, K., and Appels, A. (1997). Behavioral-neuroendocrine-immunologic interactions in myocardial infarction. *Medical Hypotheses*, 48, 209–214.

Grayston, J.T., Kronmal, R.A., Jackson, L.A., Parisi, A.F., Muhlestein, J.B., Cohen, J.D., et al. (2005). Azithromycin for the secondary prevention of coronary events. *New England Journal of Medicine*, 352, 1637–1645.

Gurfinkel, E.P., de la Fuente, R.L., Mendiz, O., and Mautner, B. (2002). Influenza vaccine pilot study in acute coronary syndromes and planned percutaneous coronary interventions: the FLU Vaccination Acute Coronary Syndromes (FLUVACS) Study. *Circulation*, 105, 2143–2147.

Hansson, G.K. (2005). Inflammation, atherosclerosis, and coronary artery disease. *New England Journal of Medicine*, 352, 1685–1695.

Ikonomidis, I., Andreotti, F., Economou, E., Stefanadis, C., Toutouzas, P., and Nihoyannopoulos, P. (1999). Increased proinflammatory cytokines in patients with chronic stable angina and their reduction by aspirin. *Circulation*, 100, 793–798.

Kapadia, S.R. (1999). Cytokines and heart failure. *Cardiology in Review*, 7, 196–206.

Kibler, J.L., and Ma, M. (2004). Depressive symptoms and cardiovascular reactivity to laboratory behavioral stress. *International Journal of Behavioral Medicine*, 11, 81–87.

Koenig, H.G. (1998). Depression in hospitalized older patients with congestive heart failure. *General Hospital Psychiatry*, 20, 29–43.

Kop, W.J. (1994). *The predictive value of vital exhaustion in the clinical course after coronary angioplasty.* Maastricht: Datawyse.

Kop, W.J. (1999). Chronic and acute psychological risk factors for clinical manifestations of coronary artery disease. *Psychosomatic Medicine*, 61, 476–487.

Kop, W.J., and Cohen, N. (2007). Psychoneuroimmunological pathways involved in acute coronary syndromes. In R. Ader (ed.), *Psychoneuroimmunology*, 4th ed. (pp. 921–943). Amsterdam, Boston: Academic Press.

Kop, W.J., Stein, P.K., Tracy, R.P., Barzilay, J.I., Schulz, R., and Gottdiener, J.S. (2010). Autonomic nervous system dysfunction and inflammation contribute to the increased cardiovascular mortality risk associated with depression. *Psychosomatic Medicine*, 72, 626–635.

Kop, W.J., Synowski, S.J., and Gottlieb, S.S. (2011). Depression in heart failure: biobehavioral mechanisms. *Heart Failure Clinics*, 7, 23–38.

Kop, W.J., Zhu, J., Doyle, M.P., Tracy, R.P., Gottdiener, J.S., Asch, F., et al. (2004). Mental stress and exercise effects on immune system and blood coagulation parameters in patients with coronary artery disease following coronary angioplasty (abstract). *Annals of Behavioral Medicine*, S069.

Krantz, D.S., Kop, W.J., Santiago, H.T., and Gottdiener, J.S. (1996). Mental stress as a trigger of myocardial ischemia and infarction. *Cardiology Clinics*, 14, 271–287.

Ladwig, K.H., Marten-Mittag, B., Lowel, H., Doring, A., and Koenig, W. (2003). Influence of depressive mood on the association of CRP and obesity in 3205 middle aged healthy men. *Brain, Behavior, and Immunity*, 17, 268–275.

Libby, P., Egan, D., and Skarlatos, S. (1997). Roles of infectious agents in atherosclerosis and restenosis: an assessment of the evidence and need for future research. *Circulation*, 96, 4095–4103.

Libby, P., and Theroux, P. (2005). Pathophysiology of coronary artery disease. *Circulation*, 111, 3481–3488.

Lichtman, J.H., Bigger, J.T., Jr, Blumenthal, J.A., Frasure-Smith, N., Kaufmann, P.G., Lesperance, F., et al. (2008). Depression and coronary heart disease: recommendations for screening, referral, and treatment: a science advisory from the American Heart Association Prevention Committee of the Council on Cardiovascular Nursing, Council on Clinical Cardiology, Council on Epidemiology and Prevention, and Interdisciplinary Council on Quality of Care and Outcomes Research: endorsed by the American Psychiatric Association. *Circulation*, 118, 1768–1775.

Linden, W., Stossel, C., and Maurice, J. (1996). Psychosocial interventions for patients with coronary artery disease: a meta-analysis. *Archives of Internal Medicine*, 156, 745–752.

Marsland, A.L., Herbert, T.B., Muldoon, M.F., Bachen, E.A., Patterson, S., Cohen, S., et al. (1997). Lymphocyte subset redistribution during acute laboratory stress in young adults: mediating effects of hemoconcentration. *Health Psychology*, 16, 341–348.

McCaffery, J.M., Frasure-Smith, N., Dube, M.P., Theroux, P., Rouleau, G.A., Duan, Q., et al. (2006). Common genetic vulnerability to depressive symptoms and coronary artery disease: a review and development of candidate genes related to inflammation and serotonin. *Psychosomatic Medicine*, 68, 187–200.

Miller, G.E., Freedland, K.E., Duntley, S., and Carney, R.M. (2005). Relation of depressive symptoms to C-reactive protein and pathogen burden (cytomegalovirus, herpes simplex virus, Epstein-Barr virus) in patients with earlier acute coronary syndromes. *American Journal of Cardiology*, 95, 317–321.

Mills, P.J., and Dimsdale, J.E. (1996). The effects of acute psychologic stress on cellular adhesion molecules. *Journal of Psychosomatic Research*, 41, 49–53.

Mittleman, M.A., Maclure, M., Sherwood, J.B., Mulry, R.P., Tofler, G.H., Jacobs, S.C., et al. (1995). Triggering of acute myocardial infarction onset by episodes of anger. Determinants of Myocardial Infarction Onset Study Investigators. *Circulation*, 92, 1720–1725.

Mommersteeg, P.M.C., and Pouwer, F. (2012). Personality as a risk factor for the metabolic syndrome: a systematic review. *Journal of Psychosomatic Research*, 73, 326–333.

Naghavi, M., Libby, P., Falk, E., Casscells, S.W., Litovsky, S., Rumberger, J., et al. (2003). From vulnerable plaque to vulnerable patient: a call for new definitions and risk assessment strategies: part II. *Circulation*, 108, 1772–1778.

Nicholson, A., Kuper, H., and Hemingway, H. (2006). Depression as an aetiologic and prognostic factor in coronary heart disease: a meta-analysis of 6362 events among 146 538 participants in 54 observational studies. *European Heart Journal*, 27, 2763–2774.

Parthenakis, F.I., Patrianakos, A., Prassopoulos, V., Papadimitriou, E., Nikitovic, D., Karkavitsas, N.S., et al. (2003). Relation of cardiac sympathetic innervation to proinflammatory cytokine levels in patients with heart failure secondary to idiopathic dilated cardiomyopathy. *American Journal of Cardiology*, 91, 1190–1194.

Pasic, J., Levy, W.C., and Sullivan, M.D. (2003). Cytokines in depression and heart failure. *Psychosomatic Medicine*, 65, 181–193.

Paterson, J., and Cottral, G.E. (1950). Experimental coronary sclerosis III. Lymphomatosis as a cause of coronary sclerosis in chickens. *Archives of Pathology*, 49, 699.

Pepine, C.J., Hirshfeld, J.W., Macdonald, R.G., Henderson, M.A., Bass, T.A., Goldberg, S., et al. (1990). A controlled trial of corticosteroids to prevent restenosis after coronary angioplasty. M-HEART Group. *Circulation*, 81, 1753–1761.

Philbin, E.F., Dec, G.W., Jenkins, P.L., and DiSalvo, T.G. (2001). Socioeconomic status as an independent risk factor for hospital readmission for heart failure. *American Journal of Cardiology*, 87, 1367–1371.

Ridker, P.M., Cannon, C.P., Morrow, D., Rifai, N., Rose, L.M., McCabe, C.H., et al. (2005). C-reactive protein levels and outcomes after statin therapy. *New England Journal of Medicine*, 352, 20–28.

Roberts, R., De Mello, V., and Sobel, B.E. (1976). Deleterious effects of methylprednisolone in patients with myocardial infarction. *Circulation*, 53, I204–206.

Robinette, C.D., and Fraumeni, J.F., Jr, (1977). Splenectomy and subsequent mortality in veterans of the 1939–45 war. *Lancet*, 2, 127–129.

Rosenman, R.H., Brand, R.J., Jenkins, D., Friedman, M., Straus, R., and Wurm, M. (1975). Coronary heart disease in Western Collaborative Group Study. Final follow-up experience of 8 1/2 years. *Journal of the American Medical Association*, 233, 872–877.

Ross, R. (1999). Atherosclerosis – an inflammatory disease. *New England Journal of Medicine*, 340, 115–126.

Rutledge, T., Reis, V.A., Linke, S.E., Greenberg, B.H., and Mills, P.J. (2006). Depression in heart failure a meta-analytic review of prevalence, intervention effects, and associations with clinical outcomes. *Journal of the American College of Cardiology*, 48, 1527–1537.

Sapolsky, R., Rivier, C., Yamamoto, G., Plotsky, P., and Vale, W. (1987). Interleukin-1 stimulates the secretion of hypothalamic corticotropin-releasing factor. *Science*, 238, 522–524.

Seeman, T.E., Singer, B.H., Rowe, J.W., Horwitz, R.I., and McEwen, B.S. (1997). Price of adaptation – allostatic load and its health consequences. Macarthur studies of successful aging. *Archives of Internal Medicine*, 157, 2259–2268.

Segerstrom, S.C., and Miller, G.E. (2004). Psychological stress and the human immune system: a meta-analytic study of 30 years of inquiry. *Psychological Bulletin*, 130, 601–630.

Smolderen, K.G., Spertus, J.A., Reid, K.J., Buchanan, D.M., Krumholz, H.M., Denollet, J., et al. (2009). The association of cognitive and somatic depressive symptoms with depression recognition and outcomes after myocardial infarction. *Circulation. Cardiovascular Quality and Outcomes*, 2, 328–337.

Stone, G.W., Rutherford, B.D., McConahay, D.R., Johnson, W.L., Giorgi, L.V., Ligon, R.W., et al. (1989). A randomized trial of corticosteroids for the prevention of restenosis in 102 patients undergoing repeat coronary angioplasty. *Catheterization and Cardiovascular Diagnosis*, 18, 227–231.

Suls, J., and Bunde, J. (2005). Anger, anxiety, and depression as risk factors for cardiovascular disease: the problems and implications of overlapping affective dispositions. *Psychological Bulletin*, 131, 260–300.

Tracey, K.J. (2002). The inflammatory reflex. *Nature*, 420, 853–859.

Verrier, R.L. (1987). Mechanisms of behaviorally induced arrhythmias. *Circulation*, 76, I48–56.

von Kanel, R., Mills, P.J., Fainman, C., and Dimsdale, J.E. (2001). Effects of psychological stress and psychiatric disorders on blood coagulation and fibrinolysis: a biobehavioral pathway to coronary artery disease? *Psychosomatic Medicine*, 63, 531–544.

Wald, N.J., Law, M.R., Morris, J.K., and Bagnall, A.M. (1997). Helicobacter pylori infection and mortality from ischaemic heart disease: negative result from a large, prospective study. *British Medical Journal*, 315, 1199–1201.

Westlake, S.L., Colebatch, A.N., Baird, J., Curzen, N., Kiely, P., Quinn, M., et al. (2011). Tumour necrosis factor antagonists and the risk of cardiovascular disease in patients with rheumatoid arthritis: a systematic literature review. *Rheumatology (Oxford)*, 50, 518–531.

White, P.D. (1997). The relationship between infection and fatigue. *Journal of Psychosomatic Research*, 43, 345–350.

Whooley, M.A., de Jonge, J., Vittinghoff, E., Otte, C., Moos, R., Carney, R.M., et al. (2008). Depressive symptoms, health behaviors, and risk of cardiovascular events in patients with coronary heart disease. *Journal of the American Medical Association*, 300, 2379–2388.

Winkleby, M.A., Jatulis, D.E., Frank, E., and Fortmann, S.P. (1992). Socioeconomic status and health: how education, income, and occupation contribute to risk factors for cardiovascular disease. *American Journal of Public Health*, 82, 816–820.

Wolfe, F., Mitchell, D.M., Sibley, J.T., Fries, J.F., Bloch, D.A., Williams, C.A., et al. (1994). The mortality of rheumatoid arthritis. *Arthritis and Rheumatism*, 37, 481–494.

Yokoya, K., Takatsu, H., Suzuki, T., Hosokawa, H., Ojio, S., Matsubara, T., et al. (1999). Process of progression of coronary artery lesions from mild or moderate stenosis to moderate or severe stenosis: a study based on four serial coronary arteriograms per year. *Circulation*, 100, 903–909.

Zhu, J., Nieto, F.J., Horne, B.D., Anderson, J.L., Muhlestein, J.B., and Epstein, S.E. (2001). Prospective study of pathogen burden and risk of myocardial infarction or death. *Circulation*, 103, 45–51.

Index

The Wiley-Blackwell Handbook of Psychoneuroimmunology, First Edition. Edited by Alexander W. Kusnecov and Hymie Anisman.

CPSIA information can be obtained
at www.ICGtesting.com
Printed in the USA
BVHW022015210123
656202BV00010B/4